Systematic Endocrinology

Systematic

Edited by

Calvin Ezrin, M.D.
Associate Professor, Departments of Medicine and Pathology, University of Toronto; Staff Physician and Director, Medical-Endocrine Clinic, Toronto General Hospital, Toronto

John O. Godden, M.D., C.M.
President, Medi-Edit Limited; Editor of Publications, The Ontario Cancer Treatment and Research Foundation, Toronto

Robert Volpé, M.D.
Professor, Department of Medicine, University of Toronto; Head, Division of Endocrinology, The Wellesley Hospital, Toronto

Richard Wilson, M.D.
Assistant Professor, Department of Obstetrics and Gynecology, University of Toronto;
Staff Obstetrician and Gynecologist, Toronto General Hospital;
Gynecologic Consultant, The Hospital for Sick Children, Toronto

Endocrinology

Medical Department
Harper & Row, Publishers
Hagerstown, Maryland
New York, Evanston, San Francisco, London

 Printed in the United States of America. For information address Medical Department, Harper & Row, Publishers, Inc., 2350 Virginia Avenue, Hagerstown, Maryland 21740.

Standard Book Number: 06-140796-8
Library of Congress Catalog Card Number: 72-83809

Dedicated to the memory
of our inspiring teacher
RAY FLETCHER FARQUHARSON
1897–1965
Distinguished and beloved physician,
medical statesman, and pioneer Canadian
clinical endocrinologist

After serving as Professor of Medicine at the University of Toronto from 1947 to 1960, he helped to establish the Medical Research Council of Canada. At the time of his death, he was Chairman of that body.

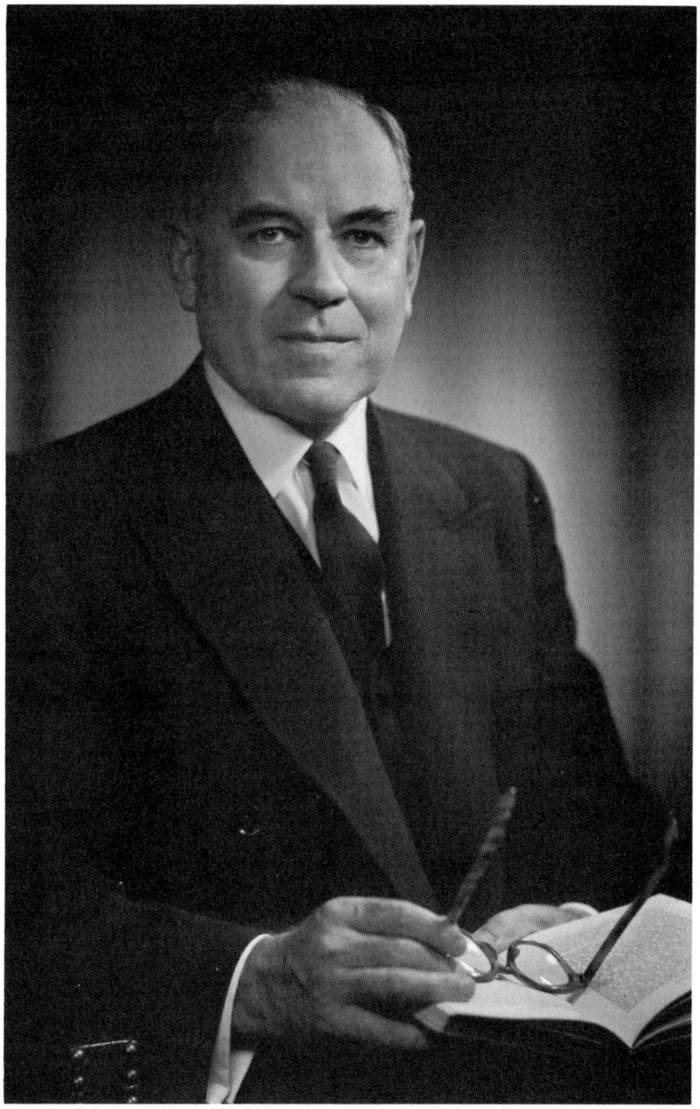

Contents

Contributors

John D. Bailey, M.D.
Head, Division of Endocrinology, The Hospital for Sick Children;
Professor of Pediatrics, University of Toronto,
Toronto, Ontario

Charles E. Bird, M.D., Ph.D.
Associate Professor, Department of Medicine and Assistant Professor, Department of Physiology, Queen's University,
Kingston, Ontario

Albert F. Clark, M.Sc., Ph.D.
Associate Professor, Departments of Biochemistry and Pathology, Queen's University;
Clinical Chemist, Kingston General Hospital,
Kingston, Ontario

Patrick Edward Conen, M.B.B.S., M.R.C.P., MC Path.
Associate Professor, Department of Pathology, University of Toronto; Associate Scientist, The Research Institute, and Senior Staff Pathologist, The Hospital for Sick Children,
Toronto, Ontario

Carol Ann Cowell, M.D.
Associate, Department of Obstetrics and Gynecology, and Assistant Professor, Department of Pediatrics, University of Toronto;
Staff Obstetrician and Gynecologist, Toronto General Hospital; Head, Division of Pediatric and Adolescent Gynecology, The Hospital for Sick Children, Toronto, Ontario

Calvin Ezrin, M.D.
Associate Professor, Departments of Medicine and Pathology, University of Toronto;
Staff Physician and Director, Medical-Endocrine Clinic, Toronto General Hospital,
Toronto, Ontario

C. Kenneth Gorman, M.D., Ph.D.
Assistant Professor, Department of Medicine, University of Toronto; Head, Department of Internal Medicine, Grace Hospital; Senior Physician, Institute for the Study of Addiction; Staff Physician, Toronto Western Hospital,
Toronto, Ontario

John C. Laidlaw, M.D., Ph.D.
Director, Institute of Medical Science, School of Graduate Studies, and Professor, Department of Medicine, University of Toronto; Senior Physician, Toronto General Hospital,
Toronto, Ontario

George Steiner, M.D.
Director, Diabetes Sub-Division, Toronto General Hospital; Assistant Director, Lipid Research Clinic, Associate Professor of Medicine and Assistant Professor of Physiology,

University of Toronto,
Toronto, Ontario

Robert Volpé, M.D.
Professor, Department of Medicine, University of Toronto; Head, Division of Endocrinology, The Wellesley Hospital,
Toronto, Ontario

Richard Wilson, M.D.
Assistant Professor, Department of Obstetrics and Gynecology, University of Toronto;
Staff Obstetrician and Gynecologist, Toronto General Hospital; Gynecologic Consultant, The Hospital for Sick Children,
Toronto, Ontario

Edmund R. Yendt, M.D.
Professor and Head, Department of Medicine, Queen's University; Physician-in-Chief, Kingston General Hospital,
Kingston, Ontario

Preface

Almost 200 years ago, Peter Mere Latham, a distinguished English physician and teacher, said, "A good book, though it be not necessarily a hard one, contains important facts, duly arranged and reasoned upon with care." The authors of SYSTEMATIC ENDOCRINOLOGY set out to write such a book. From 1966 to 1971, members of the Faculty of Medicine at the University of Toronto devised a new system-based curriculum. The material gathered to meet the demands of systems teaching was refined and elaborated to give an integrated view of endocrinology. To achieve comprehensiveness and cohesiveness, the authors of chapters on organs with overlapping or closely related functions were paired and their presentations integrated during serial revisions. Each chapter was assigned to a young authority—a well-qualified endocrinologist with considerable experience in research and practice, yet one still intimately involved in the day-to-day teaching of medical students.

The authors assume that the reader has recently completed studies of anatomy, physiology, and biochemistry, upon which any sound understanding of endocrinology depends. Therefore, only the structural, functional, biochemical, and other relationships essential to understanding endocrine function are presented. Important data and concepts not wholly essential to this understanding are summarized briefly or subordinated to the rest of the text. A great amount of supporting data is not provided except in the chapter on the adrenal.

We weighed the impact of the technical language on the learner, attempting to ascertain what ideas, terms, and definitions are common to senior medical students. Throughout we attempted to follow the principle that new learning must start with what the student already knows.

The field of endocrinology is rapidly changing, and we have made every effort to keep this book up to date. Addenda have been made where thorough understanding of the field called for additional information on current developments. These are assembled at the end of the book in an appendix. Also, to create a platform for further learning, we periodically introduced unsolved endocrinologic problems which may stimulate exceptional students to deeper thought and exploration.

In writing these chapters, we paused repeatedly to make sure that we had explained to the reader the purpose of the communication and that we had stated our objectives clearly at the outset so that the reader could adapt to them. In this, we succeeded only in part; nevertheless, the effort to do so helped us meet what we conceive to be the reader's needs.

References have been kept to a minimum to avoid distracting the student. However, each author is deeply conscious of an unacknowledged debt to his many colleagues, past and present, and the general references at the end of each chapter will direct the reader to some of the more important sources.

Most illustrations were prepared by Miss Elizabeth Blackstock and her colleagues in the Department of Art as Applied to Medicine, on the basis of material supplied by each author. I believe the illustrations testify to the success of this collaboration.

In short, SYSTEMATIC ENDOCRINOLOGY is not a compendium but a synthesis that emphasizes the alliance and interdependence of laboratory and clinic in the developments of modern endocrinology.

J. O. G.

A Special Acknowledgment

Authorship is a serious responsibility. Participation in a scientific textbook, if it is to represent a worthwhile contribution to medical education, commits the physician to a significant additional workload. Because they do not recognize this, or recognize but ignore it, many physicians fail. For this reason, the rate of "fetal wastage" in medical textbook publishing is high.

Soon after the inception of SYSTEMATIC ENDOCRINOLOGY, we recognized that we needed a manager to keep the book moving, particularly because the contributors, experienced teacher-practitioner-researchers, were already deeply committed when they accepted responsibility for their chapters. Thus, we invited Dr. John O. Godden, an internist and experienced editor, to join us. This managerial-editorial function is time consuming: The author's work is intermittent; the editor's work nearly continuous. If a chapter has been misconceived, or although properly conceived, has miscarried, the editor must persuade and assist the author, who is sometimes understandably reluctant, to begin again. In all of this, the editor, because he too is a physician, takes an active role, representing the reader and, where necessary, asking for clarification or elaboration.

In SYSTEMATIC ENDOCRINOLOGY, individual authors had from one to four chapters to worry about; John Godden had seventeen. His objective with each of us was to help the writer get his best on paper, in a form most useful to the medical students and practitioners for whom this book was written. If SYSTEMATIC ENDOCRINOLOGY is successful, it will be so because its authors contributed their best to it and because another physician saw it through.

C. E.

Systematic Endocrinology

1

Introduction to Endocrinology

Calvin Ezrin

The endocrine system is an important component of the automatic regulatory mechanisms by which the organism keeps in tune with its environment.[3] It is profitable to compare and contrast it with a similar regulating mechanism, the nervous system—a finite group of structural connections analogous to a telephone system. The endocrine glands communicate by "water travel" at a much slower rate than the nervous system. The neural and endocrine control of lactation and suckling illustrates clearly some important differences in these systems (Fig. 1-1). When an infant is put to the lactating breast, the stimulus of suckling travels by neural pathways up the spinal cord and brain to reach, in milliseconds, the secretory cells of the hypothalamic paraventricular nuclei and their neurohypophyseal connections. The release of stored oxytocin from the neurohypophysis into the circulation follows immediately. The oxytocin travels through the systemic circulation to reach, in a few seconds, the myoepithelial cells of the collecting ducts of the breast, which are filled with milk. The contraction of these cells occurs swiftly and causes the "milk let-down reaction," which expresses a small stream of milk into the infant's mouth. Often the sight of a hungry infant is enough to start milk dripping from the mother's breasts. The visual stimulus travels with the speed of light, but its effect is governed by the rate of impulse transmission from the retina to the hypothalamus and by the slower transport of oxytocin to the breast.

Prolactin, from the adenohypophysis, is the main hormone controlling the manufacture of milk in the breast that has been prepared by previous exposure to prolactin and other hormones. The factors governing the release of prolactin are manufactured in the hypothalamus. There seem to be two mechanisms operating here: (1) a tonic inhibition of prolactin secretion by a normal hypothalamic influence, prolactin inhibitory factor (PIF); and probably (2) an additional prolactin-stimulating factor (PSF), which is produced in response to suckling.

Whatever the substances concerned, they are delivered to the adenohypophysis by a two-stage neurovascular system from the hypothalamus. The first stage is a short neural pathway to the primary capillary network of the hypophyseal portal vessels in the neurohypophysis. The second stage is via the portal venous trunks to the secondary capillary network of this circulation within the adenohypophysis, which leads directly to the cell that manufactures prolactin. However, prolactin, which converts intermediary metabolites into the complex food called milk, takes much longer than oxytocin to act, as is shown by the interval required for the breast to fill up between feedings—usually a matter of 3–4 hours.

Endocrine secretion can be broken down into a

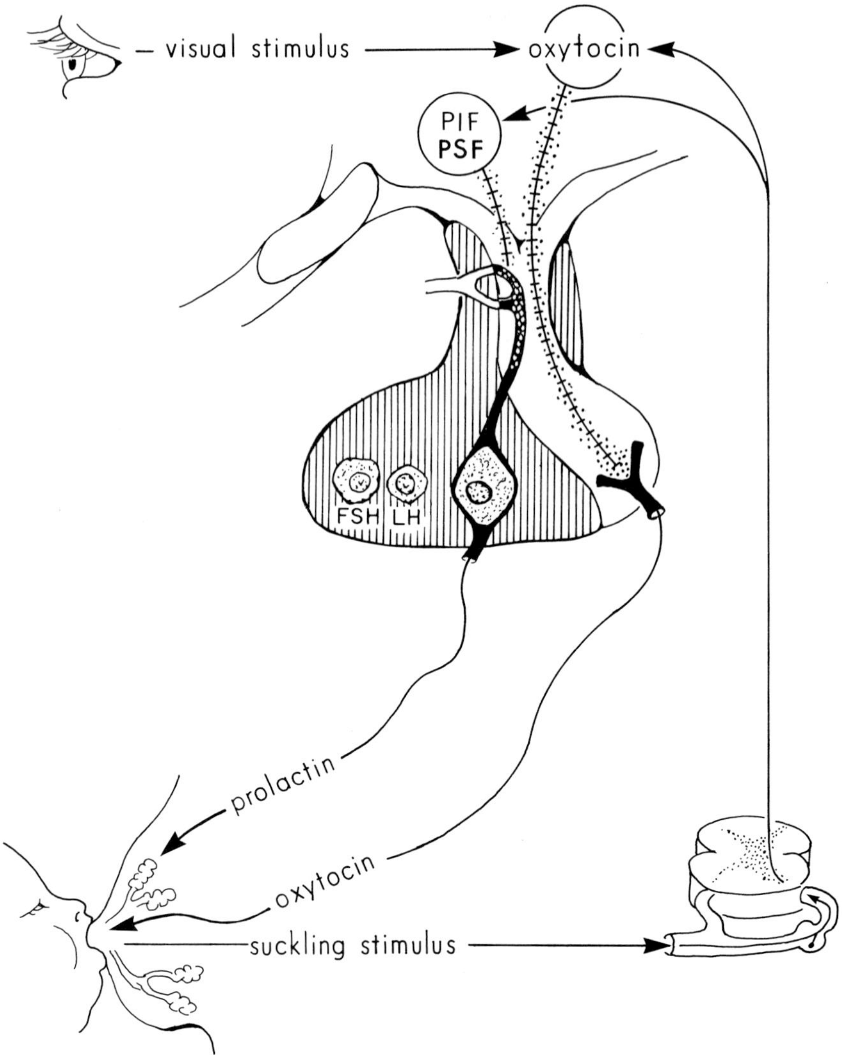

Fig. 1-1. Neuroendocrine control of suckling and lactation. Neurovascular pathways involved in milk production and secretion—hypothalamic neurohypophyseal (oxytocin) and hypothalamic adenohypophyseal (PIF-PSF prolactin)—differ from each other.

The oxytocin path, which begins with nipple stimulation (*lower left*) or visual stimulus (*upper left*), is entirely neural until hormone is delivered from neurohypophysis into veins of systemic circulation (*midright*). The prolactin path depends on secretion of hypothalamic releasing factors (hormones)—prolactin-inhibiting factor (PIF), sometimes called prolactin-inhibiting hormone (PIH), and prolactin-stimulating factor (PSF)—into primary capillary network of hypophyseal portal circulation.

The adenohypophysis contains several different cell types: possibly one for each hormone it secretes. Only three are shown here: one for follicle-stimulating hormone (FSH), one for luteinizing hormone (LH), and one for prolactin (lactogenic hormone). Only in lactation and in the last two trimesters of pregnancy does the prolactin cell contain an abundance of stored stainable granulation. The prolactin cell hyperplasia and hypersecretion in pregnancy may be due to stimulation by high estrogen levels. However, the resultant high levels of circulating prolactin are not enough to induce lactation in pregnancy in the presence of other peripheral interfering factors, e.g. excessive estrogens, which disappear at the time of delivery. Nonpuerperal lactation (galactorrhea) may result if, through the effect of disease or drugs, PIF is blocked, because the prolactin cell is normally held in check by a sustained secretion of this factor.

series of steps similar to those that occur in exocrine cells. The synthesis, storage, release, and transport of hormones are related events that can best be understood if considered separately. Synthesis of the hormones is under the control of nuclear DNA, which regulates the nucleotide sequences of RNA messengers. The amino acid sequences of the polypeptide or protein hormones are transcribed at the ribosomes; the steroid hormones are probably synthesized at the smooth endoplasmic reticulum. In most glands, the product is sufficiently electron-dense to be easily visible by electron microscopy only after it has passed from the ribosomes and their associated rough endoplasmic reticulum to the Golgi apparatus where membrane-bound granules are formed. In most endocrine glands these granules are stored within the neighboring cytoplasm. In the specialized hypothalamic neurosecretory cells of vertebrates, granules containing oxytocin or vasopressin, in association with a stainable carrier substance, pass inside the axons into terminals in the neurohypophysis, where they are temporarily stored until special stimuli induce their release into the circulation. The significance of this mode of transport may be appreciated by recalling that, from the time of its manufacture until its release into the circulation, the hypothalamic hormone is held within a controlled system analogous to sealed railway cars traveling to a storage depot.

Intact secretory granules do not escape as such from the cell. Instead, the membrane coating them partly fuses with the cell membrane and the contents are then extruded in a soluble form. Some of the hormones, such as thyroxine and cortisol, are transported in the bloodstream bound to specific carrier proteins, which limit their free entry into the tissues. Insulin and other protein and peptide hormones appear to travel to their cellular sites of action without being bound to any carrier substance.

The cell responds to a given hormone only after it is bound to a specific receptor site on the cell membrane. With the receptor the hormone may form a new entity, which is capable of generating a signal. The action of a hormone may be regarded as a specific chemical signal producing a specific adaptive response by the cell. However, a relatively nonspecific mechanism involving the ultimate production of one of the adenine nucleotides—3′,5′-adenosine monophosphate (cyclic AMP)—has been implicated in a large number of metabolic responses involving hormones.[1] Many of the hormones appear to act on their target cells by activating an enzyme system, adenyl cyclase, which is associated with binding sites on the cell membrane that can accept only the specific hormone. Adenyl cyclase converts adenosine triphosphate (ATP) to cyclic AMP.[11] Cells respond to increased levels of cyclic AMP with reactions that are characteristic of the particular tissue involved. Thus specificity of the cellular response to hormones is insured mainly by the particular binding sites that initially accept the hormone.[2] Several hormones may evoke a similar response in a tissue (e.g., lipolysis in fat cells may be induced by ACTH, glucagon and epinephrine), but the selective sites for binding of different hormones are different in each case.* There is also considerable evidence that before steroid hormones (e.g., aldosterone) act on target cells, they are bound to specific sites within the nucleus. There the hormone probably liberates or de-represses certain genetic information in the chromosomes, where the messenger RNA is synthesized.

Further details of the cellular action of the hormones will be considered in appropriate sections of the book. In general, it appears that hormones, like enzymes, do not initiate new reactions but act as powerful catalysts in a wide range of physicochemical situations. Life usually continues when a hormone is deficient, although its quality may be considerably altered. Sometimes failure of specific endocrine function, as in severe adrenal cortical insufficiency, is incompatible with life.[7] It is obvious that continuation of life to the succeeding generation depends on normal gondal function.[6]

Since this book concerns clinical endocrinology there will be little mention made of hormones of gastrointestinal origin, such as gastrin and secretin. Some attention will be paid to those hormones derived from tissues not usually considered to be glandular—e.g., the placenta and a variety of nonendocrine neoplasms. The remaining endo-

* See Appendix: Addendum to Chapter 1.

crine tissues and their hormones may be subdivided according to their physiology, as follows.

Pituitary-Target Gland Model (thyroid, adrenal cortex, and gonads)

Morphologic studies have shown that the adenohypophysis probably produces each of its seven hormones from a specific cell type. Thus the anterior pituitary may be regarded as a confederation of seven relatively independent endocrine glands over which the hypothalamus exerts higher control.[4] Under this type of control, a small change in the central regulator may produce very large peripheral effects. The hypothalamus produces, in picogram quantities, a number of releasing or governing factors that affect the anterior pituitary gland. In turn, the pituitary glands produce, in nanogram quantities, hormones that stimulate target cells, such as thyroid, to produce, in microgram quantities, hormones that have widespread effects on peripheral tissues. Another principle operating to regulate this group of endocrine glands is "negative feedback," which is easiest to observe in the control of thyroid activity[8] (Fig. 1-2). An increase above the normal level of either of the two thyroid hormones (thyroxine or triiodothyronine) reaching the hypothalamic-pituitary region will inhibit the release of thyrotropin from the adenohypophysis, either by affecting the pituitary directly or by suppressing the hypothalamic thyrotropin-releasing factor, which stimulates the cells of the anterior lobe that manufacture this hormone (Fig. 1-2**A**). Conversely, if the level of the thyroid hormones falls below normal, more thyrotropin is secreted. This drives the thyroid gland to produce and release more hormone—if it can (Fig. 1-2**B**). An enzyme defect may severely impair the synthesis of thyroid hormones in a gland that is still capable of further growth. In this case, lack of thyroid hormone is associated with continued overproduction of thyrotropin, which leads to enlargement of the thyroid gland or goiter (Fig. 1-2**C**). Such a goiter may be reduced greatly if the patient is treated early with a daily ration of thyroid hormone sufficient to inhibit the secretion of thyrotropin (Fig. 1-2**D**).

Pituitary-Peripheral Tissue Model (growth hormone, prolactin, and melanocyte-stimulating hormone)

This model is similar to the foregoing in that the effect of each of the hormones is amplified as one moves from the center to the periphery, but it differs in that a target endocrine gland does not take part in this amplification. The control is vested in the hypothalamus, which causes the pituitary to act on some or all of the peripheral tissues. This regulation is complex and depends in large measure on "tonic inhibition"—the sustained suppression of secretion that would otherwise occur, especially with regard to the production and release of prolactin. Growth hormone or somatotropin has been linked with body growth because, in its absence, growth is deficient and when it is present in excessive quantities, as in pituitary gigantism, growth is stimulated. Thus there appears to be a basal secretion of growth hormone related to growth. Also growth hormone seems to respond to other poorly understood influences that cause its secretion to fluctuate rapidly. These factors presumably operate through hypothalamic regulation and vary with age, sex, sleep, and nutritional status.[5]

Hormones Regulating Glucose

In addition to its powerful anabolic effects that are brought about in conjunction with growth hormone, insulin is the hypoglycemic hormone.[10] All the other hormone regulators of blood glucose (growth hormone, epinephrine, glucagon, cortisol and thyroxine) *raise* the glucose level by acting in homeostatic competition with insulin and thus provide an elaborate defense against hypoglycemia. Such a defense is essential because the central nervous system must have a continuous supply of glucose if the organism is to survive.

Hormones Regulating Calcium

The hormones that regulate calcium metabolism are parathyroid hormone—from the parathyroid gland, and calcitonin—from the ultimobranchial body, which is represented in part by the

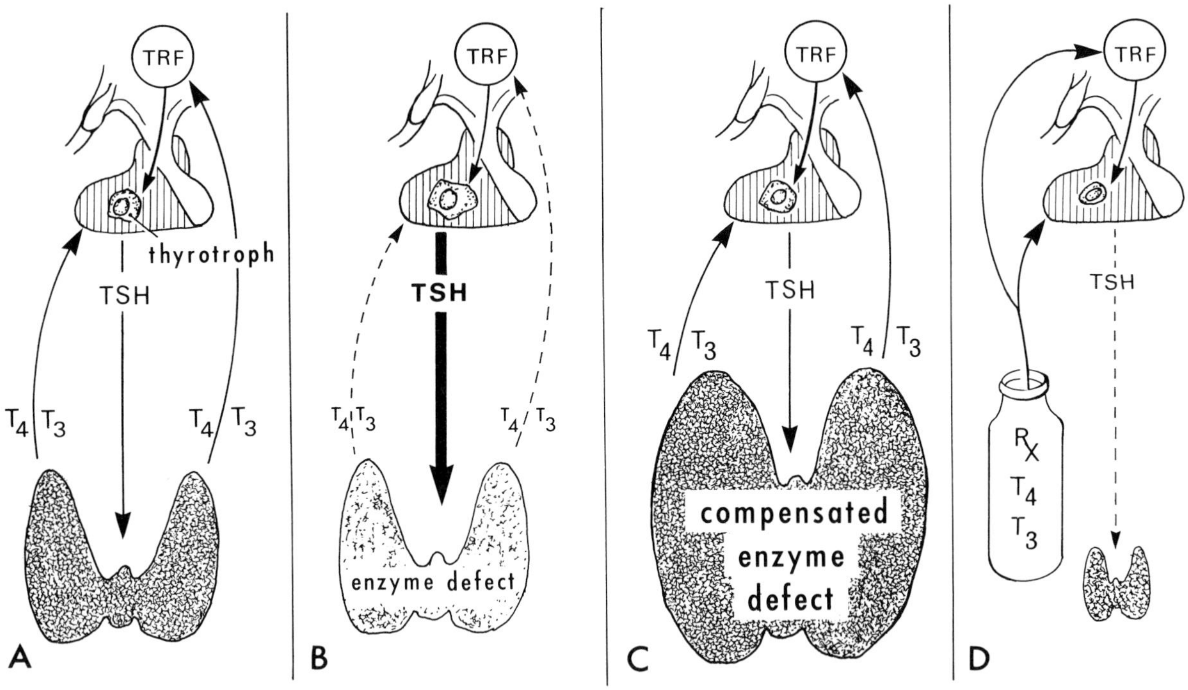

Fig. 1-2. Hypothalamic-pituitary-thyroid relationships in diffuse goiter due to enzyme defect. These figures illustrate activity of the "thyrotroph"—the cell which produces thyroid-stimulating hormone (TSH) or thyrotropin.

A. In normal individual, hypothalamic hormone—thyrotropin-releasing factor (TRF)—has stimulated release and production of TSH, which in turn acts on thyroid to increase output of two thyroid hormones: tetraiodothyronine or thyroxine (T_4) and triiodothyronine (T_3). These hormones, carried in circulation to hypothalamus and adenohypophysis, inhibit further TRF production and TSH release. (Note in **B, C,** and **D** that size of thyrotroph changes commensurate with its activity in these several situations. Variations in TSH output are indicated by arrows of various width. Broken line indicates deficiency or absence of T_4, T_3, and TSH.

B. In individual with enzyme defect, production of thyroid hormones is reduced below level needed to inhibit TSH output. (See also Chapter 4, Physiology of Hormones Produced in the Adenohypophysis.)

C. Thyroid hypertrophy will sometimes overcome effects of enzyme deficiency and raise thyroid hormone production to a level sufficient to again control TSH output. (See also Chapter 5, Goiters Due to Enzymatic Defects.)

D. Treatment of hypertrophied gland with T_4 and T_3 inhibits thyrotroph.

parafollicular cells in the human thyroid gland. The secretion of both of these hormones is regulated directly by the level of calcium ions in the blood. There is no evidence of significant pituitary control. The calcium level of the blood and tissues is also influenced by many other factors: the calcium content of the diet, the vitamin D available in the diet and from sunshine acting on the skin, intestinal absorption, renal function, and contributions from calcium stored in the bones. Because calcium is the key to many hormone-membrane interactions, its regulation is vital to all glandular functions.[9]

Hormones Made by Nervous Tissue (hypothalamic releasing factors, oxytocin and vasopressin, epinephrine and norepinephrine)

Hormones in this group are characterized by low molecular weight and rapidity of action. Compared with the other hormones, their action is rapid but is still much slower than nerve-fiber transmission. The timing of events in the neuroendocrine reflex involved in suckling illustrates this difference. The hormones of the nervous system will be dealt with more fully in the next chapter—Neuroendocrinology.

References

1. Bär, H. P., and Hechter, O. Adenyl cyclase and hormone action. I. Effects of adrenocorticotropic hormone, glucagon, and epinephrine on the plasma membrane of rat fat cells. *Proc Natl Acad Sci USA 63:*350–356, 1969.
2. Butcher, R. W., Robison, G. A., Hardman, J. G., and Sutherland, E. W. The role of cyclic AMP in hormone actions. *Adv Enzym Regul 6:*357–389, 1968.
3. Catt, K. J. ABC of endocrinology. I. Hormones in general. *Lancet 1:*763–765, 1970.
4. Catt, K. J. ABC of endocrinology. II. Pituitary function. *Lancet 1:*827–831, 1970.
5. Catt, K. J. ABC of endocrinology. III. Growth hormone. *Lancet 1:*933–939, 1970.
6. Catt, K. J. ABC of endocrinology. IV. Reproductive endocrinology. *Lancet 1:*1097–1104, 1970.
7. Catt, K. J. ABC of endocrinology. V. Adrenal cortex. *Lancet 1:*1275–1283, 1970.
8. Catt, K. J. ABC of endocrinology. VI. The thyroid gland. *Lancet 1:*1383–1389, 1970.
9. Catt, K. J. ABC of endocrinology. VII. Hormonal control of calcium homeostasis. *Lancet 2:*255–257, 1970.
10. Catt, K. J. ABC of endocrinology. VIII. Insulin and glucose homeostasis. *Lancet 2:*353–358, 1970.
11. Liddle, G. W., and Hardman, J. G. Cyclic adenosine monophosphate as a mediator of hormone action. *N Engl J Med 285:*560–566, 1971.

2

Neuroendocrinology

Calvin Ezrin

"Endocrine Hypothalamus"

The hypothalamic-pituitary relationship is the most important in neuroendocrinology.[1] The hypothalamus, a complicated collection of nerve cells and fiber tracts, participates in the regulation of many autonomic functions and body rhythms: it contributes to the control of body temperature, blood pressure, "emotional tone," hunger, thirst, sex and sleep.[10] The hypothalamus also contains cells that combine neural and secretory activity. This portion is difficult to define anatomically, but functionally it may accurately be designated as the "endocrine hypothalamus." The hormones it produces are delivered to the pituitary gland (Fig. 2-1).

The best known of the cellular aggregates of the endocrine hypothalamus are the supraoptic and paraventricular nuclei, which produce vasopressin and oxytocin, respectively. Combined with a carrier lipoprotein as stainable neurosecretion, these hormones travel within the axons of the hypothalamic-neurohypophyseal tract to the neurohypophysis, where they are stored.[9] Subsequently they are released into capillaries of the systemic circulation, in response to appropriate stimuli—e.g., changes in plasma osmolality (vasopressin) and suckling (oxytocin).

Other neurohumoral substances derived from ill-defined areas of the hypothalamus regulate the production of the various adenohypophyseal hormones and their release from their separate cells of origin. As unstainable neurosecretion, these "adenohypophysiotropic" (releasing) factors travel chiefly to the median eminence of the neurohypophysis. There they enter the primary capillary network of the pituitary portal system, which empties into the sinusoids of the anterior pituitary gland.

The production of these releasing factors may be affected by the level of pituitary hormones reaching the hypothalamus (short feedback loops) or by the level of target-gland hormones reaching the hypothalamus (long feedback loops). The cells producing hypothalamic hormones respond to stimuli from other areas of the brain or from peripheral receptors, as well as to the level of circulating hormones and probably to other changes in chemical constituents of the blood (Fig. 2-2). The details of this aspect of their function will be discussed in the next two chapters in the section dealing with physiology of the neurohypophysis and adenohypophysis. Although all of the pituitary hormones are probably under the influence of the endocrine hypothalamus, hypothalamic regulation is so important in the neuroendocrine control of the phenomena connected with reproduction that a special section

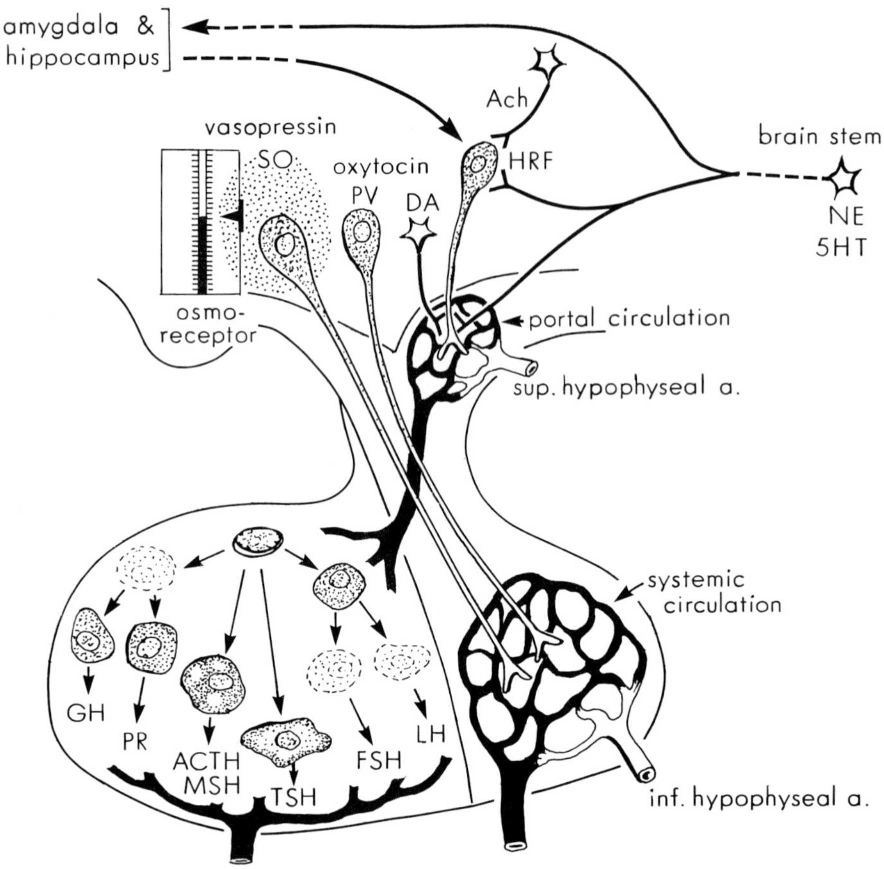

Fig. 2-1. Anatomy and Physiology of the "endocrine hypothalamus" and its relationship to the neuro- and adenohypophysis. This figure illustrates the general organization of the region in which the nervous and endocrine systems meet most intimately.

At the *upper right,* the neuron, labeled HRF (for hypothalamic releasing factors) stands for the ill-defined groups of cells which secrete a series of releasing factors (hormones) into primary capillary network of portal circulation to govern activities of anterior pituitary cells. Various neurotransmitter substances affect the activity of these neurons. Norepinephrine (NE) and 5-hydroxytryptamine (5 HT) arise in neurons with cell bodies in the brain stem. Dopamine (DA) is made in cells that are found in the basal hypothalamus. Acetylcholine (Ach) is another important regulatory neurotransmitter active in this region. The amygdala and hippocampus are important higher connections of the "endocrine hypothalamus."

Two well-defined groups of hypothalamic cells, supraoptic (SO) and paraventricular (PV) nuclei, make vasopressin and oxytocin respectively, but these hormones are not released into the systemic circulation until they have reached the neurohypophysis. The shaded area surrounding SO cell body represents the "osmoreceptor" that is responsive to changes in osmolality of the fluid perfusing it. The thermostat symbol to the left of the osmoreceptor represents the variable "set-point" concept used to explain the regulation of many hormones (see Figs. 3-3 and 4-2).

The adenohypophysis contains a variety of cell types, possibly one for each of the hormones it produces. Six are shown here: somatotropic or growth hormone (GH); prolactin (PR); adrenocorticotropic (ACTH) and melanocyte-stimulating (MSH), which are made in the same cell in the human gland; thyroid-stimulating (TSH); follicle-stimulating (FSH); and luteinizing (LH) which are depicted in broken lines because their hormones also may arise in a combined FSH-LH gonadotroph (shown in unbroken outline). (See also Fig. 4-1.)

Fig. 2-2. Endocrine hypothalamus and control of ACTH. Illustrated are the various influences that govern production and release of one of the hypothalamic releasing hormones—corticotropin-releasing factor (CRF). Similar models could be constructed for the other known and postulated hypothalamic hormones.

Increased delivery of CRF into portal circulation stimulates the corticotroph (anterior pituitary cell that makes ACTH), to release ACTH. Normally hypothalamic cells that produce CRF are inhibited by a rising level of circulating cortisol, which also directly inhibits the corticotroph (*long feedback*). *Short feedback* is inhibition induced by ACTH acting directly on cells that make CRF. The level at which these hypothalamic and adenohypophyseal cells are inhibited by cortisol is determined by the setting of a hypothetical thermostat-like control, called the *set-point.* Diurnal variations in circulating ACTH can be viewed as reflecting this fluctuating set-point. (See Chapter 4, Physiology of Hormones Produced in the Adenohypophysis.)

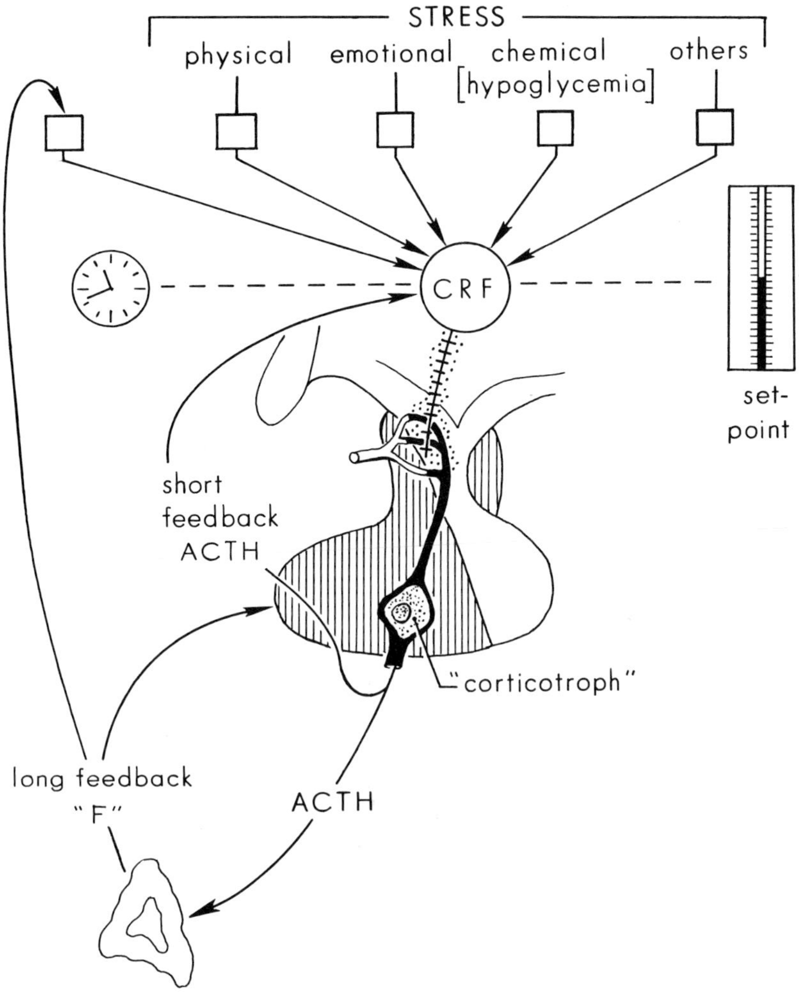

is devoted to a description of some of these interrelations.[5]

Influence of Sex Hormones on the Hypothalamus

There is experimental evidence that the hypothalami of both male and female rats tend to develop along female lines (with inherent rhythmic release of gonadotropic hormones) unless, early in life, male hormone exerts a certain "imprinting influence" on cells associated with the endocrine hypothalamus. If a newborn male rat is castrated, this portion of the nervous system is not exposed to the normal imprinting effect of androgen at this critical time. A state equivalent to castration may also be induced by implanting a minute amount of androgen-antagonist, cyproterone, in the appropriate hypothalamic region. Subsequently the hypothalamus of a male rat so treated can be shown to have retained an inherent cyclicity in its ability to release gonadotropic hormones, in particular luteinizing hormone (LH), which is necessary for ovulation. The evidence for ovulation is the appearance of corpora lutea in an ovary transplanted under a kidney capsule. Conversely, in the newborn female rat, a single injection of testosterone produces a permanent alteration in the hypothalamus that is manifested in later life by failure to ovulate spontaneously.[12] The defect appears to be in the manufacture or release of the adenohypophysiotropic hormone, LH-releasing factor (LHRF).

In rats the creation of electrolytic lesions or the

implanting of minute quantities of sex hormones in the hypothalamus has shown that the areas controlling the release of gonadotropic hormones are separate from those affecting sexual behavior. The sex hormones appear to influence sexual behavior by attaching themselves to specific receptor sites within the hypothalamus and probably elsewhere in the brain. The hormones seem to alter the threshold of nervous mechanisms, particularly those involving the limbic (hippocampal) and reticular-activating systems, which are closely related to the hypothalamus anatomically and functionally.[6]

Clinical experience has shown us that the onset of puberty is under the control of the hypothalamus. Hypothalamic disease, usually involving its posterior portion, sometimes produces precocious puberty.[2] Such premature puberty may be due to an increased "threshold of inhibition," or higher "set-point" for shutoff of hypothalamic gonadotropin-releasing factors—a condition in which low levels of sex steroids no longer inhibit the release of pituitary gonadotropin as is characteristic of the prepubertal stage. Thus the level of sex steroids can rise high enough to produce secondary sexual characteristics before inhibiting the secretion of pituitary gonadotropins by negative feedback. The feedback probably acts at both the hypothalamic and the pituitary levels.

The pineal gland appears to produce a gonadotropin-inhibiting substance (melatonin), which also delays the onset of puberty. The hypothalamus may similarly produce a gonadotropin-inhibiting substance that is responsible for delaying the onset of puberty until the normal time; hence disease of the hypothalamus would interfere with the production or delivery of this substance and thus further favor the development of sexual precocity.

With lesions of the hypothalamic area, delayed puberty is more common, presumably because the delivery of gonadotropin-releasing factors to the adenohypophysis is interfered with. Patients who have hypothalamic lesions often have associated damage to the hypophyseal-portal circulation or to the adenohypophysis itself. Hypogonadism secondary to hypothalamic and pituitary disease is discussed further in the chapter on the adenohypophysis.

Hormones and Human Behavior

Because normal function of the central nervous system depends on an adequate supply of glucose, insulin-induced hypoglycemia is usually accompanied by disturbances in behavior and consciousness. Adrenal cortical steroids also affect brain function. Chronic adrenal insufficiency (Addison's disease) may present as a paranoid psychosis. Because adrenal glucocorticoid excess (Cushing's syndrome) is sometimes associated with a severe depression, suicide is an important cause of death in this condition.

The sex steroids are responsible for some of the behavior that separates (and sometimes joins) the sexes. However, after copulatory behavior has been established, sexual responses in humans are less hormone-dependent than they are in lower mammals. In adult females, androgen excess frequently increases libido. In a study of the effect of female hormones on epileptic patients, exogenous estrogen seemed to activate abnormal electroencephalographic patterns and precipitate seizures; seizures decreased with premenstrual progesterone therapy.[8] Although the role that progesterone plays in the syndrome of premenstrual tension is still not clear, the estrogen-progesterone ratio may be important, as in premenstrual epileptic seizures.

Parathyroid dysfunction may alter behavior by its effect on the circulating level of ionized calcium. Increased calcium decreases neuromuscular activity. In hyperparathyroidism, elevated serum calcium levels may produce a neurasthenia, which is sometimes confused with psychoneurosis. Hypoparathyroidism may induce hypocalcemic tetany or, in susceptible individuals, convulsions; such patients may have chronic mental instability or even a psychosis.

Congenital absence of thyroid hormones leads to severe mental deficiency (cretinism), which may be permanent unless it is treated within the first few months of life. Thyroid underactivity may be associated with a psychosis ("myxedema madness"), which usually has paranoid features. Long untreated hypothyroidism may eventually terminate in "myxedema coma" with accompanying hypothermia. Hyperthyroidism often produces restlessness, irritability, and anxiety, some of which appears to result from the associated increased sensitivity to epinephrine and norepinephrine that is characteristic of thyroid overactivity.

Hypothalamo-Sympatho-Adrenal System

The hypothalamus contains higher integrative centers that govern the activity of the sympathetic nervous system (Fig. 2-3). It sends fibers to other centers in the brain stem from which relays descend in the intermediolateral columns of the spinal cord and emerge, as the sympathetic outflow, from the central nervous system between T1 and L2 to reach the sympathetic ganglia. The fibers that arise in the central nervous system are "preganglionic"; the fibers that take origin from the cells of the sympathetic ganglia are "postganglionic."

The adrenal medulla is a collection of sympathetic ganglia in which the ganglionic cells have lost their axons and have become specialized for endocrine secretion. Acetylcholine, released at the preganglionic nerve endings, stimulates the chromaffin cells of the adrenal medulla to secrete the catecholamine hormones—epinephrine and norepinephrine. Catecholamines are also synthesized and released from norepinephrine-producing sympathetic nerve trunks. The biosynthetic pathways involved in the production of catecholamines are illustrated in Figure 2-4. Synthesis proceeds via phenylalanine to tyrosine, then to dihydrophenylalanine (dopa); this stage is followed by dopamine (hydroxytyramine) which, by the action of a hydroxylase, becomes norepinephrine; epinephrine is then produced by *N*-methylation. The *N*-methylating enzyme is only found in high concentration in the adrenal medulla, which secretes

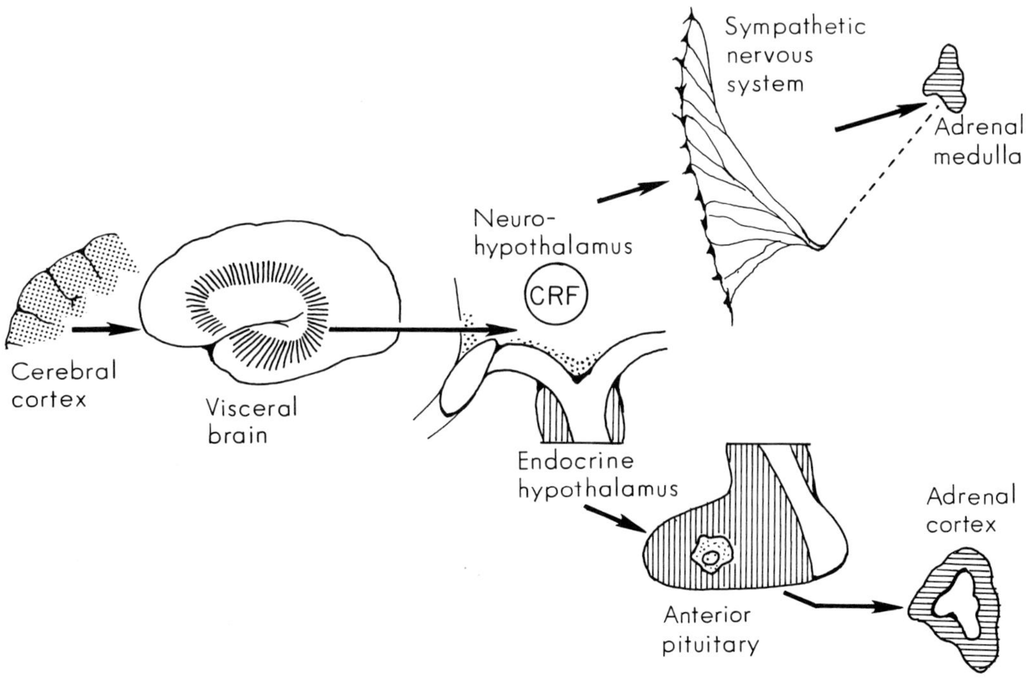

Fig. 2-3. Neuroendocrine pathways in emotional stress leading to adrenal activation. Stress activates the adrenal through the hypothalamus via both nervous (neurohypothalamus) and hormonal (endocrine hypothalamus) pathways. Nervous stimuli originating in cerebral cortex bifurcate in the hypothalamus. Some continue in direct nervous pathways to the adrenal medulla; others stimulate release of CRF and activate first the pituitary corticotroph, then the adrenal cortex.

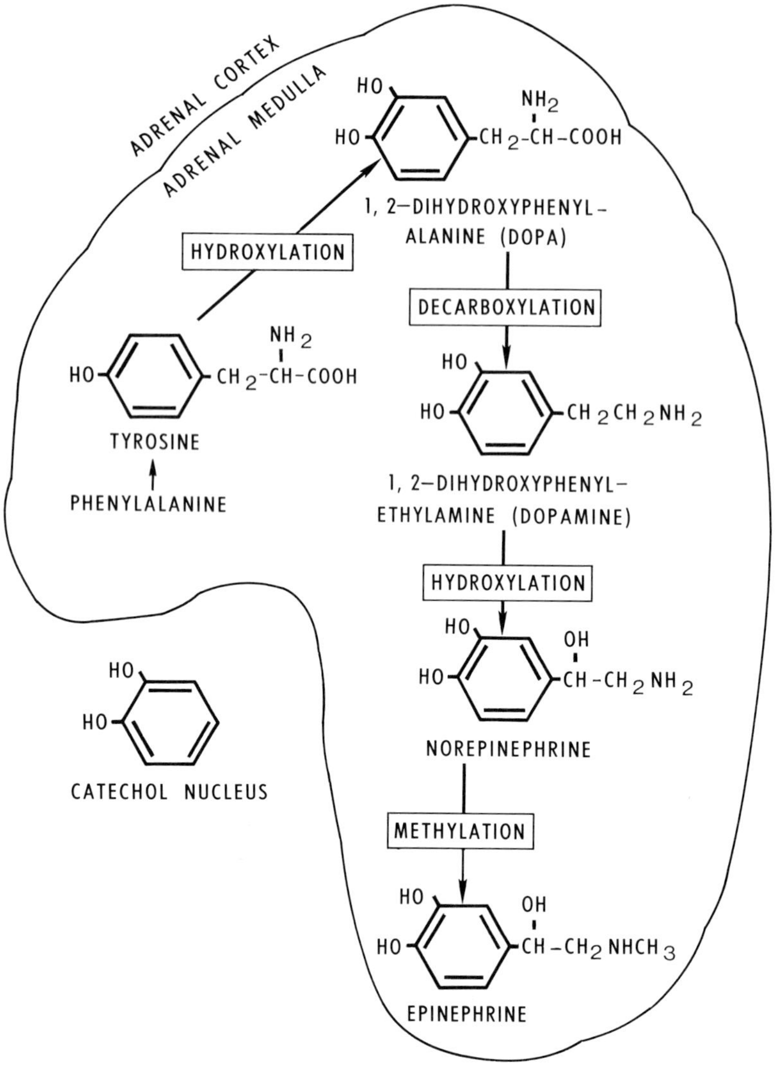

Fig. 2-4. Biosynthetic pathways of the catecholamines. See text for details.

both epinephrine and norepinephrine. In all other sympathetic neurons most of the catecholamine is norepinephrine.*

The similarity between neurosecretion of the hypothalamic neurohypophyseal system and secretion within the sympathetic nerves is illustrated by electron microscopic studies that have shown, in both, secretion granules that are transported from their site of synthesis in the cell body to distant sites of release in the axons. In the sympathetic nerves the granules are composed of catecholamines and their precursors, but they also contain a hydroxylase capable of completing the synthesis of norepinephrine. In and near the sympathetic nerve endings there is a complex circulation of the catecholamines, their precursors, and breakdown products. In this circulation, several different catecholamine "pools" or compartments appear to exist in dynamic equilibrium. In addition to being liberated or secreted, circulating catecholamines and related substances are taken up by the axonal membrane and bound by the granules in the axoplasm. Granules in the adrenal medulla may also take up the catecholamines in

* See Appendix: Addendum to Chapter 2.

such a fashion. The significance of these multiple sources of catecholamine hormones is not known at the present time, although it undoubtedly has something to do with finer regulation of the functions under sympathetic control.

Although epinephrine and norepinephrine differ considerably in other physiologic and pharmacologic effects, both are potent vasopressors. The most important lesion involving the adrenal medulla is a functioning tumor which produces excessive amounts of these catecholamine hormones. This tumor, called pheochromocytoma or chromaffinoma because of its staining qualities, usually arises in the adrenal although it may be found anywhere in the sympathetic-adrenal system. It secretes excessive quantities of catecholamines, chiefly epinephrine, and may, by intermittent release of hormone, produce paroxysmal hypertension with accompanying anxiety and irritability of the central nervous system.

The catecholamines raise the blood glucose level by activating glycogenolytic enzymes and increase the circulating level of free fatty acids by activating adipose-tissue "hormone-sensitive" lipase. This increase in the supply of easily available energy assists survival of an animal during emergencies that induce "fright, fight, or flight." This concept, which was first propounded by Cannon,[3,4] in his "emergency theory of the emotions" and called the "alarm reaction," was expanded by Selye to include secondarily increased adrenal cortical activity in the "general adaptation syndrome" during "stress." The pathways underlying this sympatho-adrenal interaction may spread from the cerebral cortex through the limbic system to ultimately involve the hypothalamus. Increased secretion of hypothalamic corticotropin-releasing factor (CRF) then leads to pituitary corticotropic activation, which in turn stimulates the adrenal cortex. Figure 2-3 shows the principal structures involved in this combined adrenal activation in response to stressful circumstances.

Disorders of the Hypothalamus

Etiology

Both congenital and acquired disease may affect the hypothalamus and neighboring areas.[2] *Hamartoma of the tuber cinereum,* a congenital reduplication of tissue, may produce precocious puberty. *Head injury* or *trauma during operation* on the pituitary may derange hypothalamic function. *Encephalitis, chronic inflammation* (tuberculosis or syphilis), and *xanthomatous granulomas* may also damage this region. The *tumors* which may be found in this area include neurofibroma, ganglioglioma, ectopic pinealoma, and craniopharyngioma. *Degenerative disorders* such as tuberous sclerosis, encephalopathy, and hydrocephalus may also produce hypothalamic disturbance. *Leukemic infiltration* sometimes involves the hypothalamus.

Clinical Features

Specific symptoms of hypothalamic involvement are those of sexual abnormality (e.g., delayed or precocious puberty [Fig. 2-5], or disturbances in ovulation or lactation) or of diabetes insipidus (polydipsia and polyuria). Common additional symptoms include obesity from hyperphagia (presumably the result of destruction of centers in the basal hypothalamus that normally inhibit the intake of food), and visual disturbances resulting from pressure on the optic chiasm, which lies below the hypothalamus. The patient may also have headaches, changes in personality, dementia, somnolence, or increased restless activity. Dysthermia, failure to maintain normal body temperature, is due to interference with the temperature-regulating mechanisms in the hypothalamus. Convulsions may occur from neurologic disease but may also be due to water intoxication, electrolyte disturbances or hypoglycemia. Hypothyroidism may result from hypothalamic disease, due to a failure of TRH production. (See also Chapter 4, Pituitary Hypothyroidism.)

Persistent postpartum lactation, usually with amenorrhea (the Chiari-Frommel syndrome) or galactorrhea with amenorrhea in women who have not been pregnant, is probably due to impairment of the normal delivery to the adenohypophysis of prolactin-inhibiting factor (PIF) and gonadotropin-releasing factors. Many of these patients have a purely functional disorder secondary to emotional disturbance related to reproduc-

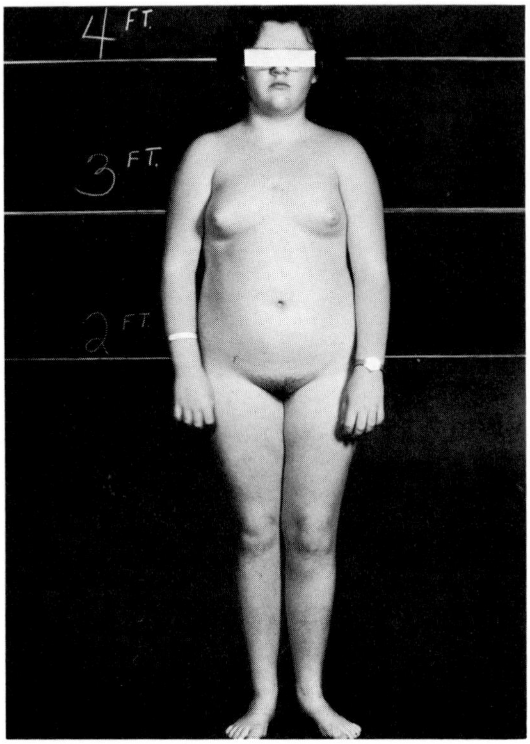

Fig. 2-5. Precocious puberty as a symptom of hypothalamic disorder. This 7-year-old girl's precocious sexual development was manifest in well-formed breasts, pubic hair, and menses. Now 18, she has been followed for 10 years, has shown no evidence of an organic hypothalamic or other glandular lesion, and hence is presumed to have "constitutional" precocious puberty. Her condition is probably due to an aberration in hypothalamic function.

tion; however, in some the syndrome is associated with a pituitary tumor. Because the adenohypophysis is so close, hypothalamic lesions may involve the anterior pituitary and produce adrenal cortical or thyroid insufficiency.

Disorders of the Hypothalamus Simulating Anterior Pituitary Insufficiency: Some hyposomatotropic midgets with associated hypothyroidism have been shown to respond to TRH with an increase in serum TSH by immunoassay. This strongly suggests that anterior pituitary is intact but is not secreting growth hormone because of a failure of hypothalamus to deliver growth-hormone-releasing factor into the portal circulation. Similar defective secretion of corticotropin-releasing factor may explain some cases of adrenal insufficiency associated with hypothalamic disease. Proof of this hypothesis awaits the availability of these releasing hormones for clinical trial in such cases.

The *diencephalic syndrome,* a condition of infancy, presents as severe wasting in spite of presumably adequate caloric intake. The infant is usually restless and overactive, which accounts for its failure to gain. Other characteristic features are a pleasant personality and nystagmoid eye movements. The results of most endocrine studies of this conditon have been normal, but abnormal responses to the administration of Metopirone (metyrapone), which normally increases the output of ACTH by interfering with the production of cortisol, suggests that this syndrome is sometimes associated with a defect in the hypothalamic-pituitary-adrenal cortical control system.[7] The disease may be caused by malignant tumors, which, for a time, may respond favorably to radiation therapy.

Frölich's syndrome is usually caused by craniopharyngioma, which produces a combination of hypogonadism and obesity; both are presumably of hypothalamic origin. Because this tumor may progress to involve other anterior pituitary functions, it is discussed more fully in the chapter on the adenohypophysis.

In the *Laurence-Moon-Biedl syndrome* (hypogonadism, mental retardation, obesity, and polydactyly) the endocrine aspects are attributed to a congenital disorder of the hypothalamus. Patients with this syndrome present with gross obesity, hypotonia, mental retardation and undescended testes. They have a characteristic facies which makes the diagnosis obvious.

Kallman's syndrome, which occurs in both sexes but is more common in males, is the association of hypogonadotropic hypogonadism with anosmia. It is probably due to a lesion of the hypothalamus or its higher connections, associated with agenesis of some portion of the olfactory pathway.

Radiographic Diagnosis

Recognition of gross hypothalamic lesions is aided by radiographs of the skull which may show regional calcification in the wall of a cystic tumor or in the substance of a solid tumor. Increased intracranial pressure may be suggested by separation of sutures or decalcification of the dorsum sellae. Pneumoencephalography may reveal distortion by the expanding lesion of the neighboring subarachnoid cisterns or the ventricular system. Angiography may reveal an abnormal vascular pattern characteristic of glioma or meningioma.

Management

Treatment and prognosis depend on the disease. Hamartomas are usually self-limited and produce only precocious puberty, with no further functional impairment. Operative treatment of tumors in this region is very hazardous because of the extreme vulnerability of the hypothalamus to grave functional derangement from slight injury. Usually only enough tissue is removed to relieve pressure on the visual pathway. Many tumors respond satisfactorily to radiation. Xanthomatous granulomas (histiocytosis) can often be controlled by radiation, particularly in children. Craniopharyngiomas may be treated successfully by a combination of cautious resection and X-ray. Investigation of pituitary disorders associated with hypothalamic lesions is considered further in the chapters on the adenohypophysis and neurohypophysis.

References

1. Association for Research in Nervous and Mental Disease. *Endocrines and the Central Nervous System.* Research publications, Vol. 43. Baltimore, Williams & Wilkins, 1963.
2. Bauer, H. G. Endocrine and metabolic conditions related to pathology in the hypothalamus: A review. *J Nerv Ment Dis 128:*323–338, 1959.
3. Cannon, W. B. The emergency function of the adrenal medulla in pain and the major emotions. *Am J Physiol 33:*356–372, 1914.
4. Cannon, W. B. *Bodily Changes in Pain, Hunger, Fear and Rage,* 2d ed. New York, Appleton, 1929, p. 404.
5. Catt, K. J. ABC of endocrinology. IV. Reproductive endocrinology. *Lancet 1:*1097–1104, 1970.
6. Glaser, G. H. Panel discussion: Recent concepts of central neurophysiology; their bearing on psychosomatic phenomena. *Psychosom Med 17:*337–346, 1955.
7. Krieger, D. T., Glick, S., Silverberg, A., and Krieger, H. P. A comparative study of endocrine tests in hypothalamic disease: Circadian periodicity of plasma 11-OHCS levels, plasma 11-OHCS and growth hormone response to insulin hypoglycemia and metyrapone responsiveness. *J Clin Endocrinol Metab 28:*1589–1598, 1968.
8. Logothetis, J., Harner, R., Morrell, F., and Torres, F. The role of estrogens in the catamenial exacerbation of epilepsy. *Neurology 9:*352–360, 1959.
9. Mylroie, R., and Koenig, H. Soluble acidic lipoproteins of bovine neurosecretory granules. Relation to neurophysins. *J Histochem Cytochem 19:*738–746, 1971.
10. Reichlin, S. Editorial: Function of the hypothalamus. *Am J Med 43:*477–485, 1967.
11. Selye, H. *The Stress of Life.* New York, McGraw-Hill, 1956.
12. Swanson, H. E., and van der Werff ten Bosch, J. J. The 'early-androgen' syndrome; Its development and the response to hemispaying. *Acta Endocrinol (Kbh) 45:*1–12, 1964.

3

The Neurohypophysis

Calvin Ezrin

The neural portion of the pituitary gland consists mainly of two specialized transportation systems:

1. A neurosecretory pathway that extends from hypothalamic nuclei where the hormones are manufactured, to the neural lobe where they are stored
2. A neurovascular pathway that runs from the endocrine hypothalamus via fiber tracts to the primary capillary plexus of the portal circulation, and from there via the bloodstream to the adenohypophysis (see Fig. 2-1)

Anatomy and Physiology

In the standard nomenclature applied to the major subdivisions of the pituitary gland, the neurohypophysis consists of 3 parts:

1. The median eminence of the tuber cinereum, which is histologically distinct from the hypothalamus
2. The infundibular stem
3. The infundibular process (neural lobe)

The infundibular stem and portions of the pars tuberalis of the adenohypophysis, forming a sheath around it, make up the hypophyseal stalk. The main nerve supply of the neurohypophysis consists of two fairly distinct parts:

1. The supraopticohypophyseal tract which runs in the anterior (ventral) portion of the median eminence. It is very superficial and hence liable to be involved by inflammations affecting the base of the brain.
2. The tuberohypophyseal tract, which runs in the posterior (dorsal) wall of the median eminence and the stalk.

Blood Supply of the Pituitary Gland

The neurohypophysis has two separate blood supplies:

1. Branches of the superior and inferior hypophyseal arteries arising from the internal carotid, which supply the neurohypophyseal tissues
2. The primary plexus of the portal system, which receives chemical messages from the fibers of the tuberohypophyseal tract and delivers them to the adenohypophysis via the portal veins

The portal venous system is the only significant blood supply to the sinusoids of the anterior lobe. Thus it may be said that "the life-blood of the adenohypophysis flows through the neurohypophysis." Postpartum necrosis of the pituitary gland usually involves mainly the adenohypophysis; the neurohypophysis is spared because of its different blood supply which makes it less vulnerable to ischemia during an *episode* of hypotension.

The hypothalamic hormones, vasopressin and oxytocin, are held in storage in the neurohypophysis, combined with a stainable neurosecretory substance; when required, they are released into the systemic circulation. They are both octapeptides; their amino acid constituents differ only in two locations. Vasopressin has considerable oxytocic potency and oxytocin has a mild antidiuretic effect. Their structural similarities explain their overlapping biologic properties.

Oxytocin exerts its physiologic effect only during labor and lactation. The neurohormonal reflex responsible for milk ejection was described in the introductory chapter (see Fig. 1-1). On the afferent side, the suckling stimulus travels from sensory nerve endings of the nipple to the paraventricular nucleus of the hypothalamus; on the efferent side of the reflex, oxytocin (which is stored in the neurohypophysis) is released into the circulation. In a study conducted on rabbits shortly after parturition, Ferguson showed that mechanical dilation of the body of the uterus, cervix, and vagina stimulates the reflex release of oxytocin, which is manifested by an increase in uterine contractions. That this reflex is also active during labor was illustrated as follows: A woman in labor who was still lactating from a previous pregnancy expelled milk from her nipples with each "labor pain," presumably in response to oxytocin. A similar ejection of milk was also observed when posterior lobe extract containing oxytocin was injected at the end of the second stage of labor.

Vasopressin, the antidiuretic hormone, is required to maintain the normal osmotic pressure of the plasma. The increase of plasma osmolality associated with dehydration stimulates "osmoreceptors" in the anterior hypothalamus; this causes the neurohypophyseal terminals of the supraopticohypophyseal tract to release vasopressin into the general circulation (Fig. 3-1). Vasopressin acts on the distal renal tubules and the collecting ducts to increase reabsorption of water.[6]

Diabetes Insipidus

Because the neurohypophysis secretes only two hormones and because there appear to be no diseases associated with oxytocin, diseases of the neurohypophysis involve only vasopressin—usually as a deficiency syndrome termed diabetes insipidus (DI). This clinical condition, characterized by a water diuresis and secondary polydipsia, is usually due to neurohypophyseal and adenohypophyseal involvement. Patients with DI often prefer ice-cold drinks—a fact that distinguishes this disorder from other types of polyuria with secondary polydipsia.

The specific gravity of the urine is usually below 1.004 except in some patients with partial insufficiency or in those who are severely dehydrated. If the thirst mechanism is depressed by associated central nervous system disease, patients with untreated DI may quickly develop serious dehydration from the combined effect of excessive loss of fluid and inadequate replacement.

If the supraopticohypophyseal tract is interrupted close to the median eminence, a characteristic pattern of transient polyuria develops, which is best studied in experimental animals. This polyuria appears in a few hours, lasts 4 to 6 days, is followed by an apparent remission ("interphase") lasting about 5 days, and terminates in permanent DI. The normal interphase is probably due to the resorption of vasopressin from the denervated neurohypophysis, which is undergoing atrophy. In man, when the tract is cut at the level of the diaphragma sellae, permanent DI does not usually develop because about 20% of the neurohypophysis is still connected to the hypothalamus and produces enough vasopressin to meet ordinary need. However, transient DI is very common after low stalk section or removal of the pituitary gland from below by the transsphenoidal route, presumably because of reversible damage to the remaining portion of the neurohypophysis. Such dysfunction usually subsides within 2 weeks.

Etiology

The known causes of DI can be divided into hereditary, traumatic, inflammatory, and degenerative. However, a large number of cases appear to be idiopathic. Hereditary DI is rare; it is thought to be due to a failure of the supraoptic nuclei to develop sufficiently to produce adequate amounts of vasopressin. The more common in-

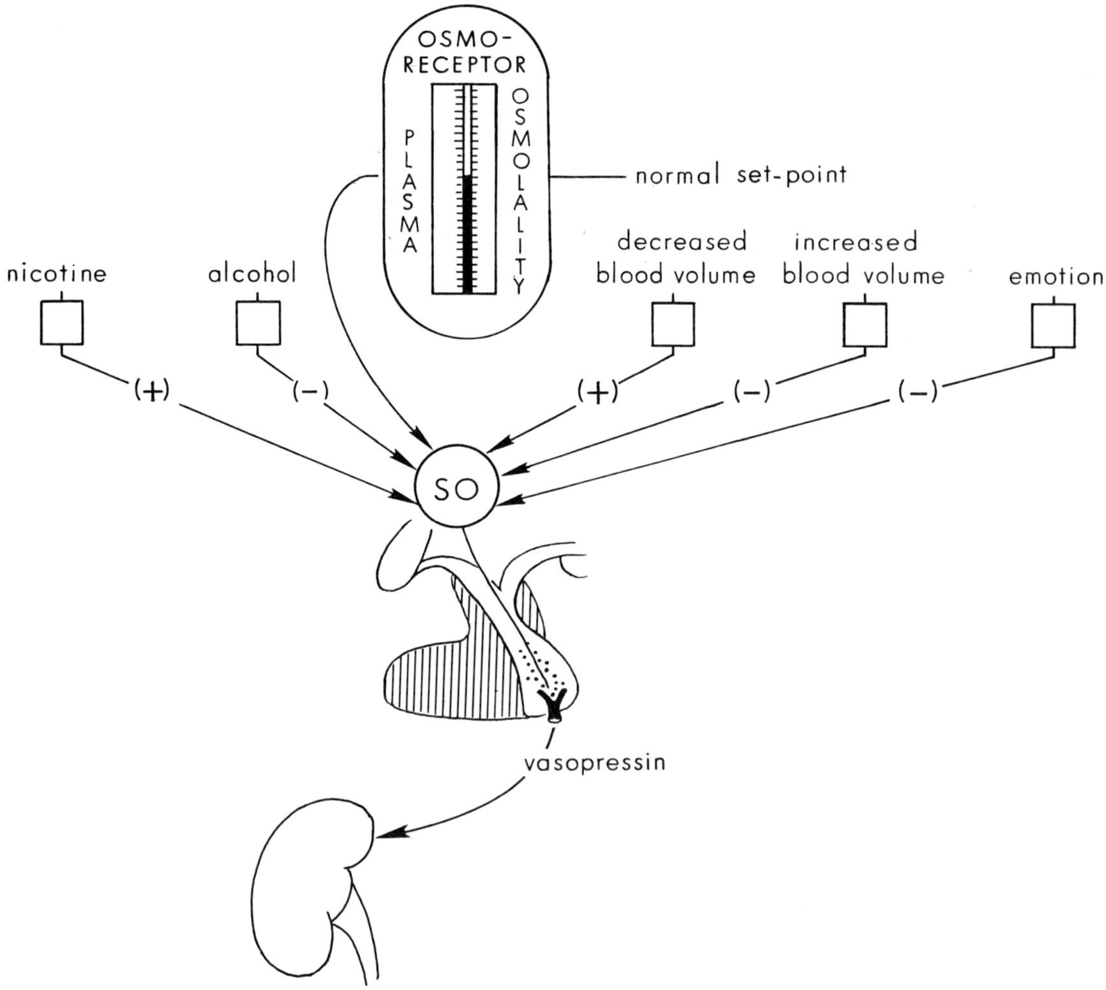

Fig. 3-1. Control of vasopression release. The normal stimulus for vasopressin release is plasma osmolality higher than the normal set-point, which is usually constant but may be altered in disease.

Vasopressin release can also be increased by severe decrease in blood volume or by administration of nicotine or its absorption from cigarette smoking.

Vasopressin release can be decreased by reduction in plasma osmolality, increase in blood volume, or by administration of alcohol.

Generally emotional stress results in decreased vasopressin release and hence produces polyuria.

herited variant—nephrogenic diabetes insipidus—results from a failure of the distal renal tubular epithelium to respond to vasopressin, even though this hormone is produced in adequate amounts.

With trauma, the most common site of the lesion is the stalk, which may be torn without any associated skull fracture. When inflammatory disease of the base of the brain causes DI, such disease is usually chronic (e.g., tuberculous meningitis or syphilis—basal meningitis of the secondary stage or gumma). In infancy and childhood, histiocytic granuloma of the Hand-Schüller-Christian variety is an important cause; in this age group, pertussis (whooping cough) either by inducing anoxia or hemorrhage may also produce DI. Sarcoidosis and Hodgkin's disease occasionally cause this syndrome in later life. Many patients develop DI after attempted removal of a pituitary tumor. Either a primary or secondary tumor may be responsible for the spontaneous development of this disorder. Metastatic lesions in the neurohypophysis or its immediate neighborhood may interfere with the production or delivery of vasopressin, or may damage the osmoreceptors so that hyperosmolality does not stimulate its secretion. However, in the rare patient with osmoreceptor failure, nicotine administration will still trigger the release of vasopressin by a nonosmotic pathway.

Differential Diagnosis of Polyuria with Dilute Urine

In the interpretation of tests for DI, three phenomena must be kept in mind:

1. Whether adequate vasopressin can be produced
2. Whether one is dealing with a failure of the osmoreceptors to respond to hyperosomolality in the presence of an adequate amount of vasopressin (this can only be demonstrated by using an alternative stimulus such as nicotine to release vasopressin)
3. Whether the kidney can respond to vasopressin

In adults the differential diagnosis involves consideration of hysterical polydipsia or compulsive water drinking; in children primary renal disorders are most likely to be confused with DI.

A history of emotional disturbance may suggest the diagnosis of psychogenic polydipsia. However, many patients with true DI have a psychogenic component to their polydipsia which may be misleading if only the history is considered. Furthermore, in some patients with psychogenic polydipsia, prolonged water intake makes the renal tubules somewhat resistant to vasopressin. This situation, which is a type of acquired nephrogenic DI, complicates the interpretation of the diagnostic tests.

In patients with polyuria the function of the neurohypophyseal-renal system can be evaluated by serial tests:

1. The most useful is water deprivation to induce hyperosmolality. Withholding fluids for 8 hours is usually sufficient to produce changes in plasma and urine osmolality that will enable the diagnosis of DI to be made.*
2. Hypertonic sodium chloride may be given intravenously to induce hyperosmolality (Hickey-Hare or Carter-Robbins tests).[5]
3. Nicotine may be injected in the rare case suspected to represent osmoreceptor failure. It stimulates the release of vasopressin by a nonosmotic pathway.
4. After water loading, vasopressin is injected to determine the response of the kidneys.

Determination of urine and serum osmolality greatly increases the accuracy of these tests and should be used more widely.[5] During fluid deprivation with normal vasopressin secretion, the serum osmolality (expressed as milliosmoles per kilogram of water) is kept at a near-constant level—about 285. If the serum osmolality rises by as little as 2 mOsm, vasopressin is released to restore the serum osmolality to normal. Its antidiuretic effect produces a hypertonic urine. The urine osmolality will rise from about 400 mOsm to 1,000 after 8 hours of fluid restriction. In true DI, the continued renal excretion of large volumes of water during fluid deprivation causes the serum osmolality to increase to 330 mOsm or more in severe cases. The compulsive water drinkers will usually have a normal response to fluid deprivation. Patients with partial vasopressin deficiency will show intermediate responses. In true DI the serum sodium does not rise greatly as long as the thirst mechanism is intact and fluid is not restricted. However, prolonged water deprivation may produce a moderate increase in serum sodium.

A useful approximation of serum osmolality may be obtained by the following formulas:

Serum osmolality =

(*1*) $2 \times \text{serum Na (mEq/liter)} + 10$

or

(*2*) $2 \times \text{serum Na (mEq/liter)} + (\text{blood glucose}/18) + (\text{blood urea}/6)$

In DI, since the polyuria is primary, the urine output is slightly ahead of the fluid intake, which leads to an increased "resting" (i.e., before fluid

* See Appendix: Addendum to Chapter 3.

deprivation) serum osmolality. However, in hysterical polydipsia, the fluid intake is slightly ahead of the urine output, which leads to some reduction in resting serum osmolality.

In normal individuals and in most patients with psychogenic polydipsia, intravenous hypertonic saline causes a decrease in urine volume; in true DI, there is no such decrease. In patients with osmoreceptor failure, nicotine injection, but not hyperosmolality, reduces the volume of urine and increases its osmolality. In nephrogenic and "nephritigenic" (secondary to chronic nephritis) DI, vasopressin does not have its normal antidiuretic effect. This latter condition is seen mainly in children who may present with polyuria. Thus renal function must be evaluated with particular care in children with suspected DI. This is done by routine urinalysis, determination of blood urea nitrogen, serum electrolytes (including calcium and phosphorus), and urea and creatinine clearance, which help to establish the renal reserve. Intravenous and retrograde pyelography may give useful information.

Treatment

The most effective treatment of DI is the intramuscular administration of long-acting vasopressin tannate in oil; 1 cc (containing 5 units) is usually given about three times a week. The vial should be warmed and shaken well before withdrawing the suspension, otherwise most of the hormone will adhere to the wall of the container. After the injection, the patient should limit fluid intake to reduce the risk of transient water intoxication. A nasal spray of lysine-vasopressin may relieve polyuria for a few hours, but the limited duration of effect is a drawback to this form of therapy. Nasal snuff containing posterior-lobe hormone in powder form has been prescribed for a similar purpose, but it is usually too irritating for long-term use.

In both nephrogenic and ordinary DI, thiazide diuretics paradoxically may act as antidiuretics, causing symptomatic improvement by a complicated effect on the renal tubules. However, after an initial improvement, patients usually become resistant to thiazides. Even when the therapy continues to be effective, the patient's need for added potassium should be remembered.

The most promising recent development in the treatment of DI is the demonstration that one of the sulfonamide antidiabetic agents, chlorpropamide, is effective in some patients with ordinary DI (but not in those with nephrogenic DI).[3] The dose varies from 125 to 500 mg. every 12 hours. Chlorpropamide appears to act by potentiating the effect of small amounts of vasopressin that otherwise would be insufficient to prevent polyuria. However, hypoglycemia may complicate the treatment, particularly in patients with associated anterior pituitary disease. A combination of chlorpropamide and thiazide diuretic may have an effect that is greater than either alone.[7] Conservative treatment still has a role to play in the management of some patients with moderate DI who refuse or cannot tolerate drugs and are willing to accept the inconvenience of some polyuria and polydipsia.

Transient DI is a recognized clinical phenomenon. It may be associated with the following events:

1. Reversible damage to the pituitary stalk at operation
2. Amelioration of DI by progressive anterior pituitary insufficiency
3. Improvement following lumbar puncture

In some patients, following pituitary ablation or resection of tumor, transient DI may be observed. Recovery follows because damage to the supraoptic neurohypophyseal tract is mild enough to be reversible. In patients with a progressive granuloma or tumor in the region of the pituitary, the onset of anterior pituitary insufficiency may be heralded by amelioration of DI (which was the first manifestation of the disease) and is probably due to moderate adrenal cortical insufficiency with reduced glomerular filtration rate (top four panels, Fig. 3-2). Sometimes latent DI due to unsuspected associated granuloma of the supraoptic neurohypophyseal tract may be unmasked by steroid treatment of a pulmonary granuloma as shown in the bottom panel of Figure 3-2. This is another example of the glucocorticoid-vasopressin antagonism.

Fig. 3-2. Functional antagonism between vasopressin and adrenal glucocorticoid hormones. When the system is in normal balance **(top panel)**, enough vasopressin is released to keep urine volume at about 1,500 cc.

A lesion of the supraoptic neurohypophyseal tract **(second panel)** has blocked vasopressin release. DI results.

When the lesion extends to involve adenohypophyseal corticotrophs **(third panel),** the resultant adrenocortical insufficiency will "relieve" DI, probably by reducing glomerular filtration rate (GFR). The patient treated by glucocorticoid replacement "relapses" **(fourth panel)** because the steroid restores GFR to normal.

In another type of glucocorticoid-induced diabetes (DI), a patient with pulmonary granuloma **(bottom panel)** and an unsuspected lesion of the supraoptic neurohypophyseal tract has no symptoms of DI until he is treated with large doses of prednisone. In this patient, GFR is presumably normal; hence there must be other sites where glucocorticoid antagonizes vasopressin—e.g., at renal tubular level, at site of release of vasopressin, and/or by glucocorticoid stimulation of thirst.

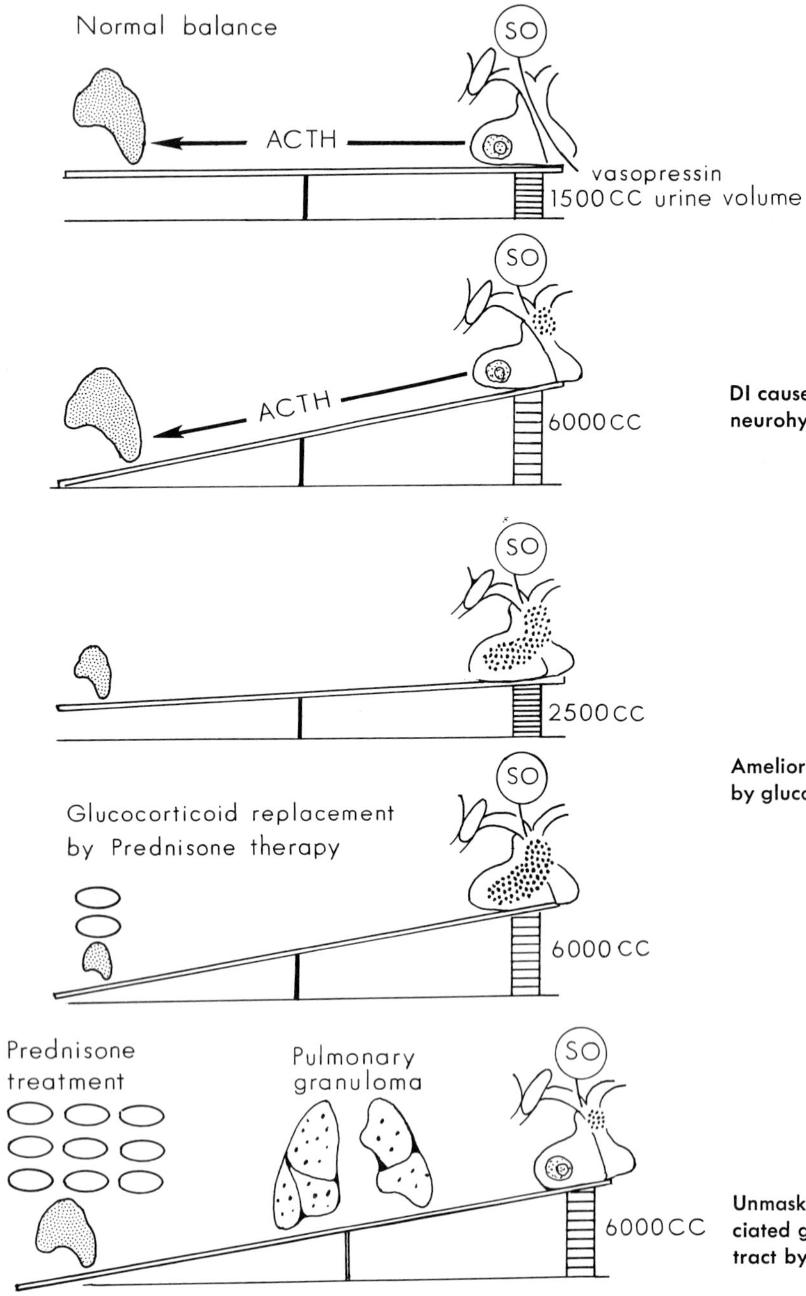

DI caused by progressive granuloma of supraoptic neurohypophyseal tract

Amelioration of the above DI and its restoration by glucocorticoid treatment of adrenal insufficiency

Unmasking of latent DI due to unsuspected associated granuloma of supraoptic neurohypophyseal tract by steroid treatment

Lumbar puncture or air encephalogram seems, on rare occasions, to "cure" DI. The mechanism is obscure, but probably these procedures somehow open up new channels for the delivery of vasopressin into the circulation.

Inappropriate Secretion of Antidiuretic Hormone

In this context, "inappropriate" secretion (or release) of antidiuretic hormone (ADH) refers to either increased delivery or secretion appearing when the serum osmolality would not normally call it forth. This leads to excessive retention of water. The clinical conditions associated with such disproportionate water retention may be either transient or sustained.[1]

Transient

The most common cause of *water intoxication* is overtreatment of DI with either vasopressin or chlorpropamide, associated with the continued ingestion of water. Occasionally after transsphenoidal hypophysectomy or pituitary-stalk section, a similar "hypervasopressinism" may develop, because of unregulated absorption of vasopressin from the denervated portion of the neurohypophysis. Such vasopressin excess produces inappropriate retention of water from ingested fluids or from administered intravenous glucose and water, and hence dilutional hyponatremia. The patient's confusion or decreased consciousness may be mistakenly ascribed to postoperative intracranial bleeding. The diagnosis of transient postoperative vasopressin excess may be suspected if attention is paid to water balance. If water intake is limited and the damage to the stalk has not been extensive, the patient rapidly returns to normal. If the damage is more severe, this improvement may be followed by permanent DI.

Sustained

In certain cases of cerebral disease, for example tuberculous meningitis, excessive secretion of vasopressin may cause water intoxication that is manifested by convulsions and an associated dilutional hyponatremia. A similar clinical and laboratory pattern may be seen in patients with malignant disease outside the cranial cavity. This syndrome of "inappropriate" secretion of antidiuretic hormone may be due also to the manufacture of a hormone with similar actions by the neoplastic tissue itself. This excessive secretion, which is characterized by hyponatremia with a persistent urinary loss of sodium, is best treated by fluid restriction to less than 1,000 cc per day. Inhibition of aldosterone secretion by the expanded intravascular fluid volume may explain the increased renal excretion of sodium, although excessive production of a natriuretic "third factor" of renal origin has also been postulated.[4]

The factors that normally control the release of vasopressin and some of the pharmacologic agents that may be used to test this system are depicted in Figure 3-1. In dealing with diseases involving the supraoptic nucleus and its connections, it is helpful to consider the concept of a normal "set-point"—the level at which a rising serum osmolality triggers the release of vasopressin. If this point is set too low, an inappropriate and therefore excessive secretion of vasopressin may result (Fig. 3-3). A similar state of affairs may occur if vasopressin or another antidiuretic hormone is manufactured in a site other than the hypothalamic-pituitary region and hence is not under the control of normal homeostatic mechanisms. The set-point may also be abnormally elevated, which would lead to chronic hyperosmolality. The thirst mechanism may also be deranged in diabetes insipidus secondary to diseases of the hypothalamus. In cases of chronic, sustained hyperosmolality, it seems likely that there is also an associated blunting of the thirst mechanism.

Although vasopressin derived its name from its influence on blood pressure of laboratory animals, it does not make a significant contribution to the maintenance of normal blood pressure in man, since hypotension is not a feature of DI. Thus the study of the syndrome of DI provides a key to the understanding of the physiology of that portion of the neurohypophysis concerned with the storage

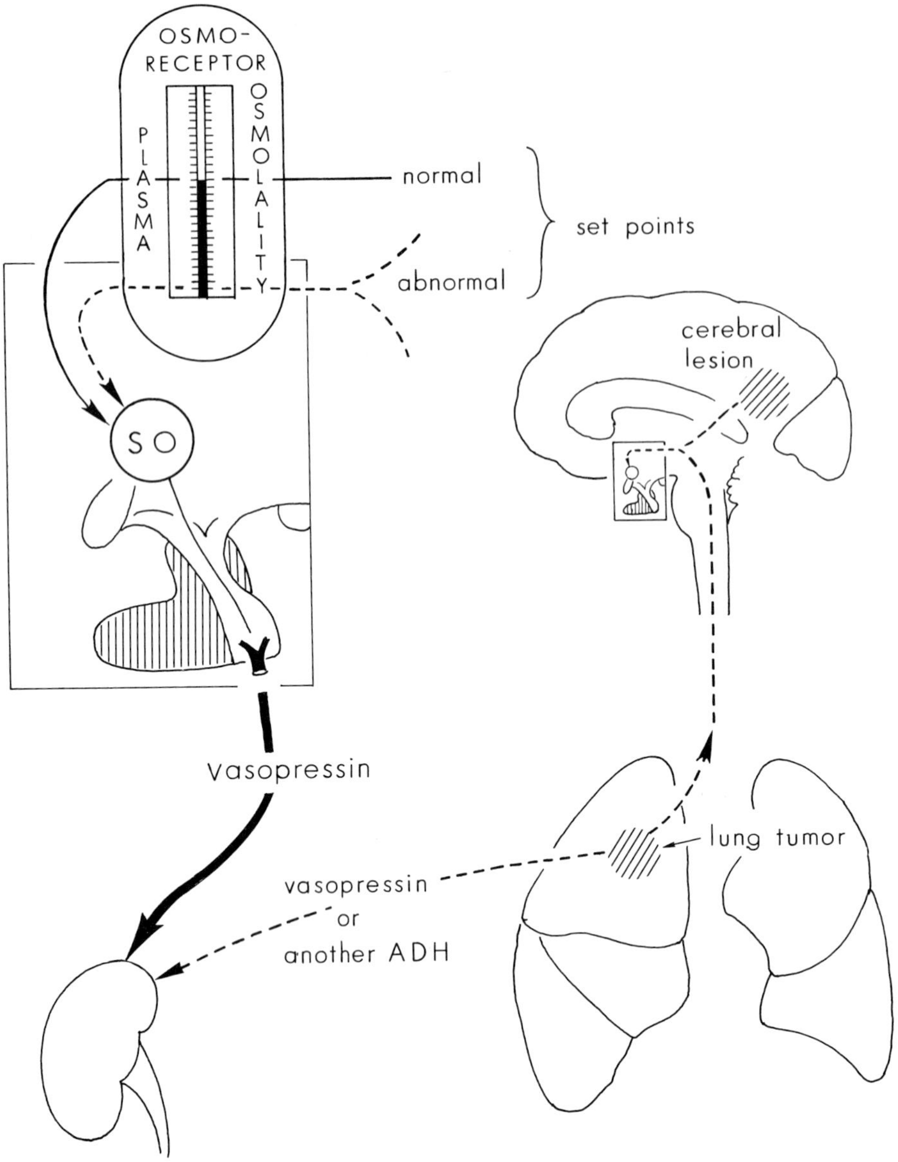

Fig. 3-3. Some factors that may lead to inappropriate secretion of vasopressin. Upper left. Osmoreceptor with both a normal and abnormally low setting for vasopressin release in response to plasma osmolality. This set-point may be abnormally low in certain metabolic diseases (e.g., hypothroidism) or secondary to organic intracranial disease (e.g., tuberculoma, etc.)

An intracranial lesion (*upper right*) may also lead to excessive vasopressin secretion, without going through osmoreceptors, by direct "irritative" stimulation of supraoptic nucleus. Lung tumor (*lower right*) may produce (1) vasopressin itself, (2) abnormal antidiuretic hormone (ADH) or (3) inappropriate reflex secretion of vasopressin by irritation of local sensory nerves.

and release of vasopressin. It is puzzling that there is no recognized clinical deficiency of oxytocin comparable to DI. In patients with DI, parturition and lactation usually proceed satisfactorily, indicating that oxytocin can be released separately in adequate amounts, or that the supply of other oxytocic factors may be sufficient to allow normal labor and milk ejection.

References

1. Bartter, F. C., and Schwartz, W. B. The syndrome of inappropriate secretion of antidiuretic hormone. *Am J Med 42:*790–806, 1967.
2. Ferguson, K. J. W. A study of the motility of the intact uterus at term. *Surg Gynecol Obstet 73:*359–366, 1941.
3. Hocken, A. G., and Longson, D. Reduction of free water clearance by chlorpropamide. *Br Med J 1:*355–356, 1968.
4. Ivy, H. K. The syndrome of inappropriate secretion of antidiuretic hormone. *Med Clin North Am 52:*817–826, 1968.
5. Price, J. E. D., and Lauener, R. W. Serum and urine osmolalities in the differential diagnosis of polyuric states. *J Clin Endocrinol Metab 26:*143–148, 1966.
6. Verney, E. B. Croonian lecture: The antidiuretic hormone and factors which determine its release. *Proc R Soc Lond* [*Biol*] *135:*25–106, 1947.
7. Webster, B., and Bain, J. Antidiuretic effect and complications of chlorpropamide therapy in diabetes insipidus. *J Clin Endocrinol Metab 30:*215–227, 1970.

4

The Adenohypophysis

Calvin Ezrin

History

Although the pituitary gland has been recognized since the time of Galen, it was regarded as a vestigial relic with no apparent function until nearly the end of the nineteenth century. Acromegaly, a syndrome of generalized overgrowth associated with a pituitary tumor, was the first pituitary disorder to be recognized; it was described clearly and named by Pierre Marie, a neurologist, in 1886. In 1901, Alfred Fröhlich published his memorable case report of tumor of the pituitary without acromegaly. He attributed the syndrome of hypogonadism and obesity to destruction of the pituitary. Later it was recognized that hypothalamic involvement accounted for the obesity and possibly the hypogonadism in such cases.

Harvey Cushing in 1908 contrasted the *hyperpituitarism* of acromegaly with the *hypopituitarism* produced by partial destruction of the gland by tumor or surgical excision. Among the earliest cases of severe hypopituitarism were those described by Morris Simmonds from 1914 to 1918. He attributed the associated atrophy of gonads, thyroid, and adrenal glands found at necropsy to puerperal infarction of the adenohypophysis.[6] From these beginnings, physiologic and clinical studies led to the modern concept of the anterior pituitary gland as the master endocrine organ controlling the activities of its three target glands, and also influencing body size, lactation, and pigmentation by the elaboration of separate hormones.

Gross Anatomy

The adenohypophysis consists of three parts: (1) the pars tuberalis, (2) the pars intermedia, and (3) the pars distalis (anterior lobe). In the human, the pars intermedia is not well defined. Purves suggests that it has been incorporated into the pars distalis. The intimate relationship of adenohypophysis, neurohypophysis, and hypothalamus has been described in the chapter on neuroendocrinology.

Anatomically the optic chiasm is the most important neighbor of the pituitary, because of its frequent compression by expanding tumor. The sella turcica, which houses the pituitary gland, is sometimes enlarged by tumors or affected so that radiologic evidence of pituitary disease may be seen on a radiograph of the skull. This matter will be elaborated upon further in the section on radiology of the adenohypophysis. Now that meningitis can be prevented with antibiotics, surgeons have taken renewed interest in the transsphenoidal approach to the pituitary fossa. However, for the usual patient with a suprasellar extension of tumor which compresses the visual pathway, the transfrontal approach to the pituitary region is still favored because the upward extension of the tumor can then be seen.

Microscopic Anatomy

In the early terminology based on staining procedures which used eosin and methyl blue to color their storage granules, the cells of the adenohypophysis were divided into red acidophils, blue basophils, and unstained chromophobes. Recently, special staining techniques, particularly modifications of the periodic acid–Schiff (PAS) procedure, have given considerable new information about pituitary histology. It now appears that the human adenohypophysis consists of at least five separate functional cell types and possibly seven, one for each of its generally accepted hormonal products (Fig. 4-1). *The Ciba Collection of Medical Illustrations,* Volume 4, *Endocrine System,* Section 1, Plate 9, pages 10 and 11, gives a detailed description of the relationship of the newer pituitary stains to older procedures.[3] At present there is general agreement about the separate identity of the growth hormone cell ("somatotroph" or "somatotrope"), prolactin cell ("lactotroph," "lactotrope" or "mammotroph"), TSH cell ("thyrotroph" or "thyrotrope"). It is still not clear whether there are separate gonadotrophs, which make FSH and LH respectively.

Fig. 4-1. Anterior Pituitary Cell Types as revealed by Special Stains. The adenohypophysis appears to be evolving toward a complete separation of cell types such that each hormone ultimately will have a separate cell of origin. At present the thyrotroph is the only cell that appears to be confined to the production of one hormone. With special stains the acidophils can be separated into growth-hormone-and prolactin-producing cells, but some acidophil tumors appear to be composed of cells that can make both hormones. Immunolocalization studies have shown that ACTH and MSH arise in the same cell. Immunostaining of the gonadotrophs indicates that FSH and LH may also have some common cell of origin along with some cells that appear to make only one or other of these gonadotropins. These cells are depicted by interrupted lines, which also indicate the presumed common cell for the production of both growth hormone and prolactin that sometimes gives rise to mammosomatotropic tumors.

The original acidophil-basophil-chromophobe classification of pituitary cell types should now be replaced with a new nomenclature based on function. Two special stains that are particularly useful in separating the various cell types are the basis for this diagram. The acidophils that make growth hormone (GH) can be distinguished from the prolactin cell (PR) acidophils by the greater affinity of the prolactin cell granules for erythrosin, leaving the GR cells to be stained only by orange G.

The remainder of the cell types, which belong more to the basophil category, can be distinguished from the acidophils and to some extent from each other by special stains involving a combination of periodic acid–Schiff (PAS) stain and either aldehyde thionin or alcian blue. The TSH cell (thyrotroph) has the greatest affinity for aldehyde thionin and therefore takes on a deep blue-purple color. The ACTH-MSH cell, with little affinity for aldehyde thionin, retains a red color derived from the PAS reaction. The FSH and LH cells usually take on a color mid-way between red and blue-purple.

(Adapted from Werner, S. C., and Ingbar, S. H., eds. *The Thyroid: A Fundamental and Clinical Text*, ed. 3. New York, Harper, 1971. Reproduced with permission.)

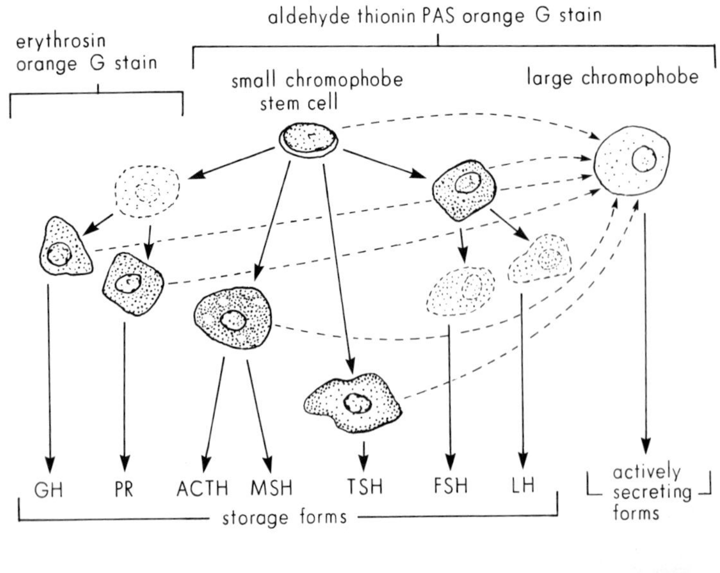

Also it seems likely that ACTH and MSH come from the same cell—the "melanocorticotroph."[17]

Cytophysiology

Description of the microscopic anatomy of the functional subdivisions of the adenohypophysis is complicated by the intermixing of the different cell types throughout the gland. However, the various cells tend to occupy fairly constant regions of the gland and can usually be readily identified by size, shape, staining reactions and responses to target-organ hormone excess or deficiency.[19] In a study of the physiology of the adenohypophysis, each of its hormones should be considered in turn.[7] We shall begin with thyroid-stimulating hormone which has already been considered in the introductory chapter defining "negative feedback" control.

Physiology of Adenohypophyseal Hormones

Thyroid-Stimulating Hormone or Thyrotropin

Thyrotropin, a glycoprotein hormone, increases the growth and activity of thyroid cells; its secretion is inhibited by rising levels of circulating thyroid hormones. The production and release of thyroid hormones is not totally dependent on thyroid-stimulating hormone (TSH). An autonomous basal secretion of thyroid hormone can be detected when circulating thyrotropin has apparently been eliminated by hypophysectomy.

A hypothalamic thyrotropin-releasing factor (TRF) has been demonstrated first by animal experiments and later in clinical studies. In 1969, when two groups of workers described the chemical structure of thyrotropin-releasing hormone (factor), we were surprised to discover that this substance consisted of only three amino acids.[2, 22] The role of TRF in maintaining the narrow normal range of concentration of circulating thyroid hormones is still not established although, compared to the influence of some of the other "adenohypophysiotropic" hormones, it is probably of relatively minor importance. It seems to mediate thyroid activation that results from prolonged exposure to cold. It also appears to be involved in the thyroid adaptation of the newborn to the relatively cold extrauterine environment. The high serum thyroxine and protein-bound iodine of the newborn represents a true hyperthyroid state that can be avoided by increasing the environmental temperature for the first few days of life.

Hypothyroidism due to target-gland insufficiency leads to increased secretion of TSH and eventually to hypertrophy and hyperplasia of the thyrotropic cells (see Fig. 1-2**B**). These "thyrotrophs" are polyhedral, PAS- and aldehyde thionine-positive basophils, which are usually found in the anteromedial portion of the gland.[4] They probably arise from relatively undifferentiated cells which would be classed as chromophobes. Although some of these precursor cells differentiate into thyrotrophs as early as the thirteenth week of human fetal life, a reserve of undifferentiated cells possibly persists into adult life. From this reserve, additional thyrotrophs or other anterior pituitary cell types can be produced under appropriate circumstances. The mechanism controlling this differentiation is still unknown. However, there is no evidence that differentiated anterior pituitary cells change from the production of one hormone to another.

Like many other hormones, TSH appears to stimulate its target cells by activating adenyl cyclase in the cell membrane.

Adrenocorticotropic Hormone or Corticotropin

Adrenocorticotropic hormone (ACTH), a polypeptide, regulates the growth and function of the adrenal cortex and is especially important in the control of the production and release of glucocorticoid hormones such as cortisol. The production of aldosterone by the zona glomerulosa is largely under the control of the renin-angiotensin system; the production of sex steroids by the zona reticularis is governed by a mechanism that is still not clear. The glucocorticoid hormones arise in the zona fasciculata which undergoes hyperplasia under the influence of ACTH. The other zones of the adrenal cortex also grow under such stimulation but to a lesser extent. The pituitary "corticotrophs" sometimes appear as lightly granulated cells, usually classed as chromophobes, or as a subtype of basophil that undergoes the Crookes' hyaline change in Cushing's syndrome. In the present state of our knowledge it seems that ACTH and melanocyte-stimulating hormone (MSH) are both produced by the same basophil sub-type (Phifer). The sequence of seven amino acids that constitutes the "active" center of MSH is also found within the corticotropin molecule and accounts for its moderate melanocyte-stimulating activity.

The release of ACTH by the corticotrophs appears to be governed by three independent mechanisms (see also Fig. 2-2):

1. *Negative feedback.* Cortisol, the principal glucocorticoid product of the adrenal cortex, inhibits ACTH release when present in the bloodstream in greater than physiologic levels. If the cortisol level falls, ACTH secretion commences through a negative feedback mechanism; the cortisol level rises again and turns off the ACTH.

2. *Diurnal rhythm.* There is a diurnal variation in ACTH secretion. In man, adrenal activation is maximal in the early morning hours; after 8 A.M., there is a gradual fall in the ACTH release and consequent cortisol secretion so that, in the afternoon, blood cortisol levels are only about one-half of the 8 A.M. value. This diurnal rhythm appears to be imposed by the nervous system, for it is abolished by certain central nervous lesions as well as by alternations in the sleeping pattern, such as in night workers. It is also lost in Cushing's syndrome.

3. *A stress-activated mechanism.* Stressful stimuli reaching the endocrine hypothalamus permit corticotropin-releasing factor (CRF) to enter the portal circulation and stimulate the corticotrophs. This stress mechanism may override both of the previously described control systems at any time. The greater the stress, the more ACTH is secreted.

The Gonadotropic Hormones

Using special staining and immunostaining, one can distinguish in the human pituitary gland 3 different cell types, which appear to produce the gonadotropic hormones: follicle-stimulating hormone (FSH), luteinizing hormone (LH), and prolactin or lactogenic hormone. The FSH and LH gonadotrophs[1] are subtypes of the basophils; the prolactin cell is a subtype of the acidophils. Some basophils make both FSH and LH.

Gonadotropins and Ovarian Function

FSH, a glycoprotein, enlarges the graafian follicle to the point of rupture. Under its influence, the follicular cells secrete estrogen. Ovulation results from the additional secretion of another glycoprotein, LH, which is necessary in small amounts to stimulate estrogen secretion from the follicular cells. To maintain its production of progesterone, the corpus luteum, at least in rodents, appears to require another pituitary protein hormone, luteotropin, which is identical with prolactin. When the fertilized ovum is implanted, chorionic gonadotropin is secreted to maintain the corpus luteum beyond its normal life span (see Fig. 4-3**A**).

Effect of Ovarian Steroids on Gonadotropins

The ovarian steroids, estrogen and progesterone, exert a negative feedback effect on both FSH and LH gonadotropin secretion. This is clearly illustrated when "castration" cells (degranulated, actively-secreting FSH and LH gonadotrophs) appear after ovariectomy in rats, or after the menopause in women, associated with increased gonadotropin levels in the blood and urine.

The complicated relationship between the pituitary gonadotropins, the ovary, and the ovary's main target tissues, the uterus and the breast, is diagramed in Figure 4-2—a simplified account of the hypothalamic-pituitary-ovarian interactions with increasing sexual maturity. There is good evidence that the pituitary of young girls puts out small amounts of gonadotropin, chiefly FSH, which in turn stimulates the ovary to make estrogen. However, the "set-point" for negative feedback inhibition of the hypothalamus is so low in early childhood that the level of estrogen never rises high enough to produce secondary sexual characteristics. Figure 4-2**A** represents the presumed balance of factors in a prepubertal girl. Puberty likely results when the hypothalamic set-point is elevated to the point where FSH can stimulate estrogen production sufficiently to produce secondary sexual characteristics before a level is reached that shuts off the secretion of FSH-releasing factor (Fig. 4-2**B**). As yet no ovulation has occurred.

Fig. 4-2. Hypothalamic-pituitary-ovarian interactions.

A. In the newborn, the pituitary secretes a small amount of gonadotropin, chiefly FSH, and the ovary responds with low level estrogen release. At this stage the hypothalamic set-point is so low that estrogen can exert negative feedback inhibition even though it exerts no demonstrable biologic effect. The sleeping moon represents the quiescent cycling center, which ultimately will trigger periodic secretion of LHRF necessary for ovulation.

B. Onset of puberty may be explained by progressive rise in the set-point level for negative feedback inhibition. With the elevated set-point, sufficient gonadotropin is secreted and enough estrogen manufactured so that secondary sex characteristics emerge. However, ovulation usually does not take place because the cycling center is still dormant.

C. The cycling center must awaken before ovulatory cycles can begin. In this situation, estrogen seems to exert positive feedback (stimulating) effect on LHRF—i.e., a rising level of estrogen from the graafian follicle stimulated by FSH will thus trigger an LH surge at midcycle that will be sufficient to induce ovulation. As shown, progesterone from the corpus luteum produces a secretory endometrium favorable to nidation.

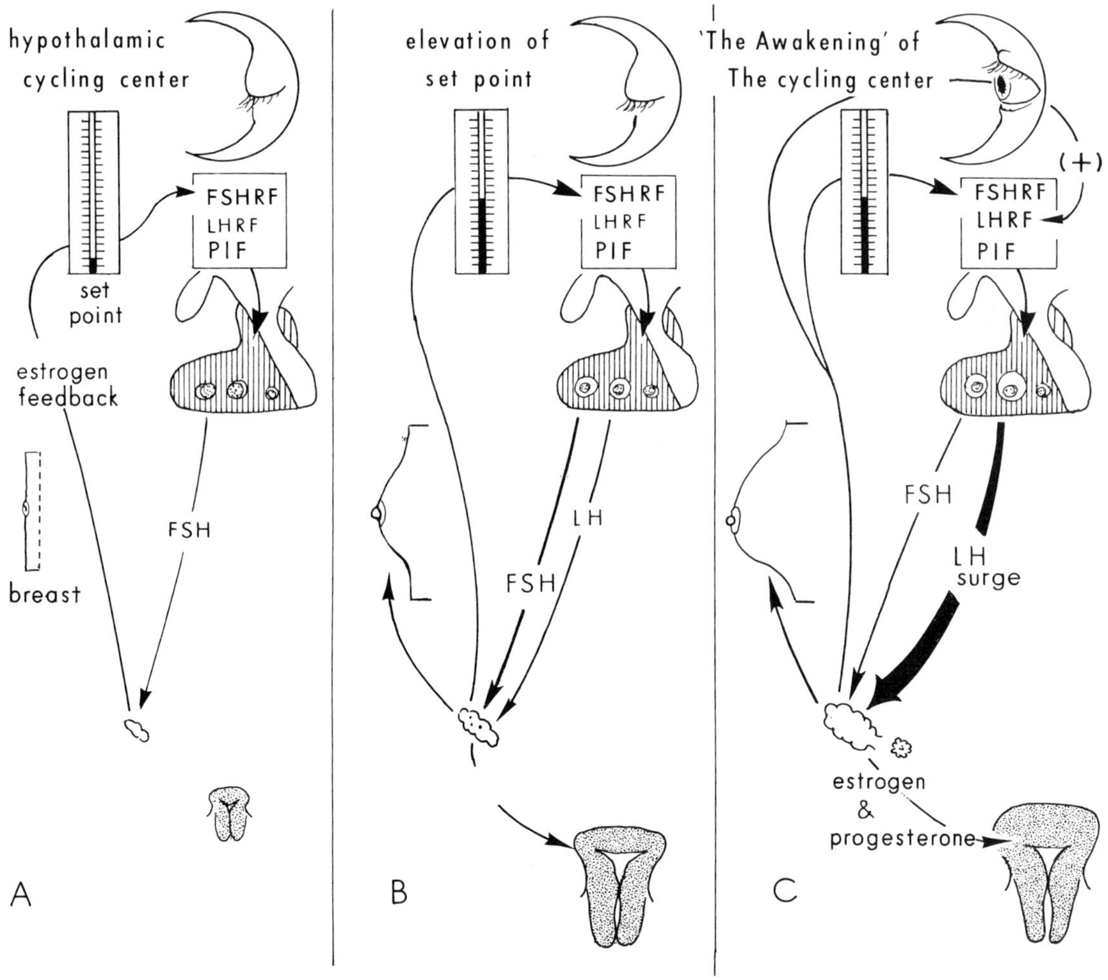

There is a "cycling" center in the hypothalamus of females that comes into operation some time after puberty. It is this center which, in rodents, seems to be affected by the early injection of androgen; in such animals ovulation never takes place (see Ref. 12, Chap. 2). The cycling center may operate on a positive feedback whereby increasing secretion of estrogen reaches a level by midcycle at which a burst of LH-releasing factor is secreted and transmitted to the adenohypophysis. This leads to a brief LH surge—the effective stimulus for ovulation (Fig. 4-2**C**).

After ovulation, the corpus luteum is formed and produces progesterone. Clinical experience has shown that estrogen administration over a prolonged period can suppress gonadotropin synthesis and release. Prolonged progesterone treatment can block ovulation, presumably by inhibiting release of the surge of LH that appears to be necessary for ovulation, without affecting basal secretion of either FSH or LH. Ovulation may occur after sudden withdrawal of either progesterone or estrogen treatment. To complicate matters, single injections of either of the ovarian steroids can induce ovulation if the ovary contains follicles that have been suitably prepared by previous FSH and slight LH stimulation. This indicates that there is a *positive* feedback circuit capable of inducing LH release in this manner. A rapid rise in circulating estrogen probably accounts for the ovulatory surge of LH during the human menstrual cycle.

Gonadotropins and Testicular Function

The gonadotropic control of testicular function is complicated. FSH stimulates spermatogenesis although, for complete development and function of the tubules, it probably requires the aid of LH and androgen. The Leydig cells are stimulated to produce androgen by LH or (as it is known in the male) interstitial-cell-stimulating hormone (ICSH). When adult male rats are castrated, gonadotropin levels in blood and urine increase and degranulated FSH and LH "gonadotrophs" appear in pituitary sections. In patients with primary hypogonadism, there are similar increases in urinary gonadotropins (which are usually measured as combined FSH and LH in bioassay), suggesting that there is a negative feedback between the testes and the pituitary. In this feedback, the role of androgen is small; it probably involves mainly ICSH, because testosterone, a potent androgen, does not appear to inhibit FSH secretion when it is administered therapeutically. Seminiferous tubular failure is usually accompanied by increased urinary gonadotropin, even when Leydig-cell production of androgen appears adequate, suggesting that another substance (designated "inhibin") made by the tubules, normally inhibits FSH secretion by negative feedback.

Prolactin and the Endocrinology of Pregnancy and Lactation

Although there is considerable similarity in the molecular structure of prolactin and growth hormone, and some overlap in biologic properties, morphologic evidence indicates that prolactin is definitely a separate hormone distinct from growth hormone. These two hormones arise from separate subtypes of acidophilic cells.[8] In the latter half of pregnancy and during lactation, the human pituitary contains large numbers of prolactin cells (Fig. 4-3, **B** and **C**). At other times in the female and at all times in the male pituitary, well-granulated prolactin cells are rare. Prolactin is one of a group of hormones necessary for breast development and milk secretion. When the breast has developed under the influence of estrogen, progesterone, prolactin, and possibly other pituitary hormones, milk secretion appears to depend on an additional pituitary secretion of prolactin.

The manufacture and release of prolactin is mediated mainly by the secretion of a hypothalamic inhibitory factor into the portal circulation. A reduced delivery of this prolactin inhibitory factor (PIF) leads to increased output of prolactin. If the pituitary is transplanted away from the region of the hypothalamus, the predominant cell type changes to the prolactin cell, presumably because of hypertrophy and hyperplasia of "chromophobes" that in the normal gland were very sparsely granulated prolactin cells. There is some evidence that the hypothalamus also produces a prolactin-stimulating factor, which in itself may

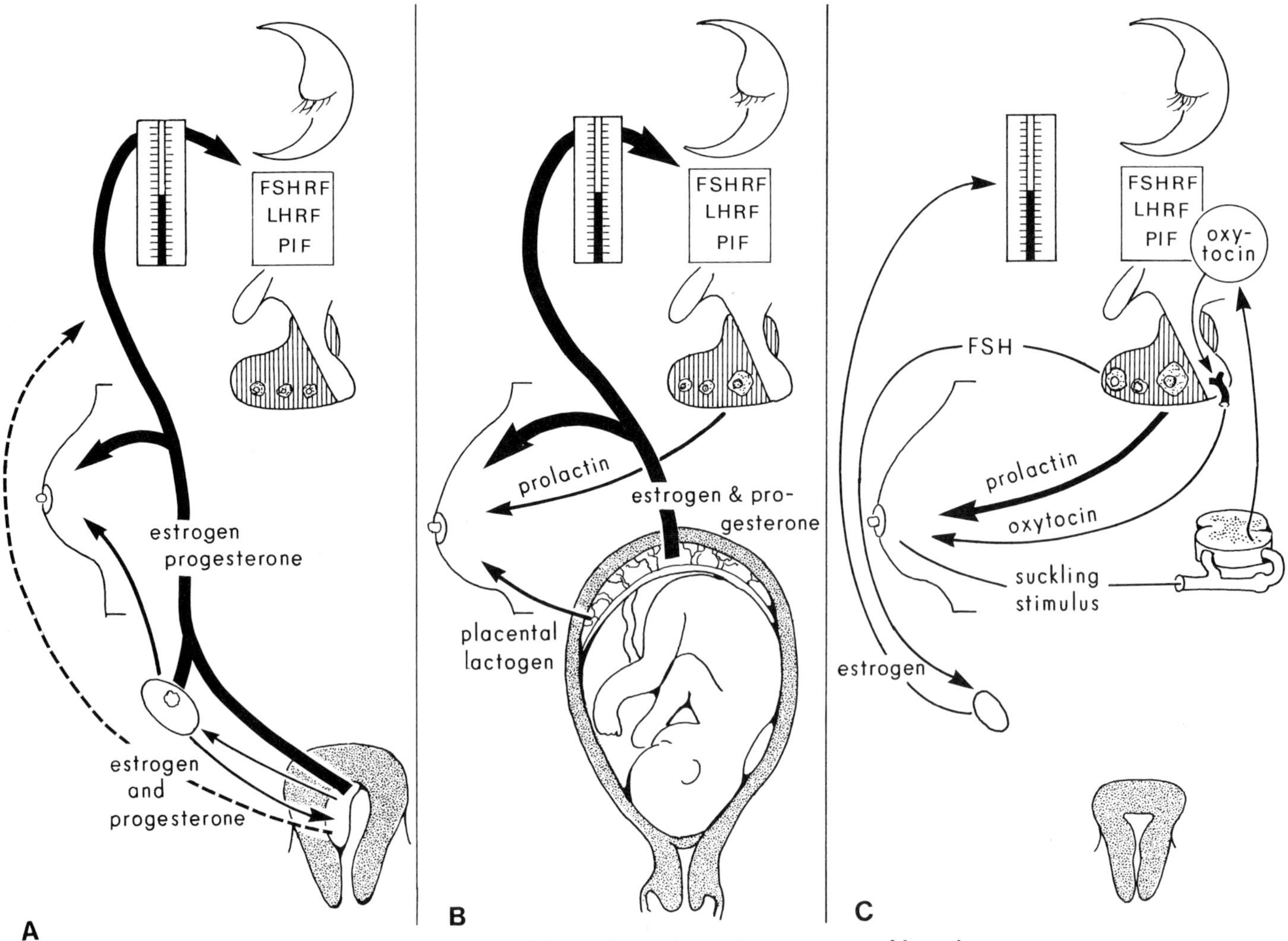

Fig. 4-3. Prolactin and the endocrinology of pregnancy and lactation.

A. In the first trimester, pituitary and hypothalamus are strongly inhibited by high levels of female hormones produced by ovary and placenta. Arrow leading from placenta to ovary (not labeled) represents chorionic gonadotropin, which maintains the corpus luteum during early pregnancy. The corpus luteum, in turn, produces large amounts of estrogen and progesterone. The breast responds to these hormones without requiring any pituitary contribution at this stage. During this period ovulation does not occur because of the strong inhibitory effect of these high levels of female hormones on the hypothalamic and pituitary gonadotropic apparatus.

B. In the third trimester, there is considerable breast development induced by combined effects of three placental hormones (estrogen, progesterone, and placental lactogen) and prolactin from the pituitary. At this time, the anterior pituitary contains an abundance of well-granulated prolactin cells that are seen only in the last half of pregnancy and during lactation.

C. After delivery, lactation is established under the influence of prolactin secretion in response to repeated suckling stimuli. This suckling also serves to empty the breast by reflex release of oxytocin (milk let-down reflex).

Here the stage appears to be set for ovulation: estrogen is being released from the graafian follicle (as in Fig. 4-2**C**). However, this estrogen does not induce ovulation, presumably because the cycling center is usually blocked during lactation. (Primitive peoples have long known that lactation has a contraceptive effect.)

be capable of increasing the secretion of prolactin (see also Fig. 1-1). The rate of prolactin secretion may be influenced by gonadal steroids, particularly estrogen. The long-term administration of estrogen may induce prolactin-secreting pituitary tumors. The short-term administration of estrogen inhibits the output of prolactin; this effect has been used clinically to terminate postpartum lactation. To produce these varied effects, ovarian steroids probably act both on the hypothalamus and the adenohypophysis.

Somatotropin or Growth Hormone

Somatotropin, a protein hormone, is made by a subtype of acidophil cell whose granules preferentially stain yellow with orange G, rather than with erythrosine or carmoisin, which stain prolactin granules red.[8] This hormone stimulates protein anabolism, releases free fatty acids by lipolysis, and induces hyperglycemia by interfering with glucose utilization. It also appears to mobilize calcium and phosphorus from the skeleton and increases temporarily the urinary excretion of calcium. Radioimmunoassay has shown that there are previously unsuspected rapid fluctuations in the circulating level of this hormone, in response to nutritional and psychic events, to sleep and to muscular exercise. A hypothalamic component undoubtedly controls the release of growth hormone (Fig. 4-4). Hypoglycemia stimulates the release of growth hormone, whereas hyperglycemia inhibits its output.

Attention should be paid to the level of insulin and glucose in the blood in considering the regulation of growth-hormone secretion. This interaction is illustrated in Figure 4-5, which shows the suppression and subsequent stimulation of growth-hormone secretion in a prolonged (6-hour) glucose tolerance test, along with the levels of blood glucose and insulin obtained in a normal subject. The hormones are measured by radioimmunoassay which may not reflect accurately the level of biologically active hormone. Free fatty acids may also be measured in such a test. Their rise in the later stages could be used as evidence that the peripheral tissues are responding to growth hormone. However, since free fatty acids rise with a falling blood glucose and a falling insulin concentration, the change in this test is not specific for growth hormone. A rise in circulating insulin is also used as an indicator of peripheral-tissue response to growth hormone.

The intravenous infusion of several individual essential amino acids increases plasma levels of both insulin and growth hormone, probably by different mechanisms. This effect is not dependent on changes in the level of blood glucose. A similar increase has been observed following the oral intake of protein. Arginine infusion, a safe reliable stimulus of growth-hormone secretion, avoids the dangers of insulin-induced hypoglycemia. Recent experience has shown that, in some normal males, arginine does not always induce the secretion of growth hormone; in such men, pretreatment with estrogen usually leads to a normal response to arginine. Thus in such patients a failure to respond to arginine must not be accepted as evidence of hypopituitarism.

Melanocyte-Stimulating Hormone

This polypeptide hormone is similar in structure to a portion of the ACTH molecule, described earlier. However, in physiologic amounts, it does not appear to have significant adrenocorticotropic effects. In the human, it can increase skin pigmentation by stimulating the dispersion of melanin granules in the melanocytes. In its absence the skin may be pallid. Melanocyte-stimulating hormone (MSH) and probably ACTH appear to be produced by a subtype of basophil that occupies a prominent place in the adenohypophysis.[17] In conditions associated with prolonged, excessive levels of cortisol, this cell undergoes Crooke's hyaline change, which is a progressive loss of granulation in a characteristic crescentic pattern.[4] The physiologic control of MSH appears to be similar to that of ACTH secretion: It is inhibited by cortisol by a negative feedback mechanism. In some animals, when the pars intermedia is separated from the hypothalamus, there is cellular overgrowth and MSH hypersecretion, which suggests that the hypothalamus may produce a factor that normally inhibits MSH output by the adenohypophysis.

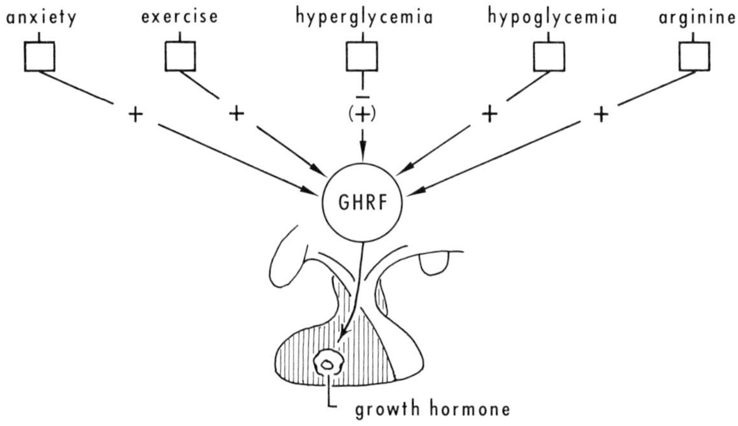

Fig. 4-4. Some influences affecting hypothalamic control of growth-hormone-releasing factor (GHRF). In some normal men, arginine will not stimulate release of GH unless the subject is pretreated with estrogen. Although hyperglycemia usually causes inhibition of GH secretion (except in acromegaly), in some normal individuals and some patients with hypothalamic or pituitary disease, paradoxical stimulation of GH has been observed following a glucose load.

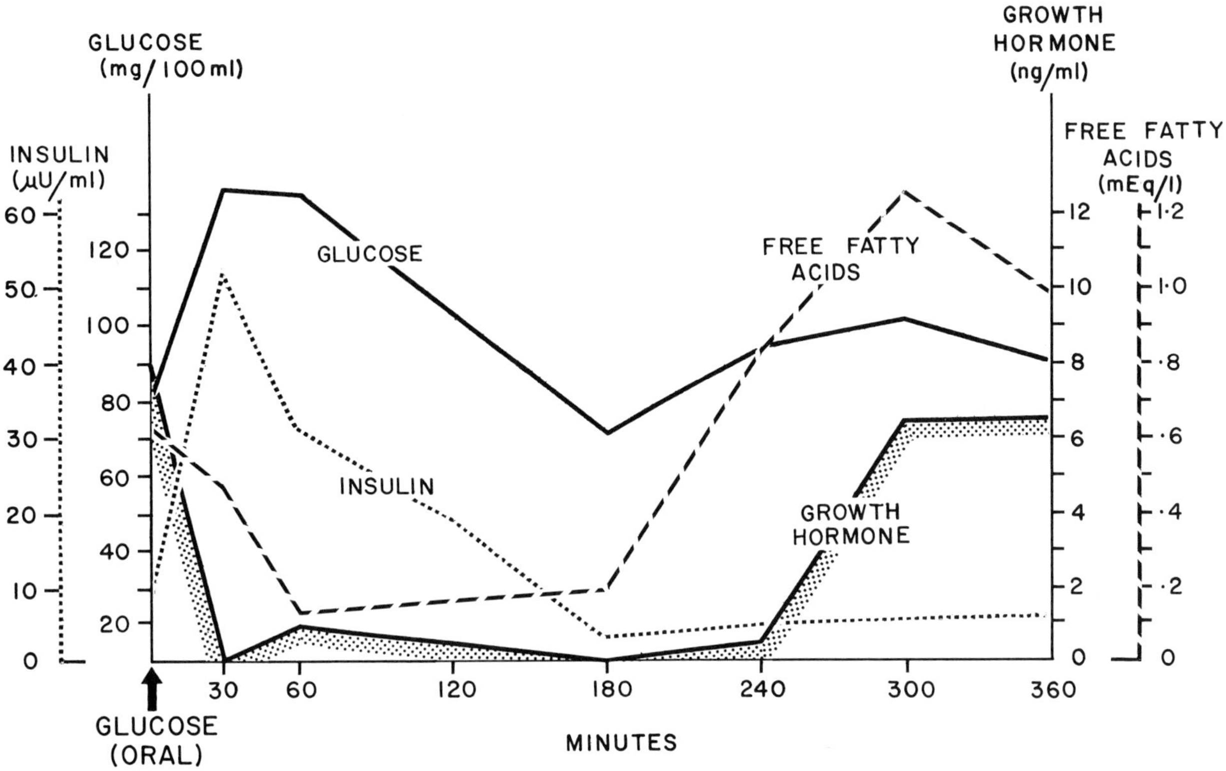

Fig. 4-5. Growth hormone secretion during prolonged glucose tolerance test. Growth hormone level (*scale on right*) is slightly increased in the fasting state—zero time (normal range, 1–5 ng/ml) and quickly falls when the blood glucose level rises.

Insulin level (*scale on left*) rises initially in response to hyperglycemia and usually rises a second time when growth hormone level becomes elevated later in test. In this patient its failure to respond the second time is somewhat unusual.

After 3 hours, free fatty acids (*scale on right*) rise *before* there is any rise in growth hormone, indicating that other lipolytic factors probably produce this elevation.

Pathology

The main lesions of the adenohypophysis are tumors, infarctions, and granulomas. The therapeutic ablation of the pituitary and congenital deficiency of one or more of the anterior pituitary hormones are also important causes of pituitary insufficiency.

Pituitary Adenomas

Chromophobe adenoma, so named because it has little or no affinity for acidophilic or basophilic stains, is the commonest intracranial tumor. It may be so small that it is only found on serial section of the pituitary or may be large enough to compress the visual pathway and other neighboring structures. Varying degrees of hypopituitarism may result from pressure on the surrounding normal gland. Hypogonadism is usually the first clinical manifestation of this functional impairment. Most chromophobe adenomas do not produce hormones, but some are associated with overproduction of somatotropin (growth hormone), thus producing acromegaly, or of corticotropin excess, causing Cushing's syndrome. The tumors associated with Cushing's syndrome often show local invasive growth with considerable pleomorphism.

In an important study of a large series of pituitary tumors employing careful fixation and special staining, McCormick and Halmi found that virtually all of them were composed of cells with specific granules.[14] Most pituitary tumors classified as non-functioning chromophobe adenomas seem to contain some acidophil granulation. In most instances there was no evidence of hypersecretion of any of the pituitary hormones. Electron microscopic studies of human and rodent pituitaries have shown that most of the cells, which would be classed as chromophobes on the basis of differential staining for light microscopy, contain enough secretory granules to allow them to be identified as specific cell types.

Using electron microscopic radioautography, Stratmann has found in the normal adult rat pituitary that the somatotroph takes up tritiated thymidine (a labeled precursor of DNA) more readily than any other cell type.[24] Because of this frequent cell division, there is probably a greater tendency to adenoma formation from such proliferating cells. Much more remains to be learned about cell turnover in the adenohypophysis.

Acidophil adenoma usually produces acromegaly and may be regarded as a tumor of somatotropin-producing cells (somatotrophoma). In some cases there is associated prolactin production with galactorrhea. Rarely, a small acidophil adenoma may be found without acromegaly. In some of these patients, a mammotropic tumor may produce excessive prolactin. In some tumors associated with active acromegaly, the cells may be mainly chromophobic—presumably because of the lack of storage of normal staining granules. In such tumors the production and release of hormone is probably so rapid that there is no stage of storage long enough to permit satisfactory staining as in the normal acidophils.

Basophil adenoma is usually associated with Cushing's syndrome although chromophobe tumors also are found with this condition. All of these tumors presumably produce a corticotropic hormone. There is a constant degranulation of some basophils in the pituitaries of all patients with Cushing's syndrome from any cause, including adrenal tumor, exogenous steroids, ACTH administration, or abnormal corticotropin production by various nonpituitary malignant tumors. This "Crooke's hyaline change," which affects the beta-1 subtype of basophil, represents a regressive effect of glucocorticoid on a specific cell type which may be the source of MSH, ACTH, or both. The hyaline change does not affect the basophils of the adenoma, even when similarly staining beta-1 cells of the surrounding gland may be involved. This indicates that the adenoma is composed of cells that respond differently to hypercortisolemia.

Pituitary Cystic Tumors

Craniopharyngiomas may be cystic or solid in varying degrees, but since most of them are cystic they will be considered here. The craniopharyngioma arises from the ectodermal craniopharyngeal canal and may affect some or all of the hypothalamic-pituitary region by an erosive compression.

The clinical picture depends on the direction of growth. There may be pressure on the optic chiasm from above if the tumor arises suprasellarly, or from below if the tumor arises within the sella. Suprasellar extension may compress the infundibulum and thus produce diabetes insipidus. Pressure on the hypothalamus may give rise to various hypothalamic syndromes such as obesity, somnolence, and, rarely, precocious puberty (see Ref. 2, Chap. 2). Patients with predominantly intrasellar tumors may present with manifestations of anterior pituitary insufficiency which include failure of growth, delayed puberty, adult hypogonadism, and thyroid or adrenal insufficiency.

Pathologically these tumors have been referred to as adamantinomas, Rathke's pouch tumors, or suprasellar cysts. Their structure varies greatly from simple cysts containing dark, oily fluid to solid tumors composed of columnar cells on a basement membrane. Sometimes squamous cells with masses of cornified tissue are found within the tumor. These tumors commonly calcify and thus give a most important diagnostic sign on radiologic examination of the sellar region.

Epidermoid cyst is rare but, in its time of onset and clinical features, may simulate a craniopharyngioma. On a radiograph of the skull, if there is calcification, it usually affects only the wall of the tumor and may present as a curved line rather than the diffuse specks characteristic of a craniopharyngioma.

Miscellaneous Pituitary Tumors

Miscellaneous tumors include glioma arising from the optic chiasm, ectopic pinealoma, meningioma, lymphoma, and secondary carcinoma. These may produce hypopituitarism by affecting either the suprasellar region or the adenohypophysis directly.

Postpartum Necrosis

In 1939, 25 years after Simmonds' original description of infarction of the anterior lobe, Sheehan reemphasized the importance of postpartum hemorrhage in the pathogenesis of postpartum necrosis.[23] Necrosis of the anterior lobe appears to be due to the spasm of some preportal arterial vessels that accompanies postpartum peripheral circulatory collapse. At term, the adenohypophysis is markedly hyperplastic and is thus more vulnerable to a sudden decrease in its portal blood supply.

In Sheehan's series, about one-half of the patients with postpartum necrosis had a lesion which involved about 90% of the anterior lobe. Lesser degrees of involvement are probably due to variations in the extent and duration of the spasm of the arterial twigs. The posterior lobe has a separate blood supply with more collaterals and thus is usually less severely affected, although mild DI has been observed, which may be aggravated by treatment of associated adrenal insufficiency with glucocorticoid hormone (see also Fig. 3-2). Women with extensive destruction of the gland do not lactate, and pubic hair shaved off before delivery does not grow back. Although amenorrhea is usual, irregular menstruation has been reported in patients with well-marked thyroid and adrenal insufficiency following postpartum hemorrhage. On rare occasions, such patients have become pregnant and seem to improve because of the hypertrophy of the pituitary remnant associated with pregnancy. In the absence of such a stimulus, there is little tendency for the remnant to regenerate after the initial damage.[12]

Hemorrhagic infarction of the pituitary gland can occur in the newborn about the time of delivery. Thus pituitary pathology in both mother and child can be related to abnormal events at term.

Granulomatous Lesions

Granulomatous lesions rarely cause severe pituitary insufficiency; more often the involvement is mild. At times sarcoidosis, histiocytosis, tuberculosis, syphilis, and actinomycosis have involved the hypophysis and neighboring suprasellar region, causing a destructive granulomatous process with subsequent fibrosis. Giant-cell granuloma involving both pituitary gland and adrenals appears to be a distinct entity. A suprasellar lesion may present with diabetes insipidus; as the disease progresses, the adenohypophysis is affected by ischemic atrophy induced by interruption of the portal circulation and the cutting-off of neuroendocrine adenohypophysiotrophic factors. As the anterior pituitary insufficiency increases, the diabetes insipidus, present at onset, may appear to regress because of the ameliorating effect of adrenal insufficiency. In such a situation, treatment with glucocorticoid hormone usually brings a return of polyuria (see also Fig. 3-2). Only the combination of severe anterior- and posterior-lobe insufficiency should be designated "panhypopituitarism."

Miscellaneous Lesions

Congenital absence of one or more of the anterior-lobe hormones has been observed, sometimes in families.[16] In some instances, the primary cause may be a disturbance in the hypothalamic control of the manufacture and release of pituitary hormones (e.g., Kallman's syndrome, a type of hypogonadotropic hypogonadism associated with anosmia. See Chapter 2, section on Disorders of the Hypothalamus). Agenesis of the adenohypophysis occurs, with or without anencephaly. Trauma at birth has been suspected as a cause of hypopituitarism in one of identical twins when the other twin appeared to be unaffected.

It has been observed that destruction of most of the anterior pituitary gland induces a remission in many patients with progressive diabetic retinopathy, although the mechanism for this remains obscure. Some patients with endocrine-sensitive metastatic mammary cancer, particularly those with severe osseous involvement, seem to be helped temporarily by surgical hypophysectomy or other forms of pituitary ablation. Thus the therapeutic destruction of the nontumorous pituitary gland is now an important cause of pituitary insufficiency.[5]

Effect of Diseases of Target Glands on the Adenohypophysis

The normal adult pituitary weighs between 500 and 600 mg; multiparous females tend to have the highest values. In primary hypothyroidism the pituitary gland is enlarged, sometimes weighing as much as 1 gm. The cell type responsible for this hyperplasia, the thyrotroph, increases in size and number when released from the inhibition normally exerted by thyroid hormones. Depending on the degree of thyroid underfunction, the range of different forms of thyrotroph contained in the adenohypophysis may extend from a well-granulated stage with intense aldehyde-thionine straining to a largely chromophobic stage with an enlarged vesicular nucleus and copious cytoplasm, indicating considerable secretory activity without much storage of stainable granulation.

Fig. 4-6. Thyrotrophs in normal state and in hypo- and hyperthyroidism. A. Previously healthy male, age 18, whose death was sudden and accidental. Note polyhedral, dark beta-2 cells (thyrotrophs). A group of beta-1 (ACTH and MSH) cells is also shown ($\times$ 500).

B. Healthy male, age 17, sudden accidental death. Note group of ovid delta cells (gonadotrophs) at lower right. A group of partially degranulated polyhedral beta-2 cells is at upper right. Some light-colored alpha (growth hormone) cells are also present ($\times$ 500).

C. Male, age 56. Hypothyroidism following ^{131}I treatment of Graves' disease in 1952. Pretibial myxedema and severe exophthalmos were still present when he was seen again in 1963; LATS was found in the serum. At time of death he was clinically hypothyroid, and the PBI was 1.5 μg/100 ml shortly before. Note many vesiculated, some lightly granulated, and two heavily granulated beta-2 cells ($\times$ 500).

D. Female, age 52, with Graves' disease, who was hyperthyroid at time of death. Note group of "regressed" vesiculated beta-2 cells with small nuclei and scanty cytoplasm containing many aldehyde thionine-positive globules ($\times$ 1200).

All photomicrographs are of pituitary sections stained with aldehyde thionine-PAS-orange G. The film used was Kodak plus X pan sheet with X 1 yellowish green filter.

(From Werner, S. C., and Ingbar, S. H., eds. *The Thyroid: A Fundamental and Clinical Text*, ed. 3. New York, Harper, 1971. Reproduced with permission.)

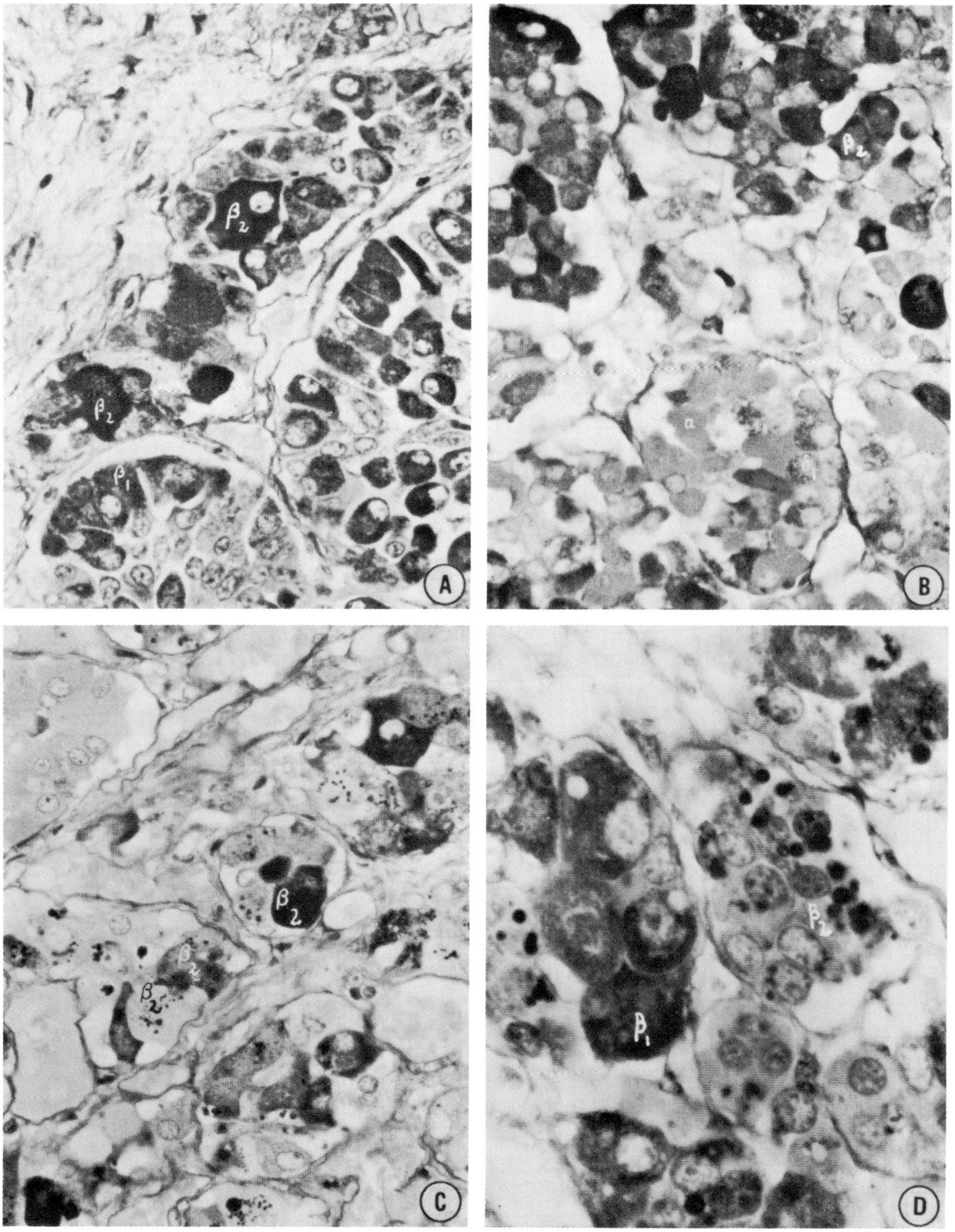
β2
β2
β1
A
β2
a
B
β2
β2
β2
C
β2
β1
D

A characteristic feature of the pituitary histology in myxedema is the presence, in these chromophobic thyrotrophs, of many PAS- and aldehyde-thionine-positive vesicles.[3] A small tumor composed of thyrotrophs (thyrotrophoma) may be found in the pituitary of patients with long-standing, untreated primary myxedema, usually of juvenile onset. This tumor may enlarge the sella turcica, as seen on the radiograph, but it does not grow large enough to press on the visual pathway. In the pituitaries of patients with hyperthyroidism the thyrotrophs appear shrunken and inhibited by the high levels of circulating thyroid hormones (Fig. 4-6). This inhibition of thyrotrophs is also seen in patients with nontoxic goiter treated with large doses of thyroid hormone (see Fig. 1-2**D**).

In pituitaries of patients with primary hypogonadism, or in women past the menopause, the gonadotropic basophils are vacuolated and appear as large chromophobes. Since the other more obvious types of basophils are not affected, this change can easily be missed unless these specific basophils are sought with special stains.

In primary adrenal insufficiency, the weight of the pituitary gland is not increased; it may even be decreased. In this condition, pituitary cytology is difficult to interpret because both the acidophils and basophils appear to be greatly reduced. In the characteristic cellular alteration in mild adrenal insufficiency, increased numbers of large chromophobes appear which are presumed to be hypersecretory degranulated corticotrophs. In Cushing's syndrome, prolonged excessive circulating levels of hydrocortisone or its analogues produce a characteristic inhibitory degranulation of the most prominent subtype of basophil, the beta-1 cell (see also Basophil Adenoma earlier in this chapter). The basophil affected by "Crooke's hyaline change" may produce MSH, ACTH, or both.

Clinical Anterior Pituitary Disorders

Hyperpituitarism

Functioning tumors of the anterior pituitary gland are usually associated with either (1) acromegaly or gigantism, or (2) Cushing's syndrome with bilateral adrenal cortical hyperplasia. Rarely, isolated excessive prolactin production from a tumor may cause galactorrhea, but such abnormal lactation is usually the result of interference with the delivery to the adenohypophysis of prolactin-inhibitory factor, causing selective hypersecretion of the prolactin cells (see Fig. 1-1).

Acromegaly

This chronic disorder of somatic growth is caused by hypersecretion of growth hormone (Fig. 4-7) and is always associated with a pituitary tumor although sometimes the tumor is not large enough to expand the sella turcica. The condition is characterized by enlargement of the extremities, coarsening of the facial features and a high incidence of impaired sugar tolerance.[9] The pituitary tumor may reduce vision by compressing the visual pathway. Gigantism, a similar disorder, begins in childhood when the limb bones are still capable of further longitudinal growth. Pituitary giants may reach a height of 8 feet and weigh over 300 lb. These individuals usually have some features of acromegaly as well. The symptoms and signs are those associated with either local effects of the tumor or its metabolic effects.

Headache, which may vary from mild to severe in different patients, is usually attributed to the expanding tumor pressing on the sensitive walls of the sella turcica. The headache may also be the result of hormonal influences. Pressure upward on the optic chiasm most commonly produces a bitemporal hemianopsia, but other visual field defects are sometimes seen. The metabolic effects of growth hormone are complex. The frequent association of diabetes mellitus with acromegaly indicates that somatotropin and insulin are antagonistic with respect to blood sugar level. The bony and soft-tissue overgrowth of acromegaly is the expression of an increased anabolism, which characterizes this condition. Hypermetabolism with heat intolerance and excessive perspiration is found in about one-third of acromegalics, although hyperthyroidism is not common (it occurs in less than 5%); in most instances the thyrotoxicosis appears to be of the primary thyroidal type and arises in a toxic adenoma. Hyperparathyroidism may also accompany acromegaly, sometimes as a feature of multiple endocrine adenomatosis, which may be familial.

Pituitary Hormones in Acromegaly

Growth Hormone. Impaired glucose tolerance is found in at least one-third of acromegalics, and one-sixth have diabetes mellitus requiring treatment. Sometimes the diabetes is resistant to insulin. Elevation of the fasting serum inorganic phosphate is an indirect measure of growth-hormone hypersecretion; it is often above 4.5 mg/100 ml. Recently a sensitive radioimmunoassay for growth hormone has become available, which may not measure the biologically active form of this material but serves as a general guide to activity. Because transient elevations of considerable magnitude appear in normal subjects, serial tests should be done. Normally the administration of glucose orally or intravenously inhibits the secretion of growth hormone. In acromegaly this inhibition does not occur, and sustained elevations of growth hormone will usually be observed in the radioimmunoassay when the samples are taken during a glucose tolerance test. Sometimes in this condition a paradoxical rise in growth-hormone secretion seems to follow hyperglycemia.

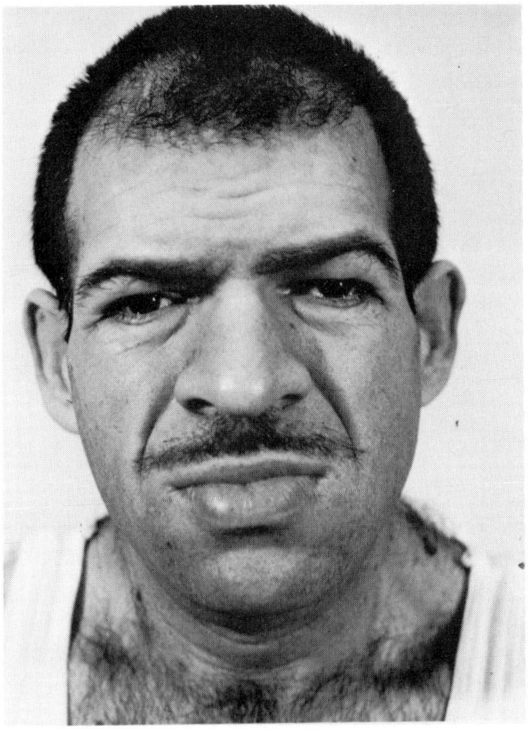

Fig. 4-7. Acromegaly and associated diabetes mellitus. This 36-year-old man's maximum serum growth hormone (GH) level was 160 ng/ml (normal, under 5). His GH did not respond to stimulation with insulin-induced hypoglycemia or arginine. Thus the pituitary adenoma was secreting maximally and GH production by remainder of the gland was suppressed by tumor.

In the normal individual, GH level falls when blood sugar level rises. In this man, as in all "active" acromegalics, the GH level did not fall during a glucose tolerance test, an indication that the tumor is relatively autonomous.

Gonadotropic Hormones. FSH and LH are sometimes absent in acromegaly because the normal gland is compressed by the tumor: In women, this results in amenorrhea; in men, it causes loss of libido and potency. In postmenopausal women, urinary gonadotropins are normally elevated. This elevation may not be found in acromegaly and in some cases gonadotropins may be absent from the urine.

Prolactin. Some patients with acromegaly have galactorrhea, probably because growth hormone and prolactin have similar molecular structures. Alternatively the tumor may be putting out a hormone with the combined effect of both substances, or it may be interfering with the delivery of prolactin-inhibitory hormone (PIH).

ACTH. Some women with acromegaly have elevated adrenal output of androgens, which is manifested by hirsutism and an increased urinary excretion of 17-ketosteroids. Because these patients have no corresponding increase in the output of adrenal glucocorticoid hormones, the adrenal disturbance probably does not reflect increased ACTH production.

TSH. Patients with untreated acromegaly rarely show evidence of hypothyroidism, although this response may follow various treatments; then it usually occurs in combination with adrenal cortical insufficiency. It may be very difficult to distinguish the clinical effects of acromegaly from those of hypothyroidism because both conditions tend to produce an overgrowth of soft tissues. In some cases even the laboratory data may be confusing since acromegaly tends to reduce thyroxine-binding globulin and this will decrease the serum thyroxine levels. Measurements of thyroxine-binding capacity, either directly or indirectly by the T_3-resin uptake, will help clarify the situation. Sometimes a therapeutic trial with thyroxine is justified in puzzling cases.

MSH. Apparently this hormone is not involved at any stage of acromegaly.

Radiologic Aspects of Acromegaly

Although the sella turcica is usually enlarged, at times a small adenoma causing acromegaly may not distort the fossa. Other changes usually found in the skeleton on radiographs are enlargement of the accessory nasal sinuses, prognathism, thickening of the inner table of the skull, spinal osteoporosis, and tufting of the terminal phalanges. Increased thickness of the skin may be demonstrated by measuring the heel pad or the subcutaneous fat layer on the radiograph.

Diagnosis, Treatment, and Prognosis

The diagnosis of acromegaly is usually not difficult. However, the choice of treatment is not easy unless the visual pathway is compressed; then an operation is recommended. In acromegaly a variety of methods have been tried to partially destroy the pituitary gland; none appear to selectively affect the hyperpituitarism. Thus successful treatment of acromegaly usually involves the production of some degree of hypopituitarism. As measured by radioimmunoassay, growth hormone is only slightly decreased by conventional X-ray and cobalt-beam irradiation. More powerful treatment—e.g., stereotactic cryosurgical destruction of the gland or high-energy-particle irradiation from a betatron or cyclotron—has been successful in expert hands. Transsphenoidal implantation of radioactive yttrium seeds is sometimes effective but may produce radiation damage to the optic nerves or leakage of cerebrospinal fluid through the sphenoid sinus and the threat of meningitis.

Prognosis for survival in acromegaly is usually good; however, slowly progressive disfigurement usually occurs unless the tumor is effectively treated. Since an amazing regression of the soft-tissue and even bony changes in acromegaly may follow successful treatment, the more radical measures might justifiably be contemplated in young women in whom the cosmetic aspects are very important. The resultant hypopituitarism may be dealt with by adequate replacement, including gonadotropic hormones to restore fertility. In patients without accompanying infertility, replacement therapy for pituitary insufficiency includes cortisone or prednisone, thyroxine, and sex steroids. Because treatment usually leads to hypopituitarism and associated infertility, it can sometimes be postponed for a few years in mild forms of acromegaly in patients contemplating marriage. This can usually be done without serious consequences, notwithstanding the somewhat increased risk of permanent diabetes.

Cushing's Syndrome

Because most of the clinical features of this disorder are the direct consequence of adrenal cortical hyperfunction, it will be considered more fully in Chapter 7 in the section on Disorders of the Adrenal Cortex. The disease is characterized by the effects of excessive adrenal glucocorticoid hormones, namely plethora, moon face, truncal obesity, osteoporosis, increased capillary fragility, and impaired glucose tolerance, with a variable degree of added androgenic effect (see Fig. 7-11). Although Cushing's first observations tended to stress the association of basophilic pituitary tumor and this syndrome, it has since become apparent that the pituitary may be involved in other ways. About 50% of patients with bilateral adrenal hyperplasia have pituitary tumors of one kind or another, but only one-third of these are predominantly basophilic in staining reaction.

Most of them are too small to distort the outline of the sella or to press on the visual pathway. Only about 10% of patients with pituitary tumor have an adenoma large enough to deform the sella; in a few of these, the visual fields are reduced. The tumor may be a chromophobe adenoma or even a carcinoma with a propensity to local invasion.

The hyaline change originally described by Crooke, which occurs in basophils of the beta-1 subtype, is now generally considered to be a regressive phenomenon induced by prolonged high levels of circulating cortisol because it is found in those who have been treated with ACTH and glucocorticoids, as well as those with spontaneous Cushing's syndrome. (See also Basophil Adenomas earlier in this chapter, and Effects of Diseases of Target Glands on the Adenohypophyses.)

The normal inhibitory mechanism (see Fig. 2-2) whereby a rising level of cortisol inhibits ACTH secretion, is deranged in every patient with Cushing's syndrome with bilateral adrenal hyperplasia, even when no ACTH-producing tumor is present; if it were not so, the disease would shut itself off. Excess ACTH has been demonstrated in the plasma of these patients by bioassay and radioimmunoassay. ACTH secretion can be inhibited in most patients with Cushing's syndrome of pituitary origin by giving them potent analogues of cortisol such as dexamethasone. However, this inhibition can only be achieved by giving higher doses of dexamethasone than would be required for inhibition in the normal patient. Two doses of dexamethasone are used in inhibition studies: a 2-mg total dose, usually given as 0.5 mg 4 times a day, and an 8-mg total dose, given as 2 mg 4 times a day. Low-dose inhibition may be seen in patients with virilizing adrenal hyperplasia who are producing excessive quantities of ACTH because of an enzyme defect in the proper synthesis of cortisol. The mechanism involved is depicted in Figure 7-3 and is discussed in more detail in Chapter 7, The Adrenals.

The differential diagnosis of Cushing's syndrome is also set out in Chapter 7. The principal tests used are dexamethasone suppression, diurnal variation of plasma cortisol and the Metopirone test.

Postadrenalectomy Pituitary Tumor

In Cushing's disease, the patient may develop symptoms and signs of pituitary tumor only after both adrenals have been removed. Probably the tumor was present from the onset of Cushing's syndrome; however, it grows more rapidly after the target glands have been removed. After operation, such patients often develop a dark brown pigmentation because part of the ACTH molecule is identical with melanocyte-stimulating hormone (MSH), and shares some of its biologic properties. (See also Melanocyte-Stimulating Hormone earlier in this chapter.) On the skull film, which is usually normal before operation, the sella turcica may now be expanded from within sufficiently to destroy the dorsum sellae and posterior clinoid processes. Most of these tumors are chromophobic adenomas or pleomorphic carcinomas; rarely they contain PAS-positive or basophilic granulation. Some patients develop only part of the postadrenalectomy syndrome—i.e., they may have excessive pigmentation but no demonstrable tumor. Such patients are treated with radiation in a dosage similar to that given for acromegaly, but because it is usually not completely effective, the pigmentation often persists.

Treatment and Prognosis

Patients suspected of harboring a pituitary tumor because they have either sellar enlargement, chiasmal compression, or excessive pigmentation should have treatment directed primarily to the pituitary gland. As in acromegaly, radiotherapy may be ineffective. If the visual pathway is affected, the tumor should be excised. However, the results of such excision are not always satisfactory; even virtually complete hypophysectomy may not suppress adrenal function. The adrenals of such patients can be inhibited by high doses of dexamethasone, indicating that a remnant of hyperfunctioning pituitary tissue persists and still controls the adrenal glands. In these resistant cases, Cushing's syndrome can be controlled only by total adrenalectomy. In young women in whom fertility must be preserved, total adrenalectomy may be chosen as primary treatment. In most patients with bilateral adrenal hyperplasia, bilateral adrenalectomy is still the treatment of choice.

Anterior Pituitary Insufficiency

The clinical picture in anterior pituitary insufficiency may vary greatly, depending on the patient's age at onset, the presence of a space-occupying lesion that may compress the visual pathway, and the number of anterior pituitary hormones affected. Clinically, gonadotropic function appears to be the most susceptible to factors that damage the pituitary. However, recent studies of growth hormone by radioimmunoassay have shown that its secretion is often impaired in mild cases of pituitary insufficiency: Sometimes it may be the only hormone affected.[20] However, in the mildest form of pituitary underfunction, usually only hypogonadism is manifested clinically; as the insufficiency increases, evidence of thyroid and adrenal cortical deficiencies appears. Although hypopituitarism is more commonly chronic, it may be acute after postpartum necrosis or after the sudden pituitary failure associated with hemorrhage into a tumor ("pituitary apoplexy"). To encourage an organized approach to the clinical problems arising from pituitary underfunction, we will describe each of the adenohypophyseal hormones in turn, considering relevant symptoms, signs, diagnosis, and treatment. When necessary for illustration and clarification, specific disease entities will be mentioned.*

Gonadotropic Hormones—FSH and LH (ICSH)

If gonadotropin production fails before sexual maturity, puberty does not take place. In growing males who lack androgenic hormone, the epiphyseal lines remain unfused, and if the secretion of somatotropic hormone is adequate, the long bones go on growing. This excess growth occurs slowly, presumably because of the lack of growth spurt normally induced by androgen. The arms and legs become disproportionately long; the individual's span exceeds his height (normally they are equal). These eunuchoid patients often have osteoporosis, presumably because testicular androgens have not produced their protein anabolic effect. They do not develop libido or become potent. The penis is small, the scrotum does not have mature rugae, the testes are tiny, and the prostate is underdeveloped. *Congenital absence* of gonadotropin seems to produce poor gonadal development with hypoplastic testes, which are often undescended; *acquired deficiency* usually permits more prepubertal development of scrotal testes. The voice is high-pitched and the larynx is not enlarged to adult size. These patients have some fine pubic hair but no coarse mature pubic hair. Axillary hair is sparse, and beard growth is completely absent. The male patients do not develop frontal baldness.

Girls with isolated hypogonadotropism have amenorrhea and develop no breast tissue. However, because pubic and axillary hair is also under the control of adrenal cortical androgens, they have a small amount of hair in these regions. If they have more severe disease with associated deficiency of other pituitary factors—chiefly corticotropin—pubic and axillary hair is completely absent. The epiphyses do not fuse at the normal time, and the women develop a eunuchoid habitus, as in males with hypogonadism.

When gonadotropin deficiency develops in adult life, the manifestations are similar, except that these patients do not have the eunuchoid habitus. The male has loss of libido and testicular atrophy. Pubic and axillary hair is decreased, and there is commonly some loss of facial hair; these patients notice that they shave less often than before. When testicular androgen production fails, hair may grow again on previously bald areas. Female patients develop secondary amenorrhea, usually with a regression of secondary sexual characteristics.

The most useful test for gonadotropin insufficiency is that for urinary gonadotropins; this differentiates between primary gonadal failure and that which is secondary to pituitary failure. Patients with pituitary failure have no urinary gonadotropins; those with primary hypogonadism have higher than normal levels of urinary gonadotropins. Urinary 17-ketosteroids may be somewhat reduced in men with any type of hypogonadism, although, because about two-thirds of these substances are derived from the adrenal cortex, the

* See Appendix: Addenda 1 and 2 to Chapter 4.

level of 17-ketosteroids may not be much below normal if adrenal cortical function remains unaffected.

Both primary and secondary male hypogonadism may be treated by replacing the androgen, which may be given as intramuscular testosterone compounds such as testosterone cyclopentylproprionate or testosterone ethanate. Linguets of methyltestosterone are also available, but this agent should be used with caution because in some individuals it produces hepatocellular jaundice. As yet, we have not been able to stimulate spermatogenesis to a degree sufficient to promote fertility by administering human pituitary gonadotropic hormones. In the adult female, sequential estrogen and progestational agents will restore secondary sexual characteristics and produce regular withdrawal menses. Such treatment will not induce ovulation or restore fertility. Infertility is treated by the sequential administration of human FSH from pituitary or menopausal urine extracts, followed by human chorionic gonadotropin which, by mimicking the action of LH, induces ovulation. This treatment may be complicated by the production of ovarian cysts, which may rupture with serious consequences. It is also frequently associated with multiple ovulation.

Hypothalamic Anovulation

On occasion, selective failure of the ovulatory surge of LH required to induce ovulation causes amenorrhea or infertility. Often this failure is associated with amenorrhea, but sometimes women who lack the LH surge continue to menstruate, although menses are usually irregular. That ovulation is not taking place can be demonstrated by basal body-temperature readings that do not show the thermogenic effect of progesterone, by endometrial biopsy showing only proliferative endometrium, and by vaginal cytology showing only estrogen effect. In these circumstances, LH radioimmunoassay may also give useful information, but because the increase before ovulation is usually transient, several daily determinations must be made around midcycle to demonstrate that the LH surge has not occurred.

The importance of psychic stimuli in the control of ovulation is apparent in these patients, who usually show excessive anxiety or unusual sensitivity to change in environmental conditions. Psychotherapy alone may be effective, but usually some form of hormone treatment is required to induce ovulation. If sequential estrogen and progestational agents are given cyclically for 3 months and then withdrawn, ovulatory cycles may sometimes begin spontaneously. Ovulation can be induced with clomiphene, an analogue of the nonsteroid estrogens. However, this form of treatment may overstimulate the ovary through excessive release of LH and possibly FSH by the pituitary, and induce ovarian cysts or multiple pregnancy.

Thyrotropin

Although thyrotropin (TSH) deficiency may produce all of the characteristic signs of myxedema—lethargy, cold intolerance, bradycardia, excessive dryness, and myxedematous infiltration of the skin, the hypothyroidism is usually less severe than in the primary form. Serum cholesterol may be increased and protein-bound iodine, serum thyroxine, T_3-resin uptake, and basal metabolic rate may be decreased. In pituitary hypothyroidism, radioiodine uptake and serum thyroxine are usually not decreased as much as in primary myxedema. A significant increase in the radioiodine uptake following one to three injections of 10 units of thyrotropin daily establishes that the diagnosis is hypothyroidism of pituitary or hypothalamic origin. In "hypothalamic hypothyroidism," serum TSH is undetectable until TRH is administered, following which there is a normal rise in serum TSH (Pittman *et al.*). In pituitary hypothyroidism, TSH is undetectable before and after the administration of TRH.[16]

As treatment L-thyroxine is better than desiccated thyroid because of its uniform potency. The initial dosage should be about one-quarter of the final maintenance dose, which, depending on body size, is usually 0.2–0.3 mg daily. The dose is doubled every 3–4 weeks to allow the body and, particularly, the cardiac muscle to adapt to the new metabolic demands. TSH deficiency rarely exists alone; it is usually accompanied by latent insufficiency of corticotropin and obvious hypogonadism.

In patients with combined deficiencies, metabolic stimulation may convert a borderline adrenal insufficiency into a life-threatening crisis. Therefore, before giving thyrotropin during investigation or thyroid as replacement to patients with suspected combined deficiencies, the physician should test ACTH reserve with metyrapone (Metopirone). If the response is unsatisfactory (or if there is not time to do the test), begin steroid replacement with prednisone, 7.5 mg daily, in divided doses. Later, if the thyroid does not respond to thyrotropin or the initial level of TSH by radioimmunoassay was elevated (i.e., if the patient has primary hypothyroidism), the steroid can be withdrawn after a few weeks of thyroid treatment.*

Corticotropin

This hormone stimulates the adrenal cortex and thus increases the production of cortisol and other steroid hormones produced in this portion of the adrenal. Aldosterone, made by the zona glomerulosa, is largely independent of ACTH control. Adrenal insufficiency secondary to corticotropin lack may produce low blood pressure, asthenia, crises of nausea and vomiting, and spontaneous hypoglycemia, although this latter symptom usually requires concomitant somatotropin deficiency. These episodes of adrenal insufficiency are often precipitated by infection or other stress. The serum electrolytes are usually normal although hyponatremia may sometimes be found, especially in patients who have been vomiting.

Patients with primary adrenal insufficiency usually have increased pigmentation; those with secondary adrenal cortical insufficiency do not. These two conditions can be differentiated by the intravenous ACTH test and the resultant response of urinary 17-hydroxycorticoids or plasma cortisol levels. Patients who have adrenal cortical deficiency secondary to hypopituitarism have a slight increase in these values on the first day after an 8-hour infusion of 25 units of ACTH; a similar infusion causes a more pronounced increase on the second day.

Patients with primary adrenal cortical insufficiency show no response. The ACTH test, however, tells nothing about the ACTH reserve of the anterior pituitary. This can be assessed with metyrapone, which, acting on the adrenal cortex, blocks the conversion of 11-desoxycortisol to cortisol and thus markedly reduces the normal cortisol inhibition of ACTH (Fig. 4-8). If the pituitary can respond by increasing its output of ACTH, there is a resultant increase in urinary and plasma 17-hydroxycorticoids derived from precursors of cortisol. In disease of the endocrine hypothalamus which affects the production of corticotropin releasing factor (see also Chapter 2, Disorders of the Hypothalamus Simulating Anterior Pituitary Insufficiency), or in pituitary disease which involves the corticotrophs, there is little or no increase in the 17-hydroxycorticoids because the pituitary cannot respond to the removal of cortisol inhibition.

Insulin-induced hypoglycemia as a "stress" stimulus has been used to test the responsiveness of the endocrine hypothalamus and the pituitary corticotrophs; during hypoglycemia, plasma cortisol levels will normally rise appreciably. Because a normal stress response to hypoglycemia may require neural pathways other than those involved in the negative feedback response to metyrapone, some patients may have a defective response to one of these tests but not the other and may still respond normally to stresses other than hypoglycemia. When he has doubt about the patient's ACTH reserve, the physician should give enough cortisone to cover the increased steroid requirements associated with operative procedures or intercurrent illness.

As a rule, patients with corticotropin deficiency secrete enough aldosterone and therefore require no salt-retaining effect. Prednisone, 2.5 mg at 8 A.M. and 4 P.M., is usually all that is required to restore appetite, normal strength, and energy. Patients who work hard or who have a larger body size may require a total of 7.5 mg daily, which, to mimic the diurnal rhythm of adrenal cortical secretion, can be given as 5 mg at 8 A.M. and 2.5 mg at 4 P.M. Steroid replacement should be increased during febrile illnesses or operations and other trauma. With respect to dose, it is safer to give too much for a short time than risk adrenal crisis. In circumstances in which corticoid

* See Appendix: Addendum 3 to Chapter 4.

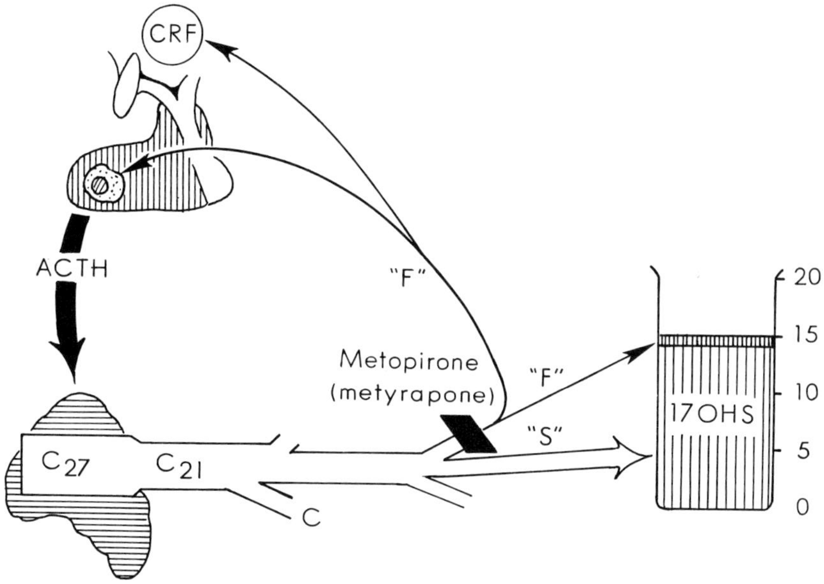

Fig. 4-8. Mechanism of the Metopirone test. Negative feedback inhibition induced by an increased plasma level of cortisol (Compound F) normally keeps the corticotroph from secreting excessive ACTH. Metopirone inhibits 11β-hydroxylation of the steroid molecule and thus decreases cortisol production. ACTH secretion increases if the hypothalamic structures associated with CRF and the pituitary corticotroph are normal. The adrenal is then stimulated to increase secretion of 11-dehydrocortisone (Compound S), the metabolite of which is measured in urine as 17-hydroxycorticoid. Thus a normal response to the Metopirone test is indicated by a rise of 17-hydroxycorticoid excretion on the day of or following Metopirone to twice the control value. When routine separation of the tetrahydro metabolites of Compounds F and S becomes possible, these changes can be followed with greater precision. C_{27} refers to the number of carbon atoms in the cholesterol molecule, and C_{21} to the number of atoms in glucocorticoid hormones (e.g., Compounds F and S).

requirements are uncertain, give the patient doses that prevent nausea, an early symptom of insufficiency, yet do not induce insomnia, the common symptom of overdosage.

Melanocyte-Stimulating Hormone

Most patients who have severe anterior pituitary insufficiency have pallor out of proportion to the moderate degree of anemia present—a striking finding. This pallor probably reflects the deficiency of melanocyte-stimulating hormone.

Somatotropin (Growth Hormone)

If the individual is to achieve normal adult body size in the first two decades he needs somatotropin (see also the section on Physiology of Adenohypophyseal Hormones earlier in this chapter for other metabolic effects). When a child lacks this hormone, growth is severely retarded; in adult life, such an individual is called a midget. If he is hypogonadal and his epiphyses remain open, he will continue to grow slowly for several decades (Figs. 4-9 and 4-10). Radioimmunoassay shows that the concentration of growth hormone in the plasma rises markedly during hypoglycemia and after the intravenous injection of certain essential amino acids (Fig. 4-4). However, we know little about the significance of these responses and the physiologic effect of growth hormone is not clear.

The preservation of normal adult organ size may depend on a continued production of growth hormone. Growth-hormone deficiency presumably produces the microsplanchnia, particularly of the heart, liver, and kidneys seen almost universally in anterior pituitary deficiency. This decrease in organ weight occurs whether these patients are emaciated, normally nourished, or even slightly overweight. Individuals deficient in growth hor-

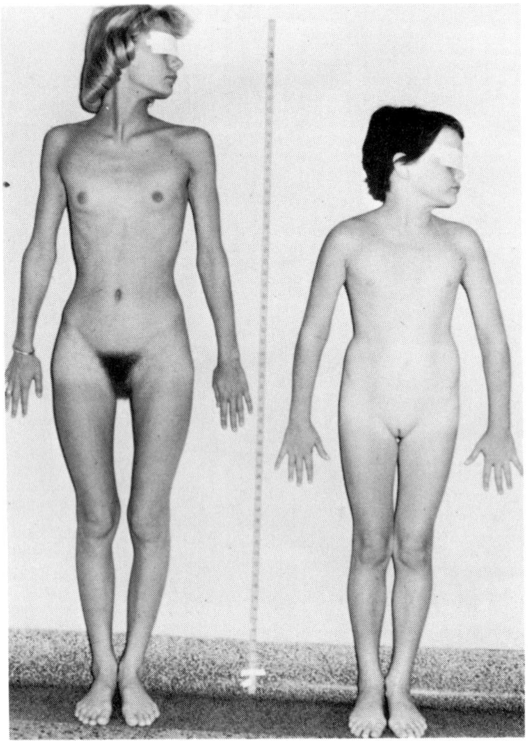

Fig. 4-9. Hypopituitarism secondary to perinatal pituitary infarction. Both these girls are 16 years old. The normal girl (*left*) is menstruating, has had her growth spurt, has developed breasts, and has pubic and axillary hair; the girl on the *right* has never menstruated, has grown only slowly, has no breast development and no pubic or axillary hair. Her skull radiographs show calcification in the pituitary fossa, presumably secondary to perinatal pituitary infarction. Her serum growth hormone is undetectable, she has no urinary gonadotropins, thyroid function is slightly reduced, and ACTH response to Metopirone is low.

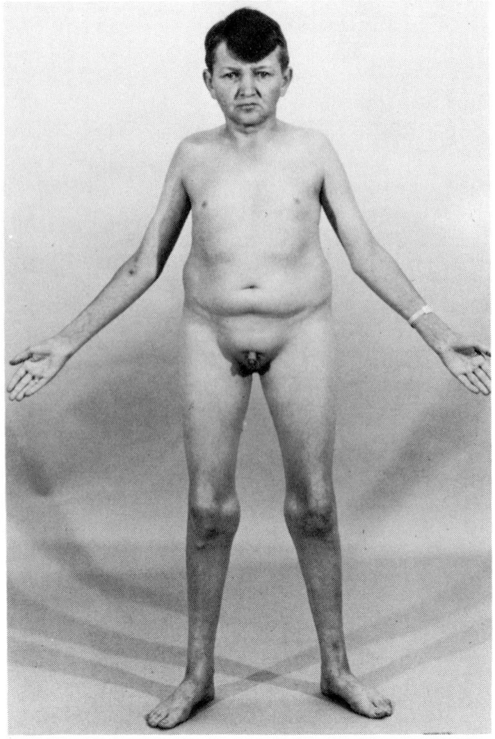

Fig. 4-10. Congenital pituitary dysplasia. The pituitary fossa of this 47-year-old man and hence the gland itself are very small. Production of GH, gonadotropins, and ACTH has long been minimal, but for some reason thyroid function appears to be normal. His face is youthful but wrinkled characteristically. He has no pubic or axillary hair, his span equals his height—i.e., he is hypogonadal but not eunuchoid (the latter state requires normal GH for long-bone overgrowth). However, in spite of lack of GH, he has continued to grow slowly and has reached a height of 5 feet 3 inches, an indication that some growth can occur in the absence of detectable growth-hormone secretion.

mone are extremely sensitive to insulin and may have episodes of spontaneous hypoglycemia, particularly if they also secrete insufficient corticotropin. After the pituitary has been destroyed to treat diabetic retinopathy, insulin requirements are usually considerably reduced—a reduction that has been attributed to growth-hormone withdrawal.[5]

Some workers suggest that growth hormone does not produce its effects directly but through some other factor which growth hormone converts into an active growth-promoting substance. One such intermediary has been designated "sulfation factor" because it increases the incorporation of radioactive sulfur in rat cartilage.* Sulfation factor is found in extracted normal plasma and in high concentration in acromegalic plasma, but only appears in the plasma of hypopituitary patients and animals after the administration of growth hormone. In the rat cartilage, growth hormone alone cannot produce the effects of the sulfation factor.

* "Somatomedin" has been proposed as a more suitable name for this substance (Daughady, W. H., Hall, K., Raben, M. S., Salmon, W. D. Jr., Van Den Brande, J. L. and Van Wyk, J. J. *Nature 235:* 107, 1972).

When assessing the adequacy of growth-hormone production, the safest and most useful test is intravenous arginine administration. Insulin-induced hypoglycemia can be used only with extreme caution because prolonged reduction in blood sugar may cause permanent intellectual impairment or even death. Failure of growth-hormone response to the administration of insulin and arginine is an early manifestation of progressive pituitary failure; such failure is usually demonstrable in patients whose only other recognizable endocrine deficiency is hypogonadism; in some patients growth-hormone failure is the only endocrine abnormality. That some normal men do not respond to arginine unless they are pretreated with estrogen suggests the hypothalamus requires some estrogen effect to allow this reaction to occur.

Selective failure of growth-hormone production has been reported in several members of certain families.[21] Sexually, these patients mature somewhat later than usual; androgenic hormones then induce epiphyseal closure. If the physician wishes to give such patients growth hormone to increase height, he must give it before the epiphyses close and must use a hormone of human or simian origin.[10] This species specificity is also seen in gonadotropic hormones; patients will not respond to hormones from other species.

Some fertile female midgets, who appear to lack only growth hormone, have babies that are of normal size at term; these mothers then lactate normally. These observations suggest that maternal growth hormone is not necessary for fetal growth and that, in the human, prolactin is a substance separate from growth hormone. Some of the children of these fertile midgets cannot themselves produce growth hormone although this is not apparent from their normal birth weights: apparently fetal growth hormone is not essential for normal fetal growth. Despite the lack of growth hormone, these midgets remain healthy and vigorous, just as hypophysectomized patients do if other important hormones are replaced, namely prednisone, thyroxine, and the sex steroids. Thus, apart from its essential role in producing normal growth, growth hormone appears to be dispensable.

Prolactin

Chemically and immunologically, prolactin was hard to separate from somatotropin in humans. Clinical and morphologic evidence suggested that these were separate hormones. The human pituitary appears to contain two types of acidophil cells: one, which increases greatly in number during late pregnancy and at the time of lactation, appears to be the source of prolactin; the other acidophil which produces growth hormone is the commonest granulated cell in all normal pituitary glands. We have not been able to extract prolactin from human pituitary glands obtained at routine necropsy, perhaps because only pituitaries of patients who die in late pregnancy or during lactation contain adequate amounts of stored prolactin. After postpartum shock causes extensive pituitary necrosis, a woman does not lactate, presumably because she secretes inadequate prolactin.

Investigation and Treatment of Patients Requiring Pituitary Surgery

Visual Field Defects

The sections dealing with acromegaly, Cushing's syndrome, and anterior pituitary insufficiency described the symptoms and signs of hormonal imbalance produced by pituitary tumors. This section deals with the general investigation of patients with pituitary problems and considers the effects of an expanding lesion originating in or near the pituitary fossa.

Because the optic chiasm lies above the diaphragma sellae, a pituitary tumor, when it extends beyond the confines of the sella turcica, often produces a visual defect by pressure on the optic chiasm: This defect, usually a bitemporal hemianopsia, results from compression of the crossing central fibers of the chiasm; the uncrossed lateral fibers are spared. The earliest changes are the enlargement of the blind spot, loss of color vision especially for red, and a wedge-shaped area of defective vision in the upper temporal quadrants, which gradually enlarges to occupy the whole upper quadrant and subsequently extends to the lower quadrant as well. Most patients with extensive visual field defects have primary optic atrophy. Although papilledema is rare, it may develop with large tumors that cause increased intracranial pressure. If the pressure on the visual pathway is relieved early enough, the visual fields usually return to normal, often dramatically a few hours after operation.

Visual field defects can be detected on gross examination by observing the angle at which an object such as the examiner's finger becomes visible to the patient looking straight ahead, but tangent screen and perimetry are necessary for exact plotting of the size and shape of the defect. In patients with long-standing amenorrhea due to slowly expanding pituitary tumor, the visual fields may be normal on initial examination; however, the test should be repeated at least every 6 months to detect the progressive compression of the visual pathway, which calls for surgical intervention.

Radiology of Pituitary Tumors

Serial films of the skull show that the tumor slowly expands the pituitary fossa and destroys or distorts the clinoid processes. Calcification in this region may point to a craniopharyngioma or epidermoid cyst and thickening of the tuberculum sella may be evidence of a suprasellar meningioma. Only by air encephalography can the physician determine the degree to which the tumor has become suprasellar.

If there is a defect in the diaphragma sellae, subarachnoid space may expand into the pituitary fossa, and the pituitary region may gradually enlarge on repeated X-ray films. This enlargement may simulate a tumor, even producing visual field defect by some unknown mechanism. Then, at operation, an "empty sella" is encountered. In these patients, the pituitary gland is flattened out on the floor of the fossa but functions normally, and usually there is no pituitary insufficiency. The "empty sella" syndrome can be diagnosed without operation, and the patient is spared the risk and trauma of exploration. These individuals suspected of having a pituitary adenoma but who, in fact, have this syndrome and in whom operation is being considered should have pneumoencephalography, which will reveal air in the pituitary fossa.

Aneurysm of the internal carotid artery may also expand the pituitary fossa from within, and such patients may need carotid angiography to exclude an aneurysm or meningioma. Pituitary tumor often distorts both the internal carotid and anterior cerebral arteries.

Preparation and Management of Patients Undergoing Procedures for Pituitary Disorders

Before a patient with a pituitary tumor is operated upon, concomitant adrenal or thyroid hypofunction must be treated. These patients should be given extra cortisone during the operation and in the immediate postoperative period. Adult patients whose endocrine function is normal need only adrenal cortical replacement immediately before and during operation. To meet the stress of operation, 50 mg of cortisone acetate is usually given intramuscularly the evening before and the morning of operation, supplemented by 100 mg of soluble hydrocortisone hemisuccinate in 1,000 cc of 5% glucose in water administered slowly over a 10-hour period, during and after operation. Intramuscular cortisone (50 mg) is then given twice daily for 3 days and oral cortisone is substituted as soon as intravenous therapy can be withdrawn. Oral prednisone is equally satisfactory.

In Cushing's disease, when body potassium stores are depleted, potassium chloride supplements should be given before operation. In diabetes mellitus, one-third of the daily dose of long-acting insulin is administered hypodermically on the morning of operation, and a liter of 5% glucose in distilled water containing 100 mg of added hydrocortisone hemisuccinate is given intravenously at the rate of 100 cc/hour. As indicated by blood glucose determinations done 4 times daily, give additional crystalline insulin.

Patients undergoing transsphenoidal procedures or implantation should receive prophylactic antibiotic therapy; ampicillin, 0.5 g 4 times daily, or tetracycline, 0.5 g 4 times daily, and penicillin, 1 million units daily intramuscularly, usually prevent meningitis. Patients undergoing chronic destruction of the pituitary gland by radioactive implants, or after radiotherapy to the gland may need steroid replacement, which is introduced gradually.

In patients with diabetic retinopathy and metastatic breast cancer, the completeness of hypophysectomy may determine the outcome of the therapy, although incomplete pituitary removal may well produce worthwhile results. The safest way to assess function of any pituitary remnant is to compare the radioiodine uptake and serum thyroxine determination 7–10 days after the operation with the preoperative values. If the operation has not produced hypothyroidism, pituitary resection has probably been incomplete.

In diabetic patients the physician can get additional information about the completeness of hypophysectomy by determining their insulin requirements after operation; in those with a satisfactory resection, these requirements should be reduced by at least 50%.[5] Adrenal function should not be assessed because, for this, replacement therapy must be withdrawn; this may be dangerous. Serum levels of growth hormone can be measured by radioimmunoassay: Levels of 1–5 mg/ml after an overnight fast are normal. If growth-hormone release is normal, the serum level should increase fivefold after arginine is injected intravenously, or hypoglycemia has been induced.

Postoperative radiation is usually recommended for patients who have pituitary adenomas that cannot be resected completely.[13] After operation for craniopharyngioma, radiation usually delays the advance of the tumor.[15]

It is extremely important that the patient with hypopituitarism be educated concerning the need for proper treatment of the adrenal insufficiency accompanying anterior pituitary failure. He should register with the Medic-Alert Association and obtain a bracelet that shows he is taking cortisone or prednisone because of pituitary insufficiency. Adjustment of steroid dosage to meet increased requirements during illness and after operation should be emphasized. Through such adaptation, patients with pituitary insufficiency can lead useful, even vigorous lives.

Differential Diagnosis

Anorexia Nervosa

Because of superficial similarities and their respective clinical features, anorexia nervosa and adiposogenital dystrophy may be mistakenly interpreted as organic pituitary disease. *Anorexia nervosa* (Fig. 4–11), seen chiefly in psychoneurotic adolescent girls, is characterized by extreme emaciation and amenorrhea in the absence of any organic disease of the endocrine or any other system. The patient usually denies that she is ill until she is wasted to a degree that is not seen in those with organic disease until they are bedridden. Until she is close to starvation she remains alert, active, restless, and hostile. Apparently the emaciation in these young women is due to an obsessive aversion to food rather than to lack of appetite. Many will admit later that they never actually lost their desire to eat but that their desire to avoid food was stronger than the physiologic hunger. If forced to eat, these people will often regurgitate immediately. They may cease menstruating early but sometimes not until they have lost considerable body weight.

When the syndrome is well developed, the body temperature is often subnormal and the pulse rate and blood pressure are low. Amenorrhea reflects some deficiency of gonadotropic hormone, and develops because the hypothalamic stimulation required for the release of LH at the time of ovulation is interfered with. Such "hypogonadotropism" may also be due to undernutrition. The patient usually does not begin to regain weight until she is removed from the home environment and placed in a hospital. Psychotherapy to reduce her conflict with the environment should be attempted only after her extreme emaciation has been overcome, because only then is the patient receptive to reason. If necessary, duodenal feeding is begun and gradually increased to 3,000–

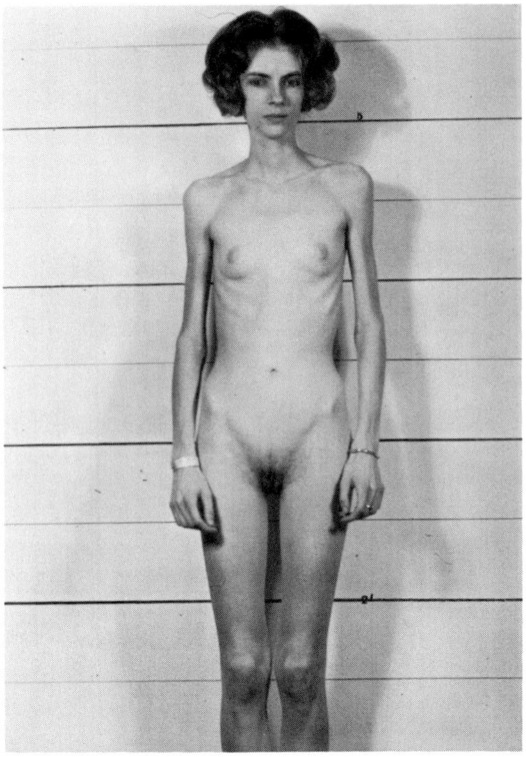

Fig. 4-11. Anorexia nervosa. This 19-year-old girl has emaciation with marked shrinkage of breast tissue and loss of pubic and axillary hair. In girls with this disorder, the associated amenorrhea may precede marked weight loss and persist long after weight has returned to normal. Apart from absence of gonadotropin in the urine, other tests of pituitary function are normal.

4,000 calories daily, the level required for weight gain. During the period of refeeding, the patient may become edematous, and may even have tachycardia and a slight elevation of temperature. These findings, which have also been observed during the same interval in volunteers undergoing starvation, are transient. They do not indicate associated complicating illness and do not call for treatment.

In general, younger patients respond more quickly; the older the patient and the longer she has had her symptoms, the more difficult and unsatisfactory is her treatment. Some of these patients become psychotic and exhibit a form of schizophrenia; in others with a strong psychoneurosis, the illness recurs after they leave the protected atmosphere of the hospital. Soon after they regain weight, the urinary gonadotropin levels rise and, somewhat later, menses usually resume. However, in occasional patients, many years may pass before menstruation becomes regular.

Adiposogenital Dystrophy

In some respects, adiposogenital dystrophy in males (Fig. 4–12) is the counterpart of anorexia nervosa. It is usually seen in emotionally disturbed prepubertal boys who are obese and have moderately delayed puberty. Individuals with true Fröhlich's syndrome, which sometimes is also called adiposogenital dystrophy, have a tumor in the neighborhood of the pituitary gland that causes hypogonadism and, by extending into the hypothalamus, may produce obesity.

When distinguishing between the two types of

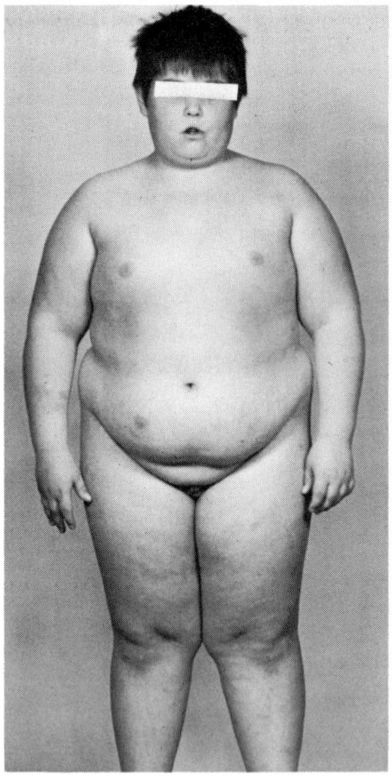

Fig. 4-12. Adiposogenital dystrophy. This boy, 16 years old when this picture was taken, has delayed puberty. The degree and distribution of his obesity makes his phallus appear small. He eventually matured sexually and fathered a child at age 23.

adiposogenital dystrophy, evidence of thyroid or adrenal insufficiency should strongly suggest organic rather than a functional disturbance, which commonly complicates sexual maturation in an emotionally disturbed boy. In the functional type of adiposogenital dystrophy, the obesity is usually associated with severe psychologic maladjustment. The boy's mother may often be oversolicitous and protective. Frequently, he has been confined to bed for a long time because of an illness which started the excessive weight gain. In these obese, adolescent boys, the genitalia often seem unduly small because the phallus is partly hidden in suprapubic fat. As treatment, they usually only require caloric restriction. These patients tend to be inactive and should be encouraged to participate in sports. Most of these boys later mature into normal fertile men. Often the obesity disappears spontaneously as they mature.

Delayed Puberty

Puberty may be delayed without associated obesity. Spontaneous sexual maturity occurs as late as age 20. A favorable prognostic sign is enlargement of the testes which may precede other signs of puberty by several months. In boys who are very sensitive about their lack of maturity, the physician may treat delayed puberty with "priming" doses of long-acting testosterone intramuscularly or by chorionic gonadotropin. After 3 months, the injections should be withheld to see if endogenous production of pituitary and testicular hormone will occur, which often happens.

Investigation and treatment of disorders of the adenohypophysis will be rational and orderly if the physician keeps in mind the concept of the seven separate adenohypophyseal glands, each with a higher hypothalamic control. Functional disturbances may be readily explained by the considerable hypothalamic contribution to the regulation of the gonadotropic hormones in particular. The diagnosis and treatment of diseases of this region must rest on a solid foundation of physiology. Clinical medicine helped to build that foundation.

References

1. Bain, J., and Ezrin, C. Immunofluorescent localization of the LH cell of the human adenohypophysis. *J Clin Endocrinol 30:*181–184, 1970.
2. Burgus, R., Dunn, T. F., Desiderio, D., Ward, D. N., Vale, W., and Guillemin, R. Characterization of ovine hypothalamic hypophysiotropic TSH-releasing factor. *Nature (Lond) 226:*321–325, 1970.
3. Ezrin, C. "The Hypophysis, the Pineal Gland." In *The Ciba Collection of Medical Illustrations,* Netter, F. H. (ed.). Vol. 4, *Endocrine System and Selected Metabolic Diseases.* Summit, N.J., Ciba, 1965, pp. 3–37.
4. Ezrin, C., and Murray, S. "The Cells of the Human Adenohypophysis in Pregnancy, Thyroid Disease and Adrenal Cortical Disorders." In *Colloque international sur la Cytologie de l'Adénohypophyse, Paris, 1963. Cytologie de l'Adénohypophyse,* Paris, 9–4 Sept. 1963. Paris, Ed. du Centre Nat. de la Recherche Scient., 1963, pp. 183–199 and plates.
5. Ezrin, C., Briant, T. D. R., and Firestone, G. The endocrine aspects of trans-sphenoidal hypophysectomy. *Can Med Assoc J 97:*72–75, 1967.
6. Farquharson, R. F. *Simmonds' Disease: Extreme Insufficiency of the Adenohypophysis.* Springfield, Ill., Thomas, 1950, p. 93.
7. Friesen, H., and Astwood, E. B. Hormones of the anterior pituitary body. *N Engl J Med 272:*1216–1223, 1272–1277, 1328–1335, 1965.
8. Goluboff, L. G., and Ezrin, C. Effect of pregnancy on the somatotroph and the prolactin cell of the human adenohypophysis. *J Clin Endocrinol Metab 29:* 1533–1538, 1969.
9. Gordon, D. A., Hill, F. M. and Ezrin, C. Acromegaly: A review of 100 cases. *Can Med Assoc J 87:* 1106–1109, 1962.
10. Henneman, P. H. The effect of human growth hormone on growth of patients with hypopituitarism: A combined study. *JAMA 205:*828–836, 1968.
11. Herlant, M., and Pasteels, J. L. Histophysiology of human anterior pituitary. *Methods Achiev Exp Pathol 3:*250–305, 1967.
12. Kovács, K. Necrosis of anterior pituitary in humans. *Neuroendocrinology 4:*201–241, 1969.
13. Kramer, S. The value of radiation therapy for pituitary and parapituitary tumours. *Can Med Assoc J 99:*1120–1127, 1968.
14. McCormick, W. F., and Halmi, N. S. Absence of chromophobe adenomas from a large series of pituitary tumors. *Arch Pathol 92:*231–238, 1971.

15. Matson, D. D., and Crigler, J. F., Jr. Management of craniopharyngioma in childhood. *J Neurosurg 30:* 377–390, 1969.
16. Miyai, K., Azukiwaza, M., and Kumahara, Y. Familial isolated thyrotropin deficiency with cretinism. *N Engl J Med 285:*1043–1048, 1971.
17. Phifer, R. F., Spicer, S. S., and Orth, D. N. Specific demonstration of the human hypophyseal cells which produce adrenocorticotropic hormone. *J Clin Endocrinol 31:*347–361, 1970.
18. Pittman, J. A., Haigler, E. D., Hershman, J. M., and Pittman, C. S. Hypothalamic hypothyroidism. *N Engl J Med 285:*844–845, 1971.
19. Purves, H. D. "Cytology of the Adenohypophysis." In *The Pituitary Gland,* Harris, G. W., ed. London, Butterworth, 1966, vol. 1, pp. 147–232.
20. Rabkin, M. T., and Frantz, A. G. Hypopituitarism: A study of growth hormone and other endocrine functions. *Ann Intern Med 64:*1197–1207, 1966.
21. Rimoin, D. L., Merimee, T. J., and McKusick, V. A.: Growth-hormone deficiency in man: An isolated, recessively inherited defect. *Science 152:*1635–1637, 1966.
22. Schally, A. V., Nair, R. M. G., Barrett, J. F., Bowers, C. Y., and Folkers, K. The structure of hypothalamic thyrotropin-releasing hormone. (Abstr.) *Fed Proc 29:*470, 1970.
23. Sheehan, H. L. Simmonds' disease due to postpartum necrosis of the anterior pituitary. *Q J Med 8:*227–309, 1939.
24. Stratmann, I. E., Ezrin, C., Sellers, E. A. and Simon, G. T. The origin of thyroidectomy cells as revealed by high resolution radioautography. *Endocrinology 90:*728–734, 1972.

5

The Thyroid

Robert Volpé

In the past, many of the opinions advanced regarding the possible functions of the thyroid gland were both imaginative and, in retrospect, amusing. For example, Wharton, who originally described the thyroid in 1656, believed that the gland was larger in women in order to give the female neck a graceful contour. Modern concepts of thyroid activity did not begin to develop until Gull in 1874 recognized the relationship of thyroid atrophy to the symptoms now known to be those of hypothyroidism.

This chapter summarizes the functions, metabolism, and disorders of the thyroid gland as they are currently understood. The treatment of each topic will not be exhaustive, but all aspects of thyroid physiology and disease are at least briefly covered. For the sake of brevity, this chapter may err on the side of dogmatism, but it fairly represents the views of the author.

Control of the Thyroid Gland

Although control of the thyroid gland by the anterior pituitary gland and hypothalamus is discussed in Chapter 4, it will be summarized briefly here.

Thyroid secretion is regulated by pituitary thyrotropin which stimulates virtually every step of intrathyroidal metabolism. The anterior pituitary (adenohypophysis) in turn secretes thyrotropin when it is stimulated by a decrease in the circulating free thyroxine, as well as by thyrotropin-releasing hormone (TRH) from the hypothalamus (see Fig. 5-3**A**). Thus lesions of the hypothalamus or pituitary gland can reduce thyrotropin secretion and produce hypothyroidism. The reverse—i.e., autonomous hypersecretion of pituitary thyrotropin in man—has been reported only once.[8] The mechanism of action of thyrotropin (TSH) on or within the thyroid cell is not fully understood, although it appears to act on the thyroid cell membrane. TSH appears to attach itself to a specific receptor site on the cell membrane and alter the calcium concentration in and around the membrane. This in turn may activate adenyl cyclase, which then increases cyclic 3′,5′-adenosine monophosphate, and relays the "message" from the cell membrane to the intracellular sites of action.

Ontogeny and Phylogeny[10]

The thyroid gland, the first endocrine gland to evolve in the vertebrate and appear in the developing mammal, begins as an invagination of the pharynx at the base of the tongue. Hence, thyroid tissue may occasionally persist at the base of the tongue, as the only such tissue in the body, or as accessory thyroid tissue. The gland is well differentiated by the fifteenth week of fetal life, and starts to produce thyroxine at this time. The thyroglossal duct, which marks the gland's downward migration into the neck, is derived from the pharynx. This duct usually atrophies completely, but occasionally may persist as a thyroglossal duct cyst.

In the most primitive vertebrates, the endostyle, a primitive salivary gland and the precursor of the thyroid gland, can trap and concentrate iodine, and produce iodotyrosines and iodothyronines. In such animals, the cells from this gland enter the gastrointestinal tract, are hydrolyzed and release free thyroxine. In these primitive vertebrates, however, thyroxine does not seem to have any real function. When animals left the sea to live on land, the iodide-concentrating mechanism had to be greatly improved to protect the organism during intervals of iodine famine. Thus an increasingly complex gland was evolved which was highly efficient in trapping and storing iodine.

The ultimobranchial body, which is discrete in some species, becomes an integral part of the thyroid gland in man, and is represented by the parafollicular or C cells.

Anatomy and Anatomical Relations of the Thyroid

The physician should understand the anatomy of the thyroid gland because goiter is a common disorder. In the average North American adult the normal thyroid gland weighs approximately 10 to 20 gm. Encapsulated in fibrous tissue, it is held around the anterior and lateral aspects of the trachea by loose connective tissue. The lateral lobes on each side of the trachea are connected by a thin band of thyroid tissue—the isthmus. The isthmus lies just below the cricoid cartilage, and occasionally a pyramidal lobe extends superiorly from the isthmus. The carotid sheath and sternocleidomastoid muscles lie laterally, and the infrahyoid muscles lie anteriorly. Generally, there are two pairs of parathyroid glands under the posterior surfaces of the lateral lobes. The recurrent laryngeal nerves lie in grooves between the trachea and the lateral lobes of the thyroid gland.

Blood for the thyroid gland comes from two superior thyroid arteries that arise from the external carotid arteries, and two inferior thyroid arteries, branches of the subclavian arteries. The right lobe of the thyroid gland has a richer blood supply than the left, is often larger, and more frequently develops nodules. The thyroid gland receives both sympathetic and parasympathetic fibers; these nerves control arterial and venous flow, but otherwise exert no direct influence on the parenchymal cells.

Structure

The gland is rubbery and homogeneous on cut section. Microscopically, it is composed of small follicles filled with colloid, which make up as much as 70% of the total thyroid mass. Each follicle is lined by a single layer of closely packed cuboidal cells, which become columnar when stimulated, and flat when inactive. The follicles, which are about 200 μ in diameter, are generally spherical, but after they are emptied by thyrotropin stimulation, they may be irregular. Lobules contain several follicles bound together with connective tissue and are supplied by a single artery. Each lobule is a functional unit, and even adjacent lobules may function at different rates and at different times.

A second type of cell, the parafollicular cell (also called the C cell or light cell) almost certainly produces calcitonin. Through the basal zone of the follicle these oval or ellipsoid cells come in contact with the basal follicular membrane. Their apical poles are directed toward the follicular lumen but are separated from it by a thin sheet of follicular parenchymatous cells.

Thyroid Hormones: Physiology and Chemistry

The thyroid gland secretes two thyroid hormones, L-thyroxine and 3,5,3′-l-triiodothyronine, which it manufactures from iodine and tyrosine. Although calcitonin (a calcium-lowering hormone) is also secreted by the thyroid gland (parafollicular cells), its function and actions will be discussed in Chapter 6, The Parathyroid and Calcium Metabolism.

Iodine Metabolism

Ingestion of iodine varies very widely throughout the world; the optimal intake is 250–270 μg/day. Many populations suffer from frank iodine deficiency, and others have only marginal iodine intake. In the modern community, most of the daily iodide is taken as iodized salt.

Iodine enters the body chiefly with food and water but can readily enter via the intact skin or lungs. Most organic iodine compounds are reduced to ionic iodide and absorbed from the intestinal tract within an hour, being transported as inorganic iodide in the circulation. Competing with the kidneys, the thyroid gland takes up between 10% and 40% of the circulating iodine; almost all of the remainder is lost in the urine. Minute amounts are also lost through the sweat and feces. Iodide is also transiently trapped and concentrated by the salivary and gastric glands, but soon returns to the circulation.

The thyroid gland withdraws iodide from the circulation and, in the "thyroid-iodide trap," concentrates it to more than 30 times the plasma levels, and occasionally even higher (Fig. 5–1). The trap appears to be within the follicle rather than in the parenchymal cells. A pumping mechanism stimulated by thyrotropin (and inhibited by perchlorate or thiocyanate) drives iodide ions from the plasma, through the follicular cells, and into the colloid.

Synthesis of Thyroid Hormones

After they reach the follicle, the iodide ions are oxidized to an active form of iodine under the influence of the enzyme peroxidase. Immediately the active iodine attaches itself to the 3-position of a tyrosine ring forming monoiodotyrosine (MIT). At this time, the tyrosine ring is already bound to a large globulin molecule (thyroglobulin) by a peptide linkage. After MIT is formed, the 5-position of the tyrosine ring is iodized to form diiodotyrosine (DIT). Coupling of 2 diiodotyrosines (still combined with thyroglobulin) produces thyroxine; alternatively, monoiodotyrosine may combine with diiodotyrosine to form triiodothyronine (T_3). Coupling enzymes are necessary for either of these alternate steps. There is now good evidence that considerable T_3 is also produced peripherally by deiodinating the 5-iodine atom from T_4.[2] The entire synthesis of thyroxine seems to take place within the follicle—a transaction between molecules of thyroglobulin, assisted only by the necessary enzymes.

The main constituent of the follicular colloid, thyroglobulin, has a molecular weight of 680,000. Under normal circumstances, only minute amounts of this large molecular protein reach the circulation. The thyroid gland contains other iodoproteins of differing properties, which have not been precisely characterized, although one of these is almost certainly an iodoalbumin and may be derived from the serum proteins. Normally, enough thyroxine is stored in the follicles to maintain normal circulating thyroid hormone levels for several months, without further production of thyroid hormone. Before thyroxine can be secreted into the bloodstream, the globulin-thyroxine complex must be split by proteolytic or mucolytic enzymes (Fig. 5-2). All of these steps appear to be stimulated by thyrotropin, although this is almost certainly by indirect means.

Each day the thyroid gland secretes about 90 μg of thyroxine; 50 μg of triiodothyronine is also produced daily, but about ⅓ of this is derived from the peripheral conversion of T_4 to T_3.* Minute amounts of other organically bound iodo-compounds are also secreted by the thyroid gland.

Thyroid Hormone Transport in the Blood

Like many hormones, thyroid hormones are largely carried in the circulation by certain plasma proteins that bind and thus transport the hormones to their sites of action.[20]

The normal plasma concentration of thyroxine is 4–11 μg/100 ml. Virtually all (normally 99.94%) of the thyroxine is bound to proteins within the plasma—i.e., thyroxine-binding globulin (TBG), thyroxine-binding prealbumin (TBPA), and albumin. TBG, an interalpha globulin (i.e., between alpha-1 and alpha-2 globulin)

* See Appendix: Addendum 1 to Chapter 5.

Fig. 5-1. Control of the thyroid. This coordinating illustration links the higher controls of thyroid function, intrathyroidal iodide metabolism and, finally, the drugs which inhibit thyroid function.

Upper third. Hypothalamic production of thyrotopin-releasing factor (TRF) is effected by (1) cerebral cortex, (2) nervous influences, and (3) circulating free thyroxine. Secretion of TSH by the thyrotroph may be stimulated directly by a falling level of circulating free thyroxine. In addition, a falling level of free thyroxine may stimulate TRF output; a rising level may inhibit this output, as it does TSH.

Box. In intrathyroidal iodide metabolism iodide (I−) and tyrosine are built up into either triiodothyronine (T_3) or tetraiodothyronine (T_4 or thyroxine). See text for details.

Bottom. The six steps below the box, which begin after iodide is transported to the gland (viz., I− trapping, organic binding, coupling, proteolysis, release, and dehalogenation), are important because enzyme defects, drugs, or goitrogens may affect these reactions.

Drugs used to reduce thyroid function are listed below the steps at which they have their principal actions.

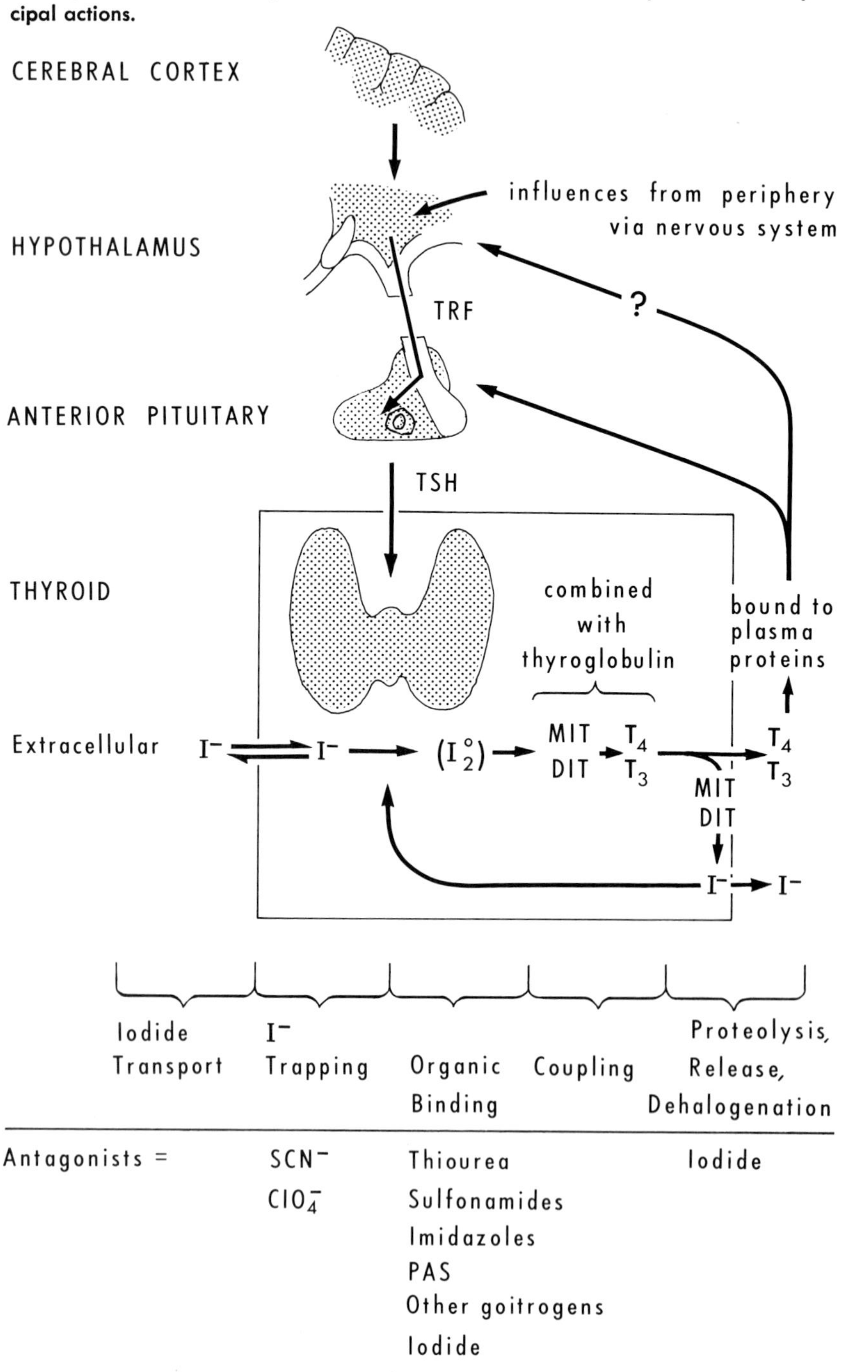

Fig. 5-2. Secretion of T_3 and T_4 by thyroid. Colloid passes from follicle into thyroid cell. In the cell, lysosomal enzymes act upon colloid, break down the globulin-thyroxine complex (proteolysis), release T_3 and T_4 into the circulation, and MIT and DIT into cytoplasm. These building blocks (MIT and DIT) lose their iodine (dehalogenation), which is used again to form more thyroid hormone. If there is not enough dehalogenase, MIT and DIT accumulate, spill over into the blood and are lost in the urine, producing iodine deficiency and goiter. Such goiter can be treated by high doses of iodine or by providing thyroxine.

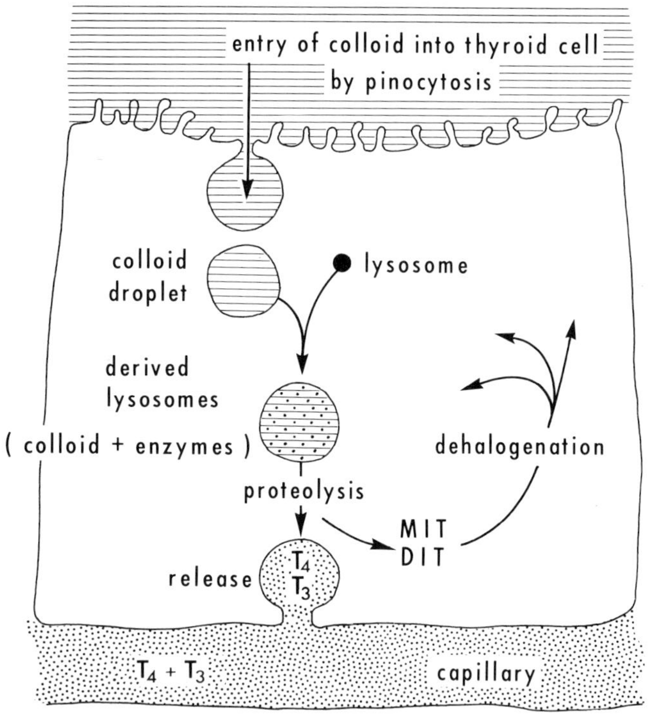

that has specific binding properties for thyroxine, is the most avid, and thus the primary carrier; normally it is one-third saturated with the thyroxine, and two-thirds unsaturated. In hypothyroidism, much less thyroxine is bound to TBG because much less thyroxine is present, hence the unsaturated TBG is increased. In hyperthyroidism, the TBG may be almost or completely saturated. The amount of TBG "binding capacity" may fluctuate spontaneously or under the influence of drugs; thus, estrogen therapy may increase TBG, while diphenylhydantoin (Dilantin) in large dosage may reduce its binding capacity. Congenital "hyperTBGemia" and "hypoTBGemia" have been reported, and are usually familial.

Compared to TBG, TBPA has a higher binding capacity but binds thyroxine less avidly. TBPA may also be altered, either by drugs such as salicylates, or during acute illnesses, cardiac arrhythmias, or surgical procedures. Albumin will also bind thyroxine, although much more loosely than either of the proteins described above.

The thyroxine bound to these proteins is not available to the tissues. Thyroxine is continuously being released from its binding sites as free thyroxine, but the concentration of this free thyroxine is exceedingly small, normally about 0.06% of the total serum thyroxine. Although T_3 binds itself to TBG in vitro, its ability to bind to TBG in vivo is much less than that for T_4; T_3 thus reaches the tissues much more rapidly than T_4 and has a much more rapid effect. It can be shown that, in the absence of TBG, T_4 and T_3 have almost identical metabolic effects, temporally and quantitatively.*

TBG seems to exert a buffering or moderating effect on thyroxine, permitting a slow, gradual response to the requirements of the body. On the other hand, T_3 is able to reach the tissues quickly, because it is bound so lightly in the plasma.

Actions of Thyroid Hormone

Both T_3 and T_4 stimulate calorigenesis, potentiate epinephrine, lower serum cholesterol, stimulate amphibian metamorphosis, and stimulate growth in humans. Thyroxine is necessary for

* See Appendix: Addendum 2 to Chapter 5.

normal central nervous system development. Whether these apparently varied actions are related to a single ("unitary") intracellular effect has not yet been determined.

Thyroxine has a very characteristic effect on amphibian metamorphosis (it causes tadpoles to grow legs and become frogs). This effect may be closely related to thyroxine-induced growth stimulation and differentiation and maturation of special tissues in humans. Thyroxine influences central nervous system development, a particularly important effect. For full brain development in the mammalian embryo, thyroxine must be present in normal amounts.

Thyroxine promotes protein synthesis and increases nitrogen retention. However, when the blood thyroxine level is elevated, protein breakdown is accelerated, and the body operates in a negative nitrogen balance. Thyroxine excess also impairs the conversion of creatine to creatinine and the formation of phosophocreatine. The wasteful creatinuria so produced results in marked muscular weakness, and increases the muscular requirement for oxygen. Thyroxine in excess also increases myocardial contraction force and heart rates. This appears to be a myocardial adjustment to the increased peripheral need for oxygen.

Thyroxine also reduces the organism's sensitivity to insulin and accelerates insulin degradation. Thus hyperthyroidism aggravates preexistent diabetes or might even precipitate diabetes mellitus in predisposed persons.

Because more calories are consumed and the effects of epinephrine are potentiated, excess thyroxine levels induce many somatic effects which will be briefly mentioned under Hyperthyroidism.

The precise mechanism by which thyroid hormone produces its cellular effects is not yet known, and it is possible that thyroxine may stimulate only a single energy-producing reaction common to most tissues.

Thyroid hormones cause swelling of the mitochondria of cells both in vivo and in vitro. Although this observation does not indicate precisely how thyroxine exerts its cellular effects, obviously it exerts some cellular action in the mitochondrial area. Oxidative phosphorylation is uncoupled in vitro by excessive concentrations of thyroxine (a possible explanation for the wasteful production of heat in hyperthyroidism), but this is not an acceptable explanation for the beneficial effects of physiologic doses of thyroxine. Furthermore, uncoupling of oxidative phosphorylation does not appear to occur in vivo even in hyperthyroidism. More recently, evidence has accumulated linking the action of thyroxine to stimulation of RNA synthesis, as well as to the synthesis of proteins. However, our exploration of this entire subject has just begun.

Current Tests of Thyroid Function*

Basal Metabolic Rate

As recently as 20 years ago, the only commonly used test of thyroid function was the *basal metabolic rate* (BMR). Unhappily, this rate was often not "basal," and even when accurately performed, was often elevated in nonthyroid diseases, such as leukemia, lymphoma, emphysema, congestive heart failure, and perforated eardrums. Similarly, the BMR was depressed in a variety of other diseases that did not affect thyroid function, such as starvation, thiamine deficiency, nephrotic syndrome, Addison's disease, and periodic catatonia. Even in the best laboratories, the BMR correlates with the final assessment of thyroid activity in only about 50% of cases, and thus is no longer widely used.

Protein-Bound Iodine

In recent years, the serum protein-bound iodine (PBI, normal range, 4–8 μg/100 ml) became the single most commonly used test of thyroid function. It measures the iodine bound to protein, which in the normal state is virtually all thyroxine iodine: hence, the PBI is usually a good measure of the amount of circulating thyroxine. However, the PBI is elevated by iodine contami-

* See Appendix: Addendum 3 to Chapter 5.

nation, particularly the organic iodine-containing dyes used in radiology. These dyes may artificially elevate the PBI for weeks, months, or even for life. Furthermore, in certain thyroid diseases, the body produces abnormal iodoproteins which, though not metabolically active, are measured as protein-bound iodine. Thus, in such instances, the PBI may be deceptively higher and not reflect true levels of serum thyroxine. The PBI is also altered by changes in thyroxine-binding proteins. Thus, when there is an increase in thyroxine-binding globulin, due either to congenital causes or to estrogen excess (e.g., pregnancy, hydatidiform moles, estrogen administration, "the pill"), the protein-bound iodine is elevated. The increased binding protein elevates the PBI by retaining more of the secreted thyroxine within the circulation.

Conversely, when the thyroxine-binding protein is reduced, either because of congenital deficiency or as a result of diphenylhydantoin or androgen therapy, the PBI is reduced. However, with either an elevation or depression of thyroxine-binding globulin, the absolute level of free (unbound) thyroxine in the circulation (see below) is within normal limits, and thus the patient remains euthyroid despite abnormal PBI values. For these reasons, therefore, the PBI may at times be misleading.

Butanol-Extractable Iodine

The butanol extractable iodine (BEI), because it does not measure iodoproteins, is a truer measure of the circulating thyroxine than is the PBI. However, it is more difficult to perform, and is also contaminated by organic iodine-containing dyes. The normal range is 3.2–6.4 μg/100 ml. This value is, of course, elevated in estrogen therapy or pregnancy. The BEI is now gradually going out of favor because methods have been introduced which measure the serum thyroxine directly.

Serum Thyroxine

The direct measurement of serum thyroxine (T_4) is much easier than the PBI and, with many available techniques, is not contaminated by organic or inorganic iodine. The Murphy-Pattee technique is currently preferable. Once again, however, an increase in TBG (estrogen therapy, pregnancy) will elevate the serum T_4. The serum T_4 techniques will probably soon supplant the PBI as the most common test of thyroid function.

Because any measurement of serum thyroxine (i.e., PBI, BEI, or serum T_4) is markedly influenced by the amount of circulating binding proteins, physicians may become confused when these levels are elevated as a result of oral contraceptive therapy, and such patients have often been incorrectly referred or even treated for hyperthyroidism. It should be reiterated that any change in the thyroxine-binding proteins is not, per se, associated with abnormalities of thyroid function or metabolism.

T_3 Resin Uptake

Fortunately the resin uptake of ^{131}I-triiodothyronine is generally available; this useful procedure complements the serum thyroxine because it measures indirectly the amount of unsaturated thyroxine-binding globulin. The resin uptake of $^{131}I\text{-}T_3$ (normal range 25–35%) has supplanted the qualitatively similar erythrocyte uptake of $^{131}I\text{-}T_3$, because it is easier to perform. When unsaturated binding sites are increased (as in myxedema, pregnancy, or estrogen therapy), the test result falls below 25%. This result indicates that most of the added triiodothyronine is retained by the thyroxine-binding globulin, leaving much less to be picked up by the resin. Conversely, when unoccupied thyroxine-binding sites are decreased (as in hyperthyroidism or in lack of TBG) the resin uptake of $^{131}I\text{-}T_3$ is elevated above 35%—i.e., there are not enough sites on TBG for the added $^{131}I\text{-}T_3$, which thus is picked up by the resin. Thus, a high serum thyroxine and a low T_3 resin test indicate an increase in thyroxine-binding globulin. On the other hand, if TBG is low, then a high T_3 resin uptake would be associated with a low PBI.*

Furthermore, the T_3 resin uptake test may be elevated in euthyroid patients when TBPA binding sites are diminished. Because thyroxine

* See Appendix: Addendum 4 to Chapter 5.

cannot bind to TBPA in this situation, more thyroxine is bound to TBG, thus reducing the number of unoccupied TBG binding sites. Since TBPA is reduced in a wide variety of nonthyroidal diseases (e.g., acute infections, operations, and cardiac arrhythmias), the T_3 resin uptake value will often be increased and thus, if taken alone, mislead the physician.

Free Thyroxine and Thyroxine-Binding Protein Determinations

Although it is now possible to determine the free thyroxine (normally about 0.06% of the total serum thyroxine), and thyroxine-binding proteins directly, these techniques are not routinely available. However, these determinations may ultimately become routine and may also be useful aids to clinical diagnosis. It must nevertheless be mentioned that free thyroxine may be elevated in conditions other than hyperthyroidism, particularly when there is a reduction in TBPA.

Determination of Total Serum Triiodothyronine

Recent attempts to measure total serum triiodothyronine have encountered many difficulties. While the immunoassay technic for T_3 appears to have won the day, there still is a considerable difference in the normal range as reported by different authors. Normal mean values vary between 0.12 and 0.22 $\mu g/100$ ml. T_3 determinations have been valuable in detecting "T_3-toxicosis," a type of hyperthyroidism in which only T_3 is elevated. Furthermore, individuals with various types of thyroid impairment maintain a euthyroid or near-euthyroid status by serum levels of T_3 that are relatively higher than the T_4 concentrations.[18]

Thyrotropin Immunoassay

The immunoassay of TSH is now widely used as a test of thyroid function,[9] chiefly in the diagnosis of primary hypothyroidism, in which it is elevated (normal range 0–6 nanograms/ml). Recently a new test of thyroid function has appeared using synthetic thyrotropin-stimulating hormone (TRH). The synthetic material is injected intravenously, and TSH measured. TSH will increase in normal persons and in patients with nontoxic goiter. It does not increase in hyperthyroidism or in pituitary disease, but will respond when hypothyroidism is due to a hypothalamic rather than a pituitary disorder.

Radioactive Iodine Uptake

Radioactive iodine uptake, a useful and common procedure, has many variations, the most common of which is the 24-hour uptake. However, uptakes at shorter periods—10 minutes, 3 hours, 6 hours, etc.—give additional information. Various other modifications of uptake studies are also well known. The normal range for the 24-hour uptake varies from locale to locale, depending largely on the average iodine in the local diet. In Southern Ontario, the 24-hour ^{131}I uptake normally ranges between 10% and 35%. Like all other tests, the results may be misleading. Uptakes may be elevated in conditions other than hyperthyroidism—e.g., iodine deficiency, rebound phases after subacute thyroiditis, or after thyroid or antithyroid drug administration, or in certain enzymatic defects of the thyroid gland. Conversely, the uptake may be suppressed in conditions other than hypothyroidism; values may be low with iodine contamination, antithyroid drugs, and thyroid administration. Further tests employing ^{131}I that measure secretion rate or incorporation of ^{131}I into the PBI (^{131}PBI) suffer from many of the same drawbacks. Radiothyroxine turnover rates have also been used as diagnostic aids.

Werner Suppression Test

In some instances, despite the wide variety of tests already detailed, a diagnosis of hyperthyroidism may still be in question. In such circumstances, a Werner suppression test with triiodothyronine may be of considerable help. This test makes use of the observation that, in normal persons or those with nontoxic goiters, the administration of triiodothyronine will suppress pituitary thyrotropin, thus suppressing thyroid function; this causes the radioactive iodine uptake to be suppressed. Thus, giving triiodothyronine in a dosage of 75–100 μg daily for 10 days will cause the radioactive iodine uptake to fall to less than 50% of its initial value within 10 days. In hyperthyroidism, however, thyroid function cannot be suppressed by triiodothyronine, and thus the uptake remains at its original level.

Kinemometry

A recent new test, kinemometry, measures the Achilles tendon reflex on electrocardiographic paper. This reflex is characteristically slowed in hypothyroidism and increased in hyperthyroidism. Although this test is simple, there is unfortunately a considerable overlap between normal persons and those with hyperthyroidism and hypothyroidism. Thus, in problem cases, the test is not definitive. It is, however, useful for follow-up purposes in individual patients.

Other Tests

Iodine metabolism can be studied in many other ways which will not be described here. Thyroid scanning will be mentioned under diseases of the thyroid, and thyroid autoantibody tests will be referred to under autoimmune thyroiditis.

Diseases of the Thyroid Gland

Nontoxic Goiter

Goiters Due to Iodine Deficiency

Although the connection between iodine and thyroid disease was first suspected in 1812, not until 1928 did Marine conclusively demonstrate that iodine deficiency produced goiter—an observation that was soon confirmed experimentally and clinically. Iodine deficiency may often be associated with other factors that induce goiter, such as increased need for thyroid hormone and/or enzymatic defects. All work together to produce goiter. At times of rapid growth or change, puberty, pregnancy, menopause, and during periods of infection, demand for thyroid hormone increases, and the need for iodine rises concomitantly. If iodide ingestion does not keep pace with the increased requirement, thyroxine synthesis is ultimately reduced. Through feedback regulation, this leads to an increase in pituitary thyrotropin secretion, which in turn causes hypertrophy and hyperplasia of the thyroid parenchymal cells. The ability of these cells to concentrate iodide increases, thus accelerating the production of thyroxine. These compensatory mechanisms are generally sufficient to maintain the patient in a euthyroid state, but occasionally, in severe iodine deficiency, the compensatory mechanisms are inadequate and the individual becomes hypothyroid.

Pathology

In the early phases, the gland is moderately and diffusely enlarged, the cut surface is reddish and homogeneous, and the tissue is somewhat rubbery. The hypertrophied and hyperplastic follicular cells contain decreased amounts of pale-staining colloid.

Later, the gland may become markedly enlarged, even huge. It is no longer homogeneous, but nodular; the nodules may vary in size, and on gross and histologic examination, may differ markedly one from another. Such nodules may remain hyperplastic, but more often they may degenerate, showing fibrosis, necrosis, dystrophic calcification, cyst formation, and hemorrhage into cysts. On the other hand, the nodules may become adenomatous, autonomous, and even toxic (see section on Hyperthyroidism).

Goiter due to iodine deficiency is common in areas where the soil is iodine-deficient and where no preventive measures are carried out. These goiters are more common and often larger in females than males. In males the incidence of goiter decreases after puberty, but in females it increases. Further increases may occur during pregnancy, lactation, and with the menopause.

A patient with an iodine-deficient goiter usually has an elevated 24-hour radioactive iodine uptake, comparable to values seen in hyperthyroidism. However, since this degree of elevation is seen in patients who are clinically and biochemically euthyroid or even hypothyroid and the serum thyroxine is normal or low, the physician should not confuse this condition with thyrotoxicosis.

Prophylaxis and Treatment

The only prophylaxis needed is iodine ingestion. In iodine-deficient areas, diet must be supplemented with iodine, generally given as table salt, which contains about 0.1% of potassium iodide. The average person taking 7 gm of such salt each day would ingest 500 μg of iodine, far more than is necessary. If such therapy is begun after nodular degeneration has occurred, such nodules will not regress markedly. However, those areas of thyroid still functioning should regress on such therapy.

Once the goiter has formed, the patient is given thyroid hormone, usually as desiccated thyroid 120–180 mg/day or equivalent doses of thyroxine, 0.2–0.3 mg/day. Thyroid hormone will benefit other types of nontoxic goiter as well, as will be described later. Most complete regression is achieved when the goiter is still diffuse, or when the goiter is small. Large, and particularly nodular, goiters respond poorly to such therapy, and only doses almost large enough to produce hyperthyroidism will achieve an optimal response. The medication must be continued indefinitely.

Goiters Due to Goitrogens

Certain "goitrogens" suppress thyroxine production and consequently increase pituitary thyrotropin secretion, thus inducing hyperplasia and hypertrophy of the thyroid. Such goiters are produced by a mechanism similar to those that operate in iodine deficiency and in the presence of enzyme defects. Goitrogens include drugs used to suppress thyroid function (antithyroid drugs) and compounds such as thiocyanate or perchlorate, which may inhibit the thyroid's ability to concentrate iodide. Various plants (e.g., the *Brassica* group—cabbages, etc.) contain goitrogens which exert an antithyroid effect. Antithyroid drugs, such as the thiourea compounds, inhibit the oxidation of iodide to iodine and later inhibit the coupling mechanism. Excessive iodide will also inhibit the oxidation of iodide to iodine, and thus may produce both hypothyroidism and a goiter. This is one of nature's paradoxes: Either iodine deficiency or excess can produce goiter, with or without hypothyroidism.

The goiters produced by these compounds have the same pathology, clinical features, and nodular complications as those caused by iodine deficiency. These goiters are treated by withdrawing the antithyroid compounds; often this is all that is required. Further thyroxine administration may also be useful.

Goiters Due to Enzymatic Defects

Five types of genetic enzymatic defects within the thyroid induce childhood goiter and sometimes hypothyroidism (Fig. 5-3, **B** and **C**). While these defects are most obvious in the large goiters of childhood, similar minor defects probably produce many sporadic adult goiters in areas where neither goitrogens nor iodine deficiency operate. Unfortunately, although the last two mechanisms can be ruled out in most sporadic adult goiters, it is often difficult to demonstrate enzyme defects in such cases. Thus, the pathogenesis of many of the adult nontoxic goiters remains unsettled.

Defect in Iodide Trapping

In this exceedingly rare genetic defect, the thyroid gland cannot concentrate iodide. The defect is not confined to the thyroid, because the salivary glands and gastric mucosa, which normally concentrate iodide, also show the same disturbance. When the intake of iodide is normal, a goiter and often hypothyroidism result. A large intake of iodide will lead to increased thyroxine production, and hence regression of the goiter. However, the goiter can be treated more effectively by thyroxine administration.

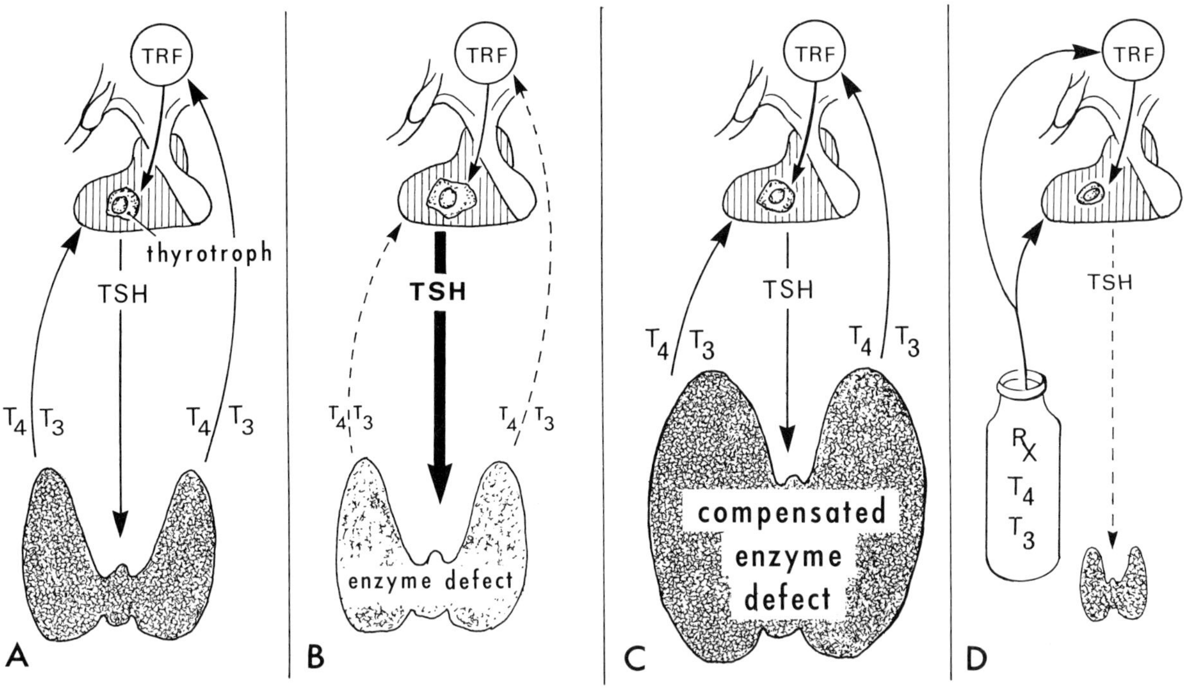

Fig. 5-3. Hypothalamic-pituitary-thyroid relationships in diffuse goiter due to enzyme defect. These figures illustrate activity of the "thyrotroph"—the cell which produces TSH or thyrotropin.

A. In normal individual, hypothalamic hormone—thyrotropin-releasing factor (TRF)—has stimulated release and production of TSH, which in turn acts on thyroid to increase output of two thyroid hormones: T_4 and T_3. These hormones, carried in circulation to hypothalamus and adenohypophysis, inhibit further TRF production and TSH release. (Note in **B**, **C**, and **D**, that size of thyrotroph changes commensurate with its activity in these several situations. Variations in TSH output are indicated by arrows of various widths. Broken line indicates deficiency or absence of T_4, T_3, and TSH.

B. In individual with enzyme defect, production of thyroid hormones is reduced below level needed to inhibit TSH output. (See Chapter 4, Physiology of Hormones Produced in the Adenohypophysis.)

C. Thyroid hypertrophy will sometimes overcome effects of enzyme deficiency and raise thyroid hormone production to a level sufficient to again control TSH output.

D. Treatment of hypertrophied gland with T_4 and T_3 inhibits thyrotroph.

Genetic Defect in Organic Binding of Iodide

The glands of patients with this type of defect trap and concentrate iodide readily but cannot convert it into iodine and thus combine it with tyrosine. Thus these patients cannot produce adequate thyroxine and often develop hypothyroidism and/or goiter. Many goitrous cretins manifest this defect.

In defective organic binding, a tracer dose of radioactive iodine will accumulate rapidly in the thyroid gland in the first few hours, but then it is gradually discharged back into the bloodstream over the next few hours; free (unbound) iodide leaves the gland, to reach equilibrium with the plasma. The defect can also be demonstrated by a potassium perchlorate "flushing" test. In this test, a tracer dose of radioactive iodine is given which accumulates within the thyroid gland over the first 2–4 hours. Then the patient is given 600 mg of potassium perchlorate by mouth, which causes a discharge of free iodide from the gland. In the normal thyroid gland, because of the rapid organic binding of the iodide, there is no such "flushing."

Probably defective binding is due to an absence or partial deficiency of thyroid peroxidase. Mild forms of this defect may account for some adult nontoxic goiters. Pendred's syndrome, a genetic disorder characterized by deafness, goiter, and often hypothyroidism, is associated with this defect.

Once again, these patients are treated with thyroxine.

Iodotyrosyl-Coupling Defect

This genetic defect, generally associated with goitrous cretinism, appears to be due to a deficiency of the coupling enzymes that combine iodotyrosines to form iodothyronines. Generally, the radioactive iodine uptake is markedly elevated, often approaching 100%. Much of the iodide is not organically bound. In most of these patients iodothyronines cannot be demonstrated in chromatograms of the thyroid tissue.

Inadequate Dehalogenase

Normally much of the monoiodotyrosine and diiodotyrosine produced in the thyroid gland is rapidly deiodinated, and the iodine so broken off is used again to form more thyroid hormone. However, in this genetic enzyme deficiency, deiodination fails because there is not enough dehalogenase. Thus, monoiodotyrosine and diiodotyrosine accumulate in the blood and urine. This accumulation produces iodine deficiency, which may improve when a patient ingests large amounts of iodine.

Production of Abnormal Iodoproteins

Some goitrous patients (with or without hypothyroidism) produce abnormal organic iodoproteins, mostly iodoalbumin. Such patients produce inadequate amounts of thyroxine. The precise cause of this disturbance has not yet been delineated. Abnormal iodoproteins are also produced in several acquired thyroid disorders, such as Hashimoto's thyroiditis, and thyroid cancer.

Summary of Nontoxic Goiter

Several mechanisms, including iodine deficiency, ingestion of goitrogens, and the genetic enzymatic defects, may produce goiters, often with hypothyroidism. In addition, thyroid enlargement may be produced by malignant thyroid neoplasms or any of the types of thyroiditis (see below).

Whether the nontoxic goiter is due to iodine deficiency, a genetic defect, or the goitrogens, the final common pathogenesis is the same in each (Fig. 5-3). Inadequate thyroxine production stimulates increased secretion of pituitary thyrotropin, with compensatory hyperplasia of the thyroid gland. If the defect is severe, hypothyroidism develops. If the defect is mild, defective thyroxine production will be offset by hyperplasia of the gland, and although the patient will have a goiter, he will be euthyroid.*

During life, we have variable requirements for thyroxine; our need increases in periods of rapid growth, puberty, menstruation, pregnancy, lactation, and the menopause. At these times, goiters enlarge further; but later will involute. Such cyclic change will ultimately lead to nodule formation, and finally a nontoxic nodular goiter.

Periods of hyperplasia followed by involution produce nodular hyperplasia that will be followed by the degenerations to which ischemic thyroid nodules are prone—fibrosis, calcification, necrosis, cyst formation, and hemorrhage into cysts. Furthermore, some nodules may ultimately become autonomous—i.e., free of pituitary thyrotropin control. Autonomous nodules may become hyperplastic enough to produce toxic nodular goiter and this autonomy also may be a factor in the pathogenesis of thyroid malignancy.

The treatment of these various nontoxic goiters is ultimately similar. Thyroxine or other forms of thyroid hormone will suppress pituitary thyrotropin and thus allow the goiter to regress. Hypothyroidism, if present, will also be controlled. However, if the goiter has already degenerated, or if

* See Appendix: Addendum 5 to Chapter 5.

autonomous nodules have already developed, the goiter will not regress.

In such instances, the nodules may be unacceptable to the patient cosmetically, or may cause symptoms by compressing or distorting adjacent structures. In such circumstances, subtotal thyroidectomy will be necessary. If the removed nodules are benign, the patients *must continue to take thyroxine thereafter,* to prevent nodule formation in the thyroid remnants.

Benign nontoxic nodular goiters are very common; in North America about 10% of adult females have one. While thyroid malignancy is not uncommon, at least in an occult, microscopic form, death from thyroid carcinoma is very uncommon. Because of this relatively good prognosis, nontoxic goiters are usually treated medically unless certain clinical considerations dictate otherwise (see section on Clinical Aspects of Thyroid Malignancy later in this chapter).*

An important diagnostic problem is that of distinguishing clinically between some thyroid malignancies and benign nontoxic goiter. Thyroid scans have been of some help in this regard, because "cold" nodules (those nodules that do not pick up radioactive iodine) are more likely to be malignant than "hot" nodules (those that pick up radioactive iodine well). About 20% of "cold" nonfunctioning nodules prove to be malignant. For this reason, most clinics recommend surgical extirpation for all "cold" nodules unless they are of exceedingly long duration, or are *obviously* benign (e.g., cysts). However, sometimes even with such diagnostic procedures we cannot exclude malignancy.

Hemorrhage into a thyroid cyst deserves special mention. These cysts may be suspected on palpation; they are hemispheric, rubbery, and smooth. They may transilluminate, but are rarely fluctuant. On aspiration, they will usually yield serous or serosanguineous fluid. Bleeding into such cysts, which may cause a sudden enlargement of a mass that may not have been noticed previously, is usually accompanied by sudden, severe pain that may simulate the symptoms of subacute thyroiditis (see below). However, the mass has the size, shape, and consistency of a cyst, and usually can be distinguished from the gland of subacute thyroiditis. Aspiration, which will yield altered blood, may relieve local pain.

* See Appendix Addendum 6 to Chapter 5.

Hyperthyroidism

Hyperthyroidism may be of several types. Graves' disease is the most common cause, and toxic nodular goiter is not uncommon, but, on rare occasions, hyperthyroidism may be due to a variety of other causes. The types of hyperthyroidism are summarized in Table 5-1.

Each of these types has different etiologies, but only Graves' disease and toxic nodular goiter will be examined at length. Hyperthyroidism is usually characterized by an increased production of both thyroxine and triiodothyronine but in at least a few instances, triiodothyronine alone is increased (T_3 toxicosis).[18]*

Graves' Disease

Definition

Graves' disease may be defined as hyperthyroidism associated with a diffusely hyperplastic goiter, although this hyperplasia may be superimposed on a previously nodular gland. Its various synonyms include exophthalmic goiter, diffuse toxic goiter, Basedow's disease, and primary

Table 5-1. Types of Hyperthyroidism

Graves' disease
Toxic nodular goiter (toxic adenoma)
Hyperthyroidism associated with acromegaly
Hyperthyroid phase of subacute thyroiditis
Hyperthyroidism due to a TSH-like substance produced by choriocarcinoma or hydatidiform mole
Hyperthyroidism in thyroid carcinoma
Due to a toxic carcinomatous nodule
Due to excessive thyroxine from widespread thyroid metastases (the tissue is not hyperfunctioning, but its total mass is very large)
Hyperthyroidism due to an autonomous struma ovarii
Hyperthyroxinemia due to excessive administration of thyroid hormone
Hyperthyroidism due to excess pituitary thyrotropin (only one case reported)

* See Appendix: Addendum 7 to Chapter 5.

hyperthyroidism. Although exophthalmos, ophthalmoplegia, pretibial myxedema, and acropathy may be seen only in Graves' disease, any one or all of these extrathyroidal features may be absent in a given case.

Etiology

Until recently, most workers believed that hyperthyroidism was probably due to a humoral substance that was stimulating the thyroid gland. Many speculated that this was increased pituitary thyrotropin. However, when thyrotropin was finally measured, no increase was demonstrated, either in the pituitary itself or in the serum of patients with Graves' disease (Fig. 5-4). (Actually only one patient with hyperthyroidism considered due to increased pituitary TSH has ever been recognized.[8])

In 1956, Adams and Purves of New Zealand showed that the serum of many patients with Graves' disease contained a substance that stimulated the thyroid gland of guinea pigs for a much longer period than did pituitary thyrotropin. Now, after more than a decade of investigation, many have accepted that Graves' disease is due to the effect on the gland of long-acting thyroid stimulator (LATS),[17] a 7S gamma globulin (IgG). This immunoglobulin may well be an antibody to a component or components of thyroid cells. Furthermore, it has been shown that the lymphocytes of patients with Graves' disease produce LATS.[17]

Thus, Graves' disease may be an "autoimmune" disease, the result of a disturbance in immunologic homeostasis. LATS may be produced because a clone of immunologically competent cells mutates and produces a "forbidden clone" that then produces the abnormal "antibody" (LATS).[22] In view of a familial predisposition to Graves' disease, it is possible that the potential patients may inherit a defect in immunologic homeostasis: that is, they cannot handle certain specific forbidden clones that might arise by random mutation. Thus, if such a clone does arise, it will not be destroyed, as in a normal person, but will persist and produce the forbidden antibody. The subsequent interaction with and liberation of the specific antigen in turn excites the replication of new daughter cells of the "forbidden" clone.

In this view, an antigen does not have to be

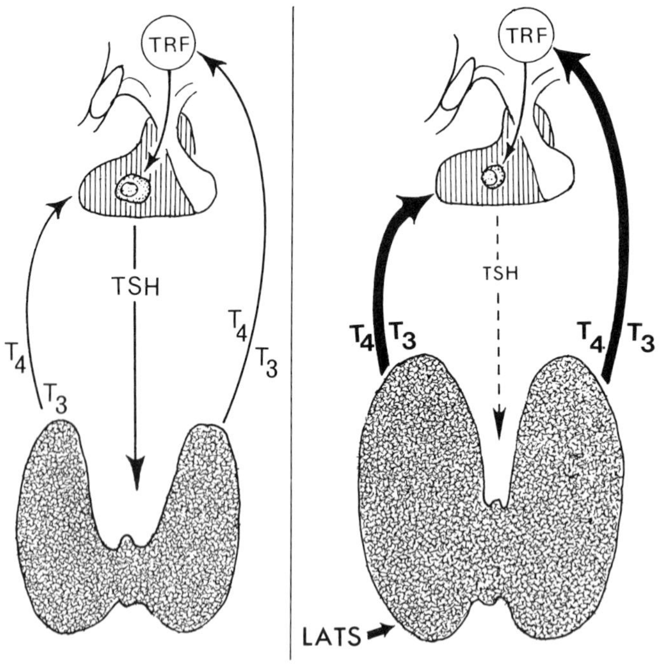

Fig. 5-4. Etiology of hyperthyroidism. In the normal person (*left*), thyroid activity is controlled by TSH, which responds to the level of tri T_3 and tetraiodo T_4 in serum.

In Graves' disease with hyperthyroidism (*right*), TSH is inhibited by high levels of thyroid hormones produced under influence of an abnormal immunoglobulin, long-acting thyroid stimulator (LATS). Unlike TSH, release of LATS is not suppressed by rising levels of thyroid hormone. We do not yet know how, in some patients, specific therapy—*viz.*, subtotal thyroidectomy, radioiodine, or prolonged antithyroid drug administration—returns the gland to TSH control.

liberated before the antibody can be produced. Kriss[13, 14] believes, however, that the thyroid must be injured and thyroid antigen released before LATS can be elaborated. He has also reported that LATS contains both kappa and lambda molecules, and therefore probably does not originate in a single clone.

However, if the "abnormal" immunologically competent cell proves to be a thymic (T) lymphocyte, which sends its specific "message" to a group of "B" lymphocytes (thymic-independent)[21] that then produces the abnormal "antibody" LATS, the fact that LATS is polyclonal does not militate against the "antibody-centered" theory of LATS production. In any event, the precise origin of LATS remains unknown.

The mode of action of long-acting thyroid stimulator is not yet understood. Its much longer action, compared to thyrotropin, may be due to its large molecular size. Current bioassay depends on mouse thyroid responses in vivo, and we have no chemical method for measuring LATS in the serum. LATS may attach itself to a receptor site on the thyroid cell identical or similar to that used by pituitary thyrotropin. This receptor site is probably on the cell membrane. Within the cell, adenyl cyclase increases the local concentration of cyclic 3′,5′-adenosine monophosphate, which converts the "stimulus" emanating from the cell membrane into increased cellular activity. We do not yet know how LATS stimulates adenyl cyclase, or whether indeed this is the only action of LATS either on thyroid cell or other cells of the body.

Recently, doubt has been cast on the hypothesis that circulating LATS has any primary role in the pathogenesis of hyperthyroidism. Recent evidence suggests that Graves' disease may be a cell-mediated immune disease, whereby local "T" lymphocytes within the thyroid gland stimulate the thyroid cells *directly*.[25] LATS may thus be an epiphenomenon, i.e., "spillover."*

The contribution of LATS to exophthalmos also remains in doubt. Although Kriss[14] has found a good correlation between the aggravation of exophthalmos after radioactive iodine therapy and LATS titers, others have not been able to demonstrate such a correlation. McKenzie and Burke, for example, could not correlate exophthalmos with LATS levels, and many patients with exophthalmos have no LATS, while others with high titers of LATS have little or no exophthalmos. There is, however, a good correlation between the presence of LATS and pretibial myxedema. Furthermore, a few patients with exophthalmos and LATS have never had hyperthyroidism (euthyroid Graves' disease). While many of these individuals ultimately become hyperthyroid, this is not inevitable.

Genetic factors operate in Graves' disease.[7, 12] Hyperthyroidism occurs in predisposed families and, genetically, is closely related to Hashimoto's thyroiditis, idiopathic myxedema, and, indeed, to pernicious anemia. These disorders tend to run in the same families. The autoimmune aspects of these various diseases will be discussed under Hashimoto's thyroiditis. Graves' disease may occur at any age, although it is most common from the second to fifth decade. Females exceed males in a ratio of about 3:1.

* See Appendix: Addendum 8 to Chapter 5.

Manifestations of Graves' Disease

Symptoms. Characteristically, Graves' disease is the most florid type of hyperthyroidism although there are many exceptions to this rule. The symptoms may commence precipitously or subtly, and sometimes seem to follow injury, a psychic disturbance, immigration to a new land, or infection. The connection between these events and the disease has not been studied carefully; hence one should reserve judgment, particularly as to their medicolegal significance.

The symptoms of hyperthyroidism include nervousness, sweating, heat intolerance, rapid heart beat, fatigue, weight loss associated with an increased appetite, thirst, dryness of mouth, dyspnea, muscular weakness, tremulousness, frequency of micturition, and diarrhea. Ocular symptoms occur less often, and these will be discussed separately below. Less common complaints include swelling of the ankles, falling hair, loss of libido in the male, and oligomenorrhea in the female, and increased headaches. Some patients become aware of their goiters, and may have local discomfort or pain.

A small number of patients have pruritus. Anorexia and nausea occur occasionally in hyperthyroidism, and surprisingly, some patients may have weight gain.

The "nervousness" of Graves' disease deserves special mention. It is associated with marked restlessness, and sometimes even agitation and manic behavior. Insomnia and difficulty in falling asleep are associated features. The tremor and feeling of muscular weakness may be quite marked.

Signs. Generally the diagnosis can be made on a brief inspection. These patients are thin, restless, hyperactive, nervous and suffused (Fig. 5-5). Eye signs (to be discussed separately below) are common but not invariably present. The thyroid mass (goiter) is almost always present although few patients may have a gland of normal size. Characteristically, however, the goiter is diffusely enlarged, although it may be asymmetrical. The enlargement may be slight to marked. The gland is moderately firm to firm and smooth and moves with swallowing. The trachea is not usually deviated. Over either lobe of the thyroid, a bruit is heard in about one-half of such patients. The heart is generally of normal size although it may be enlarged, particularly in older patients who have atherosclerotic heart disease (unrelated to hyperthyroidism). Tachycardia is characteristic, and approximately 10% of patients have auricular fibrillation; this is most common in older patients. A loud M1 and P2, and basal ejection-type systolic murmurs are likewise quite common. The pulse pressure is wide, and occasionally bruits can be heard over the peripheral arteries. Peripheral pulsations are marked, and the skin vessels are often dilated with capillary pulsations. Congestive heart failure may also occur in hyperthyroidism, most commonly in older patients. Although the liver is only occasionally enlarged in the absence of congestive heart failure, the spleen is enlarged in about 10% of patients. Lymph node enlargement is uncommon. The skin is warm and moist. Palmar erythema may be present, as well as arteriolar cutaneous "spiders," and occasionally gynecomastia in the male. Onycholysis ("Plummer's" sign) is fairly common, and clubbing of the fingers occurs in about 5% of cases. A fine tremor of the outstretched fingers is characteristic; there may be moderate or marked muscular weakness (particularly of the quadriceps) and reflexes are characteristically increased.*

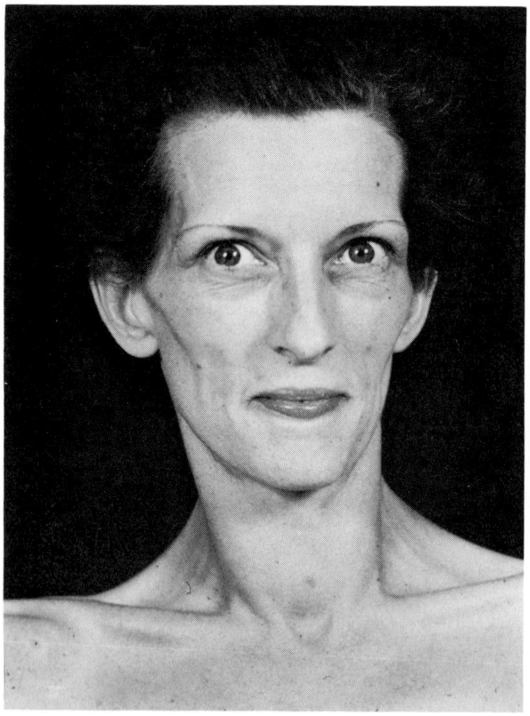

Fig. 5-5. Signs of Graves' disease. This 35-year-old woman shows obvious weight loss, diffuse goiter, widened palpebral fissure, and some puffiness of her upper lids.

Pretibial myxedema. A small percentage of patients with Graves' disease have localized (pretibial) myxedema, a unique swelling of the skin and subcutaneous tissues, commonly over the tibia of one or both legs (Fig. 5-6). The lesion is usually localized to this area, although occasionally it may be seen on the hands. Histologically, however, the lesion is widespread even when it appears to be localized clinically. The cutis is edematous, and deposited between the collagen bundles is a material that stains like mucin. This microscopic finding, as well as the gross appearance, gives rise to the term "myxedema," although it has no relationship to hypothyroidism. The cause of the pretibial myxedema is unknown

* See Appendix: Addendum 9 to Chapter 5.

although these patients tend to have the highest LATS assays. Furthermore, it is seen almost invariably in patients who have some degree of exophthalmos.

There is no permanent treatment for pretibial myxedema although large doses of systemic corticosteroid, or localized corticosteroid ointments bring at least temporary relief. The lesion is coated with the ointment and the leg may be wrapped in Saran Wrap. Sometimes this treatment is unsuccessful even for short intervals, particularly when there is already widespread lymphatic obstruction and fibrosis.

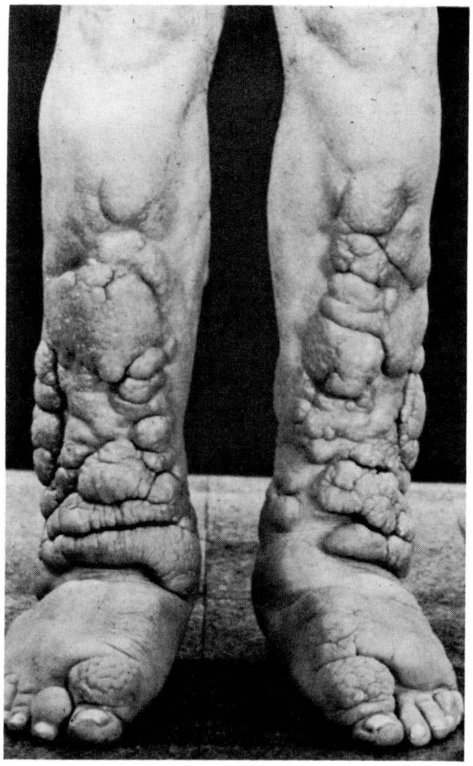

Fig. 5-6. Unusually severe pretibial myxedema. Mucopolysaccharide has gathered in locules giving the appearance of elephantiasis. This patient had had hyperthyroidism 18 years before and had moderate pretibial myxedema at that time. He was treated with radioactive iodine, and became euthyroid. However, over the years his pretibial myxedema slowly increased. He also has moderate exophthalmos and clubbed fingers. The titer of plasma LATS was very high.

Ocular manifestations. About 70% of patients with Graves' disease have some ocular manifestations, but severe hyperthyroidism may occur without any eye changes. Conversely, endocrine exophthalmos may develop without hyperthyroidism (euthyroid Graves' disease). The eye changes vary considerably from patient to patient, and even from time to time in a single patient. Symptoms may include changes in the physical appearance, with undue prominence of one eye or both, excessive lacrimation, pain or discomfort in the eyes, recurrent infections, frequent headaches, aching, blurring of vision, or occasional prolapse. The minimal eye signs in Graves' disease include proptosis, a staring expression, and widening of the palpebral fissures. There is weakness of convergence and, when the eyes are rotated downwards, lid lag.

These ocular manifestations are commonly divided into two types: those characterized by protrusion, and those in which infiltrative manifestations are most pronounced. In both types, there may be periorbital edema, which may be marked even without measurable proptosis. Proptosis can be measured by a variety of exophthalmometers, and may be considered abnormal when over 18 mm. Infiltrative exophthalmos is characterized by considerable orbital edema, congestion, chemosis, and conjunctival injection. Discomfort may be pronounced. In this type, lacrimation and a feeling of "sand in the eyes" are very common.

If the exophthalmos becomes very marked (malignant exophthalmos), the cornea may ulcerate (Fig. 5-7). Panophthalmitis may then develop and blindness may result. A variety of extraocular muscle palsies (exophthalmic ophthalmoplegias) have been observed in patients with exophthalmos. Weakness of convergence is most common, and least important. Failure of upward gaze due to superior rectus weakness is serious, and other extraocular muscles are variably affected.

On analysis of the orbital contents, such patients have an increase in muscle fiber bulk, with degeneration of muscle fibers, infiltration with lymphocytes and macrophages, and increased acid mucopolysaccharide, fat, and water content.

The cause of either the proptotic or infiltrative form of ocular manifestation is not known. We once believed that the infiltrative type was due to pituitary stimulation, while the more benign type

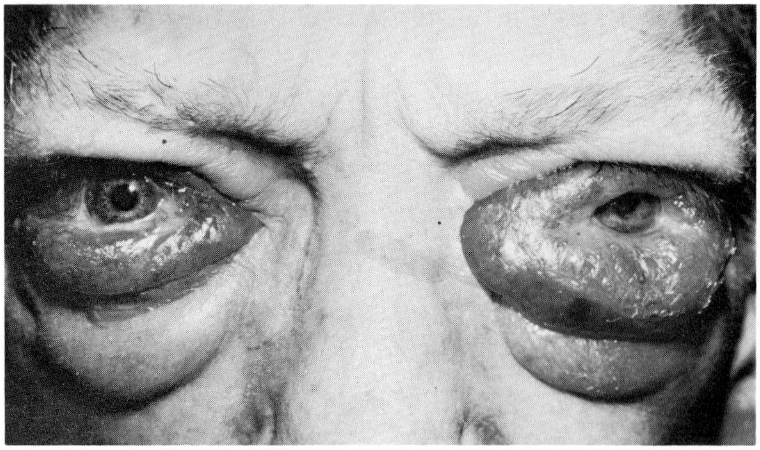

Fig. 5-7. Ocular manifestations in Graves' disease. This man has advanced ophthalmopathy ("malignant exophthalmos"). His severe conjunctival edema obscures the moderate exophthalmos.

was related to the hyperthyroxinemia. However, there is no good evidence to support either of these suppositions. The pituitary does not seem to play an important role because exophthalmos of either type may develop after pituitary removal. Because exophthalmos sometimes progresses for a short time after radioactive iodine therapy in conjunction with the temporary rise in LATS titers, Kriss[14] suggests that LATS is responsible. However, McKenzie, Burke, and others could not confirm these observations. As noted before, there is no good correlation between the presence or titer of LATS and the degree, type, activity, or course of the exophthalmos. The serum of many patients with exophthalmos contains an "exophthalmos-producing" substance (EPS)which is of pituitary origin. However, this substance is present in many other conditions, and it probably does not cause exophthalmos in Graves' disease.

One current speculation is that the exophthalmos may be produced by a form of cell-mediated (delayed hypersensitivity) immunity, or an immunoglobulin other than LATS, which may coexist or be closely related to LATS. However, as yet, there is no proof for this suggestion.*

The treatment of exophthalmos, which is empiric, leaves much to be desired. Fortunately, in many patients, the exophthalmos spontaneously improves to some degree and may need no treatment. In other instances, the infiltration becomes pronounced and even intolerable. Local steroid-antibiotic ointments, and systemic corticosteroids in large doses improve the symptoms of such infiltrations. Some have suggested total surgical and/or radioablation of the thyroid gland to relieve the exophthalmos because this would hopefully reduce the levels of LATS by removing all of the thyroid antigen. However, no one has confirmed the efficacy of total thyroid ablation,[22] and although this mode of therapy has its advocates, it has not been widely accepted. Pituitary irradiation, either with an external source or with yttrium-90 implants, and hypophysectomy have also been used. However, pituitary ablations are not effective in the control of exophthalmos.

Direct operations on the eye, most notably lateral decompression of the orbit, give cosmetic and physical relief, but do not produce a "cure." Operation to relieve extraocular muscle palsies may bring considerable improvement. Because hypothyroidism aggravates exophthalmos, thyroid replacement therapy is most important.*

Neuromuscular System. The nervousness and tremulousness of hyperthyroid patients have already been noted. Muscular weakness may become profound, and may even stimulate progressive muscular atrophy. This weakness will disappear when thyrotoxicosis is treated. Myasthenia gravis, occasionally associated with hyperthyroidism, also does not disappear when hyperthyroidism is treated.

* See Appendix: Addendum 10 to Chapter 5.

* See Appendix: Addendum 11 to Chapter 5.

Natural Course of Graves' Disease

This disease is now rarely left untreated, but from older literature, it appears that many of these patients go into spontaneous permanent remission; others have temporary remissions and relapses. However, in another group, the disease remains constant. Because we cannot accurately predict each patient's course, the disease should at least be suppressed in all patients.

Thyroid Storm

The term "thyroid storm" describes the crises that result from severe hyperthyroidism. The storm often occurs following subtotal thyroidectomy or other operations, or other types of stresses—infections, trauma, etc. Thyroid storm is seen most commonly in those who have been very ill and are then suddenly exposed to marked hyperthyroxinemia.

The patients develop marked hyperpyrexia; their temperatures sometimes reach or exceed 106° F. The skin is often dry, and the patients generally have marked tachycardia, prostration, and restlessness, although later they may become apathetic or delirious.

Fortunately, thyroid storm is rare, and can generally be avoided by giving the patient antithyroid drugs before operation. Further specific treatment will be discussed below under Therapy.

Toxic Nodular Goiter (Toxic Adenoma)

Toxic nodular goiter (Plummer's disease) has a different pathogenesis from Graves' disease. The manifestations of hyperthyroxinemia are similar, but exophthalmos or pretibial myxedema is not seen in toxic nodular goiter. In contradistinction to Graves' disease, the patient with toxic nodular goiter usually has had a nontoxic goiter for years before hyperthyroidism develops. For this reason, toxic nodular goiter is regarded as a late complication of long-standing nontoxic nodular goiter. Experimentally, long-standing thyrotropin stimulation may lead to the formation of adenomas that initially are thyrotropin-dependent but later become autonomous.

The serum of patients with solitary hyperfunctioning thyroid adenomas does not contain LATS; it is thus believed that LATS is *not* involved in the pathogenesis of toxic nodular goiter. Likewise, TSH is suppressed in this condition. The hyperfunctioning adenoma produces excess thyroxine, which suppresses pituitary thyrotropin secretion. Thus the thyroid parenchyma surrounding the "hot" nodule will involute, and there will be virtually no uptake of radioactive iodine. Since the hyperfunctioning adenoma is autonomous, it cannot be suppressed by additional exogenous thyroid hormone; thus, in the Werner suppression test (see above) triiodothyronine will not suppress radioactive iodine uptake, just as in Graves' disease.

Patients with toxic nodular goiter tend to be older than those with Graves' disease. Because a nontoxic mass evolves slowly to a toxic nodular goiter, the manifestations of hyperthyroidism develop slowly and subtly, in contradistinction to their florid presentation in Graves' disease. Furthermore, in toxic nodular goiter, thyroid hyperfunction is usually less pronounced, and manifestations and biochemical changes are much less marked than in Graves' disease. Plummer's disease may go on for long intervals unrecognized and, in elderly patients with organic cardiac disease, may produce cardiac arrhythmias, auricular fibrillation, and congestive heart failure.

Hyperthyroidism Due to Substance Produced by Choriocarcinoma

Patients with choriocarcinomas or hydatidiform moles sometimes develop a mild form of hyperthyroidism.[19] The manifestations may be minimal or may go unrecognized, even when tests of thyroid function are obviously abnormal. The choriocarcinoma or hydatidiform mole elaborates a polypeptide that has an action similar to that of pituitary thyrotropin but has different immunologic characteristics. This TSH-like substance is distinct from the gonadotropins that may be elaborated in excess by the same tumor, and it has no relation whatever to long-acting thyroid stimulator. When the underlying tumor is treated, the mild hyperthyroidism usually ameliorates.

Diagnosis of Hyperthyroidism

Tests of thyroid function have already been discussed earlier in this chapter. Generally the combination of elevated serum thyroxine (or protein-bound iodine), triiodothyronine resin test and the radioactive iodine uptake will confirm the diagnosis. Other tests can be employed, but are rarely required. The Werner suppression test deserves particular emphasis because it is often valuable in borderline cases: triiodothyronine (75–100 μg/day for 10 days) suppresses thyroid function in normal persons but cannot suppress function in hyperthyroid patients. Thus, in normal persons or those with nontoxic goiters, the radioactive iodine uptake falls to 50% or less of its initial value but will not fall, or falls only insignificantly, in hyperthyroidism. Occasionally, the serum thyroxine will be normal, but serum triiodothyronine will be elevated ("T_3-thyrotoxicosis").[18]

Therapy for Hyperthyroidism

Therapy is generally directed to the thyroid hyperfunction. Although Graves' disease has an extrathyroidal cause (presumably immunological) and has other manifestations, we have no way to attack the immune mechanism directly and thus remove the cause. Thus we must be content to control those manifestations of hyperthyroxinemia which may endanger the patient's life.

Iodine

Iodine was the first truly beneficial medication for hyperthyroidism. In the recent past, large doses of iodine (120–300 mg daily) were used either as preoperative treatment or even as maintenance therapy. This iodine was usually given as potassium iodide or Lugol's solution, a saturated solution of potassium iodide and iodine.

Iodide causes a rapid amelioration of the manifestations of hyperthyroidism by directly inhibiting the thyroid cells. Initially thyroxine release is inhibited and colloid is stored. Subsequently, thyroxine synthesis is reduced, because iodide therapy reduces the organic binding of iodide to iodine—an early intrathyroidal step in the formation of thyroxine.

We now know that the dosages used were much larger than those actually required. While such doses generally led to rapid improvement, the patient often "escaped" within several days, and became even more hyperthyroid than before. Furthermore, toxic reactions to iodide—severe rashes, pyrexia, hepatitis, and parotitis—occasionally occurred.

Smaller doses, as little as a few milligrams per day, gave almost the same improvement and avoided most of the side effects. Before newer and more effective agents were developed, preoperative iodide therapy greatly increased the benefit of thyroidectomy. However, such therapy may have contributed to postoperative thyroid storm, a not uncommon event in that era.

Iodide therapy has now largely been superseded by other forms of therapy but is still useful in rare episodes of thyroid storm.

Nonspecific Measures

Bed rest is often valuable in the general treatment of hyperthyroidism, although its mechanism of action has never been explained. Perhaps by diminishing the release of catecholamines, to which these patients are sensitive, rest may ameliorate the manifestations of hyperthyroidism. Similarly, reserpine and sympathetic blocking agents such as propranolol often produce a dramatic clinical improvement, usually without biochemical change.

Antithyroid Drugs

The antithyroid drugs thiourea and 2-thiouracil were introduced in 1943 and greatly improved the treatment of hyperthyroidism. Currently, propylthiouracil, methimazole (Tapazole), carbimazole (Neomercazole) and methylthiouracil are most commonly employed. These drugs cross the placenta and are secreted in the milk. Their action is limited to a few hours and the dosage of each depends on the response of the individual. The daily doses are as follows: propylthiouracil, 600 mg., methylthiouracil, 300 mg; and carbimazole and methimazole, about 60 mg, divided into equal amounts every 8 hours. Patients with large, firm goiters generally require larger doses than those with smaller softer goiters. After the patient has improved, the drug can be gradually reduced, and many patients can be maintained on much smaller doses. The time required to produce remission varies considerably, although the patient usually begins to improve within a few weeks. Previous iodine therapy will delay the response to the antithyroid drug, because large amounts of colloid have been stored. Sometimes the patient's response to the drug is so pronounced that he develops temporary hypothyroidism; this can be avoided, particularly in pregnancy, by giving concomitant thyroxine therapy.

After long-term antithyroid therapy, about 50% of patients go into permanent remission by a mechanism that is not understood. The remainder relapse sooner or later.

The indications for antithyroid therapy vary widely. In general, prolonged therapy with these drugs is the treatment of choice in childhood and adolescent hyperthyroidism, and in pregnant women. Many clinics use such agents for most hyperthyroid patients of all ages. In clinics where it is *not* considered the best therapy, it should be used before other more definitive therapy in elderly patients who are extremely ill with hyperthyroidism or other associated disease—e.g., heart or chest disease. Because patients with very large or toxic nodular goiters are not likely to achieve remission even after prolonged antithyroid therapy, some definitive therapy should be selected early in the course of the disease.

Each of the potent antithyroid compounds produces toxic side reactions. Agranulocytosis develops in 0.1–0.8%. Other reactions—fever, rashes, leukopenia, malaise, headaches, myalgia, arthralgia, abdominal pains, nausea, vomiting, swelling of salivary glands, hepatitis, thrombocytopenia, and mental disturbances—have been reported in 1.9–13.8% of these patients.

The agranulocytosis usually develops suddenly, often 4–6 weeks after therapy has been started. Because it develops so suddenly, routine leukocyte counts are of little value. Generally the agranulocytosis begins with severe pharyngitis, fever, and malaise. The drug is, of course, immediately discontinued.

Subtotal Thyroidectomy

Subtotal thyroidectomy is still preferred as definitive treatment in many centers, although in Toronto we believe it is the treatment of choice only in selected patients, particularly children or adolescents. The patient should be prepared with an antithyroid drug, and rendered euthyroid before operation. If the patient has other associated disorders, these must be appropriately treated (e.g., a patient with cardiac disease should be digitalized, and arrhythmias corrected or controlled before operation). Diabetes mellitus, if present, should also be properly controlled. In the last few days before operation, in addition to the antithyroid medication, iodine is given to promote the storage of colloid and cause involution. These changes reduce vascularity, and decrease the technical difficulties during surgery.

The surgeon must remove all but a small amount of thyroid tissue to keep recurrence at a minimum. If he takes too much tissue, the gland will not regenerate enough to produce a euthyroid state, and myxedema will develop. The surgeon must carefully isolate the recurrent laryngeal nerves and parathyroid glands to avoid injuring these structures.

Subtotal thyroidectomy is attended by a variety of complications: recurrence or persistence of hyperthyroidism, postoperative myxedema (which may be either mild or severe, and may occur soon after operation or years later), hypoparathyroidism, vocal-cord palsies, and even death (Table 5-

Table 5-2. Major Complications of Subtotal Thyroidectomy

Complication	%
Recurrence or persistence of hyperthyroidism	5–15
Postoperative myxedema	2–43
Permanent overt hypoparathyroidism	1
Occult hypoparathyroidism	5–10
Vocal cord palsy	1
Death	0–1

2). In addition, minor complications may develop, such as local infection, bleeding, phlebitis, and so on.

Thyroid storm, which now is extremely rare, should not occur at all if the patients are prepared carefully for subtotal thyroidectomy.

Paralysis of one vocal cord causes an initial loss of voice, and subsequently, chronic hoarseness. However, paralysis of both cords produces spastic airway obstruction and may require tracheotomy.

Hypoparathyroidism. At times, even when the parathyroids have been identified and left in situ, the patient may develop *hypoparathyroidism* because of ischemia of all parathyroid tissue. On the other hand, one normal parathyroid gland will prevent tetany. Furthermore, hypoparathyroidism due to surgical trauma may be transient if the blood supply ultimately returns to normal. Following subtotal thyroidectomy, permanent hypoparathyroidism with obvious tetany develops in about 1% of patients, but an additional group, perhaps 5–10% have occult hypoparathyroidism without obvious tetany. One can demonstrate that these patients have no parathyroid tissue reserve, especially after challenge with ethylenediaminetetraacetate (EDTA). This material is a chelating agent which binds calcium, thus reducing it in the bloodstream, and hence stimulating the parathyroid glands. It is not clear whether patients with occult hypoparathyroidism will develop late complications, or whether this "latent" hypoparathyroidism is of no real concern. Overt hypoparathyroidism, at least, must be treated as discussed in Chapter 6, The Parathyroid and Calcium Metabolism.

Myxedema. Permanent myxedema may be seen within the first 3 postoperative months. However, transient postoperative hypothyroidism is not uncommon, clearing as a result of the increased secretion of pituitary thyrotropin (Fig. 5-8). In some patients, however, myxedema may develop years after thyroidectomy; for this reason, all patients should be followed at least annually to detect such late recurrences. The rate of late myxedema after subtotal thyroidectomy is about

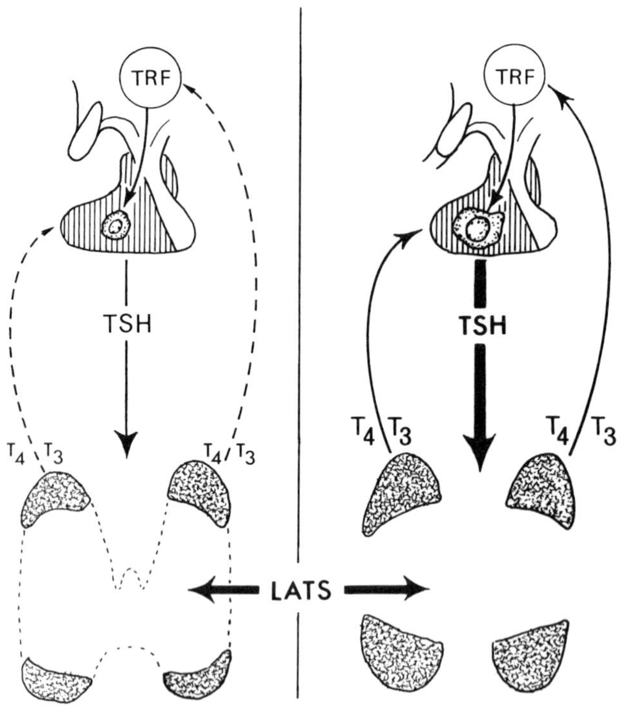

Fig. 5-8. Transient hypothyroidism after subtotal thyroidectomy. *Left.* The major portion of the thyroid has been removed. If LATS cannot stimulate the remaining gland to normal activity, secretion of pituitary TSH will resume.

Right. The "thyrotroph" is enlarged, secreting an increased amount of TSH. Under its influence, the gland will be brought back to normal function. The degree to which the hypertrophied thyroid remnant is under TSH control can be determined by a Werner T_3 suppression test. If radioiodine uptake cannot be well suppressed, the physician can assume that to some degree the thyroid is still under the influence of an abnormal stimulator.

1.7% per year.[5] Patients who have transient hypothyroidism after operation are particularly prone to develop permanent myxedema later. Coexistent Hashimoto's thyroiditis acts as an aggravating factor and increases the incidence of postoperative myxedema. If hyperthyroidism persists or recurs, the patient should not be operated on again; this is a clear indication for radioactive iodine therapy.

Radioactive Iodine

Radioactive iodine was suggested for the treatment of hyperthyroidism because thyroid is the only tissue that retains iodine, whether radioactive or not. ^{131}I (half-life, 8 days) has been the isotope of choice since 1946. ^{131}I is largely a beta emitter; only about 10% of its effect is derived from gamma emissions. Because the beta rays travel only about 2 mm, the ^{131}I within the thyroid does not damage surrounding structures, and considerable radiation can be applied within the gland without damaging adjacent tissues.

Since radioactive iodine was introduced more than two decades ago, it has been used increasingly as a therapeutic agent and, in many centers, is the treatment of choice for adult hyperthyroidism. It has many advantages: The treatment is usually definitive, it is convenient, and generally it can be administered without admitting the patient to hospital. It rarely causes local reaction within the neck, produces no morbidity other than that related to the hyperthyroidism, and there is no surgical scar.

With one exception, hypothyroidism, the hazards of radioactive iodine have been largely hypothetical. The increased incidence of leukemia predicted following the use of radioactive iodine in hyperthyroidism has not materialized. Actually, it is extremely unlikely that the dosage given to the average patient with hyperthyroidism would cause any significant increase in leukemia. Nor has gonadal radiation increased the incidence of mutations, possibly because the dose of radioactive iodine usually employed in hyperthyroidism is so small.

Similarly, radioactive iodine has not produced carcinoma of the thyroid; the incidence of such carcinoma in patients so treated is extremely low. However, chromosomal abnormalities have been demonstrated in the lymphocytes of patients treated with radioactive iodine; these usually involve breakage of one or more of the autosomes. These changes, however, have not been related to any clinical abnormalities, and their significance remains to be demonstrated.

The one real complication is hypothyroidism, particularly since it may develop gradually years after ^{131}I therapy. As many as 40% of patients treated with radioactive iodine became hypothyroid within a decade. This figure applies chiefly to patients with Graves' disease; the incidence of post-^{131}I hypothyroidism in toxic nodular goiter appears to be much lower (Fig. 5-9). Late myxedema also follows subtotal thyroidectomy and, although the exact incidence of this complication after surgery is not known, it may be quite high.

The indications for radioactive iodine therapy vary considerably from center to center. In Toronto, most adult nonpregnant patients over the age of 25 are treated with radioactive iodine. In some other centers all patients over 40 years of age are so treated, while elsewhere radioactive iodine is reserved for patients who do not respond to other forms of therapy.

The dosage of radioactive iodine needed to produce optimal results cannot be estimated precisely, and the appropriate dosage has been estimated by a variety of techniques. Commonly, the dosage is based upon an estimate of the gland size, derived from palpation and thyroid scanning. In Toronto, we give 100 μc per estimated gram of thyroid tissue, when the 24-hour radioactive iodine uptake is approximately 50%. If the radioactive iodine uptake is considerably higher than this, the dosage is reduced somewhat. If the uptake is lower than 50%, the dosage is increased slightly. Generally, physicians tend to overtreat small goiters, and increase the incidence of hypothyroidism. Large goiters are often undertreated.

Some physicians are now employing smaller doses of ^{131}I in Graves' disease because of the high incidence of late hypothyroidism. Some have recommended that one should give 80 μc per estimated gram of thyroid tissue, which will leave the patient mildly hyperthyroid, and then follow this treatment with long-term antithyroid or iodine therapy.[5] By this regimen, they hope to reduce

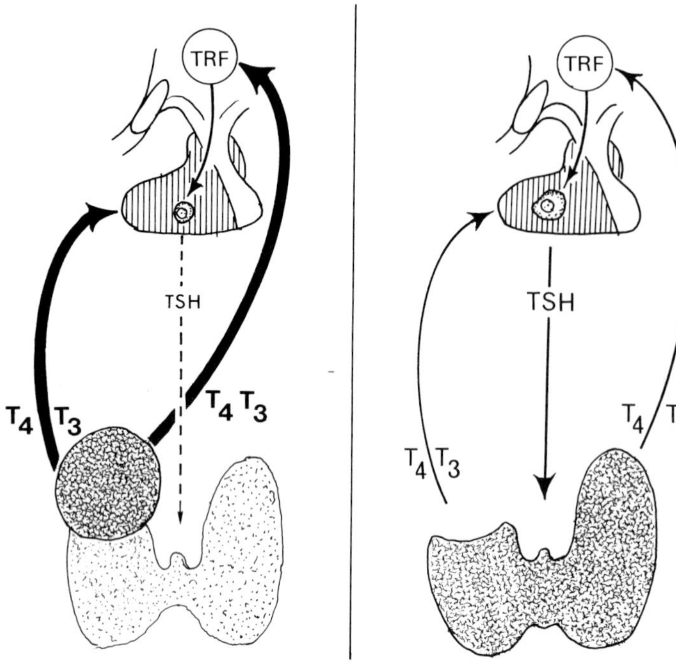

Fig. 5-9. Treatment of Solitary Hyperfunctioning Nodule (Toxic Nodular Goiter). *Left.* The hyperfunctioning thyroid nodule has suppressed TSH secretion (note the small thyrotroph); for this reason, the remaining parenchyma (*light shading*) does not pick up radioiodine. Because only the nodule is affected during radioiodine therapy, subsequent myxedema is rare.

Right. The nodule has been destroyed or resected. Normal negative feedback control has been reestablished and the now-active parenchyma (*darker shading*) takes up radioiodine.

the high incidence of late myxedema. Most previous schedules have used somewhat higher doses.

All these considerations relate only to Graves disease. Because the remaining parenchyma is suppressed and has no radioactive iodine uptake, patients with solitary hyperfunctioning nodules can be given a much larger dose of radioactive iodine, 15–30 mc, which will usually ablate the hyperfunctioning nodule but will not be picked up by the surrounding resting, suppressed parenchyma. After the serum thyroxine declines, the increase in pituitary thyrotropin will restore the suppressed parenchyma to normal function, after the radioactive iodine has disappeared (Fig. 5–9).

Although, in most patients, the hyperthyroidism does not worsen after radioactive iodine, some patients with severe hyperthyroidism or elderly patients with associated cardiovascular disease or diabetes mellitus may have such exacerbations or, rarely, even go into thyroid storm. For this reason, these patients should be rendered euthyroid with antithyroid agents before radioactive iodine is given.

Results of ^{131}I Treatment. Because radioiodine may take many months to produce its effect, patients with cardiac or psychiatric complications may need other antithyroid drugs to control the disease in the interval. Most patients become euthyroid within 3 months. However, about a quarter of our patients have little or no improvement from the first dose of radioactive iodine and need a second dose. Generally, larger doses are given on the second occasion. A few patients are resistant to radioactive iodine and require quite large doses before the hyperthyroidism is truly cured. Hypothyroidism may develop quickly within a few months in a small percentage, and, as mentioned above, many patients may become and remain euthyroid for years after ^{131}I, only to become hypothyroid ultimately. Aside from occasional thyroidal pain and rare exacerbations of hyperthyroidism that occur 7–12 days after therapy, there are no other clinical side effects from radioactive iodine.

Therapy for Other Aspects of Graves' Disease

Ophthalmopathy

This has been discussed in the section on Ocular Manifestations of Graves' Disease earlier in this chapter.

Hyperthyroidism in Children

We have no really satisfactory treatment for hyperthyroidism in a child. Subtotal thyroidectomy in children is attended by increased complications. Long-term antithyroid therapy is perhaps the best treatment, although many children do not adhere to such programs, and some are not truly controlled by these drugs. Physicians have not yet accepted radioactive iodine therapy in childhood, because of the possible threat of carcinogenesis and genetic abnormalities. For the present, therefore, a combination of long-term antithyroid drugs and/or subtotal thyroidectomy appears to be the best treatment for children.

Hyperthyroidism in Pregnancy

Radioactive iodine is contraindicated during pregnancy because the fetal thyroid picks up iodine after the fourth month and because of possible fetal whole-body radiation. Here in Toronto, we generally recommend antithyroid therapy throughout pregnancy. Because the antithyroid drugs cross the placental barrier, the dosage is decreased to a minimum in the last trimester to prevent fetal goiter. These patients may thus be mildly hyperthyroid during this interval, but this causes little trouble. Although the patient may be given thyroid therapy to prevent (maternal) hypothyroidism, such therapy does not protect the fetus from goiter; the amounts usually given (e.g., thyroxine, 0.3 mg daily) do not cross the placenta adequately. However, triiodothyronine crosses the placenta more readily and should be used instead of thyroxine in these situations; the dose is 25 μg 3 or 4 times a day. Generally no form of thyroid hormone is employed, however.

Subtotal thyroidectomy, a very acceptable therapy, may be performed in the second trimester after several weeks of antithyroid drug therapy. The hyperthyroid mother aborts more frequently; however, it is not yet known whether this frequency is greater in those treated surgically than in those treated with antithyroid drugs. In this center, we use antithyroid drugs throughout and immediately after pregnancy. After delivery, the mothers do not nurse, because the antithyroid drugs are excreted in the milk. Also, infants of these mothers should be examined for evidence of hyperthyroidism, because LATS crosses the placenta passively and in the newborn may produce transient Graves' disease.

In considering the differential diagnosis of hypermetabolism, the physician should remember that the PBI (or serum thyroxine) is normally elevated during pregnancy, as is the BMR. The PBI (or serum thyroxine) elevation is due primarily to an increase in thyroxine-binding globulin (a result of the increase in endogenous secretion of estrogen), although the normal placenta also elaborates a small amount of a TSH-like substance. In normal pregnancy, the T_3 resin uptake is greatly reduced on testing, but in patients who have hyperthyroidism during pregnancy, the T_3 resin uptake usually rises to normal or even higher.

Treatment of Thyroid Storm

Thyroid storm is very rare and can generally be avoided entirely by judicious therapy. It occurs most commonly after subtotal thyroidectomy or, on rare occasions, after radioactive iodine therapy. Occasionally it may occur spontaneously after infections and other stresses. Treatment consists of electrolyte and water replacement, alcohol sponge baths, oxygen, corticosteroid therapy, intravenous potassium iodide, and an antithyroid drug. In addition, a sympathetic blocking agent such as propranolol may produce dramatic improvement.

Thyroid Malignancy

Little is known about the cause of thyroid malignancy, but excessive thyrotropin secretion probably plays an important part. Some workers have reported that patients with carcinoma of the thyroid have increased amounts of pituitary thyrotropin in their serum. Experimentally, thyroid malignancy develops in animals after prolonged antithyroid medication has produced sustained excessive thyrotropin secretion. Most human thyroid carcinomas probably begin as thyroid carcinomas, and do not arise from benign thyroid nodules.

Thyroid cancer is found in approximately 0.1%

of routine autopsies, but the incidence is much higher in individuals with nontoxic nodular goiters. The incidence is said to be even higher (up to 12%) in Hashimoto's thyroiditis; however, this has been disputed at least in patients with *diffuse* Hashimoto's thyroiditis. Commonly, however, a focal form of thyroiditis may develop adjacent to thyroid malignancies, perhaps representing an immune response to the tumor. X-ray radiation to the thymus or neck in growing children may increase the incidence of carcinoma of the thyroid. Curiously, no increase has been demonstrated after radioactive iodine therapy for hyperthyroidism.

At times, it may be very difficult to determine on a histologic basis whether a given thyroid tumor is benign or malignant. The diagnosis is usually based on the abnormal appearance and lack of differentiation of cells, the presence of mitotic figures, and the invasion of the thyroid capsule. Some pathologists consider that, in addition, the lesion should show invasion of blood vessels.

The American Thyroid Association divides thyroid cancer into 4 main groups:

1. Papillary carcinoma
2. Follicular carcinoma
3. Solid (medullary) carcinoma with amyloid stroma
4. Anaplastic carcinoma

Papillary Carcinoma

The papillary carcinoma, the most common type, accounts for approximately 60% of all thyroid cancers. Most common in the young, and in females (over two-thirds), it is usually slow-growing. This tumor spreads primarily to regional lymph nodes through lymphatics. The lesions are often bilateral and the nodal metastases may be more extensive than the primary malignancy. When, in rare instances, the tumor spreads beyond the neck, it usually goes into the lungs.

Histologically, there is papillary arrangement of tall columnar epithelial cells, with very little colloid. In some thyroid carcinomas, there may be much variation in the cell pattern; in a papillary tumor, for example, one area may show follicular features. Occasionally anaplastic areas may be seen—a poor prognostic sign. Some tumors may show psammoma bodies, which contain small amounts of calcium. Generally, the prognosis in papillary carcinoma is good; 90% of these patients will still be alive 10 years after diagnosis.

Follicular Carcinoma

About 20% of thyroid carcinomas are follicular. These patients are somewhat older than those who have papillary carcinomas. The follicular tumors often show wide histologic variation, with microfollicles and other areas that closely resemble normal thyroid tissue. Elsewhere, tumor cells may appear in solid sheets. Blood vessels are invaded early, and hence, metastases to lungs and bones are fairly common. Because Hürthle cells are occasionally prominent, Hürthle cell carcinomas are placed in a separate subgroup. The prognosis for patients with follicular carcinoma is distinctly worse than for those with papillary carcinoma.

Solid (Medullary) Carcinoma with Amyloid Stroma

This type of tumor, which accounts for only 6% of thyroid carcinomas, spreads into regional lymph nodes and quickly invades the bloodstream, producing distant metastases to lungs and bones. These tumors produce calcitonin, and their principal cellular constituent is the parafollicular cell. These tumors also occasionally produce prostaglandins and ACTH. Histologically, they are composed of small or round cells in no distinct pattern, and have no elements resembling papillary or follicular carcinoma. The abundant stroma stains for amyloid. These tumors occasionally coexist with pheochromocytomas and may reflect a familial predisposition. The prognosis is even worse than that for follicular carcinoma, but many patients survive for several years.

Anaplastic Carcinomas

Anaplastic thyroid carcinomas contain many cell types—spindle cells, giant cells, and various other configurations. These undifferentiated cells extend rapidly into blood vessels and metastasize quickly to lungs, liver, and bone.

Clinical Aspects

Patients with papillary or follicular carcinoma often have a long history of goiter, although those with anaplastic cancer usually do not. Thus, physicians should become concerned when long-standing goiters enlarge rapidly or become painful or if the patient develops associated dysphagia, cough, dyspnea, or change in voice.

The age of onset is important; single nodules in young persons are malignant until proved otherwise, but the diagnosis of cancer often cannot be made clinically in a homogeneous thyroid mass. Advanced thyroid cancer is stony hard and irregular and may adhere to adjacent structures. However, chronic thyroiditis or Riedel's struma may also present with this clinical picture. Symptoms or signs of recurrent laryngeal nerve compression suggest thyroid carcinoma but may also accompany other types of goiter.

Solitary nodules are regarded as malignant, unless one can clearly identify a specific benign lesion such as hemorrhage into a cyst. Here, the thyroid scan contributes to the differential diagnosis because about 20% of "cold" nodules are malignant. However, most scanning devices do not pick up very small thyroid cancers. Conversely, some thyroid cancers concentrate radioactive iodine and thus appear as "warm" nodules. Nevertheless, despite these exceptions, the thyroid scan is a helpful screening procedure.

If the patient has obvious lymph-node involvement, or if biopsy of a pathological bone fracture has yielded a histologic diagnosis, the thyroid malignancy will be self-evident. If the chest film shows a suspected lesion, the possibilities of thyroid cancer will at least be considered. However, because most thyroid cancers are difficult to diagnose, most "cold" solitary thyroid nodules are removed. Finally, many thyroid malignancies are "occult"—i.e., tiny microscopic lesions that are found incidentally—and may never become clinically apparent.

We do not yet have good treatment for the various types of thyroid carcinomas. Therapy is largely empiric, and until we know a great deal more about these tumors, we will have to employ such measures.

Treatment of Thyroid Malignancy

Thyroidectomy should only be done when thyroid malignancy is strongly suspected on the basis of clinical or laboratory data. It should *not* be performed in most common nontoxic nodular goiters. We have no evidence that removing benign thyroid nodules will prevent the subsequent development of thyroid cancer. Moreover, only a few people (six per million per year) will die of thyroid cancer. We have not yet determined whether (total) thyroidectomy is an effective treatment for many thyroid cancers, although it may cure low-grade carcinomas. Reliable evidence is difficult to obtain because papillary carcinomas are slow-growing, and in any event, some of these tumors may not be true cancers. Even in malignancies with moderate growth rates, we have little objective evidence because controlled studies are so rare. Finally, operation is of doubtful value in anaplastic thyroid carcinoma.

Nevertheless, in Toronto, as in most centers, the thyroid is removed when malignancy is finally suspected. When he has a tissue diagnosis, the surgeon will do a total or almost-total thyroidectomy because malignancy is commonly bilateral. Generally, the entire lobe is removed on the side of the tumor, and almost all of the contralateral lobe as well. Total thyroidectomy is frequently associated with hypoparathyroidism and recurrent laryngeal palsy. After operation, the patient will require further medical therapy and close surveillance.

The surgeon should remove lymph nodes in the immediate area and obvious metastases in the neck. Radical resections are rarely advisable, except when a slow-growing cancer has involved surrounding tissues.

Administration of Thyroid Hormone

After the primary lesion has been removed, all patients should be given thyroid hormone in high, subtoxic doses, to completely inhibit the secretion of pituitary thyrotropin. Because pituitary thyrotropin aggravates thyroid malignancy, and at least some thyroid cancers are partly dependent on thyrotropin, the secretion of thyrotropin must be suppressed as completely as possible. It should be added, however, that this suppression appears to be of no importance whatever in the treatment of medullary carcinoma of the thyroid, which is not under even partial control of thyrotropin. Furthermore, in many cases, such therapy will not prevent recurrence, but since this cannot be predicted accurately, thyroxine therapy should be continued indefinitely.

Radioactive Iodine

Radioactive iodine is also given after operation to certain patients with metastatic carcinoma but only to those with metastatic lesions which concentrate the iodine. Radioactive iodine has no place in the primary treatment of thyroid malignancy because, with rare exceptions, the cancer does not take up enough radioiodine. Operation thus remains the prime mode of treatment.

Metastases from follicular carcinomas are most likely to pick up radioactive iodine, but sometimes it is necessary to give exogenous thyrotropin to increase iodine uptake. After such preparation, large doses of ^{131}I are administered, in the order of 100–200 mc, and the leukocyte count is followed for some weeks thereafter. Stimulation of endogenous thyrotropin with propylthiouracil treatment or letting the patient become hypothyroid after a total thyroidectomy is not advisable because this permits wider extension and more rapid growth of metastases than does short-term administration of thyrotropin.

If the lesions concentrate it well, the radioactive iodine may destroy or damage all of the metastases. More often, ^{131}I only produces moderate destruction even with good pick-up. In high dosage, radioactive iodine therapy will ultimately produce a variety of side effects, including pulmonary fibrosis and radiation sickness.

Irradiation may be used to treat anaplastic carcinomas; some respond rapidly, although many are radioresistant. X-ray therapy has little value in other types of thyroid malignancy.

Table 5-3. Classification of Thyroiditis

Infectious thyroiditis
Suppurative (acute or chronic)
Nonsuppurative (acute or chronic)
Subacute nonsuppurative thyroiditis (probably viral)
Autoimmune thyroiditis
Hashimoto's thyroiditis (struma lymphomatosa)
Chronic thyroiditis
Lymphocytic thyroiditis of adolescence and childhood
"Idiopathic" myxedema
Riedel's struma
Miscellaneous
Radiation thyroiditis
Traumatic
Sarcoidosis

Thyroiditis

In current usage, "thyroiditis" embraces not only diseases that are inflammatory, but also disorders characterized by fibrosis or lymphoid infiltration.[23] Since the etiology of many of these disorders remains doubtful, treatment is often empiric. For the same reason, this group is difficult to classify, but Table 5–3 indicates the varieties of disease considered under this term and provides an approximate etiologic classification.[24]

Infectious Thyroiditis

Although a variety of bacterial organisms may attack the thyroid gland, these infections are rare compared to other types of thyroiditis. In our clinic, we have seen only 10 patients with bacterial thyroiditis in the past decade. (In the same interval, we saw 71 patients with subacute [nonsuppurative] thyroiditis, and over 130 with Hashimoto's thyroiditis.) These infections are most commonly due to *Pneumococcus, Staphylococcus,* and *Escherichia coli,* although other organisms have been isolated. The gland often suppurates, and usually only one lobe is involved. It becomes exquisitely painful and tender. Hyperpyrexia is common, and local lymph nodes are usually enlarged.

Chronic bacterial infections have also been reported, notably tuberculosis and syphilis, but these are very rare. Even rarer are mycotic or parasitic infections.

In the early stages, suppurative bacterial thyroiditis may prove difficult to differentiate from subacute (nonsuppurative) thyroiditis. However, only one lobe is involved, the local lymph nodes are often enlarged (unlike subacute thyroiditis), and there are signs of suppuration (e.g., redness); all these are evidence against subacute thyroiditis. Serum protein-bound iodine is rarely elevated in suppurative thyroiditis, and radioactive iodine uptake is rarely suppressed, again in contrast to subacute thyroiditis.

Once it is recognized, suppurative thyroiditis is drained and appropriate antibiotic therapy begun. Treatment of chronic, mycotic, or parasitic thyroiditis is that of the underlying infection.

Subacute Thyroiditis

Subacute thyroiditis may be defined as an acute, subacute, or occasionally even chronic, generally self-limiting, nonbacterial inflammation characterized by painful, tender thyroid enlargement that usually goes on to complete recovery after weeks or months. Although unproved, it is assumed to be due to one or more viruses. This entity is separate and distinct from Riedel's struma or Hashimoto's thyroiditis. Although Hashimoto's thyroiditis may occasionally present with similar clinical manifestations, histologically proved subacute thyroiditis rarely culminates in chronic thyroiditis. Subacute thyroiditis has a variety of synonyms: acute thyroiditis, simple thyroiditis, DeQuervain's thyroiditis, giant-cell thyroiditis, granulomatous thyroiditis, and pseudotuberculous thyroiditis.

Etiology

A variety of clinical features suggest that this condition is of viral etiology. Subacute thyroiditis is often preceded by an upper respiratory infection, or it may have a prodrome characterized by muscular aches and pains, and upper respiratory symptoms. Furthermore, during the acute phase, the patient often has pyrexia and other systemic manifestations, although without neutrophilia. This condition may occur at the time of specific viral epidemics. Finally, complete recovery after weeks or months, almost as a rule, suggests a benign viral disease.

Subacute thyroiditis has been observed in epidemics and in individual cases associated with either specific viral diseases or with antibodies to certain viruses—the common cold, influenza, mumps, measles, infectious mononucleosis, cat scratch fever, Coxsackie infections, and adenovirus (Fig. 5-10). However, positive viral cultures have been obtained in only one patient, and viral inclusion bodies have never been found in sections of thyroid tissue.

Subacute thyroiditis is probably not an autoimmune disease. Circulating autoantibodies to thyroid antigens appear in a minority of patients with subacute thyroiditis; they appear in low titers after several weeks, and usually disappear completely after several months. In most patients, however, they are absent throughout the course of the disease. These observations suggest that the thyroid autoantibodies are secondary to the inflammation, and do not produce the disease.

Pathology

In subacute thyroiditis, the gland is only slightly or moderately enlarged, but one lobe may be more involved than the other. Although the inflammation does not spread beyond the capsule, there may be minimal adhesions between the capsule and the surrounding tissues. Microscopically, the follicles are completely disrupted and the follicular cells are necrotic. There is a marked cellular infiltration of the interstitial tissues and the follicles themselves, initially with polymorphonuclear leukocytes but subsequently with histiocytes and lymphocytes. There is also marked interstitial edema. Histiocytes surround the colloid within the follicles and imitate giant cells (pseudo-giant cells). Some of the colloid leaks into the interstitial tissue, where it is surrounded by histiocytes, once again resembling giant cells. Most of the colloid may ultimately disappear. As the gland recovers, the follicles seem to re-form, with flattened cuboidal epithelium and pale colloid. The edema gradually subsides, although chronic small-cell infiltration may persist for a long time. The

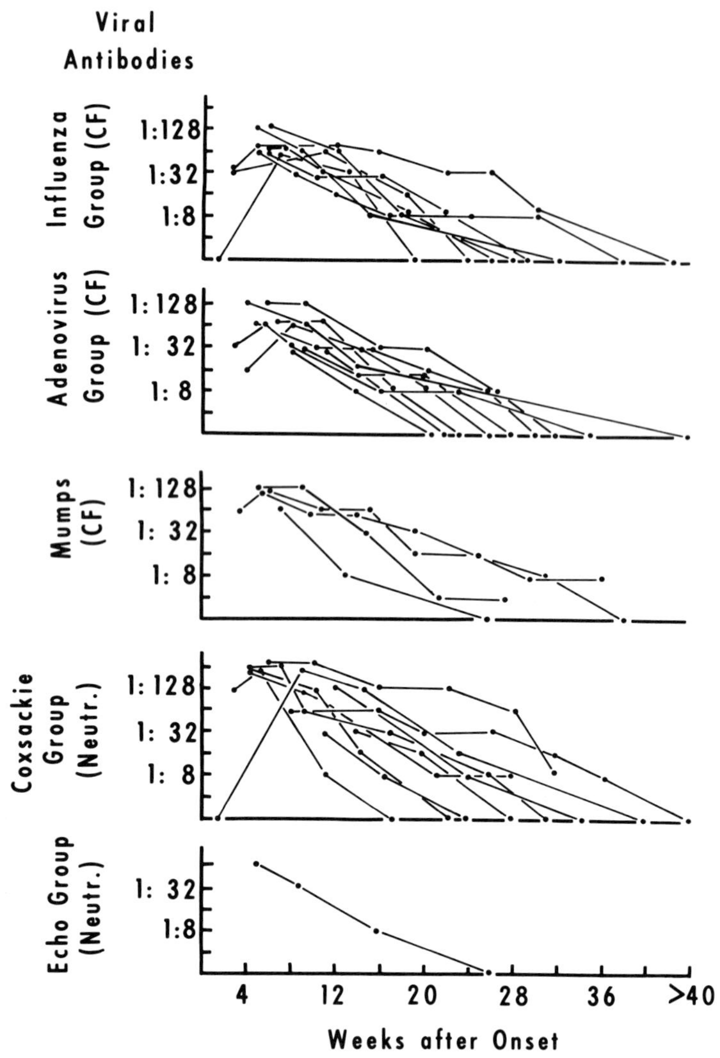

Fig. 5-10. Viral antibodies in subacute thyroiditis. This graph depicts changing titers of significant viral antibodies in 32 patients with subacute thyroiditis; in an additional 58 patients with this condition, viral antibodies did not show significant changes in titer or were not demonstrated throughout the course of their illnesses. It may be noted that the most common significant viral antibodies were from the Coxsackie antibody group, and the titers were highest in this group also. (From Volpé, R., Row, V. V., and Ezrin, C. *J Clin Endocrinol Metab* 27:1275, 1967. Reproduced with permission.)

variable amount of fibrosis, which persists permanently, occasionally may be extensive.

Clinical Aspects

Subacute thyroiditis is most common in young and middle-aged women, and is seen only occasionally in men. It may be preceded by a prodrome of malaise and fever, or even an upper respiratory infection. The patients then complain of moderate or severe pain in the thyroid, commonly over one or both lobes. The pain often radiates to the angle of the jaw and to the ear on the involved side. If one lobe is involved initially, the other lobe may be involved later (creeping thyroiditis). Coughing, swallowing or turning the head may aggravate the pain. Many patients are aware of a tender lump in the neck. Systemic complications are common—malaise, fatigue, and mild feverishness. In addition, many patients complain of nervousness, tremulousness, some weight loss, heat intolerance, and rapid heart beat.

On examination, most of these patients appear flushed and uncomfortable, but not seriously ill. Fever is common, although rarely extreme. The thyroid gland is slightly or moderately enlarged, one lobe often being larger than the other. The larger lobe is usually very firm or hard and quite tender. Occasionally the tenderness is exquisite. In addition, the patient often shows signs of hyperthyroidism.

If not treated, the disease may persist for weeks or months; occasionally, the patient may have exacerbations over 1–2 years. In the late phase, about one-quarter of these patients may become hypothyroid because the gland becomes depleted of colloid; this may last a few weeks to several months. Permanent myxedema is very rare, and most of these patients recover completely. Rarely the disease may recur some years later, again with full recovery.

Laboratory Findings

In the early phase, serum PBI is elevated, and this may be quite marked (Fig. 5–11). The difference between PBI and butanol-extractable iodine (BEI) is also increased, indicating the presence of an iodoprotein. However, the serum thyroxine is also often elevated, apparently because of colloid leakage. This leakage may explain the mild clinical manifestations of hyperthyroidism. The PBI is elevated, but the radioactive iodine uptake is usually depressed by the disruption of parenchymal cells, quite often to zero. The erythrocyte sedimentation rate is markedly elevated. The thyroglobulin is only modestly increased, and most of the iodoprotein present is probably iodoalbumin. About 40% of these patients produce thyroid autoantibodies, which appear after several weeks. These usually reach only a modest titer, and tend to subside completely.

Treatment

Treatment is empiric, but effective. A corticosteroid, generally prednisone or a similar analogue, is prescribed in pharmacologic doses—e.g., prednisone, 10 mg. q.i.d. This dose is gradually decreased over a 1-month period. The remission is usually rapid and, when the dose is decreased, the thyroiditis usually does not recur. However, some patients do have exacerbations and are treated again with larger doses. Occasionally repeated exacerbations occur.

The corticosteroid apparently acts as an anti-inflammatory agent, allowing the disease to run its course to recovery at a subclinical level. When the patient has repeated exacerbations, thyroxine or triiodothyronine may bring considerable benefit, although there is no clear rationale for such therapy. Presumably pituitary thyrotropin is suppressed by this medication, although in those who have a high PBI, the pituitary TSH is suppressed already.

Roentgen therapy has been used in the past with considerable success but is no longer popular. Analgesics do not seem to control symptoms as effectively as corticosteroids. Antibiotics are generally useless. There is no indication for thyroidectomy because recovery is the rule.

Permanent hypothyroidism following subacute thyroiditis is rare. Surprisingly, however, six patients have been described who became hyperthyroid after subacute thyroiditis.

Autoimmune Thyroiditis

"Autoimmune thyroiditis" covers a group of closely related diseases considered due to autoclastic (self-destructive) mechanisms. Currently this group contains four clinical or pathological entities: Hashimoto's thyroiditis (struma lymphomatosa), chronic thyroiditis, lymphocytic thyroiditis of childhood and adolescence, and "idiopathic" myxedema, although these may represent only variants of the same process. It is not yet known why some glands atrophy, as in idiopathic myxedema, while others undergo hypertrophy and remain so, as in classic Hashimoto's thyroiditis, or why one gland will fibrose (chronic thyroiditis) and another will be infiltrated with lymphocytes. As will be seen below, although there is considerable evidence that these variants represent autoimmune disorders, there is no final proof.

Pathology

In Hashimoto's thyroiditis, the thyroid is usually enlarged, very firm, lobulated, or even nodular. Both lobes are usually involved. Histologically, the acinar cells are usually degenerated, and follicles are reduced or almost completely absent.

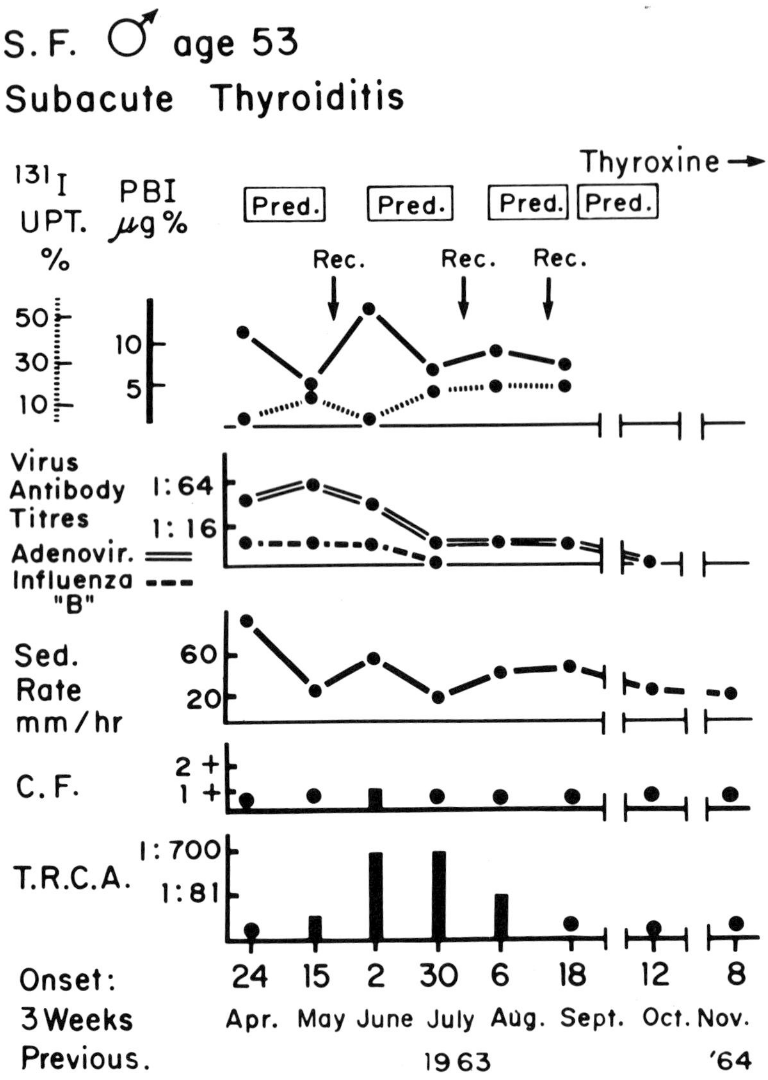

Fig. 5-11. Laboratory work in patient with recurrent subacute thyroiditis.

Pred., prednisone; *Rec.*, recurrence; *C.F.*, complement fixation test for the antibody against the intracellular microsome component of thyroid cells; *T.R.C.A.*, tanned red-cell agglutination test for antithyroglobulin.

Initially, this 53-year-old man responded well to prednisone, 10 mg q.i.d., with rapid amelioration of his pain, tenderness, and thyroid enlargement. In addition, his mild signs of hyperthyroidism and fever subsided very quickly, with a marked fall in erythrocyte sedimentation rate. The PBI fell, and radioactive iodine uptake began to rise. The dosage of prednisone was gradually reduced and finally discontinued altogether after 3 weeks. The patient had no symptoms for about 4 days after prednisone was stopped completely, but they soon recurred. Within 7–10 days, symptoms had become severe again but were quickly relieved once more by another course of prednisone. After prednisone was discontinued the second time, subacute thyroiditis recurred. For the third time he was given prednisone, and when the dosage declined to only 5 mg daily, he again developed mild symptoms of subacute thyroiditis. Prednisone was accidentally discontinued for 1 day by the patient, but then was started again in a dosage of 10 mg t.i.d. Thyroxine, 0.3 mg/day, was given with the prednisone. On this final occasion, we decreased the prednisone over 4 weeks and discontinued it altogether without any further recurrence. The patient continued on thyroxine for 1 year, at which time it was decreased gradually and then discontinued. He has had no further recurrence.

Note viral and thyroid autoantibody response in this patient. (From Volpé, R. *Mod Treat* 6:474, 1969. Reproduced with permission.)

Oxyphilic changes in the cytoplasm of follicular cells are common. Some areas may show considerable acinar cell hyperplasia. The gland is infiltrated with lymphocytes and plasma cells, and germinal centers may be prominent. There is marked though variable fibrosis. Although these changes may be diffuse or local, Hashimoto's thyroiditis should be considered as an entity, separate from focal lymphocytic infiltration.

Lymphocytic thyroiditis, seen most commonly in adolescent girls, differs only slightly from Hashimoto's thyroiditis. The adolescent variety contains no oxyphilic cells, but these oxyphilic (Hürthle) cells are common in Hashimoto's disease.

The term chronic thyroiditis is applied when fibrosis predominates, and when lymphocytic infiltration is much less marked than in Hashimoto's thyroiditis. In idiopathic myxedema, the gland is markedly atrophic but histologically indistinguishable from either Hashimoto's thyroiditis or chronic thyroiditis.

We believe that, despite the gross and microscopic differences among the members of this group, all have a similar pathogenesis.

Etiology

Until a decade ago, Hashimoto's thyroiditis was a disease of unknown etiology. However, considerable evidence now suggests that autoimmune mechanisms underlie Hashimoto's thyroiditis and the other conditions listed above. This evidence is summarized as follows.

1. The histologic appearance suggests an immunologic lesion.
2. Circulating antithyroid antibodies are found most consistently and in the highest titer in Hashimoto's disease.
3. Thyroiditis can be produced in animals by injecting thyroid autoantigen with Freund's adjuvant.
4. Experimental thyroiditis can be transferred by leukocytes.
5. Thyroglobulin induces a skin reaction in patients with Hashimoto's thyroiditis.
6. About 50% of relatives of patients with Hashimoto's thyroiditis have circulating antithyroid antibodies in their serum.
7. Hashimoto's thyroiditis often appears in association with other "autoimmune" disease—e.g., rheumatoid arthritis, Addison's disease, pernicious anemia, diabetes mellitus, and Sjögren's syndrome. There is also a close association with Graves' disease.

Thyroid Autoantibodies

Patients with Hashimoto's thyroiditis and other forms of autoimmune thyroiditis produce a variety of thyroid autoantibodies. These include an antibody against thyroglobulin (demonstrable by the tanned red-cell hemagglutination test, by the precipitin test, and by Coon's immunofluorescent technique); an antibody against the intracellular microsome component of thyroid cells (demonstrated by a complement fixation test, by the immunofluorescent technique, and by a cytotoxic effect in tissue culture); an antibody against a colloid component other than thyroglobulin (demonstrated by precipitating antithyroglobulin and removing it from the circulation, and then using an immunofluorescent technique); and an antinuclear factor. Except for the last of these, the antibodies are all organ-specific and display a narrow range of species specificity—i.e., they are confined to primate thyroid tissue.

Exceedingly high titers for thyroglobulin antibodies can be demonstrated in Hashimoto's thyroiditis: dilutions of one in several million are common. The various other antibodies may also be present in high dilutions. However, a small group of patients with Hashimoto's disease have no demonstrable circulating thyroid autoantibodies, and many others have low titers. These observations suggest that the circulating autoantibodies are not themselves the cause of the Hashimoto's disease. Furthermore, thyroid autoantibodies, usually in low titers, appear in many conditions other than autoimmune thyroiditis: in subacute thyroiditis and nontoxic goiters, and in patients with angina who are given radioactive iodine to destroy normal thyroid tissue. These antibodies are also seen in about 50% of *relatives* of patients with either Hashimoto's disease or Graves' disease, most of whom have no clinical evidence of thyroid disease. They are present in the circulation of many patients with other "autoimmune" diseases—Sjögren's syndrome, rheumatoid arthritis, and particularly, pernicious anemia. Most of these persons also have no clinical evidence of thyroid disease. The incidence of thyroid autoantibodies is also increased in certain chromosomal disorders, such as Turner's syndrome and mongolism. Finally, a few normal, particularly older, persons have circulating thyroid autoantibodies.

Many patients with Graves' disease also have thyroid autoantibodies, often in high titer; this may be explained by coexistent Hashimoto's disease and Graves' disease ("Hashitoxicosis").

It may be that whenever these antibodies appear, there also is lymphocytic infiltration, at least in focal areas of the thyroid gland. However, very high titers of thyroid antibodies occur only in autoimmune thyroiditis and in Graves' disease, for the reasons mentioned.

Experimental Immunological Thyroiditis

Although a lesion similar to the human Hashimoto's thyroiditis can be produced in animals by the injection of thyroid autoantigen with Freund's adjuvant (a mixture of killed tubercle bacilli in oil), there are a number of fundamental differences between the experimental disorder and the human disease. In the human, liberation of thyroid autoantigen (after radioactive iodine therapy; in subacute thyroiditis; or after surgical trauma) rarely leads to Hashimoto's thyroiditis. Thyroglobulin leakage was initially blamed for initiating Hashimoto's thyroiditis by inducing antibodies to the thyroglobulin that had been released from the follicle. This, however, seems unlikely because thyroid injury does *not* lead generally to Hashimoto's disease. Furthermore, we now know that some thyroglobulin leakage is normal. Thus, there is no good evidence that an antigenic stimulant is initially necessary to initiate the antibody development that later leads to Hashimoto's thyroiditis. Freund's adjuvant appears to confer a tuberculin-like antigenicity on the thyroid autoantigen; without this adjuvant, lesions will not usually develop in the experimental animal. There is no apparent counterpart to the experimentally induced effects of Freund's adjuvant in the human disease.

Studies in Human Thyroiditis

In many studies Hashimoto's thyroiditis has been associated with other "autoimmune" diseases such as rheumatoid arthritis, Addison's disease, Sjögren's syndrome, diabetes mellitus, and disseminated lupus erythematosus, but Masi and his associates have disputed this association after a variety of epidemiologic studies. In Toronto, about 10% of our patients with Hashimoto's thyroiditis have other autoimmune diseases.

In this category, pernicious anemia deserves special mention. Irvine and his coworkers demonstrated an association between pernicious anemia and either primary hypothyroidism, Hashimoto's thyroiditis, or Graves' disease. Furthermore, patients with either Graves' disease or Hashimoto's thyroiditis commonly have antibodies to gastric intrinsic factor or to gastric parietal cells. Conversely, patients with pernicious anemia more often have thyroid autoantibodies than members of the general population.

Genetically, autoimmune thyroiditis and hyperthyroidism appear to be linked.[6,7] If the propositus has Hashimoto's thyroiditis, there appears to be as much chance of hyperthyroidism or myxedema appearing in his family as of Hashimoto's thyroiditis. Conversely, Hashimoto's thyroiditis often appears in family members of the patient who has hyperthyroidism. Both Graves' disease and Hashimoto's thyroiditis have been reported in twins, and recently twins were described who had combined Hashimoto's disease and Graves' disease.[12]

There is considerable evidence that the circulating thyroid autoantibodies do not themselves cause the lesions of Hashimoto's thyroiditis. In tissue culture, thyroid cells may be damaged by the complement-fixing antibody, which acts as a cytotoxic factor, but in vivo, the passive transfer of thyroid autoantibodies does not produce thyroid lesions. Some have suggested that the transfer of antibodies across the placenta might produce human cretinism. However, such transfer across the *animal* placenta did not damage fetal thyroid; furthermore, patients with Hashimoto's thyroiditis bear normal children. It has been established that when lymphocytes are transferred from animals with experimentally induced thyroiditis, their recipients develop thyroiditis.

If the circulating thyroid autoantibodies are not themselves autoclastic, the lesions may be due to fixed tissue antibodies that cannot be demonstrated. There is thus considerable circumstantial evidence suggesting that autoimmune thyroiditis is a disorder of delayed hypersensitivity. While it has yet to be established beyond doubt that an "autoimmune" reaction causes autoimmune thyroiditis, all current evidence supports such a mechanism.*

We believe that autoimmune thyroiditis represents an abnormal "antibody-centered" response, and that thyroid tissue injury is not a necessary predisposing factor. Hashimoto's thyroiditis may well arise from a mutation of an immunologically competent cell which then produces a new "forbidden" clone. Either this mutation or, more likely, the subsequent failure to eliminate it—a failure in immunologic surveillance—leads to the production (by the forbidden clone) of an antibody directed toward previously normal thyroid tissue. It may be normal for immunologically competent cells to mutate at random and the disease may arise when, because of an inherited defect in surveillance, specific single forbidden clones (or closely related clones) are not eliminated when they appear by chance. Once such a clone appears by chance in an individual who cannot eliminate it, this clone produces an antibody that interacts with thyroid tissue; this then causes further elaboration of thyroid antigens, further excitation and replication of clonal cells, and further production of autoantibodies. The defect appears to be inherited, although the factors governing such inheritance are not completely understood. The above concepts are based on the clonal selection theory of Burnet. Such a hypothesis might equally well explain the pathogenesis of Graves' disease[25] and has been discussed in the section on hyperthyroidism.

Clinical Aspects of Hashimoto's Disease or Thyroiditis

Hashimoto's thyroiditis commonly affects women in their fourth and fifth decades; they often have a family history of goiter, myxedema, or Graves' disease. Occasionally, they may present with mild pain in the thyroid region but more commonly have no local symptoms. They may, however, have noted a goiter for variable intervals. These patients may complain of malaise and fatigue, and have symptoms of hypothyroidism.

The gland is often two or three times normal size, is usually very firm or even hard, and tends to be lobulated and diffusely involved. Although hyperthyroidism may coexist with Hashimoto's disease, the thyroiditis does not cause hyperthyroidism, but it often leads to hypothyroidism.

Laboratory Tests

Thyroid autoantibody tests have already been discussed. The PBI may be normal or somewhat low; however, the BEI is often considerably lower than the PBI. The PBI-BEI difference indicates the presence of an iodoprotein. The BEI or serum thyroxine is commonly low, a result of the reduced production of thyroxine. Patients with Hashimoto's thyroiditis have a variety of enzymatic defects of the thyroid gland secondary to cell damage.

In addition, the sedimentation rate may be elevated and the gamma globulin increased. Because of the hypergammaglobulinemia, various precipitation tests (e.g., the cephalin-cholesterol flocculation test) tend to be abnormal.

Relationship to Carcinoma and Treatment

Certain studies suggest that patients with Hashimoto's thyroiditis have a high incidence of carcinoma of the thyroid—up to 12%. In autopsy studies, however, the incidence of thyroid cancer has been low. Here in Toronto, we followed 140 patients with Hashimoto's thyroiditis who were treated with thyroxine. In virtually all, the goiters regressed at least partially and, for as long as 10 years, did not enlarge further or become malignant. In only six of these patients did the thyroid gland enlarge while they were taking thyroxine; in these, thyroidectomy was performed. None of these six had a thyroid cancer.

We believe that most patients with Hashimoto's thyroiditis can be treated with thyroxine and that this should be continued indefinitely. With this therapy, the goiter regresses at least partially, and symptoms of hypothyroidism are relieved. In patients on long-term thyroxine therapy, the titer of thyroid autoantibodies often declines. Thyroidectomy is only rarely indicated.

* See Appendix: Addendum 12 to Chapter 5.

Riedel's Thyroiditis

In Riedel's thyroiditis, an extremely rare disorder, the thyroid is woody hard and adherent to adjacent structures, although not to the skin. Microscopically, there is widespread fibrosis that extends beyond the capsule to involve adjacent structures—muscles, vessels and nerves; this fibrosis may even extend into the mediastinum. Parts of the gland may be spared, although this is variable. Rarely this form of thyroiditis may be associated with diffuse inflammatory fibrosis elsewhere—e.g., cholangitis, retroperitoneal fibrosis, mediastinitis.

The etiology is unknown. It is probably not an end-stage of Hashimoto's thyroiditis, because many patients with the latter have been followed for long intervals without developing such a complication. The symptoms—dyspnea, hoarseness and dysphagia—reflect compression of surrounding structures. These patients rarely become hypothyroid, an indication that at least some thyroid parenchyma has been preserved. Thyroid autoantibodies are either absent or low, and only occasionally do these patients show the high titers seen in Hashimoto's thyroiditis.

Conservative treatment is unsatisfactory. Significant pressure symptoms are treated by local wedge thyroidectomy. More widespread surgical extirpation should not be attempted because it is exceedingly difficult and dangerous to vital structures. Thus, the surgeon should not attempt to remove an entire lobe from its bed of fibrous involvement with surrounding structures.

Hypothyroidism

Hypothyroidism, an inadequate output of thyroid hormone, may develop at any time of life, even in utero.* The inadequate production may be due either to disorders of the thyroid gland itself, or to anterior pituitary insufficiency (Table 5-4). The term "myxedema," often used as a synonym for hypothyroidism, has another connotation: the presence of mucinous edema, which can be demonstrated clinically. Because many patients with hypothyroidism do not show marked organic changes, the term "myxedema" should be applied only to those with severe disease and specific tissue alterations.

* See Appendix: Addendum 13 to Chapter 5.

Table 5-4. Etiology of Hypothyroidism

Marked reduction in thyroid parenchymal cells
Thyroid agenesis or hypogenesis
Autoimmune thyroiditis
Irradiation
Thyroidectomy
Cancer
Types due to normal or hyperplastic thyroid gland
Genetic enzyme deficiency
Iodine deficiency
Goitrogens
Decrease in stimulation of thyroid gland (deficiency of thyrotropin) due to pituitary or hypothalamic disease

Cretinism

Etiology

Cretinism results from an inadequate output of thyroid hormone during uterine and neonatal life. It may be endemic, generally associated with an enzymatic defect within the thyroid gland, and a goiter—goitrous cretinism. The more uncommon sporadic cretinism is usually not associated with a goiter; indeed, many such patients have no demonstrable thyroid tissue—athyreotic cretinism. The causes of cretinism may be classified as follows: thyroid aplasia or hypoplasia, iodine deficiency, genetic enzyme defects, and excessive maternal intake of goitrogens.

The various genetic enzyme defects have already been discussed. Some cretinism may be due to thyroiditis, but if there is such a relationship, the number of cases must be exceedingly small.

Clinical Aspects

Thyroid hormone is essential during embryonic life for the growth and development of many tissues, especially brain tissue. The infant deprived of thyroxine during fetal life will be mentally retarded, although the retardation can be partially reversed if thyroxine is begun immediately. Most of the other clinical manifestations, however, are readily and completely reversible. The cretin is dwarfed and has short limbs. The nose is broad, the eyelids puffy and wrinkled, the tongue thick, the voice husky, and the forehead short (see Fig. 16-9). The teeth appear late. The fontanels also close late. The hands and feet are short, broad, and puffy. The skin is coarse and dry, and the hair is sparse and dry. The abdomen usually protrudes, and umbilical hernias are common. The mental retardation is obvious, and cretins are slow to crawl, sit, or stand. Their movements are slow. The physician should suspect cretinism in infants who show marked retardation of development, sluggishness, dwarfism, delayed bony development, bradycardia, and often hypothermia.

Diagnosis

Circulating thyroxine levels (serum protein-bound iodine or serum thyroxine) establish the diagnosis. Roentgenograms reveal such abnormalities of osseous development as delayed ossification, delayed closure of fontanels, delay in appearance of epiphyseal centers, delayed bone age, and retarded growth of the base of the skull. Ossification centers often have an unusual stippled appearance, because several small subcenters unite to form an irregular center.

Cretinism may occasionally be confused with mongolism, but mongoloids, although they are retarded, are active and have hyperextensible joints and fine features. They display no evidence of retarded ossification, and their growth is usually normal.

Treatment

These infants are treated by thyroid replacement. (For details, see Chapter 16, section on Management of Patients with Short Stature—Hypothyroidism.) Here it should be noted that children require almost the same amount of thyroid as adults. The initial dosage in a newborn is 15 mg of desiccated thyroid per day (or 0.025 mg of thyroxine daily), later increasing gradually to 180 mg of desiccated thyroid (or 0.3 mg of thyroxine) daily. This therapy, which is continued throughout life, markedly improves the mental retardation although it rarely restores the child to normal. Otherwise, these children return to normal growth and development, and if properly treated, can expect to attain normal stature and normal sexual maturation.

Childhood and Adult Hypothyroidism

Hypoplasia of the thyroid gland is an uncommon cause of hypothyroidism beginning in childhood. Acquired hypothyroidism is more common and is due to milder genetic enzymatic defects, thyroiditis, and medical or surgical interference—subtotal thyroidectomy or ^{131}I therapy. Less commonly, goitrogens, iodine deficiency, and malignant destruction of the thyroid may produce hypothyroidism.

Iodide-induced myxedema is of considerable interest; it results from the prolonged ingestion of moderate or large doses of iodide, usually in the form of an expectorant mixture. The proprietary drugs used in the treatment of asthma—e.g., Felsol or Bethiodyl—also contain large amounts of iodine. Only persons who are especially responsive to the inhibitory effects of iodide will develop goiters and/or hypothyroidism under such prolonged therapy. Some of these patients have thyroid autoantibodies and perhaps had previous thyroid abnormalities, such as Hashimoto's thyroiditis, which predisposed to this excessive response to iodide; hence the development of goiter and/or hypothyroidism. In any event, the iodide acts directly on the thyroid and prevents the organic binding of iodide to iodine (see Fig. 5-1). This blocks further synthesis, reduces the amount of thyroxine, and increases pituitary thyrotropin secretion. The thyroid then hypertrophies and may overcome the iodide-induced block, but if the block is severe, the individual will become hypothyroid. The process, of course, can be stopped by discontinuing the iodide.

Thyroxine deficiency causes a wide variety of disturbances: It decreases the metabolic activity of virtually all body cells and allows mucinous interstitial fluid to accumulate. Pathologically, the heart is enlarged; the myocardium is pale and flabby. The myocardial fibers, which are swollen, are separated by an accumulation of mucinous material. Similar material may accumulate on the serous surfaces. Occasionally, these patients may go into failure. The skin shows similar changes.

The patients complain of lethargy, fatigue, mild weight gain, cold intolerance, dryness of hair and skin, puffiness of face and body, decreased sweating, muscular aches and pains, constipation, bloating, hoarseness, dyspnea, menorrhagia, deafness, difficulty in concentration and lapses in memory. These symptoms may develop so subtly and gradually that the patients do not seek medical attention. Gradually they decline into a vegetative existence, and may die in coma after decades of myxedema.

Severe myxedema is usually self-evident. The patients are sluggish and slow to react. Scalp hair is dry and coarse. Periorbital edema and loss of the outer third of the eyebrows is common. The face appears pallid and puffy. The voice is slow, low-pitched, and hoarse. The tongue is commonly enlarged. The thyroid gland may be either impalpable or enlarged. The heart is commonly enlarged, and the heart sounds may be distant. Signs of heart failure may be present. The abdomen often seems distended. The skin is dry, thick, and cold; fingernails are brittle. On neurological examination, mentation is slow, comprehension poor, tendon jerks reduced, and pseudomyotonia (myedema) may be present. A few have peripheral neuropathy and cerebellar ataxia. Deafness is common. More severe cases may be stuporous or comatose. Patients with milder deficiencies may have almost none of these symptoms and signs; fatigue and muscular aching may be the only manifestations.

Diagnosis

The diagnosis in most patients is obvious but can be confirmed by demonstrating reduced values for PBI, serum T_4, and radioactive iodine uptake. The T_3 resin (Triosorb test) may be reduced, but here hypothyroidism and euthyroidism overlap. When the hypothyroidism is due to autoimmune thyroiditis, thyroid antibodies may be present.

The differentiation of primary from secondary hypothyroidism has been discussed in Chapter 4 under "Anterior Pituitary Insufficiency—Thyrotropin" and also in the Appendix of Chapter 4 under "Thyrotropin Deficiency." However, it should be noted that if the patient has a goiter and thyroid autoantibodies, pituitary hypothyroidism is virtually excluded. Furthermore, in primary hypothyroidism, the PBI does not generally increase when exogenous thyrotropin is administered. Currently available techniques for measuring human thyrotropin in the serum by immunoassay may be helpful; in primary hypothyroidism, these values are very high, whereas in pituitary hypothyroidism they are low.

The serum cholesterol, which is generally elevated, has no value as a differential test. The electrocardiogram shows bradycardia and low voltage; and radiographs of the chest may show cardiac enlargement.

In the differential diagnosis of hypothyroid patients, the physician should consider such conditions as nephrotic syndrome when the physical appearance suggests thyroid deficiency; appropriate tests of renal and thyroid function will rule this out. Severe pernicious anemia may present with similar manifestations and may coexist with myxedema. The differential diagnosis may be difficult because hypothyroidism produces moderate to severe anemia and, on occasion, macrocytosis, although this is not associated with a megaloblastic marrow. Here studies of vitamin B_{12} absorption may be helpful; a normal absorption rules out pernicious anemia. Patients who have primary myxedema and who are also slowly developing pernicious anemia may have circulating antibodies to gastric constituents—i.e., parietal cells and intrinsic factor—and may even have defective B_{12} absorption without megaloblastic anemia.

Treatment

The treatment is thyroid hormone. If patients have severe myxedema or are elderly, or have angina pectoris, one should start them at a very low dose (e.g., thyroxine, 0.025 mg daily), and in such patients it may not be possible to increase this dosage much further. However, if there are no other nonthyroidal complications, the dosage may be increased at intervals of 3–4 weeks. Too rapid increase may aggravate angina or even induce congestive heart failure. However, occasionally angina pectoris seems to be ameliorated by cautious use of small doses of thyroid hormone, suggesting that hypothyroid heart disease was a factor in its production. Younger patients, however, can tolerate an initial dose of 0.1 or 0.2 mg of thyroxine per day (or desiccated thyroid, 60–120 mg/day). Triiodothyronine has a faster but shorter action than thyroxine, but has no particular advantage. Patients should gradually improve and should reach a euthyroid state. Maintenance dose in uncomplicated cases is kept between 0.15 and 0.3 mg of thyroxine per day or its equivalent in desiccated thyroid.

In older patients with angina, the dose is kept at a suboptimal level, and may have to be titrated against the severity of the angina. The therapy is continued for life.

Once patients are stabilized on a maintenance dose of thyroxine, the dosage should not be adjusted to meet the patient's various complaints, because most of these complaints are functional. Periodic tests of thyroid function are unnecessary because the doctor can rely on his clinical judgment in estimating function. When patients take thyroxine as maintenance, the PBI tends to be elevated; when desiccated thyroid is used, the PBI may vary; with triiodothyronine, the PBI is low. A new preparation which combines thyroxine and triiodothyronine keeps the PBI within normal limits on a full maintenance dose, but this is its only advantage.

Developmental Defects

Lingual Thyroid

On rare occasions, thyroid tissue does not migrate from its usual site of origin at the base of the tongue. In such instances, all of the thyroid tissue remains in the lingual region, where it is observed during childhood as a reddish, fleshy lump at the base of the tongue. Children with lingual thyroid, who are usually euthyroid, are treated with desiccated thyroid or thyroxine to suppress the lingual thyroid and cause it to regress. If left untreated, goiters might develop in the lingual thyroid and produce airway obstruction. These patients are kept on maintenance therapy for life.

Thyroglossal Duct Cyst

Occasionally the thyroglossal duct, which leads from the pharynx to the thyroid, may not atrophy completely and may give rise to a thyroglossal duct cyst. Such cysts may erupt onto the skin and discharge periodically; if so, they are excised. This, however, is difficult because the entire tract must be removed. Furthermore, in some of these patients, thyroid tissue extends along the course of the duct; hence the amount and site of other thyroid tissue should be determined before operation.

Summary

The thyroid gland seems to represent a "prototype" for the target endocrine organs (thyroid, adrenal cortex, testes, ovaries) that are under the control of the adenohypophysis. The regulation and control of thyroid secretion has parallels in these other glands, so that an understanding of thyroid physiology and control is helpful when one studies the other target endocrine glands. Similarly, disorders of the thyroid gland are usually quite clear-cut, and also have their analogies in the other endocrine organs. Nevertheless, there are many dissimilarities between the various endocrine glands, and these analogies should not be carried too far. The thyroid gland thus must be considered as a unique tissue, sharing some qualities with its sister glands, and having a complex relationship with them. The foregoing chapter has presented current concepts of thyroid disorders, but these views may have to be drastically altered as thyroid studies progress and fill the many gaps in our knowledge.

References

1. Adams, D. D., and Purves, H. D. Abnormal responses in the assay of thyrotrophin. *Dunedin, N Z Univ Otago Med Sch Proc 34:*11–12, 1956.
2. Braverman, L. E., Ingbar, S. H., and Sterling, K. Conversion of thyroxine (T_4) to triiodothyronine (T_3) in athyreotic human subjects. *J Clin Invest 49:* 855–864, 1970.
3. Burke, G. Dissociation between thyroid injury and formation of long-acting thyroid stimulator in thyrotoxicosis. *Ann Intern Med 67:*349–355, 1967.
4. Burnet, F. M. *The Clonal Selection Theory of Acquired Immunity*. Cambridge, Univ. Press, 1959, p. 208.
5. Editorial. Treatment of hyperthyroidism. *Can Med Assoc J 98:*462–464, 1968.
6. Fialkow, P. J. Genetic aspects of autoimmunity. *Progr Med Genet 6:*117–167, 1969.
7. Fraser, G. R. The genetics of thyroid disease. *Progr Med Genet 6:*89–115, 1969.
8. Hamilton, C. R., Adams, L. C., and Maloof, F. Hyperthyroidism due to thyrotropin-producing pituitary chromophobe adenoma. *N Engl J Med 283:*1077–1080, 1970.
9. Hershman, J. M., and Pittman, J. A. Control of thyrotropin secretion in man. *N Engl J Med 285:* 997–1006, 1971.
10. Ingbar, S. H., and Woeber, K. A. "The Thyroid Gland." In *Textbook of Endocrinology* (4th ed.), Williams, R. H., ed. Philadelphia, Saunders, 1968, pp. 105–286.
11. Irvine, W. J., Davies, S. H., Delamore, I. W., and Williams, A. W. Immunological relationship between pernicious anaemia and thyroid disease. *Br Med J 2:*454–456, 1962.
12. Jayson, M. I. V., Doniach, D., Benhamou-Glynn, H., Roitt, I. M., and El Kabir, D. J. Thyrotoxicosis and Hashimoto goitre in a pair of monozygotic twins with serum long-acting thyroid stimulator. *Lancet 2:*15–18, 1967.
13. Kriss, J. P. Inactivation of long-acting thyroid stimulator (LATS) by anti-kappa and anti-lambda antisera. *J Clin Endocrinol Metab 28:*1440–1444, 1968.
14. Kriss, J. P., Pleshakov, V., Rosenblum, A. L. Holderness, M., Sharp, G., and Utiger, R. Studies on the pathogenesis of the ophthalmology of Graves' disease. *J Clin Endocrinol Metab 27:*582–593, 1967.
15. Marine, D. Iodine in the treatment of diseases of the thyroid gland. *Medicine (Baltimore) 6:*127–141, 1927.
16. Masi, A. T., Sarrwell, P. E., Hartmann, W. H., and Shulman, L. E. Hashimoto's disease; a study of the consistency of its histopathological diagnosis. *J Chronic Dis 18:*1–57, 1965.
17. McKenzie, J. M. Humoral factors in the pathogenesis of Graves' disease. *Physiol Rev 48:*252–310, 1968.
18. McConnon, J., Row, V. V., and Volpé, R. Simultaneous comparative studies of thyroxine and triiodothyronine distribution and disposal rates. *J Endocrinol 51:*17–30, 1971.
19. Odell, W. D., Bates, R. W., Rivlin, R. S., Lipsett, M. B., and Hertz, R. Increased thyroid function without clinical hyperthyroidism in patients with choriocarcinoma. *J Clin Endocrinol Metab 23:*658–664, 1963.
20. Oppenheimer, J. H. Role of plasma proteins in the binding, distribution and metabolism of the thyroid hormones. *N Engl J Med 278:*1153–1162, 1968.
21. Roitt, I. M., Greaves, M. F., Torrigiani, G., Brostoff, J., and Playfair, J. H. L. The cellular basis of immunological responses. *Lancet 2:*367–371, 1969.
22. Volpé, R., Desbarats-Schonbaum, M. L., Schonbaum, E., Row, V. V., and Ezrin, C. The effect of radioablation of the thyroid gland in Graves' disease with high levels of long-acting thyroid stimulator (LATS). *Am J Med 46:*217–226, 1969.
23. Volpé, R., "Thyroiditis." In *The Thyroid: A Fundamental and Clinical Text* (3rd ed.), Werner, S. C. and Ingbar, S., eds., New York, Harper, 1971.
24. Volpé, R. Treatment of thyroiditis. *Mod Treat 6:* 474–496, 1969.
25. Volpé, R., Edmonds, M. W., Clarke, P. V., and Row, R. R. A viewpoint regarding the nature of the emergence of long-acting thyroid stimulator of Graves' disease. *Acta Endocr Panamericana 1:*155–170, 1970.

General Reference

Werner, S. C., and Ingbar, S., eds. *The Thyroid: A Fundamental and Clinical Text,* 3rd ed. New York, Harper, 1971.

6

The Parathyroids and Calcium Metabolism

Edmund R. Yendt

Role of Calcium Ion in Biologic Processes

The calcium ion, an important constituent of biologic membranes, exerts a major but not yet completely understood effect upon their function. The permeability (tightness) of membranes varies indirectly with the calcium-ion concentration (Ca^{++}) of the extracellular fluids. Elevation of extracellular calcium-ion concentration reduces membrane permeability and the transport rate of various ionic (particularly sodium and potassium) and nonionic substances across the membrane. Conversely, a reduction in calcium-ion concentration increases membrane permeability.

The calcium ion has an important effect upon the electrical properties (excitability) of membranes, which may be a direct consequence of its action on membrane permeability. The relationship between membrane excitability and extracellular fluids (Ca^{++}) is an inverse one: hypocalcemia increases membrane excitability and vice versa. In nerve tissues, reduction in calcium-ion concentration leads to membrane depolarization and increased neuromuscular excitability so that the excitability of motor nerve fibers is enhanced and the threshold of peripheral sensory nerve receptors is lowered.

Calcium plays an essential role in the contraction of all types of muscle; specifically, it appears to act as a coupling factor between excitation and contraction. The first event in muscle contraction is that the excitatory process depolarizes the membranes of the cell and its microsomes; this is followed by a movement of calcium from specific intracellular binding sites or from the extracellular fluid to actomyosin which thereupon contracts (in the presence of ATP). Magnesium ions antagonize this effect of calcium upon the contractile process.

Calcium ions are also involved in the release of preformed hormones from endocrine and exocrine glands and in secretion of transmitter substances at synapses by a mechanism analogous to the "excitation-contraction" coupling mechanism of muscle. It has been postulated that the secretagogue initiates hormone release by interacting with the plasma membrane of the receptor cell so as to alter the permeability characteristics of the membrane to various ions, in particular to calcium ions, with a resultant influx of calcium into the cells. The resultant increase in intracellular calcium (or redistribution of intracellular calcium) in some way provokes hormone release—possibly by causing intracellular contractile tubular systems to discharge stored hormone granules into the circulation.

The intracellular calcium-ion concentration also appears to be a critical factor in the complex series of events by which a variety of hormones alter the function of their target cells.[33,36] These hormones ("first messengers"), upon arrival at specific receptor sites on the cell membrane, cause the release into the cytoplasm of a membrane-bound enzyme, adenyl cyclase. Adenyl cyclase catalyzes the conversion of ATP to the "second messenger," 3′5′-adenosine monophosphate (cyclic AMP), which alters intracellular function by activating enzymes known as protein kinases, which in turn activate certain other enzyme precursors by catalyzing their phosphorylation—these activated enzymes catalyze the biochemical processes that enable the target cell to perform its specific biologic function. An increased concentration of cytoplasmic calcium appears to be required for the activation of the phosphorylated proteins or enzymes produced as a result of protein kinase action. The concentration of calcium within the cytoplasm or cytosol is controlled not only by its leak through the cell membrane from the extracellular fluid but also by its release from certain intracellular organelles such as mitochondria which have a remarkable ability to concentrate calcium and thus to act as intracellular storehouses of this ion. The transfer of calcium from extracellular fluid to cytosol is facilitated by the action of the hormone or "first messenger" upon the cell membrane. The "second messenger" cyclic AMP also promotes the transfer of calcium from intracellular organelles to the cytosol.

Calcium ions are essential to the adhesiveness that binds cells together in tissues and organs and are required in enzyme activation, blood coagulation, and fertilization.[1, 37]

Normal Calcium Metabolism

The total calcium content of the body of a normal adult man (70 kg) is 1000–1100 gm.[19–21] Of this amount, 99% is in the bones and teeth; the calcium in the entire extracellular compartment does not exceed 900 mg, and all the remaining tissues contain only 10 gm.

State of Calcium in the Blood

Table 6-1 gives the mean values for the various fractions of calcium in normal adult serum. The normal range for total serum calcium in adult man varies slightly from laboratory to laboratory; in our own laboratory, it is 8.9–10.3 mg/100 ml. The narrowness of this range deserves emphasis; with older, less precise techniques, considerably wider ranges were reported (e.g., 9–11.5 mg/100 ml). However, it is now quite clear that the methods the clinician uses to measure serum calcium must provide a normal range that does not exceed 1.5 mg/100 ml and must also be reproducible with minimal deviation—0.1–0.2 mg/100 ml, from this range. In many patients with primary hyperparathyroidism, the serum calcium level may only exceed the upper limit of "normal" by as little as 0.1 mg/100 ml. Blood taken for serum calcium determinations should be drawn in the fasting state and a tight tourniquet should not be applied for more than a few seconds or the blood exposed to cork stoppers; either may cause spurious elevation of the serum calcium. The upper limit of normal for total serum calcium is slightly lower (about 0.1–0.2 mg/100 ml) in women than in men. This difference is clinically important because it may help the physician to recognize mild hypercalcemia in women whose serum calcium levels would fall within a normal range determined in a mixed population. Normal serum calcium values in children are slightly higher than in adults.

Table 6-1. State of Calcium in Blood

	Amount (mg/100 ml)
Total serum Ca	9.5
Bound to protein	4.0
Non-protein bound (ultrafiltrable)	5.5
Ionized Ca	4.5
Diffusible Ca complexes (with citrate, phosphate, bicarbonate, etc.)	1.0

Almost one-half the calcium in serum is bound to protein—chiefly to albumin. Altered serum albumin concentrations correspondingly alter the protein-bound serum calcium, a change that is reflected in the total serum-calcium levels. For example, total serum calcium is frequently low in the nephrotic syndrome and hepatic cirrhosis, conditions usually associated with hypoalbuminemia. However, such alterations are of no clinical concern because the nonprotein-bound fraction of the blood calcium, which includes all of the ionized Ca, is unchanged. Alterations in serum globulins do not change total serum calcium concentrations significantly. Hypercalcemia develops in certain conditions associated with hyperglobulinemia—e.g., sarcoidosis and multiple myeloma—but in these instances, other mechanisms are responsible for increased calcium levels.

Because nonprotein-bound serum calcium can pass through the capillary wall into the interstitial fluids or through a membrane with ultrafine pores such as cellophane, this fraction is frequently referred to as the "ultrafiltrable" calcium. The measurement is performed in many research laboratories by analyzing that component of serum which can be forced by pressure through a cellophane membrane. Since it is unaffected by variations in serum protein concentrations, the ultrafiltrable calcium reflects the level of ionized calcium in the blood more closely than the total calcium level. The major portion of the serum ultrafiltrable calcium is ionized, but a small fraction (approximately 1 mg/100 ml) persists as soluble, diffusible but un-ionized complexes with phosphate, citrate, and bicarbonate.

It is the level of ionized calcium in the blood that really interests the clinician because only this fraction affects biologic processes; it is this fraction that the parathyroid glands and all the other homeostatic mechanisms work to keep normal. Until now, however, we could not measure ionized calcium in blood easily and accurately enough to serve the clinician; he had to be content with total serum calcium and use this as a reasonably close reflection of ionized levels. Recently, however, new ion-sensitive glass electrodes have been introduced which may offer a routine measurement of ionized calcium levels.

Calcium in the Diet

The chief dietary sources of calcium are milk and milk products (cheese, ice cream) and green leafy vegetables. One liter of fresh, whole milk contains approximately 1,100 mg. calcium. The average daily intake of calcium of adults in North America is 600–1,000 mg. The calcium content of diets from which dairy products and green leafy vegetables are eliminated is approximately 300 mg.

Intestinal Absorption of Calcium

Dietary calcium is absorbed along the entire length of the duodenum, jejunum, and ileum. Although the rate of absorption is considerably greater in the duodenum than in the jejunum or ileum, the bulk of dietary calcium is probably absorbed in the jejunum and ileum because of the greater intestinal surface involved and the increased transit time in this part of the gut. Vitamin D is necessary for normal intestinal absorption of calcium. Absorption is enhanced by conditions which increase the body's need for calcium such as growth, pregnancy, lactation and previous dietary lack. We do not know what signal stimulates greater calcium absorption under these conditions but it does not appear to be parathyroid hormone. Nicolaysen suggested that an as-yet-unidentified substance, which he termed "endogenous factor," is released by the skeleton during periods of increased bone mineralization. Other factors that enhance intestinal calcium absorption include acidification of the gut contents, high protein diets, dietary lactose, and certain amino acids such as lysine. Calcium is best absorbed when given as chloride; calcium lactate is absorbed more efficiently than calcium gluconate and calcium carbonate is absorbed least well.

Intestinal absorption of calcium is diminished by alkalinization of the gut contents and by dietary factors such as oxalate and phytate (hexaphosphoinositol, a constituent of bran), which form insoluble salts or complexes with calcium. Magnesium and calcium appear to share a common transport system in the intestine so that the administration of either of these salts leads to diminished absorption of the other. Diseases associated with impaired intestinal absorption of calcium include the various causes of diarrhea and steatorrhea and the nephrotic syndrome.

Calcium gains access to the gut lumen as a normal constituent of the various gastric and intestinal juices as well as via the diet. It has been estimated that approximately 600 mg calcium is secreted into the gut in this form each day—an amount almost equal to the dietary intake. The calcium content of the intestinal juices appears to be fairly constant and is independent of the amount of calcium in the blood or in the diet.

Consequently when the dietary calcium intake is very low, as in starvation, calcium loss in the stools may actually exceed the amount ingested. Calcium secreted in the intestinal juices is partially reabsorbed in the same fashion as dietary calcium.

The net intestinal absorption of calcium equals the dietary calcium minus the quantity lost in the feces. Each day this amounts to 100–200 mg, which is roughly equivalent to the daily loss in the urine. [Net intestinal Ca absorption = dietary Ca (800 mg) − fecal Ca (600 mg) = 200 mg] However, it is obvious that the amount of calcium actually absorbed by the gut each day exceeds this figure by an amount equal to the quantity of calcium in the intestinal juices. Thus total intestinal absorption of calcium = dietary Ca (800 mg) + Ca in intestinal juices (600 mg) − fecal Ca (600 mg) = 800 mg.

Fecal calcium consists of unabsorbed dietary Ca plus unabsorbed intestinal-juice Ca; the latter fraction is sometimes referred to as "endogenous fecal calcium." When the ability of the gut to absorb calcium is impaired, as in the steatorrheas, there are excess fecal losses of both dietary and intestinal-juice calcium. This is another situation in which the loss of calcium in the stools may actually exceed the amount ingested.

Renal Handling of Calcium

Only the portion of plasma calcium that is not bound to protein (ultrafiltrable calcium) passes through the glomerular capillaries. Thus the concentration of calcium in the glomerular filtrate is approximately 5.5 mg/100 ml. In an adult human with a glomerular filtration rate of 100 ml/minute, the filtered calcium equals 5.5 mg/minute or approximately 8 gm/24 hours. Of this amount, approximately 98% is reabsorbed by the renal tubules and only 100–200 mg is lost each day in the urine. The normal daily urinary loss of calcium depends upon a wide variety of factors which are discussed below, but generally urinary calcium excretion is excessive when it is greater than 300 mg in males or 250 mg in females ingesting average diets.

Although there is some correlation between dietary calcium intake and urinary calcium excretion, in most normal subjects excretion changes little despite fairly wide variations in dietary intake. For example, increasing the calcium intake from 300 to 1,500 mg does not increase urinary calcium excretion in most people by more than 100–150 mg. However, there is a fairly wide range in the individual response to variation in dietary calcium, and in a few people, especially those with idiopathic hypercalciuria, a dietary calcium increase of this magnitude could increase urinary calcium excretion by 300–400 mg.

Changes in urinary calcium excretion are due to changes in the filtered load (of calcium) or to altered renal tubular handling, or to simultaneous changes in both factors. The filtered load is a function of the glomerular filtration rate (GFR) and the calcium level of the plasma ultrafiltrate. Thus hypocalciuria results when the GFR is reduced, as in chronic renal insufficiency, or when plasma calcium levels fall, as in hypoparathyroidism. Calcium virtually disappears from the urine when serum levels fall below 7.5 mg/100 ml. On the other hand, urinary losses of calcium become excessive when the filtered load of calcium is increased in various disorders which increase blood calcium levels.

The reabsorption of filtered calcium at various sites along the nephron is proportionately similar to that of sodium; approximately two-thirds of the filtered load is reabsorbed by the proximal tubule, 20–25% in the loop of Henle, 10% by the distal convoluted tubule, and the remainder in the collecting tubule. However, present evidence suggests that, unlike sodium, the proximal renal tubule does not reabsorb calcium actively—i.e., against an electrochemical gradient. Proximal reabsorption of calcium is passive—down a concentration gradient created by the active proximal reabsorption of salt and water. Much evidence indicates that the tubular reabsorption of calcium and sodium are closely linked, particularly at the level of the proximal tubule. This is a direct relationship so that factors which increase the proximal reabsorption of sodium also increase the proximal reabsorption of calcium, resulting in decreased urinary excretion of calcium. Factors which tend to expand extracellular fluid volume, such as NaCl ingestion, saline infusion, and chronic mineralocorticoid administration, also depress the proximal reabsorption of sodium, thereby diminishing the proximal tubular reabsorption of calcium, giving rise to hypercalciuria. On the other hand, factors that contract the extracellular fluid volume, such as dietary NaCl restriction or the administration of thiazide diuretics, enhance proximal reabsorption of sodium and calcium so that urinary calcium excretion is diminished. The urinary excretion of calcium and magnesium are linked in a manner that is as yet unclear. The oral or parenteral administration of magnesium salts increases the urinary excretion of calcium, and vice versa.

Many hormonal agents affect urinary calcium excretion, most importantly parathyroid hormone, which increases calcium reabsorption by the tubule. This action of the hormone is discussed at greater length later in this chapter. Urinary calcium excretion is increased by the administration of growth hormone but is diminished by the gonadal hormones. The exact mechanism of these effects is uncertain.

Urinary calcium excretion increases markedly in metabolic acidosis associated with the administration of ammonium chloride or acetazolamide, or in diabetic acidosis. Respiratory acidosis, on the other hand, does not produce hypercalciuria. The effect of metabolic acidosis seems to be due to depressed tubular reabsorption of calcium and is not due to changes in parathyroid hormone secretion because it has been observed in patients with hypoparathyroidism. The metabolic acidosis of chronic renal insufficiency does not produce hypercalciuria. As mentioned previously, patients with renal insufficiency have decreased urinary calcium as a result of the decreased glomerular filtration rate.

Composition of Bone

Bone consists of cells—osteogenic cells, osteoblasts, osteocytes, and osteoclasts—and intercellular substance. The composition of the intercellular substance (on a dry-weight basis) is roughly one-third organic matrix or *osteoid,* and two-thirds inorganic bone crystals. The organic bone matrix or osteoid is largely composed of collagen fibrils (90%) embedded in a ground substance composed of a number of poorly defined proteins, and a group of acid mucopolysaccharides and mucoproteins.

Formation of Bone Matrix

As the first step in the synthesis of collagen, the osteoblast forms a large soluble intracellular collagen precursor molecule, called "protocollagen." The amino acids, proline and lysine, which have been incorporated into this precursor molecule are then hydroxylated to form hydroxyproline and hydroxylysine. As a result of this biochemical event and others such as the addition of one or more carbohydrate moieties (e.g., glucosamine), the protocollagen molecule is converted to soluble collagen and extruded into the extracellular space to undergo further maturation and conversion to insoluble mature collagen. Hydroxyproline and hydroxylysine are found only in collagen. Note that proline and lysine are hydroxylated after their incorporation into the protocollagen molecule; this implies that there is no precursor pool of hydroxyproline and consequently the bulk of the hydroxyproline appearing in plasma and urine must be derived from degradation of collagen. For this reason, an increased rate of bone resorption is reflected by an increased excretion of hydroxyproline in the urine. However, an increased excretion of hydroxyproline in the urine is not necessarily due to increased bone resorption because many tissues besides bone contain collagen.[35]

Mineralization of Bone Matrix

Newly formed bone matrix matures for 5–10 days before it calcifies; during this interval certain biochemical changes, particularly the appearance of phospholipid, occur at the "calcification front" between calcified and uncalcified matrix where mineralization begins. Mineralization of osteoid is an orderly process of crystallization, not a haphazard precipitation of calcium phosphate in bone matrix. The bone mineral has been identified by X-ray diffraction as hydroxyapatite—$Ca_{10}(PO_4)_6(OH)_2$. Crystal deposition begins within the collagen fibril at specific sites, the gaps between the ends of the subunits of the fibrils. The calcium/phosphorus ratio of bone mineral is not constant but varies from 1.3:1 to 2.0:1, because hydronium ions (H_3O) can replace calcium ions in the crystal lattice, and excess phosphate can be absorbed onto the surface of the crystals. In addition, bone mineral contains many ions other than calcium, phosphate, and hydroxyl (e.g., carbonate, magnesium, sodium, potassium and fluoride).

Hydroxyapatite crystals bind water, producing the "hydration shell" on the crystal surface. Certain other ions found in bone are held in this hydration shell while others substitute with the calcium, phosphate, or hydroxyl ions on the surface or within the depths of the crystal: magnesium, lead, strontium and sodium ions can substitute for calcium in hydroxyapatite, chloride and fluoride ions can substitute for the hydroxyl ion, and carbonate can replace phosphate.

The presence of ions other than calcium and phosphate in bone mineral is of more than academic interest: Approximately 50% of the total body magnesium is in the skeleton, and there is enough sodium and carbonate in bone to contribute to acid-base regulation.

In the test tube and in bone, hydroxyapatite crystal formation from solutions containing calcium and phosphate ions is preceded by a stage in which the calcium phosphate is in a colloidal, noncrystalline (amorphous) state; as much as one-third of the calcium in mature bone may be in this form. Initial mineralization of bone is a rapid process; 70% of the total is deposited within a few hours. During this process, much of the water in bone matrix (which initially occupies about 50% of the matrix volume) is replaced by mineral. The final 30% of mineralization takes place much more slowly—over a period of weeks—perhaps because mineral diffusion is impeded when the water is displaced.

When the Ca $\times$ P ion product in extracellular fluids is reduced, osteoid calcification does not take place normally. Large amounts of osteoid are poorly mineralized or not mineralized at all, producing rickets in children and osteomalacia in adults. This suggests that there is some sort of direct relationship between the calcium and phosphate content of extracellular fluid and the fluid milieu of bone. However, the tissue fluid which bathes osteoid is not identical to extracellular fluid nor is it in direct contact or exchange with it, as formerly thought. It now appears likely that bone has an "internal milieu" of its own and that the fluid bathing it is in a closed compartment. Moreover, the exchange of mineral ions between this closed compartment and the bulk phase of the extracellular fluid is likely an active process mediated by bone cells. The walls of the bone-fluid compartment appear to be osteoblasts, which line all of the bony surfaces and are closely aligned to form an effective membrane separating this compartment from the extracellular fluid. Osteoblasts lining the bone surfaces have tiny cytoplasmic processes extending through the canaliculi of bone and communicating with similar processes of other osteoblasts and of the osteocytes buried deep in the bone substance.

The exact events which initiate the calcification of bone matrix are not clearly understood, although a number of theories have been proposed: first, that phosphorylation of specific sites within collagen fibrils forms the basic template upon which the hydroxyapatite crystal is formed; another, that destruction (by the enzyme pyrophosphatase—an alkaline phosphatase) of a calcification inhibitor, such as pyrophosphate, within collagen allows mineralization to proceed. At any rate, cellular (osteoblastic) activity is almost certainly a prerequisite for these initial events and for the formation of the primary crystals. However, once orderly crystal formation has begun, further mineralization probably proceeds in the presence of normal extracellular calcium and phosphorus concentrations.[17,35]

Bone Remodeling

Although there is little net bone growth or increase in skeletal mass after age 20, turnover or remodeling of the skeleton continues so that older bone is constantly replaced by new. This remodeling or renewing of bone takes place at three surfaces: (1) periosteal, (2) endosteal, and (3) the haversian canal surface.

Remodeling is thought to improve the mechanical resilience of bone, to promote nutritional exchange, and to repair the microdamage of normal life. The sequence of remodeling appears to be the same at all sites: Initially there is osteoclastic resorption of bone in discrete, circumscribed areas; later osteoblasts appear in these localized areas and fill in the erosion with osteoid, which subsequently calcifies to become mature bone.

In the mature individual the net effect of these opposing forces differs at the three surfaces. At the periosteal surface the rate of new bone formation slightly exceeds the rate of destruction so that new bone is added, slightly increasing the outside diameter of the bone. However, the bone cortex does not become thicker because, at the endosteal surface of the cortex and in the trabeculae, the rate of resorption slightly exceeds the rate of new bone formation, and the marrow cavity expands. In fact, the amount of new bone added to the periosteal surface of a long bone is slightly less than the net loss of bone at the endosteal surface so that, as a person grows older, a small but inevitable loss of bone mass is reflected in the thinning of the cortex and loss of trabecular bone.

Bone remodeling takes place within the depth of the cortex as well as at its periosteal and endosteal surfaces, and the sequence of events is basically the same as that at these surfaces. As a result of osteoclastic activity, longitudinal resorption cavities 150–250 μ in diameter develop in the cortex. When the resorptive activity has subsided, osteoblasts appear along the walls of the cavities and form concentric layers of new osteoid so that the initial cavity becomes progressively smaller until it becomes a small central canal carrying small blood vessels that nourish the cells of the newly formed bone. The unit of new bone formed within these resorption cavities is known as an "haversian system" or "osteon."

At some surfaces, bone neither forms nor resorbs; these are referred to as resting surfaces. The surfaces of resting bone are covered by flattened "osteogenic" cells—the stem cells of the bone and cartilage cell family. Under appropriate stimuli, these cells can differentiate into osteoblasts, chondroblasts, or osteoclasts.

Factors Influencing Bone Formation

The rate of bone formation responds directly to a few factors such as growth hormone, adrenal glucocorticoids, and the phosphate ion; however, bone formation is more likely to be altered secondarily in response to changes in the rate of bone resorption. As will be discussed later, in the phenomenon referred to as "coupling of bone formation and resorption," a change in the rate of either formation or resorption is followed by a secondary change in the rate of the other process in the same direction. For example, parathyroid hormone affects bone primarily by increasing resorption, but there is usually a secondary increase in bone formation as well so that the whole process of bone turnover is speeded up.

Growth hormone appears to be the major physiologic stimulus to bone formation. Mechanical stresses and strains may exert a similar effect, but as will be seen later, their principal effect is to inhibit resorption. The phosphate and fluoride ions also stimulate the formation of new bone. The adrenal glucocorticoids profoundly depress bone formation; in addition, they have a direct inhibitory effect upon bone resorption in tissue culture.

Bone Resorption

When bone is resorbed, its mineral content dissolves and its organic matrix digests almost simultaneously. In the process, bone releases into the extracellular fluids, calcium and phosphate and the products of collagen digestion such as hydroxyproline. Bone resorbs at all three surfaces referred to previously—i.e., periosteal, endosteal, and that in the cortical resorption cavities. With resorption in these areas, osteoclasts appear, but we do not yet know whether these cells initiate the resorptive process or appear in response to it. Parathyroid hormone increases the number of osteoclasts and the osteolytic activity of individual osteoclasts. Recent work suggests that the osteocyte may also play an important role in bone resorption by promoting dissolution immediately adjacent to the osteocyte lacunae. With this type of bone resorption, referred to as *osteolysis,* osteoclasts do not appear, and presumably the osteocyte itself initiates the biochemical events (including the secretion of collagenolytic enzymes) that dissolve the bone mineral and digest the matrix. The osteocytic lacunae enlarge during periods of active bone resorption but return to normal size after the resorptive stimulus has ceased, an observation which suggests that the osteocyte can redeposit bone it has previously resorbed.

Factors Influencing Bone Resorption

Parathyroid hormone (PTH) stimulates bone resorption strongly but cannot exert this effect in the complete absence of vitamin D, which plays an important permissive role in the process. In addition to its role as an important cofactor for PTH-induced bone resorption, in physiologic doses, 25-hydroxycholecalciferol and 1,25-dihydroxycholecalciferol which are metabolites of vitamin D_3, directly stimulate bone resorption in tissue culture, and pharmacologic doses may speed up the resorptive process so much that blood calcium rises to toxic levels.

A number of other substances besides PTH and vitamin D stimulate bone resorption: Heparin may produce osteoporosis if large doses are given for prolonged periods. Heparin may reduce the stability of lysosomal membranes and release stored proteolytic enzymes such as collagenases; also, in tissue culture, it enhances the resorptive response to a given dose of PTH. Vitamin A also has a profound effect upon membrane stability and may increase bone resorption by a mechanism akin to heparin-induced resorption—i.e., by releasing lytic enzymes from lysosomes. Thyroid hormone also increases the rate of bone resorption, probably by stimulating cellular metabolism rather than through specific action on bone. This effect is independent of the parathyroid glands.

Calcitonin, mechanical stresses and strains, estrogens and androgens, glucocorticoids, glucagon, inorganic phosphate, and fluoride all reduce bone resorption. The inhibitory effect of calcitonin on bone resorption is discussed in greater detail later in this chapter, in the section on Calcitonin. Mechanical forces such as weight-bearing normally retard bone resorption, and when these forces cease as during periods of immobilization, bone breakdown increases so markedly and rapidly that a decrease in bone mass can be seen on the radiograph within a short period. Parathyroidectomy markedly retards this breakdown; this suggests that mechanical forces do not affect bone directly but modify its response to systemic stimuli such as parathyroid hormone. How mechanical forces communicate with the bone cells is not known, but they may induce electrical fields within bones which affect cellular behavior.

Estrogens and androgens inhibit bone resorption either by a direct hormonal effect or as a consequence of an altered responsiveness of bone to endogenous parathyroid hormone. The adrenal glucocorticoids directly inhibit bone resorption in tissue culture and also reduce the resorptive effects of parathyroid hormone and 25-hydroxycholecalciferol in tissue culture; these adrenal hormones depress bone formation to an even greater degree so that during long-term administration the net effect is a decrease in bone mass. Glucagon may inhibit bone resorption by a twofold mechanism; it has a direct inhibitory effect in tissue culture but also appears to stimulate the production and release of calcitonin. Inorganic phosphate inhibits PTH-induced bone resorption in tissue cultures.[34] In this regard, phosphate may govern or regulate bone resorption because the phosphate released during bone dissolution would immediately retard the process unless phosphate was rapidly excreted, as it is in PTH-induced bone resorption. Fluoride ion, when incorporated into the hydroxyapatite crystal, makes the crystal larger and less soluble so that the bone mineral becomes less reactive to body fluids.

Coupling of Bone Formation and Resorption

The student attempting to master the intricacies of calcium metabolism and metabolic disease of bone often finds the data confusing and contradictory; for example, he may be told that parathyroid hormone increases new bone formation while, at the same time, he knows that its primary effect is to increase the rate of bone resorption, which inevitably must decrease skeletal mass. He may also be told that the rate of new bone formation slows down when osteoporotic patients are given sex hormones in an effort to reduce the rate of bone resorption.

We can resolve these seeming contradictions by examining the phenomenon of "coupling" (of bone formation and resorption).[17]

When substances such as parathyroid hormone

or thyroid hormone speed up the rate of bone resorption, bone formation increases too, so that the whole process of bone turnover or remodeling accelerates. However, the increment of newly formed bone does not quite equal the extra bone resorbed, and the net effect is a decrease in bone mass. Conversely when substances such as calcitonin or the sex hormones slow down the rate of bone resorption, bone formation secondarily decreases; however, the degree to which bone resorption is inhibited is slightly greater than the secondary depression of bone formation, so that the net effect of such substances is to reduce the rate of decline of skeletal mass. The phenomenon of "coupling" should come as no surprise because in the preceding section on bone remodeling, we noted that in the adult all new bone formation takes place at surfaces where bone has previously been broken down; therefore, when bone resorption is speeded up the skeleton provides additional surfaces at which new bone can be formed, and vice versa.

The Parathyroid Glands and Parathyroid Hormone

Only vertebrates have parathyroid glands; these vary in number from two to six in different species. They are derived from the entoderm of the third and fourth branchial pouches. Humans normally have four glands, but the number may vary from two to six. The upper glands are usually located on the posterolateral aspect of the thyroid glands at the junction of their middle and upper thirds, but the lower glands (normally located adjacent to the lower poles of the thyroid lobes) can migrate to aberrant locations such as the thymus gland or the anterior and posterior mediastinum, or they may become embedded within the substance of the thyroid gland. The normal adult parathyroid is about the size of a split pea and weighs 30–40 mg.

Normal humans have two main types of parathyroid cells—the chief cell and the oxyphil cell. The chief cell, which is present in all species, synthesizes and secretes parathyroid hormone. The oxyphil cell, which is absent in certain species, has no known function; the number of oxyphil cells increases with age, particularly in humans, and these may represent involutional forms. In some species, including man, the parathyroid glands may also contain some calcitonin-producing cells derived from the ultimobranchial gland.

Parathyroid hormone is a polypeptide. The purified bovine hormone, which has a molecular weight of 9,000–10,000, contains 84 amino acids. The exact amino-acid sequence of the hormone has recently been determined, and its first 34 amino-acid sequences have been synthesized and shown to have all the biologic activity of the natural hormone.

The regulation of parathyroid activity is simpler than that of many other endocrine glands; it does not seem to be influenced by a trophic hormone produced by the pituitary or any other gland. The level of ionic calcium in the blood governs its secretion through a negative feedback system: When the blood calcium drops below the normal level, secretion increases, and when blood calcium exceeds the normal level, secretion stops. For many years, we have had strong indirect evidence for this negative feedback system, but direct evidence was obtained only recently by perfusing the isolated parathyroid gland of the sheep with blood of varying calcium content. A slight decrease in plasma calcium increases the plasma level of parathyroid hormone within a few minutes; in humans, a calcium decrease of 1.5 mg/100 ml may lead to a fourfold increase in plasma hormone concentration. The duration, as well as the magnitude, of the change in blood calcium levels has a bearing on parathyroid hormone secretion. Animals depleted of calcium secrete more hormone in response to a given degree of hypocalcemia than do normal animals, presumably because, during the period of calcium deficiency, the glands have become hyperplastic after prolonged stimulation.

The concentration of magnesium in the plasma also appears to regulate parathyroid hormone secretion; hypomagnesemia suppresses and hypermagnesemia stimulates hormone secretion, but this is probably not important under normal conditions. Plasma phosphate level has no direct influence on parathyroid hormone secretion, but hyperphosphatemia will indirectly stimulate parathyroid hormone secretion because it suppresses bone resorption, thereby lowering blood calcium levels.

As its most important function, parathyroid hormone maintains a normal level of ionic calcium in the blood through its effect on three target organs—bone, gastrointestinal tract, and kidney. The skeleton is the most important of these target sites; here the hormone promotes bone resorption and liberates calcium (and phosphorus) into the extracellular fluids. The hormone's action on the renal tubule increases resorption of calcium from the glomerular filtrate, an effect which also contributes effectively to its ability to raise plasma calcium levels. The student may have difficulty reconciling this action with the well-known observation that parathyroid-hormone excess leads to hypercalciuria. However, the hypercalciuria induced by parathyroid-hormone excess results from increased filtered loads of calcium secondary to raised plasma calcium levels. If it were not for the effect of parathyroid hormone upon the renal tubule, bone resorption induced by the hormone would be considerably less effective in raising blood calcium levels because a much greater proportion of the calcium released from the bone would spill over into the urine. Parathyroid hormone also enhances the absorption of calcium from the gastrointestinal tract but is much less potent in this regard than vitamin D; this effect is probably not important in maintaining normal blood calcium levels.

Parathyroid hormone has another effect upon the renal tubule: It promotes the excretion of phosphate in the urine and, as a result, lowers levels of inorganic phosphate in the blood. The hormone probably diminishes phosphate reabsorption by the proximal renal tubule. The reader should note that this effect upon phosphorus metabolism contributes greatly to its ability to maintain blood calcium levels. Without this action, parathyroid-hormone excess would lead to hyperphosphatemia because phosphorus (as well as calcium) is released from the skeleton into the extracellular fluids. This, in turn, would increase bone formation and also would oppose the action of parathyroid hormone on the resorptive mechanism. In hyperparathyroidism, serum phosphorus levels are lower than normal because of the altered renal tubular handling of phosphate; hence the action of the hormone upon bone is greatly enhanced. As previously mentioned, parathyroid hormone is unable to resorb bone in the complete absence of vitamin D, but only minute amounts of the vitamin are required to restore this effect. The phosphaturic action of parathyroid hormone, on the other hand, does not require vitamin D.

Resorption induced by parathyroid hormone removes both the organic and mineral phases of bone, but we do not know whether this occurs simultaneously or in some specific sequence. Removal of the organic phase is essentially a degradation of collagen brought about almost certainly through enzymatic action. Experimental evidence suggests that parathyroid hormone not only induces the synthesis of the necessary enzymes but may also activate latent enzymes and control the rate of enzymatic activity. Osteoclasts proliferate and accumulate at the site of bone resorption, but this response might be secondary to bone resorption rather than the primary event. Bone resorption can occur in the absence of osteoclasts. It has been recently demonstrated that mature osteocytes play an important role in bone resorption and that this process is stimulated by parathyroid hormone and antagonized by calcitonin.

Parathyroid hormone acts upon target cells through the adenyl cyclase-cyclic AMP system described in the section on Role of Calcium Ion in Biologic Processes, earlier in this chapter. The hormone stimulates adenyl-cyclase activity and increases the concentration of cyclic AMP in its target tissues. Furthermore, cyclic AMP mimics the effect of parathyroid hormone in kidney and bone. As mentioned previously, an increased cytoplasmic calcium concentration is required to activate the enzymes which catalyze the biochemical processes, which enable the target cells to perform their specific biologic functions. The "first messenger" parathyroid hormone facilitates the leak of calcium across the cell membrane from extracellular fluid to cytosol, whereas the "second messenger" cyclic AMP promotes the transfer of calcium to cytosol from intracellular storehouses such as the mitochondria.

Vitamin D

Although both vitamin D and parathyroid hormone play important roles in the maintenance of normal skeletal structure and function and in the regulation of blood calcium levels, vitamin D is the more essential of the two. We can maintain patients with parathyroid-hormone deficiency in good health by providing extra vitamin D and calcium. However, we cannot prevent the injurious effects of vitamin D deficiency by increasing parathyroid hormone. The fall in blood calcium levels associated with vitamin D deficiency stimulates increased secretion of parathyroid hormone (secondary hyperparathyroidism). Although this response tends to diminish the hypocalcemia, it does not ameliorate the skeletal disease; indeed, increased amounts of hormone may aggravate it.

There are three major D vitamins: vitamin D_2, vitamin D_3, and vitamin D_4. Vitamin D_2, ergocalciferol (formerly calciferol), is produced by the irradiation of ergosterol. Vitamin D_3, cholecalciferol, the naturally occurring form of vitamin D, is formed by the activation of its precursor, 7-dehydrocholesterol, in the skin by the ultraviolet radiation of sunlight. Vitamins D_2 and D_3 have equal antirachitic activity in humans and rats, but in chickens, vitamin D_2 has only one-tenth the antirachitic activity of vitamin D_3. Vitamin D_4 (22,23-dihydroergocalciferol) is not used as a therapeutic substance in man; it has only 50% of the activity of vitamin D_3 in chickens. The early literature described vitamin D_1, thought to be distinct from the other D vitamins, but this term was abandoned when the substance was found to be an addition product of vitamin D_2 and lumisterol.

Vitamin D is absorbed in the jejunum and ileum and, from there, is rapidly carried in the chylomicrons of the lymphatics to the liver; bile is essential for its absorption. The liver converts vitamin D to a number of metabolites, some of which are biologically active and some biologically inactive. The most important of the biologically active metabolites of vitamin D_3 has recently been identified as 25-hydroxycholecalciferol (25-HCC); 25-hydroxyergocalciferol is the metabolically active form of ergocalciferol.

The vitamin D story is still unfolding. Recently it has been demonstrated that 25-HCC undergoes further metabolic transformation in the kidney to 1,25-dihydroxycholecalciferol (1,25-DHCC) before it can stimulate calcium transport by the intestinal mucosa. Both 25-HCC and 1,25-DHCC directly stimulate bone resorption in tissue culture. A number of other vitamin D metabolites have recently been identified but as yet their biologic significance is unknown.

The main target sites for the active vitamin D metabolites are the intestine and bone. In the intestinal mucosa, vitamin D stimulates the active absorption of calcium, perhaps by inducing the formation of a protein in the intestinal mucosal cell which forms a tight complex with calcium.

In addition, a vitamin D-stimulated, calcium-dependent ATPase has been demonstrated in the brush borders of the mucosal cells of the small intestine. The vitamin D-induced ATPase may facilitate the mucosal uptake of Ca^{++} by a transport system requiring ATP. The calcium ions are then transported across the cell by the calcium-binding protein where they are extracted at the basement membrane. In physiologic doses, vitamin D also has a direct resorptive effect upon bone which liberates calcium into the extracellular fluids.[7, 8]

Vitamin D may be looked upon as an essential cofactor for parathyroid hormone because the hormone cannot induce bone resorption when there is an extreme deficiency of the vitamin. Consequent upon this and its essential role in the intestinal absorption of calcium, vitamin D is essential for the maintenance of normal levels of calcium (and phosphorus) in the blood. Because mineralization of cartilage and bone matrix requires a normal blood level of both calcium and phosphorus ions, vitamin D may be considered essential for calcification. However, we have no proof that vitamin D directly affects calcification although some authorities believe it may be necessary for the proper maturation of cartilage and osteoid, thereby enabling it to undergo calcification. Vitamin D also appears to affect bone formation rates; when vitamin D is deficient, new-bone formation slows down and increases when the deficiency is corrected. We do not yet know whether this is due to a direct effect of the vitamin on the osteoblasts and matrix synthesis or to an indirect effect related to local changes in calcium-ion concentration. Neither vitamin D_2 nor vitamin D_3 stimulates intestinal calcium transport or bone resorption in vitro, but physiologic amounts of the active metabolites of vitamin D_3 have these effects in in-vitro preparations. Another action of vitamin D has been demonstrated at the subcellular level; it is essential for the uptake of calcium by mitochondria, an active process requiring energy.

Pharmacologic doses of vitamin D stimulate bone resorption to such a degree that the blood calcium rises, an effect used in the treatment of hypoparathyroidism. Pharmacologic doses of vitamin D may also inhibit renal tubular reabsorption of calcium because, when administered to normal subjects, it sometimes produces hypercalciuria before an effect on intestinal absorption of calcium or elevated serum calcium levels can be demonstrated. However, it is more likely that the vitamin D–induced mobilization of bone mineral suppresses the parathyroid even though no change in serum calcium levels has been detected; this would produce hypercalciuria because parathyroid hormone increases the reabsorption of calcium by the renal tubule. When given to patients with hypoparathyroidism, large doses of vitamin D increase urinary excretion of phosphorus and lower serum phosphorus levels. Originally these effects were attributed to the "phosphaturic" action of vitamin D, which was thought to directly inhibit the renal tubular conservation of phosphate in a manner similar to parathyroid hormone. However, in hypoparathyroid patients, when serum calcium levels are raised by prolonged infusions of calcium, a similar phosphaturia and fall in serum phosphorus levels occur—an indication that the level of calcium in the blood directly alters the renal tubular handling of phosphate. Therefore, the "phosphaturic" action of pharmacologic doses of vitamin D seems to be an indirect one. Physiologic doses of vitamin D administered to D-deficient animals or humans has an opposite effect on phosphate metabolism; tubular reabsorption of filtered phosphate increases and serum phosphorus levels rise. However, this is an indirect rather than a direct action of vitamin D because, when the vitamin D deficiency is corrected, the associated secondary hyperparathyroidism is also corrected.[48]

Calcitonin

Before 1961, we thought that parathyroid hormone was the only hormone involved in the fine regulation of plasma calcium levels and that the only hormonal response to hypercalcemia was the cessation of parathyroid-hormone secretion. However, in that year, Copp demonstrated that hypercalcemia also triggered the release of a hitherto unidentified hormonal substance, which actively lowered plasma calcium levels. Copp originally suggested that this substance, which he named calcitonin, was derived from the parathyroid glands, but subsequently other workers showed that, in mammals, the thyroid rather than the parathyroids was the main source of this hormone, which they then named "thyrocalcitonin." However, the original term "calcitonin" is more appropriate because, in lower forms (fish, reptiles, and birds), the hormone is secreted by the ultimobranchial glands, derived from the last branchial pouch. The calcitonin-secreting cells are not of entodermal origin but migrate into the ultimobranchial gland from the neuroectodermal crest. In mammals, the ultimobranchial gland cells fuse with thyroid during embryonic development and become the thyroid C (parafollicular) cells, which differ in structure and function from the thyroxine-secreting epithelial cells of the thyroid follicle. In man, the thymus and the parathyroid glands may also secrete some calcitonin.

Pure calcitonin, derived from a number of different species (including humans), has been isolated, structurally analyzed, and synthesized. All are 32-amino-acid polypeptides; although the whole molecule is required for biological activity, the amino acid sequence varies considerably in the different molecules. This variation indicates that the specific action of the hormone depends on certain critical factors of the amino acid sequence (common to all species) rather than on the structure as a whole. Salmon calcitonin is 40 times more potent than that derived from other species because it is more resistant to degradation by an inactivating factor in normal plasma.

Calcitonin reduces plasma calcium levels by a direct, rapid, and transient inhibition of bone resorption; this effect appears to be nonspecific because the hormone antagonizes a variety of bone resorptive agents including parathyroid hormone, vitamin D, and vitamin A. Moreover calcitonin exerts this effect in parathyroidectomized vitamin-D-deficient animals. Furthermore, calcitonin does not antagonize the renal or gastrointestinal effects of parathyroid hormone. After calcitonin administration, the urinary excretion of phosphate also increases, resulting in decreased serum phosphorus levels, but this may reflect increased parathyroid-hormone secretion secondary to the hypocalcemia, rather than a primary effect of calcitonin upon the renal tubule. Calcitonin also temporarily increases urinary sodium chloride excretion and, in man (but not in some species such as the dog), it increases urinary calcium and magnesium excretion.

Hypercalcemia is probably the major stimulus for calcitonin secretion, but elevation of blood magnesium levels (as well as the administration of glucagon, gastrin, and pancreozymin) has also been shown to promote calcitonin secretion in the experimental animal.

The biochemical basis of calcitonin action is not known. It does not prevent parathyroid hormone from increasing the concentration of cyclic AMP in bone, but it does block the bone resorption induced by cyclic AMP and blocks the resorptive action of parathyroid hormone. Certain experimental evidence suggests that the intracellular basis for calcitonin action may be decreased calcium-ion concentration of the cytoplasm, possibly by activating a membrane-bound "pump," which extrudes calcium from the cell. (It will be recalled that parathyroid hormone is thought to increase the cytoplasmic calcium-ion concentration.)

The entire contribution of calcitonin to human physiology is as yet unclear. Whether the hormone can be detected in normal human plasma is still being debated. Possibly its secretion may be limited to emergency situations of calcium overloading. During acute calcium loading, hypothyroid subjects adjust less well than do normal subjects and may develop serious hypercalcemia. This hypercalcemia might be due to calcitonin deficiency although the hypothyroid patient is not necessarily calcitonin deficient since human parathyroid and thymus glands may secrete calcitonin. Whether calcitonin is necessary for the development and maintenance of a normal skeleton is also still unclear.[6, 37]

Disorders of Calcium Metabolism

Hypocalcemia

The causes of hypocalcemia are listed in Table 6-2. Hypocalcemia due to diminished protein levels does not give rise to symptoms because the levels of ionized calcium in the plasma remain normal. Hypocalcemia in hypoparathyroidism, pseudohypoparathyroidism, vitamin D deficiency, and following parathyroidectomy or infarction of a parathyroid adenoma, is discussed later in this section.

Hypocalcemia Due to Hyperphosphatemia

An increase in serum phosphate concentration reduces serum calcium levels primarily by inhibiting bone resorption, but increased formation of bone and deposition of calcium phosphate in soft tissue may possibly contribute to this effect. Hypocalcemia secondary to hyperphosphatemia is frequently encountered in acute and chronic renal insufficiency. The infusion of inorganic phosphate to correct hypercalcemia may not only restore calcium levels to normal but may induce hypocalcemia and tetany.

Hypocalcemia in Neoplastic Disorders

Hypocalcemia sometimes occurs in patients who have tumors of the lung, breast, and prostate that are associated with widespread osteoblastic metastases. Increased skeletal avidity for calcium most likely explains this and also accounts for the excessive retention of infused calcium, the rapid skeletal accretion of radioactive calcium or strontium, and the increased intestinal absorption of calcium observed in normocalcemic and hypocalcemic patients with osteoblastic metastases. A

Table 6-2. Causes of Hypocalcemia

Hypocalcemia due to hypoproteinemia (diminished protein-bound calcium with normal ionized calcium)
Nephrotic syndrome
Hepatic cirrhosis
Hypocalcemia due to diminished ionized calcium
Parathyroid hormone deficiency (hypoparathyroidism)
Parathyroid hormone insensitivity (pseudohypoparathyroidism)
Vitamin D deficiency
Dietary
Malabsorption secondary to small bowel disease
Malabsorption secondary to neomycin administration
Anticonvulsant drugs
Hyperphosphatemia
Acute and chronic renal insufficiency
Phosphate infusions
Neoplastic disorders
Increased skeletal avidity due to osteoblastic metastases
Calcitonin-secreting tumors
Following parathyroidectomy in primary hyperparathyroidism or infarction of a parathyroid adenoma
Adrenal corticosteroid excess
Neonatal tetany
Acute pancreatitis
Magnesium deficiency
Renal tubular acidosis
Miscellaneous
EDTA infusions and citrate intoxication
Hypernatremic dehydration in infants
Glucagon administration
Mithramycin administration
Osteopetrosis
Porphyria with inappropriate secretion of ADH

similar mechanism probably accounts for the occasional occurrence of hypocalcemia during successful therapy of breast carcinoma, when there is regression and healing of osteolytic metastases.

In 1968, Melvin and Tashjian first described a calcitonin-secreting tumor associated with hypocalcemia (6.4 mg/100 ml) in a patient with medullary thyroid carcinoma. Extracts of this patient's tumor as well as his plasma caused hypocalcemia when injected into rats; the serum levels of immunoassayable parathyroid-hormone were also elevated, indicating that the chronic hypocalcemia had produced secondary hyperparathyroidism. The serum phosphorus was low normal, as would be expected with calcitonin excess, but there was no evidence of osteosclerosis. This patient also had a pheochromocytoma. Patients have also been reported with calcitonin-secreting thyroid medullary carcinoma without hypocalcemia.

Hypocalcemia Due to Corticosteroid Excess

Corticosteroids do not regulate plasma calcium directly, but they do influence bone formation and resorption as well as the absorption, metabolism, and action of vitamin D.[3] (See the section on Factors Influencing Bone Formation earlier in this chapter.) The mild, asymptomatic hypocalcemia sometimes observed in Cushing's syndrome indicates that glucocorticoid excess may lower serum calcium levels.

Hypocalcemia in Neonatal Tetany

In the newborn, hypocalcemic tetany is probably triggered by the high phosphate content of cow's milk during the infant's period of physiologic hypoparathyroidism—a time when he is abruptly cut off from the maternal parathyroid hormone. During the first 3 weeks of life normal infants frequently have mild hypocalcemia even though calcium levels of cord blood are normal; this finding reflects a period of temporary parathyroid hypofunction.

Hypocalcemia in Acute Pancreatitis

In acute pancreatitis, hypocalcemia, which may be associated with tetany, has been ascribed to the fixation of calcium by fatty acids liberated from necrotic mesenteric fat deposits, but there may be other contributory mechanisms that are, as yet, undefined.

Hypocalcemia Due to Magnesium Deficiency

Hypocalcemia is a well-documented complication of magnesium deficiency secondary to intestinal malabsorption, alcoholism, primary hypomagnesemia in infants, or deliberate restriction of dietary magnesium. The hypocalcemia is refractory to vitamin D administration and usually to parathyroid hormone administration as well, but serum calcium levels return to normal when the magnesium deficiency is corrected. Since a strongly positive calcium balance has been demonstrated during the hypocalcemia, it appears that the low calcium levels are due to disturbed blood-bone equilibrium with inadequate release of calcium from bone.

Miscellaneous Causes of Hypocalcemia

Hypocalcemia has been reported during hypothermia in association with major operations and following glucagon administration. Ionized (but not total) calcium level also falls with EDTA infusion and when citrate is infused rapidly enough to exceed the body's ability to metabolize it.

Hypocalcemia may also complicate hypernatremic dehydration in infants. Experimental studies of this phenomenon in the rat suggest that an increase in body sodium produces a temporary hypocalcemia if there is a concomitant deficiency of potassium.

Clinical Manifestations of Hypocalcemia

Hypocalcemia does not always give rise to dramatic symptoms and signs. Some patients develop symptoms with mild hypocalcemia (e.g., below 8.5 mg/100 ml), particularly when the serum calcium has fallen rapidly, whereas others with marked chronic hypocalcemia (5–6 mg/100 ml) have no tetany and no symptoms of any sort. Hypocalcemia in the presence or absence of tetany may be associated with a variety of nonspecific complaints such as vague ill health, weakness, fatigue, or emotional disturbances, which are erroneously attributed to psychoneurosis. (See also Chapter 2, section on Hormones and Human Behavior.)

Tetany

Diminished calcium-ion concentration in extracellular fluid increases the excitability of motor nerve fibers and lowers the threshold of peripheral sensory nerve receptors to excitation—an effect which is antagonized by magnesium and enhanced by potassium. If the disturbance is severe enough, spontaneous activity occurs, giving rise to paresthesias, and spasm of smooth and skeletal muscle. The resultant symptom complex, tetany, is characterized by paresthesias, carpopedal spasm, positive Chvostek and Trousseau signs, and changes in the electrical excitability of peripheral nerves. Laryngeal muscles may be involved, producing stridor. Sensory changes tend to precede motor symptoms. Patients may complain of numbness and tingling or a "pins and needles" sensation, which is most noticeable in the hands, feet, circumoral region, and tongue. Muscle spasm, occurring either spontaneously or induced by ischemia (Trousseau test), is most readily demonstrated in the forearm and hand, where it gives rise to the characteristic "main d' accoucheur," in which the elbow and wrist are flexed and the metacarpophalangeal joints are flexed and adducted across the palm (Fig. 6-1). Involvement of the respiratory and jaw muscles may produce dyspnea and inability to talk. Rarely, severe spasm of the glottis may produce a choking sensation, a struggle for breath, and cyanosis. The chief visceral manifestations of tetany are intestinal, but any smooth muscle or sphincter may be involved, to produce symptoms such as biliary colic or bronchospasm.

Other manifestations of increased neuromuscular excitability include Chvostek's sign (unilateral contraction of the facial muscles on percussion of the facial nerve anterior to the ear) and the Trousseau test (carpal spasm induced by tourniquet ischemia which augments the enhanced neuromuscular excitability of hypocalcemia). These clinical tests are not entirely reliable. In its incomplete form, Chvostek's test involves only the muscles of the upper lip, but such a reaction can be elicited in as many as 30% of normocalcemic subjects. An extensive response including contraction of the eyelid muscles nearly always indicates tetany. On the other hand, Chvostek's sign is absent in many patients with hypocalcemia. Trousseau's test, which is usually performed by applying a sphygmomanometer and raising the pressure above the systolic levels for 3 minutes, is negative in about one-third of patients with latent tetany and positive in 4% of the normal population.

Symptoms of tetany are more pronounced when there is pressure on a motor nerve, as when

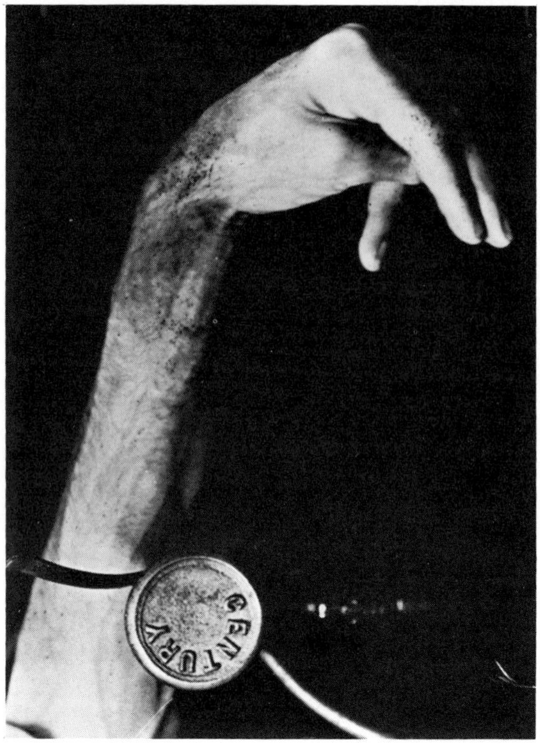

Fig. 6-1. Manifestations of hypocalcemia. Trousseau's sign is elicited in a patient with hypoparathyroid tetany.

the arm is allowed to rest over a chair, or when the patient sleeps on an arm, or when the legs are crossed. Exercise, excitement, and emotional trauma may precipitate tetany, possibly because of the alkalosis produced by the associated hyperventilation or because of concurrent epinephrine release. Factors such as virus infections, menstruation, and pregnancy, and the administration of potassium may also exacerbate tetany.

Other Neurological Manifestations

Epileptiform seizures, most often of the grand-mal type, but also jacksonian, are not uncommon in hypocalcemia, especially in hypoparathyroidism. The tendon reflexes tend to increase with moderate hypocalcemia but may disappear with profound hypocalcemia.

Mental Disturbances

Hypocalcemia may produce a variety of emotional disturbances, including irritability, emotional lability, depression, impairment of memory, confusion, delusions, and hallucinations. For this reason, patients with alleged psychoneuroses and psychoses should have serum calcium determinations. Prolonged hypocalcemia in children may produce mental retardation, which may improve considerably when normal calcium levels are restored.

Ectodermal Lesions

In long-standing hypocalcemia, as in hypoparathyroidism, abnormalities of the skin, hair, nails, teeth, and ocular lens are common. The skin may be coarse, dry, and scaly, and associated skin disorders such as eczema and psoriasis may be aggravated. Moniliasis, a frequent complication of idiopathic hypoparathyroidism, has also been described in the hypocalcemia associated with steatorrhea.

Hypocalcemic patients may have thin and patchy scalp hair, scanty eyelashes and eyebrows, and absent axillary and pubic hair. When involved, the nails are thin, brittle, and deformed by transverse grooves, and tend to split at the free edges.

Teeth that develop during a period of hypocalcemia may erupt late and fall out prematurely because the dentine and enamel are hypoplastic. The hypoplastic teeth have defects in the enamel, giving rise to yellow spots and horizontal grooves, and on X-ray, the roots of the molar teeth may be blunted—a diagnostic sign of some importance.

The patient may develop cataracts within 1 year of the onset of hypocalcemia. Cataracts are most common in hypoparathyroidism but may occur in hypocalcemia due to other disorders, notably sprue. Characteristically these bilateral cataracts consist of punctate opacities arranged in a lamellar fashion, involving both the anterior and posterior subcapsular areas of the lens. They usually do not resolve after the hypocalcemia is corrected.

Miscellaneous

Occasionally patients with hypoparathyroidism may present with severe diarrhea and may have malabsorption of fat and vitamin B_{12} as well. Other gastrointestinal symptoms include constipation and abdominal pain.

Abnormalities of Electrical Laboratory Tests

The electrocardiogram is usually normal except for prolongation of the Q-T interval, but low voltage and T-wave abnormalities have occasionally been reported. The electroencephalogram may be normal or show a variety of nonspecific abnormalities, which are usually abolished when the serum calcium is restored to normal. The electromyographic pattern, which consists of double or repetitive multiple discharges, is not diagnostic of hypocalcemia but is also seen in hyperventilation, hypomagnesemia, injuries of the anterior horn cell, and polyneuritis.

Differential Diagnosis of Tetany

Tetany may occur in individuals with normal serum calcium levels as a complication of alkalosis, either metabolic or respiratory, which reduces the calcium-ion concentration of extracellular fluid. Tetany due to respiratory alkalosis is most often encountered in patients who hyperventilate spontaneously, but the hyperventilation may not be apparent to the patient or the examiner. Certain individuals, especially anxious young women, are particularly susceptible to the effects of overbreathing and may develop tetany after exceedingly brief periods of hyperventilation. In healthy subjects, hyperventilation usually does not produce tetany until the pCO_2 has fallen below 21 mm Hg, whereas in susceptible patients, symptoms develop when the pCO_2 is considerably higher, indicating increased neuromuscular excitability. Although there is no precise explanation for this increased excitability, it has been suggested that catecholamine overproduction, which has been demonstrated in anxious subjects, may be important. This susceptibility to hyperventilation tetany can be blocked by the administration of guanethidine. Hyperventilation regularly is associated with a rise in plasma potassium levels, a point of considerable interest because a sudden rise in plasma potassium may, in itself, produce tetany.

Tetany is a rare manifestation of primary aldosteronism. Its pathogenesis in this condition is not fully understood although alkalosis (hypokalemic) and magnesium deficiency are probably important factors.

Treatment of Acute Hypocalcemia

The symptoms of acute tetany are relieved by the intravenous injection of 10–20 ml of a 10% solution of calcium gluconate, which contains 9% elemental calcium. The injection rate should not exceed 2 ml/minute and the physician should exercise particular care if the patient has been receiving digitalis, which sensitizes the myocardium to the actions of calcium ions. In the average-sized adult with severe tetany, 100 ml of 10% calcium gluconate may be infused over a 4-hour period in 1,000 ml of 5% dextrose in distilled water. This will provide 15 mg elemental calcium per kilogram of body weight. Calcium chloride solutions should not be infused intravenously because this solution, which is extremely irritating, may produce necrosis and sloughing of tissues if it escapes from the vein.

Oral calcium salts should be started as quickly as possible. When indicated, as in the treatment of hypoparathyroidism, pharmacologic doses of vitamin D should also be administered. However, vitamin D acts slowly, and many days may elapse before it produces a significant elevation of serum calcium levels and its maximum effect may not be attained for 6 weeks. Dihydrotachysterol is preferable to vitamin D when a more rapid action is required. (See section on Treatment of Hypoparathyroidism.)

Hypercalcemia

The causes of hypercalcemia are as follows:

1. Hyperparathyroidism
2. Neoplastic disorders
3. Hypervitaminosis D
4. Sarcoidosis
5. Milk-alkali syndrome
6. Immobilization
7. Hyperthyroidism
8. Hypothyroidism
9. Adrenocortical insufficiency
10. Infantile hypercalcemia
11. Hypophosphatasia
12. Recovery phase of acute renal failure
13. Generalized periostitis
14. Use of calcium ion-exchange resins in hemodialysis

Hypercalcemia in hyperparathryoidism will be discussed later in this chapter.

Hypercalcemia in Neoplastic Disorders

Hypercalcemia may complicate almost any malignant disorder but is particularly frequent in carcinoma of the breast, lung, kidney, and in multiple myeloma and lymphomas, including leukemia. It may develop in more than one-third of patients suffering from breast cancer. Measures such as radiation or specific hormone therapy, which cause regression of the tumor, will partially or completely correct the hypercalcemia, but if the wrong agent is chosen, stimulation of tumor growth by estrogen or androgen administration may induce or aggravate existing hypercalcemia.

A number of different mechanisms may produce the hypercalcemia found in these disorders. In multiple myeloma and in many other types of cancer, elevated serum calcium probably reflects bone destruction at the site of osseous metastases, with release of calcium into the extracellular fluids more quickly than it can be excreted by the kidney. This event does not necessarily involve direct action by the malignant cell upon bone but may result from a change in the functional activity of the mesenchymal cells in that area.

Hypercalcemia in neoplastic disease frequently occurs in the absence of radiographic or histologic evidence of osseous metastases. Furthermore, it is often accompanied by hypophosphatemia and may disappear when the primary tumor is removed, both in man and in experimental VX-2 carcinoma in the rabbit. These observations suggest that certain tumors produce a parathyroid hormone-like substance. This has been confirmed by finding, in tumor extracts, substances which behave immunologically like PTH and by demonstrating elevated levels of immunoassayable PTH in the blood of normocalcemic and hypercalcemic cancer patients. Attempts to isolate PTH from tumor extracts by bioassay have been inconclusive, probably because of technical problems. The usual primary sites for nonendocrine PTH-secreting tumors are the bronchus, kidney, ovary, and colon.

Hypercalcemia Due to Hypervitaminosis D

Overdosage with vitamin D_2 (ergocalciferol), vitamin D_3 (cholecalciferol), Hytakerol (AT-10 or dihydrotachysterol) may produce hypercalcemia.[48] Vitamin D intoxication may be encountered in vitamin D-treated patients with hypoparathyroidism, refractory rickets, or azotemic osteodystrophy. There is great individual variation in susceptibility to the effect of vitamin D.

Symptoms of overdosage may appear with as little as 25,000 I.U. daily, but in most cases, the daily dose has been 50,000 I.U. or more. Evidence of vitamin D toxicity has appeared as early as 12 days or as late as 6 years after administration was begun. The hypercalcemia is due mainly to increased resorption of bone induced by pharmacologic doses of vitamin D although increased intestinal absorption of calcium may contribute. Most hypervitaminosis D would be prevented or detected more quickly if proper precautions were taken when prescribing pharmacologic doses of this vitamin (see section on Treatment of Hypoparathyroidism).

Hypercalcemia in Sarcoidosis

Hypercalcemia occurs in 10–30% of patients with sarcoidosis, and hypercalciuria without hypercalcemia is about three times as common. This complication is due not to skeletal involvement by sarcoid, which is rare, or to increased binding of calcium as a result of elevated serum globulins, but to hypersensitivity to exogenous and endogenous vitamin D. When vitamin D is administered to patients with sarcoidosis, they frequently develop toxicity with doses that the general population tolerate well. Furthermore, the incidence of hypercalcemia in patients with sarcoidosis is greater during the summer months. Calcium and phosphorus balances in these patients resemble those of hypervitaminosis D, and, as in hypervitaminosis D, they generally respond well to treatment with corticosteroids.

Hypercalcemia in the Milk-Alkali Syndrome

In 1936, Cope first described hypercalcemia in patients with peptic ulcer who had ingested large amounts of absorbable alkali. The term "milk-alkali syndrome" arose when Burnett and his colleagues described six patients in whom hypercalcemia was associated with metastatic calcification, renal insufficiency (with normal or low urinary calcium excretion), and alkalosis. An earlier stage of this disorder, in which metastatic calcification is absent, is probably encountered much more frequently than is the full-blown syndrome. In a review of 3,300 patients treated for peptic ulcer, Wenger *et al.* found unequivocal evidence of this condition in 1%. The exact pathogenesis of the disorder is not clear, but it can apparently develop with an excessive intake of calcium carbonate alone so that hypercalcemia due to an excessive calcium intake is probably the factor of major importance. Many of these patients have a history of previous renal disease. Symptoms may begin within 10 days of beginning therapy for peptic ulcer. After withdrawal of the milk and alkali, serum calcium levels may promptly fall to normal, but in other cases, months may elapse before normal calcium levels are restored. Corticosteroid administration may hasten the return to normocalcemia.

Hypercalcemia in Immobilization

Mechanical forces exert a profound influence on both bone formation and resorption, possibly by inducing electrical fields within bone which modify the behavior of bone cells. The primary change produced by disuse is increased resorption, but bone formation is also reduced. The resultant osteoporosis of disuse is markedly retarded by parathyroidectomy, suggesting that local mechanical factors modify the response of bone to systemic stimuli. In other words, bone subjected to mechanical forces may be less sensitive to systemic homeostatic forces, such as parathyroid hormone, than unstressed bone. In any rapid turnover of bone (as in childhood, adolescence, or in disorders such as Paget's disease), the amount of calcium released into the extracellular fluids as a result of the increased resorption induced by immobilization may exceed the kidney's excretory capacity and hypercalcemia may result.

Hypercalcemia in Hyperthyroidism

The precise incidence of hypercalcemia in thyrotoxicosis is unknown but may be greater than is commonly supposed because it is not usually looked for. Stanbury estimates that it occurs in 10% of such patients. It is due to increased bone turnover, with relatively greater resorption than formation. This effect of thyroid hormone appears to be part of its general influence on cellular metabolism rather than a specific action on bone and is independent of the parathyroid glands. There is no correlation between serum calcium levels and the severity of the hyperthyroidism. The hypercalcemia abates after successful antithyroid therapy.

Hypercalcemia in Hypothyroidism

Hypercalcemia is a rare complication of cretinism or myxedema. In patients with myxedema, because less than a normal amount of calcium is used in bone formation and the homeostatic response to a calcium load is sluggish, the administration of ordinary doses of calcium salts may produce quite severe hypercalcemia.

Hypercalcemia in Adrenocortical Insufficiency

Hypercalcemia may be a complication of experimental adrenalectomy in animals and, in man, of adrenocortical insufficiency due to Addison's disease, of adrenalectomy for Cushing's syndrome, or of pituitary insufficiency. It responds dramatically to replacement doses of corticosteroids. The relationship of glucocorticoids to serum calcium regulation is not entirely understood but is, at least partially, independent of the parathyroids because adrenalectomy in parathyroidectomized animals may produce hypercalcemia.[27] Glucocorticoids have a direct inhibitory effect upon bone formation and bone resorption and also interfere with the absorption, metabolism and action of vitamin D.

Idiopathic Hypercalcemia of Infants

Mild infantile hypercalcemia, which has its onset between 3 and 7 months of age, is associated with gastrointestinal symptoms and failure to thrive. The infant's response to treatment is generally good and his long-term prognosis is excellent. The "severe" form develops earlier; these infants may have a characteristic "elfin" facies, are retarded mentally and physically, and have renal impairment and osteosclerosis. The prognosis in the severe form of the disease is bad; many of these children die and those who do survive are mentally retarded and may also have irreversible cardiac and renal damage. There are suggestive but not conclusive data that this disorder is probably due to excessive vitamin-D ingestion either by the mother during pregnancy or by the infant in the form of vitamin-D supplemented cow's milk.[48]

Miscellaneous Causes of Hypercalcemia

Hypercalcemia may occur in hypophosphatasia, during the recovery phase of acute renal failure, and in generalized periostitis. In uremic patients on regular hemodialysis, calcium ion-exchange resins may also produce hypercalcemia.

Clinical Manifestations of Hypercalcemia

The level of serum calcium at which symptoms develop varies greatly in different individuals. Mild hypercalcemia is less likely to produce symptoms in primary hyperparathyroidism than in the other disorders that cause hypercalcemia. Patients with only slight elevations of serum calcium may be in great distress, whereas other patients with levels of 15 mg/100 ml or higher may be disturbed very little.

General Symptoms

These consist of easy fatigability, lethargy, weakness, headaches, and increased thirst. The acutely ill patient with hypercalcemia is generally severely dehydrated.

Renal Manifestations

The earliest renal manifestations are polyuria and impaired concentrating ability. Nephrolithiasis may result from the associated hypercalciuria and, in advanced hypercalcemic nephropathy, there is nephrocalcinosis and uremia.

The renal concentrating defect in both experimental animals and patients appears to depend more on the duration of the hypercalcemia and the degree of nephrocalcinosis than on the exact level of serum calcium. In experimental hypercalcemic nephropathy, the failure to achieve high medullary osmolality is probably due to a defect in sodium transport by the loops of Henle. The increased calcium-ion concentration may interfere with the energy systems that transport sodium across the renal tubular cell membranes by forming a tight complex (Ca-ATP) with intracellular ATP. This complex is a potent inhibitor of Na-K-ATPase, the enzyme responsible for ATP hydrolysis and for providing energy for sodium transport.

In metastatic renal calcification, the early destructive lesions develop in the medulla, the site of maximal concentration of calcium. Calcification first appears in the collecting ducts and in the ascending limb of Henle's loop, where it is initially confined to intracellular or intratubular sites. The cells become necrotic and calcified and then slough away, forming calcific casts, which obstruct the tubular lumen. As regenerating epithelial cells grow into or around the intraluminal casts, interstitial calcification appears. Intrarenal hydronephrosis due to tubular obstruction, a characteristic feature of hypercalcemic nephropathy, probably contributes to the azotemia that may develop before histologic evidence of glomerular damage. Another feature of hypercalcemic nephropathy is thickening and calcification of the basement membranes of proximal tubules. Infection and hypertension commonly complicate hypercalcemic nephropathy, and the affected kidneys often show evidence of chronic pyelonephritis and/or nephrosclerosis.[10]

Gastrointestinal

The most common gastrointestinal manifestations are anorexia, nausea, and vomiting, with weight loss and constipation. Patients with pancreatitis may have either elevated or depressed calcium levels because pancreatitis may develop secondary to the hypercalcemia, and as was noted earlier, severe pancreatitis may induce hypocalcemia (Table 6-2). The incidence of duodenal ulcer seems to be increased in primary hyperparathyroidism, probably because hypercalcemia stimulates gastric secretion.

Psychiatric

Hypercalcemic patients have a high incidence of psychiatric disturbances (see also Chapter 2). With lesser degrees of hypercalcemia, patients show only mild changes in affect and energy. Memory may be impaired. When the serum calcium exceeds 16 mg/100 ml, acute psychoses usually follow in the form of disorientation, delirium, confusion, paranoia, and hallucinations. Disturbances of consciousness—lethargy, drowsiness, stupor, and coma—develop with more severe degrees of hypercalcemia but may also be seen when the serum calcium is as low as 12–13 mg/100 ml, particularly in the elderly.

Neuromuscular

Hypercalcemia produces decreased neuromuscular excitability—muscle weakness, hypotonia, and depressed or absent tendon reflexes—as opposed to the increased excitability seen in hypocalcemia. About 50% of patients with hypercalcemic nephropathy have hypertension, but it is also encountered when there is no overt nephropathy. The blood pressure may return to normal when the hypercalcemia is corrected.

Metastatic Calcification

This is less common in primary hyperparathyroidism than in disorders such as the milk-alkali syndrome and vitamin D intoxication, in which higher serum phosphorus levels and alkalosis favor deposition of calcium salts in the tissues (Fig. 6-2). In hyperparathyroidism, metastatic calcification is most likely in the cornea, conjunctiva, or kidney.

"Band keratopathy," the corneal change associated with hypercalcemia, consists of hazy, grayish, granular epithelial and subepithelial opacities running concentrically with the limbus. The opacity is most dense at the periphery, fading out centrally, and it can often be detected only by slit-lamp examination. The conjunctival lesions appear as small glass-like particles within the conjunctiva of the palpebral fissure.

Metastatic calcification may involve many organs, but those most likely to be affected are the lungs, stomach, arteries, and myocardium.

Acute Hypercalcemic Crisis

When the serum calcium rises above 18 mg/100 ml, the patient's condition may deteriorate rapidly and he may die. The dominant clinical features are intractable vomiting, severe dehydration, and a disturbed mental state or impaired consciousness. Azotemia is present, and the

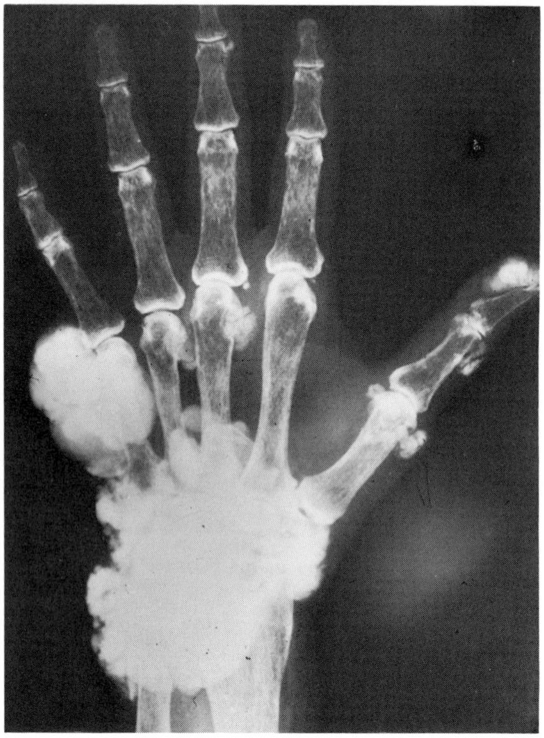

Fig. 6-2. Metastatic calcification in hypercalcemia. Periarticular soft tissue is calcified in hypercalcemia due to hypervitaminosis D.

serum phosphorus will rise to normal or elevated levels even if initially below normal. Death is associated with widespread tissue necrosis and metastatic calcification.

Laboratory Findings in Hypercalcemia

Serum phosphorus levels are usually normal or elevated but are occasionally diminished in vitamin D intoxication, multiple myeloma, hyperthyroidism, milk-alkali syndrome, and sarcoidosis. Low serum phosphorus levels are frequent in primary hyperparathyroidism and the hypercalcemia associated with neoplastic disorders, presumably because the tumor is producing some parathyroid hormone-like material. Serum alkaline phosphatase levels are nearly always elevated in patients with primary hypoparathyroidism who have clinically evident bone disease, and are frequently elevated in those with hypercalcemia secondary to neoplastic disorders and in sarcoidosis associated with granulomatous infiltration of the liver.

Whereas the plasma bicarbonate is normal or low in primary hyperparathyroidism, it is frequently elevated in patients with other kinds of hypercalcemia. The cause of this metabolic alkalosis is uncertain. In primary hyperparathyroidism, serum chloride levels nearly always exceed 102 mEq/liter, whereas, in hypercalcemia due to other causes, serum chloride levels are usually lower than 102 mEq/liter. The electrocardiogram of some patients with hypercalcemia shows shortening of the QT interval and depressed T waves.

Treatment of Hypercalcemia

The important therapeutic measures in the management of hypercalcemia can be summarized as follows:

1. Treatment of the underlying disease
2. Adequate hydration
3. Correction of associated disturbance such as hypokalemia, hypomagnesemia, acid-base disturbance, and renal failure
4. Restriction of calcium intake
5. Adrenal steroids
6. Management of the acute emergency

The treatment of the underlying disorder, such as primary hyperparathyroidism, is often all that is necessary. In mild cases of hypervitaminosis D, withdrawal of the vitamin and reduction of calcium intake frequently restores serum calcium levels to normal promptly. Similarly in adrenocortical insufficiency, corticosteroid replacement dramatically corrects the hypercalcemia; the hypercalcemia in thyrotoxicosis responds rapidly to appropriate antithyroid therapy. In malignancy, estrogens or androgens, which may have precipitated the hypercalcemia, should be withdrawn and appropriate chemotherapeutic measures instituted.

When the foregoing measures fail to alleviate hypercalcemia or when the severity of the clinical situation demands prompt and effective treatment, calcium intake should be restricted to 200 mg/day. Treatment with hydrocortisone, 40 mg every 8 hours, will nearly always correct the hypercalcemias of vitamin D intoxication and sarcoidosis within 10 days and is often effective in those associated with multiple myeloma, thyrotoxicosis, the milk-alkali syndrome, and immobilization. Occasionally, when this dose is ineffective, much larger doses of corticosteroids (e.g., 100 mg prednisone per day) will lower serum calcium levels. However, corticosteroids are usually ineffective in primary hyperparathyroidism and frequently fail to lower the serum calcium levels in neoplasia.

Management of the Acute Hypercalcemic Emergency

When an acute hypercalcemic crisis exists or threatens, the serum calcium levels should be lowered promptly in conjunction with measures to correct dehydration and associated electrolyte disturbances. The following measures can be used to lower serum calcium levels under these circumstances:

1. Oral or intravenous inorganic phosphate administration
2. Calcitonin administration
3. Infusion of sodium sulfate
4. Peritoneal dialysis
5. Cellulose phosphate administration
6. Mithramycin administration

Use of Inorganic Phosphate

Inorganic phosphate lowers serum calcium levels by diminishing bone resorption and by increasing bone formation, and perhaps by facilitating deposition of calcium salts in soft tissues. Thus it is contraindicated in hypervitaminosis D, in which it increases the danger of metastatic calcification.

Inorganic phosphate should be given orally rather than intravenously except in patients in coma or in those with intractable vomiting. Normocalcemia may be achieved within 24 hours, although the maximum effect of phosphate infusion may be delayed for as long as 5 days and some effects may persist for as long as 6–15 days. A suitable formula for intravenous use consists of 0.081 mole NaH_2PO_4 and 0.014 mole KH_2PO_4 dissolved in 1 liter of distilled water. This solution has a pH of 7.4 and an osmolality of 240 mOsm/kg, and each liter contains 100 mM (3.1 gm) of elemental P, 162 mEq Na and 19 mEq K. Five hundred milliliters of this solution may be infused over a 6–8 hour period. Only one infusion should be given in 24 hours and it is usually not necessary to continue treatment for more than 2 days.

A suitable solution for oral phosphate administration may be prepared as follows:

Na_2HPO_4 (anhydrous)	3.66 gm
$NaH_2PO_4 \cdot 2\ H_2O$	1 gm
Orange syrup	16 ml
Purified water to	60 ml

Sixty milliliters of this solution contains 1 gm of elemental P and the dosage is 20–60 ml every 8 hours. The larger doses may induce diarrhea or vomiting. One to three days generally elapse before there is any substantial drop in serum calcium levels, and normal serum calcium values are generally achieved within 1–10 days, after a cumulative dose of 1–20 gm phosphorus.

With this treatment, patients with poor renal function are particularly prone to marked hypocalcemia with tetany and, for this reason, the physician should exercise particular caution when giving phosphate to such patients. If the intravenous route is used, a dose of 0.5–1.0 gm P is given over a 24-hour period, and the amount of oral phosphate should not exceed 1 gm per day.

Calcitonin

This hormone lowers serum calcium levels in hypercalcemia due to vitamin D intoxication, parathyroid adenoma and cancer, idiopathic hypercalcemia, thyrotoxicosis, and neoplastic disorders.

Sodium Sulfate Infusions

These markedly increase urinary calcium excretion and lower serum calcium levels in a variety of hypercalcemic states. This form of therapy is less effective than phosphate administration and may produce hypomagnesemia and hypokalemia. Furthermore, the large quantities of infused water and sodium may precipitate heart failure and cause severe hypernatremia.

Peritoneal Dialysis

Dialysis has been used on several occasions for correction of hypercalcemia with good results.

Cellulose Phosphate

Oral cellulose phosphate in a dose of 10–20 gm/day lowers serum calcium and may be associated with fewer undesirable side effects than inorganic phosphate. Its interference with gastrointestinal absorption of calcium appears to contribute to its serum calcium-lowering effect.

Mithramycin

Small doses of this drug have been quite effective in the emergency treatment of hypercalcemia due to malignancy. This drug, an actinomycin-D-like antitumor agent, lowers serum calcium by inhibiting RNA synthesis, a process which is essential for bone resorption.

Idiopathic Hypercalciuria

Idiopathic hypercalciuria, the most common metabolic abnormality in patients with calcium stones, is present in 25 to 50% of those referred for investigation and treatment. Because the disorder is much more common in males, the incidence of hyperparathyroidism in hypercalciuric males with kidney stones is only 10%, but it is about 50% in hypercalciuric females with kidney stones. Generally, hypercalciuria is defined as a 24-hour urinary excretion of calcium greater than 300 mg in the male, and 250 mg in the female on unrestricted diets. The absence of hypercalcemia distinguishes idiopathic hypercalciuria from hyperparathyroidism.

Etiology

The cause of idiopathic hypercalciuria is obscure. It may be an inherited disorder because many of these patients have a strong family history of renal stones.

Since the calcium levels in the plasma ultrafiltrate are normal in idiopathic hypercalciuria, the hypercalciuria must be due to reduced renal tubular reabsorption of filtered calcium. The basis for the reduction in tubular calcium reabsorption is as yet unclear, but a popular theory is that it is secondary to overabsorption of dietary calcium. A primary defect in renal tubular function has also been postulated. Indeed, idiopathic hypercalciuria may represent several different pathogeneses.

Treatment

Urinary calcium excretion can usually be greatly reduced by 50 mg hydrochlorothiazide twice daily. This produces a sustained reduction in urinary calcium excretion and a sustained increase in urinary magnesium excretion and prevents the recurrence of calcium stones. Occasionally, patients presumed to have idiopathic hypercalciuria develop sustained hypercalcemia while taking thiazides. In our experience, these patients have parathyroid adenomas and previously undetected latent hyperparathyroidism.[47,52] The oral administration of inorganic phosphate (in amounts sufficient to supply 1.5–3.0 gm elemental phosphorus per day) is also effective in lowering urinary calcium excretion and preventing calcium stones.

Disorders of the Parathyroids

Hypoparathyroidism

The causes of hypoparathyroidism (Table 6-3) should be viewed in the context of the age of onset and the presence of associated disease. Transient hypoparathyroidism in the newborn may result from maternal hypercalcemia due to hyperparathyroidism or other disorders. In some instances, the mother's disease is first suspected when the newborn has hypocalcemic convulsions. Pregnancy in women with hyperparathyroidism carries a 25% risk of fetal death, and 50% of the liveborn babies develop tetany during the first 3 weeks of life. Physiologic hypoparathyroidism ap-

Table 6-3. Classification of Hypoparathyroidism

Neonatal
Physiologic
Maternal hyperparathyroidism
Maternal hypercalcemia of other etiologies
Idiopathic
Familial early-onset hypoparathyroidism
Congenital absence of parathyroids and thymus (III and IV pharyngeal pouch syndrome)
Idiopathic hypoparathyroidism
Surgical
After thyroid surgery
After parathyroid surgery
Pseudohypoparathyroidism and pseudo-pseudohypoparathyroidism

pears to be a feature of the neonatal period and may contribute to the hypocalcemic tetany seen in some newborn infants with high phosphate intake from cow's milk.

Idiopathic Hypoparathyroidism

Hereditary hypoparathyroidism begins in the first year of life and occurs predominantly in males. The infants tend to be mildly affected and generally survive, although they may die in convulsions. They do not have other congenital malformations or associated adrenal cortical insufficiency.

A distinctly different form of hypoparathyroidism in the newborn is due to congenital absence of the parathyroid and thymus glands. There appears to be no hereditary basis for these cases, which occur sporadically, with equal sex incidence. The term "III and IV pharyngeal pouch syndrome" has been suggested for the entity, but congenital malformations often involve other developmental areas as well. These infants, who usually die early, have a characteristic clinical picture consisting of failure to thrive from birth, hypocalcemic fits, intractable diarrhea, progressive lymphopenia, and susceptibility to infection.

Most idiopathic hypoparathyroidism begins later in life and some appears to be hereditary. Idiopathic hypoparathyroidism is frequently associated with adrenocortical insufficiency in children, and in some instances, this association has been familial. Many of these patients have cutaneous moniliasis. Idiopathic hypoparathyroidism and pernicious anemia may also exist on an autoimmune basis.

Surgical Hypoparathyroidism

Hypoparathyroidism occurs after thyroid or parathyroid surgery in up to 3% of cases[31] and probably is more common after complete thyroidectomy. It is temporary in one-third to one-half the cases, and these patients return to a euparathyroid state during the first or second year after surgery.

Clinical Manifestations

The symptoms and signs of hypoparathyroidism are largely attributable to hypocalcemia. However, these manifestations, which have been described earlier, may be absent despite marked hypocalcemia. In postoperative hypoparathyroidism, the patient may be symptom-free for as long as 30 years. Furthermore, symptoms of tetany after thyroid or parathyroid surgery may subside spontaneously after several weeks, even though serum calcium levels remain as low as they were in the symptomatic stage. Idiopathic hypoparathyroidism in children or adolescents may retard growth or cause dwarfism. The basal ganglia calcify in 14% of patients with idiopathic hypoparathyroidism.

Laboratory Findings

Hypocalcemia is accompanied by hyperphosphatemia, although in postoperative hypoparathyroidism the rise in serum phosphorus may be delayed for many days. Serum alkaline phosphatase levels are normal. The urinary excretions of calcium and phosphorus are both diminished, and the percentage of filtered phosphate which is reabsorbed by the renal tubules is abnormally high. Hypomagnesemia has been described.

The association of hypoparathyroidism and intestinal malabsorption of fat and/or vitamin B_{12} is well documented.[16] Treatment with parathormone or vitamin D corrects these abnormalities. Untreated patients may also have histamine-fast achlorhydria, but gastric acid secretion is restored when serum calcium levels are raised by calcium infusions or vitamin D administration. The electroencephalogram is frequently abnormal, thereby heightening the resemblance between hypoparathyroidism and idiopathic epilepsy.

Diagnosis

Hypoparathyroidism must be distinguished from the various causes of hypocalcemia and tetany, which have been discussed previously. In addition, these patients are frequently thought to have psychoneurosis, psychosis, or epilepsy, and the serum calcium should be measured routinely in these conditions as well as in all patients who have had a thyroidectomy. Recognition of both idiopathic and postoperative hypoparathyroidism is often delayed for years because of the complete absence of tetany.

Occasionally it is difficult to differentiate idiopathic steatorrhea from hypoparathyroidism. Although patients with hypocalcemia secondary to steatorrhea usually have normal or low serum phosphorus levels, occasionally they may have hyperphosphatemia. On the other hand, hypoparathyroid patients occasionally present with severe diarrhea and impaired absorption of vitamin B_{12} and fat. Consequently, it may sometimes be necessary to biopsy the small intestine to distinguish between these conditions.

Treatment

Parathyroid extract is ineffective when administered by mouth. Hence replacement hormone therapy is not practicable because it would require frequent intramuscular injections, which are inconvenient, painful, and prohibitively expensive.

The treatment of hypoparathyroidism with vitamin D, though effective, is hazardous because the patient's condition may so easily slip over into serious hypercalcemic toxicity.

In all forms of hypoparathyroidism, the physician attempts to correct the hypocalcemia by providing vitamin D and calcium supplements. The patient generally requires less vitamin D when he is taking large calcium supplements. Hence we frequently give 2–4 gm of elemental calcium each day. This is easily and inexpensively provided as an aqueous solution of calcium chloride, which contains 100 mg of elemental calcium per milliliter. The usual dose is 5–10 ml three or four times daily. The medication should be well diluted in water, milk, or fruit juice and, to minimize gastric upset, should not be taken on an empty stomach.

Patients who cannot tolerate calcium chloride may be given an equivalent amount of calcium in some other form. Calcium lactate powder contains 13% elemental calcium, and 4–8 gm four times a day supplies 2–4 gm of elemental calcium each day. The powder may be dissolved in hot water and then given in milk. Calcium lactate in pill form may be inefficiently absorbed. Effervescent calcium gluconate tablets, containing 500 mg of elemental calcium, are convenient but expensive.

Occasionally serum calcium levels can be maintained close to normal levels with calcium supplements alone, and if the patient's symptoms are not severe, the physician may withhold vitamin D for a week or two to determine the effect of the calcium supplements. This measure is especially useful after thyroid surgery when parathyroid deficiency may be only temporary.

The dose of vitamin D needed in hypoparathyroidism varies from 25,000 to 200,000 I.U. daily (0.625–5.0 mg), which is usually administered as vitamin D_2 (ergocalciferol). Many adults need only 50,000 I.U. of ergocalciferol daily (1.25 mg), and I prefer to start with this dose rather than the much larger amounts that are frequently recommended. Vitamin D acts slowly and should not be relied upon to treat severe acute tetany. If tetany is a problem initially, it can be relieved by intravenous calcium gluconate (see section on Treatment of Acute Hypocalcemic Emergency), and if need be, parathyroid extract can also be administered for a few days, although this is rarely necessary. Physicians commonly adjust vitamin D dosage too frequently during the first few weeks, not realizing that the maximum effect of a given dose of ergocalciferol may not be evident for 5–6 weeks. (Fig. 6-3). At best this practice lengthens the time necessary to establish maintenance requirements and at worst it increases the danger of vitamin D intoxication. If necessary, the dose of ergocalciferol may be in-

Fig. 6-3. **Hypoparathyroidism after thyroidectomy.** Effects of vitamin D_2 (ergocalciferol) and dihydrotachysterol on serum calcium and phosphorus levels are charted in a patient who experienced hypoparathyroidism after thyroidectomy. The important point is that the maximum serum-calcium raising effect of either agent was not achieved for at least 5½ weeks, and a similar period of time elapsed before these effects were dissipated.[11] (From Yendt, E. R. *International Encyclopedia of Pharmacology and Therapeutics*, Rasmussen, H., ed.[48] Reproduced with permission.)

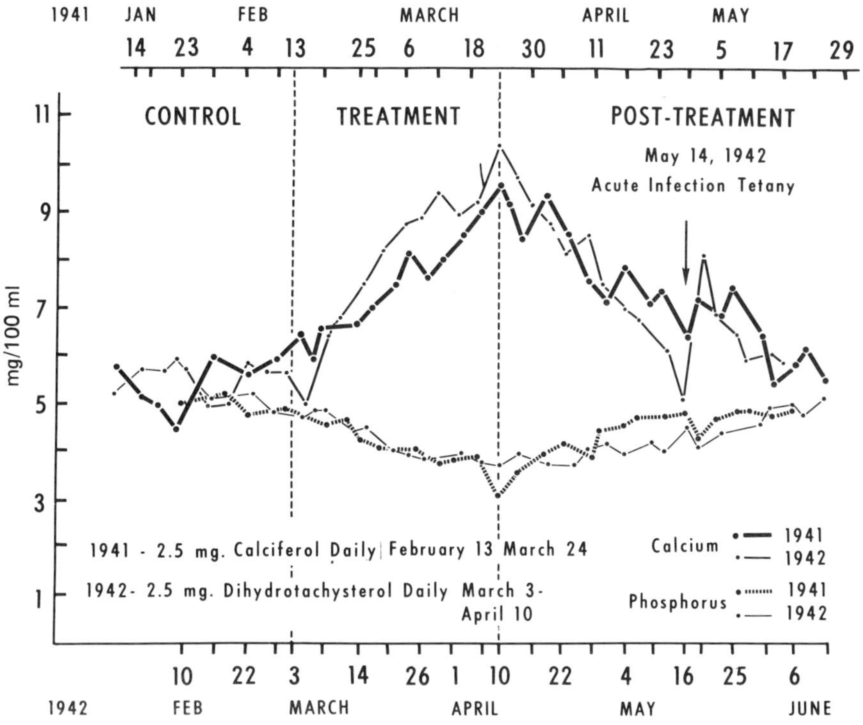

creased by 50,000 I.U. daily at 6- to 8-week intervals. Daily doses in excess of 100,000 I.U. are rarely necessary.

The effectiveness of treatment is gauged by frequent determinations of serum calcium. To minimize the degree of hypercalciuria, serum calcium levels should be maintained in the low normal range; such levels effectively alleviate symptoms. Some patients are quite comfortable even when slightly hypocalcemic (8.5–9.0 mg/100 ml), and if so, there is no harm in allowing this situation to continue. Serum phosphorus levels frequently remain in the high normal range or are slightly elevated even when serum calcium levels are normal. The practice of adjusting vitamin D dosage solely by measuring urinary calcium excretion with the Sulkowitch test has no place in modern therapeutics. Hypercalciuria may be marked when serum calcium is normal or even below normal; therefore, if one relies solely on the Sulkowitch test, it is difficult to know when the patient is being undertreated or overtreated.

Rarely, the physician encounters patients who are extremely resistant to conventional therapy and remain hypocalcemic even after immense doses of vitamin D, as high as 1.5 million units daily. Such vitamin D resistance is sometimes associated with magnesium deficiency and can be corrected by magnesium administration.[50] Another cause of vitamin D resistance may be defective synthesis of 25-hydroxycholecalciferol, the active metabolite of vitamin D; this was demonstrated in a hypoparathyroid patient who was markedly hypocalcemic despite large doses of vitamin D_2, vitamin D_3, dihydrotachysterol, and supplementary calcium. She had a prompt rise in serum calcium with doses of 25-hydroxycholecalciferol ranging from 1,200 to 2,000 units per day.

Hypervitaminosis D is a frequent complication of the treatment of hypoparathyroidism. Serious vitamin D toxicity is preventable, and most cases would not occur if the physician took proper precautions when prescribing pharmacologic doses. The following points are worthy of emphasis:

1. Patients for whom pharmacologic doses of vitamin D are prescribed should be warned of its dangers and told that they need close medical supervision as long as they receive this agent,

whether it be days, months, years, or decades. The physician must stress the importance of reporting unusual symptoms promptly.

2. All patients receiving pharmacologic doses of vitamin D should have blood-calcium determinations at least 3–4 times yearly during the entire period of treatment, and more frequently if dosage is being adjusted. As noted earlier, the practice of adjusting vitamin D dosage by assessing urinary calcium excretion with the Sulkowitch reaction is dangerous and has no place in modern practice.

3. Vitamin D intoxication may develop suddenly in patients who seemingly have been well controlled for years on a constant dose of vitamin D.

4. Even slight degrees of hypercalcemia due to vitamin D overdosage may induce serious toxicity and irreversible renal damage. In this regard it should be pointed out that the normal range for serum calcium is considerably narrower than the oft-quoted 9–11 mg/100 ml. One of our patients who developed severe irreversible renal damage never had a serum calcium greater than 11 mg/100 ml.

5. Patients recovering from an episode of vitamin D intoxication may be exquisitely sensitive to vitamin D for many months even though their serum calcium levels have returned to normal, or, in hypoparathyroid patients, are below normal. In the latter, it may be better to maintain normocalcemia by calcium supplements rather than reinstituting treatment with vitamin D at an early date. At this stage, they may also be quite sensitive to supplementary calcium.

Pseudohypoparathyroidism

This syndrome, also known as *Albright's hereditary osteodystrophy* and first described in 1942, consists of hypocalcemia and hyperphosphatemia usually associated with developmental skeletal abnormalities, mental retardation, and soft-tissue calcifications.[1] Albright and Reifenstein pointed out that the phosphaturic and hypercalcemic responses to exogenous parathyroid hormone were markedly diminished, and they postulated that the biochemical abnormalities were due to diminished end-organ sensitivity to the hormone. This syndrome proved to be the prototype of endocrine conditions that are due to end-organ unresponsiveness—e.g., nephrogenic diabetes insipidus. This resistance to parathyroid hormone has been repeatedly demonstrated, even when it is given by the subcutaneous or intramuscular routes for periods of up to 17 days. When given parathyroid hormone, patients with pseudohypoparathyroidism do not show the normal increase in the renal excretion of an important intracellular mediator of hormone action—3′5′-adenosine monophosphate (cyclic AMP). The parathyroid glands are either normal or hyperplastic in this disorder, and plasma levels of parathyroid hormone, as measured by the radioimmunoassay technique, are either normal or elevated. These observations also tend to confirm Albright's original hypothesis and suggest that there is no defect in the secretion of endogenous parathyroid hormone.

In pseudohypoparathyroidism, females outnumber males two to one, and at least one-third of the reported patients have this disorder on a genetic basis. Genetic transmission is probably through an X-linked dominant gene. These patients tend to be short, thickset, and obese. Abnormalities of the cranial and facial bones produce a round face, and the base of the nose may be flattened (Fig. 6-4). Brachydactyly, largely due to premature closure of the metacarpal and metatarsal epiphyses, is common. The first, fourth, and fifth metacarpals are commonly involved, but the second digits tend to be spared. The hands are involved more commonly than the feet. This feature is usually readily recognized when the fist is clenched, thereby causing a dimple over the head of the affected metacarpals (Albright's sign). Other commonly associated abnormalities are mental retardation, exostoses, widespread subcutaneous calcification and ossification, calcification of the basal ganglia, cataracts, and delayed dentition. There may be coexistent hypertension, and hypothyroidism due to TSH deficiency.

Although initially hypocalcemia was considered to be a fundamental feature of this syndrome, it is now clear that hypocalcemic and normocalcemic phases may occur at different times in the same patient. Hence, the diagnosis is made by demonstrating the characteristic signs. Care must be taken not to confuse this disorder with Turner's syndrome, which may be associated with many features of pseudohypoparathyroidism, including resistance to parathyroid extract. Other developmental disorders that may simulate some of the abnormal features of pseudohypoparathyroidism are myositis ossificans progressiva, familial brachydactyly, epiphyseal dysplasia, and hereditary multiple exostoses. Refractoriness to exogenous parathyroid hormone is an important diagnostic test. Because it is frequently difficult to interpret the response to a single dose of parathyroid hormone injected intravenously (Ellsworth-Howard test),[2] the response to repeated subcutaneous or intramuscular doses of the hormone at 6-hour intervals (600–800 units per day) is greatly preferred as a diagnostic procedure. In patients with postoperative or idiopathic hypoparathyroidism, repeated injections will promptly double the 24-hour urinary phosphorus excretion, serum phosphorus levels will fall to normal, and serum calcium returns to normal. However, the speed of the latter response is variable; it usually occurs within 3 days but at times may be delayed for as long as one week. In pseudohypoparathyroidism, the phosphaturic response, if any, is extremely small and there is little, if any, change in serum phosphorus levels; the maximum reported rise in serum calcium is 1.5 mg/100 ml, and in most patients, the rise does not exceed 0.6 mg/100 ml.

Fortunately patients with this disorder respond to pharmacologic doses of vitamin D in much the same manner as patients with true hypoparathyroidism.

Pseudo-Pseudohypoparathyroidism

The term, pseudo-pseudohypoparathyroidism, was also introduced by Albright *et al.* in 1952 to describe patients who were distinguishable from those with pseudohypoparathyroidism only because they had normal serum levels of calcium and inorganic phosphate. Both pseudohypoparathyroidism and pseudo-pseudohypoparathyroidism have also been observed within the same families. For this reason, pseudo-pseudohypoparathyroidism can be regarded as a modified

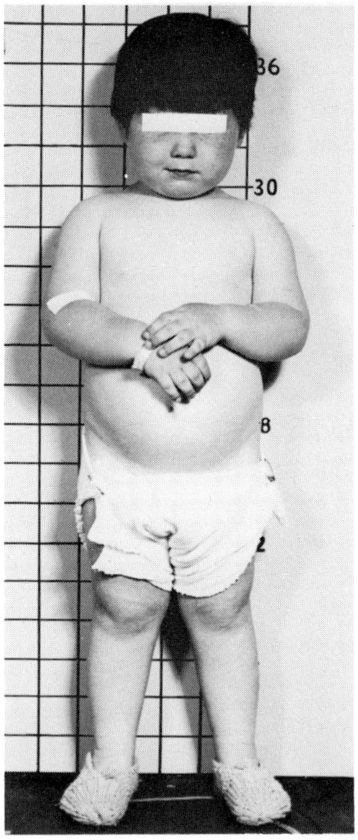

Fig. 6-4. Pseudohypoparathyroidism. Note thickset obese body habitus, round face, and short metacarpals in this 6-year-old girl.

expression of the same genetic disorder as pseudohypoparathyroidism. The student need only remember that "pseudo-pseudo" is "pseudo" with normal serum calcium.

Hyperparathyroidism

In *primary* hyperparathyroidism, the normal feedback control of parathyroid-hormone secretion is lost and excessive hormone production continues despite elevated plasma-calcium levels.

In *secondary* hyperparathyroidism, which is encountered in such conditions as chronic renal insufficiency, vitamin D deficiency or resistance, and pregnancy, chronic hypocalcemia is a stimulus to increased secretion of parathyroid hormone, and associated hyperplasia of the parathyroid glands. However, the hypocalcemia may not always be evident because the parathyroid response may have effectively corrected it. The degree and duration of secondary hyperparathyroidism is usually not great enough to produce serious clinical consequences, except in chronic renal insufficiency, in which it may present a serious therapeutic challenge. Secondary hyperparathyroidism does not generally lead to hypercalcemia because the normal feedback-control mechanism regulates hormone secretion. Occasionally, however, normal feedback control is lost and hypercalcemia does develop, perhaps because of adenoma formation within the hyperplastic glands—a situation referred to as "tertiary" hyperparathyroidism. In chronic renal disease, however, the occasional occurrence of hypercalcemia is usually related to the enormous increase in cells in the hyperplastic parathyroid tissue. Even though the secretion rate of each cell is reduced to the minimum, the total output of parathyroid hormone may be greatly increased.

Primary Hyperparathyroidism

Etiology and Pathology

Single *adenomas* of the parathyroid glands account for more than 80% of reported cases of primary hyperparathyroidism;[5] approximately 5% of these patients have multiple adenomas. Adenomas involve the inferior parathyroid more frequently than the superior, and approximately 10% of them occur in aberrant locations in the mediastinum or within thyroid tissue; they may be very small, barely larger than a normal parathyroid gland.

Hyperplasia of all four parathyroid glands accounts for 10% of primary hyperparathyroidism. This hyperplasia is of two types: (1) primary *wasserhelle* (water-clear) cell hyperplasia, a rare condition, in which the cells are large, clear, and hypernephroma-like; and (2) more commonly, primary chief-cell hyperplasia, in which the hyperplastic glands contain numerous small nodules of small or large chief cells. Chief-cell hyperplasia cannot be distinguished from parathyroid adenomas in the gross, and even on histologic examination, it may not be possible to differentiate the two entities, except when a compressed rim of normal or atrophic parathyroid tissue surrounds the adenoma. Even this criterion is open to misinterpretation because in nodular chief-cell hyperplasia, compressed, relatively less hyperplastic tissue may closely simulate such a remnant, and more often than not, the rim of normal tissue is lacking around a single adenoma. In view of these difficulties and the higher incidence of chief-cell hyperplasia in recently reported series, it is probable that, in the past, many instances of chief-cell hyperplasia have been misdiagnosed as single or multiple adenomas. It has been said that the identification of at least one normal parathyroid excludes any form of hyperplasia, but in some instances of primary chief-cell hyperplasia, one parathyroid gland is of normal size.

Hyperfunctioning *parathyroid carcinoma* is a rare cause of hyperparathyroidism; only 46 cases have been reported in the literature. All of these tumors had metastasized or were invading contiguous structures.

There are several syndromes in which hyperparathyroidism is associated with other diseases. In one of these, multiple endocrine adenomatosis, hyperparathyroidism coexists with adenomas of the pituitary and pancreatic islets and often is associated with severe peptic ulceration and sometimes with adrenal tumors as well. Hyperparathyroidism also is associated with pheochromocytoma and medullary thyroid carcinoma.[42] In the latter syndrome, hyperparathyroidism is by far the least frequent manifestation of affected families. Each of these entities may occur on either a sporadic or familial basis and, in the latter event, are inherited as genetically distinct autosomal dominants. In both syndromes, the parathyroid lesion is usually primary chief-cell hyperplasia. In the familial forms, one endocrine gland appears to be predominantly involved in each kindred, but associated endocrinopathies are frequent. Familial hyperparathyroidism that is not associated with other endocrine abnormalities has also been reported; once again, the pattern of inheritance appears to be an autosomal dominant with incomplete penetrance. There is a high incidence of multiple gland involvement and chief-cell hyperplasia although, in certain families, the lesion appears to be a single parathyroid adenoma. These cases may be examples of incomplete expression of the syndrome of multiple endocrine adenomatosis. In primary hyperparathyroidism, there also appears to be an increased incidence of papillary thyroid adenocarcinoma and thyroid lesions in general.

Clinical Manifestations

The clinical picture of primary hyperparathyroidism is exceedingly variable but, in most patients, is related to renal calculi, skeletal disease, or hypercalcemia. The symptoms and signs of hypercalcemia have already been described. Occasionally the disease may present in a variety of other forms, or symptoms may be absent and the diagnosis may be made fortuitously.

Renal Calculi. Over 75% of patients with primary hyperparathyroidism seek medical attention because of urinary stones or renal calcifications. Many of these patients have no other clinical manifestations. The incidence of hyperparathyroidism in all patients with renal calculi is difficult to determine but has been estimated at 1–3%. Patients referred to "stone clinics" (usually with multiple or recurrent stones) have a much higher incidence of hyperparathyroidism—approximately 10–15%. The stones may be composed of calcium oxalate, calcium phosphate, or a mixture of these two substances. If the stones have been complicated by urinary tract infection, the outer layers of the stone may consist of triple phosphate. Many patients have a history of multiple stones, and only one kidney may be involved.

Skeletal Disease. The incidence of clinical, radiologic, or laboratory evidence of bone disease varies in different reports, but probably, of the patients now being diagnosed, only one-third or fewer have such evidence.

The classic form of bone disease in hyperparathyroidism is *osteitis fibrosa cystica generalisata.* Histologically, this lesion is characterized by bone resorption, invasion of haversian canals and marrow spaces by a highly cellular fibrous tissue, and increase in Howship's lacunae containing osteoclasts. Radiologically, these patients have multiple cysts or giant cell tumors (osteoclastomas), diminished bone density, pathologic fractures, erosion of the inner and outer tables of the skull, and subperiosteal resorption. However, the only roentgenographic manifestation of bone disease may be giant cell tumors, which produce discrete, punched-out areas, particularly in the jaw and facial bones.

Subperiosteal resorption, which is best demonstrated in the middle phalanges of the hands (particularly on their radial aspects), is almost invariably present when there is roentgenographic evidence of generalized osteitis fibrosa (Fig. 6-5). For practical purposes, these changes can be ac-

Fig. 6-5. Subperiosteal resorption in hyperparathyroidism. Such resorption is pathognomonic. The frayed, irregular periosteal surface of the bone is particularly marked on radial aspect of middle phalanx of second finger. Punched-out lesions seen at the base of this phalanx and in terminal phalanx of third finger are due either to cyst formation or osteoclastomas. The cortices of all phalanges are abnormally thin.

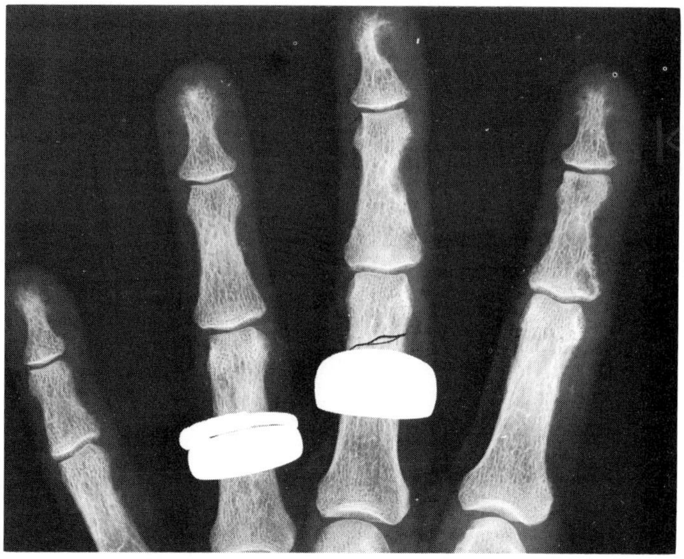

cepted as diagnostic of primary or secondary hyperparathyroidism and may be the only radiologic evidence of bone disease. The articulations of the distal end of the clavicle, the symphysis pubis, and the sacroiliac joints may also show early subperiosteal cortical erosion.

Disappearance of the lamina dura, the cortical bone lining the tooth sockets, is a common radiographic abnormality, but this sign is not pathognomonic of hyperparathyroidism because it may also be found in osteomalacia and pyorrhea. Furthermore, the lamina dura may be intact when there is clear-cut subperiosteal resorption in the phalanges. At times the radiographic picture in hyperparathyroidism is indistinguishable from osteoporosis, but in such cases, hyperparathyroidism may be an aggravating factor rather than the primary cause of the disease.

The principal clinical manifestation of osteitis fibrosa—bone pain—may be either local or diffuse. In severe lesions, the bones become tender to palpation and the pain may become incapacitating. Pathologic fractures may occur through areas weakened by cysts, tumors, or generalized resorption. Patients with less evident radiographic bone disease may be symptom-free.

Signs and Symptoms. The signs and symptoms of hypercalcemia may be associated with other manifestations of hyperparathyroidism and are found in approximately one-third of patients. They may provide the sole clue to diagnosis in 7–10% of patients; for example, 10–30% of these patients have duodenal ulcer. An increased incidence of pancreatitis has been reported in hyperparathyroidism, particularly in patients with acute hyperparathyroidism and markedly elevated serum calcium levels. It has been postulated that the high calcium content of pancreatic juice accelerates the calcium-dependent conversion of trypsinogen to trypsin, with resultant inflammatory changes in the pancreas. Other important clinical features of hyperparathyroidism include manifestations of arthritis, including the syndrome of pseudogout and muscle weakness and atrophy simulating myopathy.

Parathyroid Crisis. "Parathyroid crisis" describes the symptom complex associated with acute and progressive hypercalcemia. This complication is occasionally precipitated by hemorrhage into or infarction of a parathyroid adenoma. This complication constitutes a serious medical and surgical emergency; the overall mortality in 82 cases reported in the English literature was 57%.

Hypocalcemia and Tetany. This rare complication of hyperparathyroidism results from infarction of a parathyroid adenoma.

Laboratory Findings

Hypercalcemia is the most consistent biochemical abnormality in hyperparathyroidism. However, the degree of hypercalcemia may be slight, and as many as one-third of such patients have serum calcium levels persistently below 11 mg/100 ml. With more precise methods of calcium determination, we have defined normal ranges for serum calcium which are much narrower than the previously accepted range of 9–11 mg/100 ml, and we can now detect minor deviations from that range. EDTA photometric techinques, flame-photometry techniques that use the blue calcium emission rather than the primary calcium emission in the red, which is subject to sodium interference, or atomic absorption spectrophotometric techniques, which eliminate protein and phosphate interference have all proved satisfactory. With these methods, the upper normal limit for serum calcium is in the neighborhood of 10.3–10.5 mg/100 ml. Furthermore, serum calcium levels are slightly lower in women so that values in the high normal range for men may actually indicate hypercalcemia in women[51] (Fig. 6-6).

Although *normocalcemic* hyperparathyroidism has been reported, many of these patients probably had mild degrees of hypercalcemia that were undetected because inadequate methods were used to measure calcium or an excessively wide range of normal was accepted. Of 40 such cases studied by the new techniques, all but one had persistent, nonfluctuating hypercalcemia despite "normal" serum calcium values found elsewhere. Notwithstanding these objections, true normocalcemia may exist in patients with proven primary hyperparathyroidism in the absence of associated

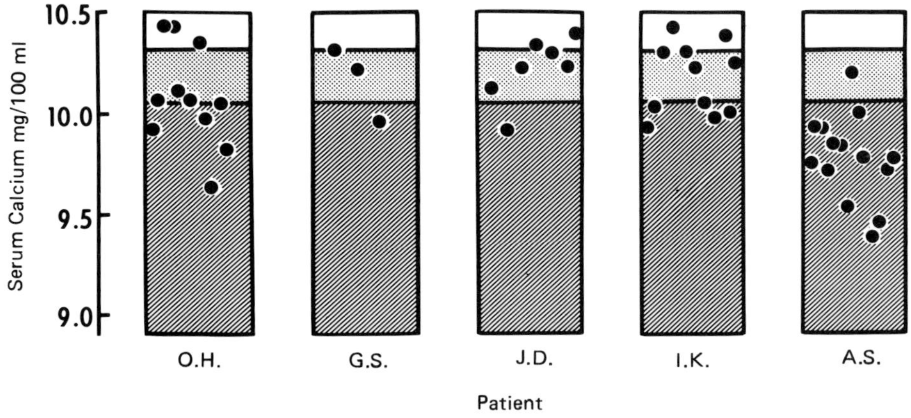

Fig. 6-6. Serum calcium values in primary hyperparathyroidism. The black dots in each block are individual total serum-calcium values obtained in each of five women with proven parathyroid adenomas. Solid lines at top of the two cross-hatched areas indicate upper limit of normal for adult population of mixed sex (10.3 mg/100 ml) and a lower upper normal limit for adult females (10.05 mg/100 ml). Unless we had recognized that women have their own distinctive normal range, these patients would all have been considered to have normal calcium levels, whereas four of the five had hypercalcemia.

conditions such as intestinal malabsorption, pancreatitis, nephrosis, infarction of a parathyroid adenoma, or a high phosphorus intake, which could have lowered serum calcium levels. Some of these patients have had elevated levels of ionized calcium, ultrafiltrable calcium, or circulating parathyroid hormone in their plasma.

Hypophosphatemia commonly accompanies the hypercalcemia, but serum phosphorus levels may be normal or elevated in the presence of associated conditions such as renal insufficiency or acromegaly. In the absence of such associated disorders, serum phosphorus levels are normal in approximately 20–50% of patients with hyperparathyroidism, but the mean serum phosphorus level rarely exceeds 3.5 mg/100 ml.

Serum alkaline phosphatase levels usually correlate well with clinical and/or radiographic evidence of bone disease.

Serum chloride levels almost always exceed 100 mEq/liter and are above normal in approximately one-quarter of these patients. This point may aid in distinguishing hyperparathyroid patients from those with hypercalcemia due to other causes. Hypomagnesemia sufficient to produce symptoms and to require magnesium replacement is occasionally encountered, especially after parathyroidectomy in patients with overt skeletal disease.

Although renal function may be moderately or seriously impaired in patients with primary hyperparathyroidism, most patients do not show such impairment, even those with long histories. Fewer than 10% of our patients had elevated serum creatinine levels.[51]

The urinary excretion of calcium is usually elevated but rarely exceeds 600 mg in 24 hours. Hypercalciuria is absent in almost one-quarter of the patients with good renal function and in a higher proportion of those with renal insufficiency.

Special Tests

Radioimmunoassay of Circulating Human Parathyroid Hormone (PTH). Assay of human PTH has proved to be unusually difficult because of the technical problems encountered in preparing antibody. Circulating human PTH has been successfully measured in only a few research laboratories.[4] Berson and Yalow, who first successfully adapted the immunoassay technique to the measurement of human PTH, frequently could not detect PTH in euparathyroid subjects and found a considerable overlap between euparathyroid and hyperparathyroid serums. Using a modified technique and a different antibody, Reiss and Canterbury[38] clearly separated euparathyroid from hyperparathyroid serums. These investigators also differentiated adenoma and primary chief-cell hyperplasia on the basis of suppression of serum PTH levels by calcium infusion in the latter condition. Immunoassay of PTH in multiple blood samples obtained by selective catheterization of the major veins draining the neck and thorax has been used in the preoperative localization of parathyroid tumors. Levels of immunoassayable PTH are also elevated in hypercalcemia due to malignant disorders and in secondary hyperparathyroidism associated with chronic renal insufficiency.

Corticosteroid Test. Changes in serum calcium following the administration of cortisone (50 mg every 8 hours for 10 days) or hydrocortisone (40 mg every 8 hours for 10 days) may help to differentiate hyperparathyroidism from other causes of hypercalcemia.[9] The serum calcium usually returns to normal in sarcoidosis and vitamin D poisoning and often does so in multiple myeloma and cancer. Rarely in sarcoidosis, cortisone either may not correct the hypercalcemia or may take an unusually long time to do so. A response to corticosteroid has also been observed in the milk-alkali syndrome, and in the hypercalcemia associated with immobilization and thyrotoxicosis. Patients with hyperparathyroidism usually show no response to corticosteroid administration.

Percentage of Tubular Reabsorbed Phosphate (%TRP). The percentage of filtered phosphate reabsorbed by the renal tubules largely depends upon the dietary phosphate intake; reported normal ranges on ad libitum diets vary from 78% to 97%. However, %TRP cannot be relied upon to differentiate hyperparathyroidism from other disorders associated with hypercalcemia because low values are not uncommon in the latter and in normocalcemic patients with kidney stones, renal insufficiency, osteomalacia, renal tubular disorders, and gout.

Phosphate Deprivation. Occasionally, restriction of the daily phosphate intake to 350 mg or less for at least 3 days will be followed by a rise in serum calcium levels and may aid in unmasking hyperparathyroidism with initially normal or borderline serum calcium values. The test is most useful in patients with azotemia and phosphate retention. Phosphate deprivation can be enhanced by administering aluminium hydroxide or carbonate gels, which decrease the gastrointestinal absorption of phosphate. During this test, the diet must be normal in calcium content and provide adequate calories.

Parathyroid Hormone Infusion Test. In normal subjects, % TRP tends to fall more than 10% below control values after the intravenous administration of PTH, whereas there is less change in %TRP in many patients with hyperparathyroidism who presumably are relatively refractory to exogenous hormone. However, the usefulness of these observations in diagnosis is limited because of the marked overlap between euparathyroid and hyperparathyroid individuals.

Calcium Infusion Test. This procedure assumes that elevation of the blood calcium inhibits parathyroid secretion in normal subjects but does not do so in primary hyperparathyroidism, in which the normal feedback control of parathyroid secretion is lost. Parathyroid hormone secretion has been assessed indirectly by measuring changes in urinary phosphate excretion or the tubular reabsorption of phosphate. In this test, with the subjects on a constant diet, elemental calcium (as calcium glucoheptonate), 15 mg/kg body weight, is infused over a 4-hour period, and the 24-hour urinary phosphate excretion is compared on the preinfusion day, the infusion day, and the postinfusion day. Normally, urinary phosphorus excretion decreases 21% or more on the day of the calcium infusion with a "rebound" rise of 12% or more on the day after the infusion. This test does not differentiate primary hyperparathyroidism from other causes of hypercalcemia, which also may show abnormal responses. Furthermore, it is of doubtful value in detecting hyperparathyroidism in persons with normal or borderline serum calcium levels because, although the test is nearly always positive in hyperparathyroidism, there is a high incidence of false positive tests in euparathyroid patients with kidney stones.

Diagnosis

There are three important steps in the diagnosis of hyperparathyroidism:

1. Keep a high index of suspicion in a wide variety of clinical disorders. The serum calcium should be determined routinely in patients with calcium-containing renal stones, nephrocalcinosis, generalized skeletal rarefaction, peptic ulcer, pancreatitis, renal insufficiency of uncertain cause, generalized weakness, and in relatives of patients with multiple endocrine adenomatosis and primary parathyroid hyperplasia. This practice is also indicated in patients with vague symptoms suggesting psychoneurosis.
2. Establish the presence of hypercalcemia.
3. Demonstrate that the hypercalcemia is due to hyperparathyroidism.

Although some writers have stressed the frequency of intermittent hypercalcemia in hyperparathyroidism, our own experience suggests that intermittent hypercalcemia is a rare manifestation of hyperparathyroidism. Nonetheless, when the physician suspects the disorder, he should do at least three determinations of serum calcium before he dismisses the diagnosis of primary hyperparathyroidism.

The importance of being able to establish the presence of minimal degrees of hypercalcemia has already been stressed. If serum calcium levels are normal or borderline, the indirect parameters of parathyroid function such as %TRP, calcium infusion, and the PTH infusion test are as likely to mislead as to help. Measurement of plasma ultrafiltrable or ionized calcium occasionally helps in these difficult diagnostic problems. In azotemic patients or those who have had excessively high phosphate intakes, reduction of dietary phosphate may induce a rise in serum calcium levels. When the technique becomes generally available, radioimmunoassay for PTH may greatly assist in diagnosis, but its role cannot be assessed with any accuracy as yet.

Careful clinical and laboratory evaluation usually enables the physician to differentiate hyperparathyroidism from other diseases associated with hypercalcemia. When he cannot, the patient's response to corticosteroids may help him to arrive at a final diagnosis. He should remember that primary hyperparathyroidism is most unlikely when the mean serum phosphorus level is above 3.5 mg/100 ml in the absence of renal insufficiency or acromegaly, or when serum chloride levels are below 102 mEq/liter. The diagnosis may be particularly difficult when hyperparathyroidism coexists with other disorders that cause hypercalcemia, such as sarcoidosis or hyperthyroidism.

The possible diagnosis of primary hyperparathyroidism is considered most often in patients with calcium-containing kidney stones, and it may be difficult to differentiate this disorder from idiopathic hypercalciuria (see the discussion earlier in this chapter).

Treatment

The only effective treatment of hyperparathyroidism, excision of the hyperfunctioning parathyroid tissue, is indicated in all symptomatic patients unless there are clear contraindications to operation. Opinion differs as to whether surgery should be performed on asymptomatic patients with mild hypercalcemia and normal renal function. However, since nearly all patients with hyperparathyroidism have evidence of abnormal skeletal metabolism, an operation seems indicated in, at least, the young and middle-aged patients who fall into this category. As a general rule, exploration should be done only when the diagnosis of hyperparathyroidism has been firmly established before operation. If the preoperative diagnosis is in doubt, exploration should be delayed until the patient has been evaluated by experienced physicians who have access to the refined laboratory techniques necessary to confirm this diagnosis. If the diagnosis is still in doubt after such evaluation, the gravity of the clinical situation may warrant an exploratory procedure.

Parathyroid surgery should be performed only by surgeons who are experienced in this procedure, because it may be exceedingly difficult to locate normal and abnormal parathyroid tissue.

Fewer than 15% of patients have a palpable neck mass which proves to be an enlarged parathyroid gland at surgery. As has been noted earlier, parathyroid adenomas have been localized before operation by measuring blood PTH levels by radioimmunoassay while the main veins draining the neck and thorax are catheterized.

During the exploration, the surgeon must attempt to identify all four parathyroid glands before he excises any tissue. Grossly enlarged glands are removed entirely, but if all the glands are enlarged a small remnant of one should be left behind. If all four parathyroid glands are identified and appear to be normal, a small piece of each should be examined microscopically. Because it may be difficult to distinguish parathyroid tissue from small lymph nodes and collections of fat, all excised tissue should be identified by frozen section.

At operation, the location of a parathyroid adenoma may be facilitated by noting the relative size of the inferior thyroid arteries (these may be distinctly larger on the side of an adenoma), and by following a sizeable branch of the inferior thyroid artery on the involved side (these branches, when followed, may often lead to the adenoma, including those located in ectopic sites). Adenomas in the mediastinum can usually be located by exploring the anterior superior mediastinum through a neck incision; sternotomy is only rarely necessary. Occasionally the serum calcium returns to normal after an unsuccessful exploration, presumably because the procedure interrupted the vascular supply to an adenoma. In view of this, at the time of an unsuccessful neck exploration it is probably wise to defer sternotomy in the hope that such a response will occur. On rare occasions, parathyroid adenomas occur deep within the thyroid gland or in a very deep fold of the thyroid capsule; consequently subtotal thyroidectomy is probably warranted if no enlarged parathyroid glands are found after a thorough exploration.

The high incidence of persistent hypercalcemia in patients who had two abnormal glands thought to be adenomas suggests that many of them had primary chief-cell hyperplasia rather than adenomas.

Occasionally primary hyperparathyroidism should be treated medically when thorough exploration of the neck and mediastinum has failed to locate hyperfunctioning parathyroid tissue. Long-term phosphate administration may alleviate symptoms, lower serum calcium levels, return elevated serum alkaline phosphatase levels to normal and produce radiologic healing of bone lesions.

Postoperative Management. After successful parathyroidectomy, serum calcium levels usually fall to normal within 24 hours. Patients without clinical or radiographic evidence of bone disease may subsequently develop mild and transient hypocalcemia for a few days, but associated symptoms are usually slight or absent, and usually they do not need vitamin D or calcium salts. The plasma calcium usually falls to its lowest level 4–10 days after operation. More severe and persistent hypocalcemia in patients without bone disease is probably due to temporary or permanent hypoparathyroidism and should be treated as such. Patients with severe bone disease are subject to marked and sustained hypocalcemia in the postoperative period and may require large amounts of calcium salts and vitamin D for weeks or months. Large doses of vitamin D may be particularly necessary in the postoperative management of patients with renal insufficiency because, in them, intestinal absorption of calcium may be impaired.

Serum phosphorus levels often remain low for long periods after operation. Hyperphosphatemia in the postoperative period, in the absence of renal failure, suggests temporary or permanent hypoparathyroidism. Serious magnesium deficiency may be encountered after an operation, even when preoperative serum magnesium levels were normal, especially in patients with bone disease. The likely explanation of this is that magnesium was sequestrated in the healing skeleton. Acute pancreatitis may also develop in the postoperative period.

Diseases of Bone

Osteoporosis

Definition and Pathology

The essential feature of osteoporosis, sometimes called "osteopenia," is a reduction in bone mass. In compact bone, this change is characterized by increased porosity due to widening of resorption cavities. The process begins on the endosteal surface of cortical bone and eventually leads to progressive enlargement of the bone marrow cavity and cortical thinning. In cancellous bone, the trabeculae are diminished in number and thickness (Fig. 6-7). On light microscopy, osteoporotic bone appears to be mineralized normally, and its chemical composition is normal. With advancing age, an increasing number of osteocyte lacunae are found to be devoid of osteocytes and some haversian canals, together with their blood vessels, become obliterated by basophilic calcified material. These changes, which are present in all aging bone, do not appear to bear any special relationship to osteoporosis.

Some of the secondary osteoporoses may show additional histologic abnormalities when they are associated with changes in the rate of bone turnover. In Cushing's syndrome, in which bone turnover is markedly reduced, there is diminished osteoblastic activity. In hyperthyroidism, on the other hand, bone turnover is accelerated and the osteoid seams may be wider than normal. This reflects an increased rate of bone formation in response to an increased rate of bone resorption. Histologically, hyperthyroid patients may have osteitis fibrosa resembling that seen in hyperparathyroidism.

Classification of the Osteoporoses

Osteoporosis is not a specific or single disease entity but is the end result of a variety of factors

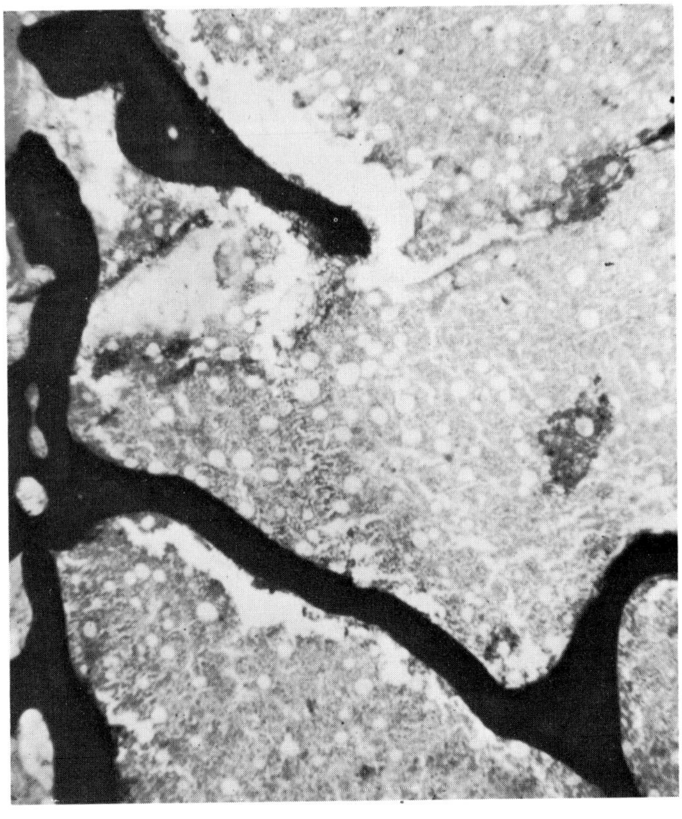

Fig. 6-7. Histopathology of undecalcified bone in osteoporosis. Mineralized areas of bone stain dark brown or black. Trabeculae are completely mineralized but are abnormally thin and diminished in number. Von Kossa stain.

Table 6-4. Causes of Osteoporosis

Diffuse osteoporoses
Primary
Senile
Postmenopausal
Idiopathic
Secondary
Steroid therapy
Cushing's syndrome
Hyperthyroidism
Intestinal malabsorption
Rheumatoid arthritis
Long-term heparin administration
Hepatic cirrhosis
Hypogonadism
Vitamin C deficiency
Gastrectomy
Local osteoporoses
Immobilization
Denervation
Fracture
Inflammation
Trauma

and/or diseases that act on the skeleton either singly or in combination. Table 6-4 gives a classification of the osteoporoses. In the primary osteoporoses—the senile, postmenopausal, and idiopathic varieties—there is no evidence of other underlying disease. The term "idiopathic" refers to those patients who have primary osteoporosis that is not senile or postmenopausal. Juvenile osteoporosis, an extremely rare form of idiopathic osteoporosis, occurs in children who are apparently perfectly well until just before puberty, when they present, after minimal trauma, with fractures of one or more long bones.

Pathogenesis of the Primary Osteoporoses

All forms of osteoporosis represent a long-sustained imbalance between bone formation and resorption in favor of resorption, regardless of the rate of either process.[46] The degree of imbalance need only be slight because a calcium loss of 30 mg/day for 30 years will produce clinically detectable osteoporosis. Such imbalance can occur at any rate of bone remodeling and can develop in a variety of ways: (1) diminished bone formation, resorption being unchanged; (2) diminished formation and increased resorption; or (3) normal formation with increased resorption. In addition, formation and resorption could both be diminished or increased but to an unequal degree favoring resorption. Bone biopsies from patients with senile and postmenopausal osteoporosis studied by quantitative microradiography and tetracycline labeling indicate that bone resorption is usually increased and bone formation is either normal or reduced.

Age, Sex, and Race

A decline in bone mass appears to be an inevitable and universal accompaniment of aging. Bone mass increases from childhood to maturity, remains steady throughout the third decade, and thereafter begins to decline. Whether clinically significant osteoporosis develops as a result of this process depends upon the maximum bone mass achieved at maturity and upon the rate of decline.

Race appears to affect one or both of these factors because Negroes tend to have a greater bone mass at any age than whites, and have a lower incidence of hip fractures resulting from osteoporosis. Anglo-Saxon women have a higher incidence of osteoporosis than other Caucasians and more than Puerto Ricans living in Puerto Rico.

Women not only have a smaller bone mass at maturity, but the decline in bone mass begins earlier and proceeds faster than in men, particularly after the menopause. These findings account for the higher incidence of osteoporosis in women —30% have this disorder after age 60, compared to 15% of men in that age group. Others have found an even higher incidence of osteoporosis; Smith and Rizek found vertebral atrophy in nearly 50% of women over age 45. The cause of this age-related loss of bone mass is unknown but the slow decline in physical activity with age, and the low level of physical activity in modern society may be important factors.

Gonadal Hormone Deficiency

Skeletal mass declines sharply and the incidence of osteoporosis increases after the menopause. Although the changes could be due to aging alone, there appears to be a much better relationship between diminished bone mass and years after the menopause, than age per se. The more rapid decline in bone mass after the menopause is probably related to estrogen deficiency and can be slowed or prevented by estrogen therapy.

Calcium Deficiency

It has been proposed that calcium deficiency with a secondary increase in bone resorption is a major etiologic factor in osteoporosis. However, no one has demonstrated a difference between the age-related loss of bone in populations with high and low dietary calcium intakes.[14]

Pathogenesis of the Secondary Osteoporoses

Cushing's Syndrome and Steroid Therapy

Patients with Cushing's syndrome and those receiving steroid therapy have a high incidence of osteoporosis, which is predominantly due to a marked impairment of bone formation. On histologic examination, the bones of these patients have diminished numbers of osteoblasts without any obvious increase in osteoclastic activity.[40]

Hyperthyroidism

Hyperthyroidism sometimes produces extremely severe osteoporosis that is due to increased bone resorption; at times this may be a major clinical manifestation of that disorder. When the other manifestations of hyperthyroidism are minimal, the true diagnosis may not be suspected. This situation has grave consequences for the patient because, if the hyperthyroidism is detected and treated, the symptoms promptly remit and the osteoporosis progresses no further.

Immobilization

Disuse has powerful effects upon the skeleton and on calcium metabolism. Curiously the hypercalciuria of immobilization is much more prominent in young men than in young women. Calcium balance may be strongly negative—up to 600 mg/day—because, in addition to the hypercalciuria, there is impaired absorption of dietary calcium and hence high fecal calcium excretion, which at times exceeds the dietary intake. Thus a young man with a fractured femur who is kept in bed for 3 months may lose as much as 5% of his total body calcium. There is no evidence that this calcium is replaced after the patient is remobilized.

Miscellaneous Causes of Osteoporosis

Osteoporosis as well as osteomalacia is a common complication of the malabsorption syndrome and the two bone disorders often occur together.[29] Other causes of osteoporosis include gastrectomy, liver disease, long-term heparin therapy and vitamin C deficiency. Factors that may contribute to the increased incidence of osteoporosis in rheumatoid arthritis include steroid therapy, immobility, increased vascularity of bone near affected joints, aging, and perhaps some direct effect of rheumatoid arthritis itself.

A causal relationship between the following disorders and osteoporosis is doubtful.

Acromegaly

Growth hormone is a potent stimulus to bone formation, but because there is an associated increase in bone resorption, the whole process of skeletal remodeling is speeded up. In acromegaly, the characteristic skeletal change is increased periosteal bone formation. New bone formation on the anterior surfaces of the vertebrae increases their anteroposterior diameter. Osteoporosis has been described in acromegalics, but it must be a rare manifestation of this disorder. Growth hormone increases the urinary excretion of calcium but also enhances its intestinal absorption so that the calcium balance does not become negative unless the intake is low. The high incidence of hypercalcemia in acromegaly is frequently due to hyperparathyroidism but sometimes serum calcium levels return to normal after the disorder is treated.

Pregnancy

Occasionally the symptoms of idiopathic osteoporosis appear during or soon after pregnancy and some have speculated that pregnancy might be a cause of the osteoporosis. Although the onset of symptoms may be related to pregnancy, pregnancy is probably not a major factor in the production of osteoporosis because the newborn fetus contains only about 20 gm of calcium, which is not an appreciable drain on maternal stores. Furthermore, osteoporotic women whose first symptoms appeared in relation to pregnancy have undergone subsequent pregnancies without apparent deterioration.

Clinical Manifestations

The chief clinical manifestations of osteoporosis arise from vertebral compression and susceptibility to fractures, particularly of the femoral neck, ribs, and lower end of the radius. Fractures of other long bones are common in juvenile osteoporosis. With vertebral compression, there may be loss of height, kyphosis, horizontal creases of the skin of the lower abdomen, and the ends of the lower ribs may ride on the iliac crests, giving rise to severe pain (Fig. 6-8). On examination, loss of height may be confirmed by finding that the standing height is less than the span and that the crown-pubis length is significantly less than the pubis-heel length. The bones are not usually tender except at the site of recent fracture. Many patients may have no symptoms, but back pain is a common complaint. Pain from a recent compression fracture is usually of sudden onset, sharp, localized over a vertebra, and aggravated by movement. It often subsides completely in 3–4 weeks or may be replaced by a dull, aching, diffuse pain; occasionally, the pain is severe, persistent, and disabling.

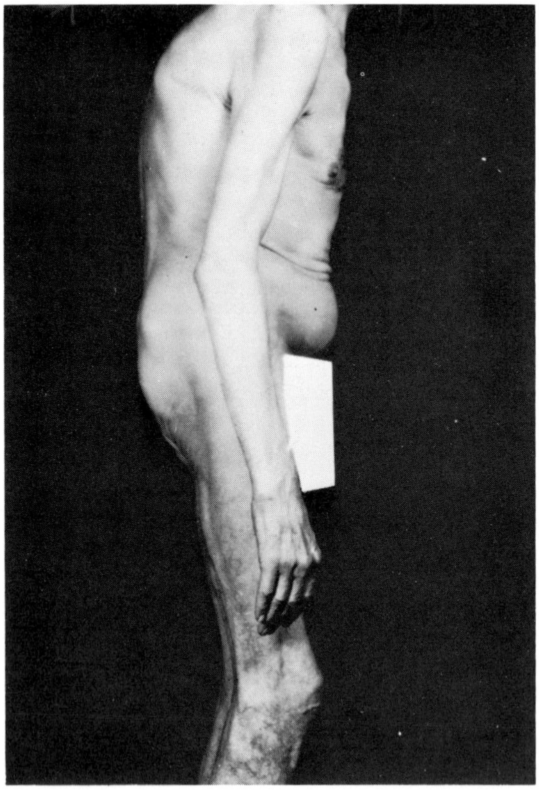

Fig. 6-8. Osteoporosis in an elderly man. Note dorsal kyphosis resulting in loss of height and transverse abdominal creases.

Radiographic Features

At least 25% and possibly 60% of bone mineral must be lost before changes in bone density are visible in ordinary roentgenograms. Radiographically, osteoporosis is most evident in the spine, pelvis, ribs, and upper femurs, but is also apparent in the appendages. The earliest changes consist of a loss of density of the vertebrae, with accentuation of the vertical trabeculae, but later these patients may develop vertebral biconcavity, Schmorl's nodules due to herniation of the nucleus pulposus into the bone substance, and anterior vertebral collapse, giving rise to wedge-shaped vertebrae. In severe lesions, the density of the vertebral bodies may not exceed that of the discs. Osteoporosis of the long bones is evident chiefly as diminished cortical thickness.

Laboratory Findings

Serum calcium, phosphorus, and alkaline phosphatase are within the normal range in postmenopausal, senile, and idiopathic osteoporosis.

Urinary calcium excretion is usually normal in ambulatory patients with postmenopausal, senile, and idiopathic osteoporosis.[39] Urinary calcium excretion is likely to be increased in immobilization, thyrotoxicosis, and Cushing's syndrome. High fecal calcium, sometimes exceeding dietary intake, is characteristic of juvenile osteoporosis and osteoporosis secondary to disuse and hyperthyroidism. In any event, fecal calcium is usually raised to some degree in osteoporosis of any etiology.

Diagnosis

The diagnosis of osteoporosis cannot be made with certainty on clinical, radiologic, or laboratory grounds, and should be arrived at only after the exclusion of other disorders which may present a similar radiographic picture, such as multiple myeloma, metastatic malignancy, acute leukemia, primary hyperparathyroidism, osteomalacia, osteogenesis imperfecta, the xanthomatoses, urticaria pigmentosa, and sickle-cell anemia.[26]

In osteogenesis imperfecta, a heritable systemic disease, a generalized defect of collagen maturation produces a variety of clinical abnormalities involving the eyes (blue sclerae), ears (otosclerosis with progressive deafness), skeleton (osteoporosis and multiple fractures), joints (loose jointedness), and skin. The bone disease, which resembles osteoporosis, is due to a defective matrix produced by osteoblasts which, in contrast to their paucity in the primary osteoporoses, are present in normal or increased numbers. In this disorder, reticulin fibers do not mature into normal collagen. Typical forms of this disease are easy to diagnose, but those of late onset—osteogenesis imperfecta tarda—are not always accompanied by features such as blue sclerae and may be difficult to distinguish from osteoporosis.

The possibility that osteoporosis is secondary to disorders such as malabsorption, hyperthyroidism, Cushing's syndrome, and hepatic cirrhosis should be carefully considered, even when symptoms and signs do not strongly suggest these diseases, because hyperthyroidism, Cushing's disease, and malabsorption may produce incapacitating osteoporosis when other clinical evidence is minimal.

Osteoporosis in children is extremely rare. It may be idiopathic but is usually secondary to liver disease, malabsorption, steroid therapy or Cushing's syndrome. In children, the effects of acute leukemia may closely resemble osteoporosis.

Treatment

Many treatments have been proposed for osteoporosis on the basis that they relieve symptoms, produce positive calcium balance, arrest the progress of the disease, or diminish the imbalance between bone formation and resorption. However, with the possible exception of fluoride administration, no method of treatment has been conclusively demonstrated to increase bone mass. Even in osteoporosis secondary to Cushing's syndrome or thyrotoxicosis, we cannot demonstrate increased bone mass radiographically after the underlying disease has been corrected, although, in growing children, new bone of normal density may be deposited around the thin bone.

Relief of symptoms is not a reliable index of therapeutic efficacy because the natural history of osteoporosis is characterized by frequent spontaneous remissions and the medications have a strong placebo effect. Standard techniques have not given convincing radiologic evidence of increased bone density even when patients have been followed for long periods. Standard radiologic techniques can detect only gross changes in bone density; however, recent developments in bone densitometry may provide more sensitive means of demonstrating the efficacy of individual therapeutic measures. Many forms of treatment, including estrogen therapy, high calcium intakes, and fluoride have been reported to produce positive calcium balance. However, in some of these studies, the discrepancy between the extremely marked calcium retention and the absence of radiologic improvement suggests that the balance techniques are faulty.

Several general therapeutic measures are most important in the treatment of osteoporosis. Patients should be informed of the generally favorable course of this disease. They should be encouraged to remain as active as possible and should take to bed only when they have acute pain from vertebral compression. They should be encouraged to sit erect in a straight-backed chair. An active program of physical therapy should be instituted. They should avoid movements and activities that might precipitate vertebral compression, such as carrying or lifting heavy objects, and should stoop to pick up objects rather than bending at the hips and knees. Corsets and braces are poorly tolerated by most patients and should be prescribed only for persistent pain or to hasten the patient's mobilization after painful vertebral fracture; care must be taken to ensure that prosthetic or supportive devices fit properly. Obese patients should be encouraged to lose weight.

Calcium Intake

Patients should receive an adequate intake of calcium (a minimum of 800 mg/day) because when the intake is less than this, calcium balance is usually negative. Calcium is absorbed better as milk than as certain calcium salts (milk has the added advantage of providing an adequate intake of protein and phosphate). The patient should be able to consume between 1.0 and 1.5 gm calcium per day as milk (it provides about 1 gm of calcium per quart), milk products such as cheese and whey, and the green leafy vegetables. Supplementing the diet with calcium salts initially results in strongly positive calcium balances, diminished bone resorption as measured by tracer kinetics, and a gradual cessation of bone pain. Because calcium supplementation carries little risk of renal calculi or metastatic calcification, it is reasonable to provide extra calcium—to give a total calcium intake of 2.0–2.5 gm/day. One gram of elemental calcium is provided by 3.5 gm calcium dibasic phosphate U.S.P. ($CaHPO_4$), 8 gm calcium lactate, 11 gm calcium gluconate, or two effervescent calcium tablets (Sandoz). With prolonged high-calcium intake, calcium balance becomes progressively less positive.

Estrogens

Although estrogens do not appear to increase bone mass, they probably prevent osteoporosis or retard its progress. Several workers have demonstrated that bone density is greater in postmenopausal or castrated women who had received estrogen replacement than in those who did not receive hormones,[24] and have reported that sex hormones arrest further loss of height in osteoporotic women. Estrogens may be administered as stilbestrol, 1–2 mg/day; conjugated equine estrogens (Premarin), 1.25–2.50 mg/day; or ethenyl estradiol, 0.1–0.2 mg daily. These agents should be administered in a cyclic fashion on the first 24 days of each calendar month. Estrogen therapy may be contraindicated if there is a personal or family history of breast or genital malignancy or thromboembolic disorders.

Androgens and Anabolic Hormones

Although androgens diminish bone resorption and improve calcium retention at least temporarily, their use in women is limited by their virilizing properties. In any event, there appears to be little advantage in giving osteoporotic women androgens in addition to estrogens. Osteoporotic men may be given androgens in the form of sublingual methyltestosterone, 25–50 mg daily (this may produce hepatocellular jaundice), or 400 mg testosterone ethanate intramuscularly once a month instead of estrogens.

Fluoride

Endemic fluorosis occurs in areas of India, China, and Japan, where the drinking water contains 8–16 ppm of fluoride. The predominant and almost universal feature of this syndrome is mottling of the tooth enamel. Skeletal changes, which are less frequent but more serious, consist of osteosclerosis and abnormal ossification of extraskeletal structures such as ligaments, tendons, and interosseous fasciae. In the most severe disease, ankylosis of the spine and flexion deformities of the hips and knees are combined with neurologic changes in the extremities due to exostoses pressing on the spinal cord. In advanced disease, the bones are brittle. In individuals with adequate nutrition, these abnormal skeletal changes do not occur; in Britain and the United States, mottled teeth and a marked reduction in dental decay are the only evidence of fluorosis in areas with 8–16 ppm fluoride in the water supply. In advanced skeletal fluorosis, there is evidence of increased new-bone formation and wide osteoid borders, as well as markedly decreased bone resorption. Fluorine substitutes for surface hydroxyl ions in the crystal lattice of hydroxyapatite, leading to the formation of fluorapatite crystals, which are larger and less soluble in body fluids and therefore less subject to resorption.[32]

Fluoride stimulates new bone formation in osteoporotic patients, but the newly formed bone is of increased fragility and it is not always normally mineralized[22] unless extra calcium and vitamin D are also provided. In any event, it remains to be established that long-term sodium fluoride administration is a safe and effective treatment for osteoporosis.

Calcitonin

Although it has been suggested that calcitonin may be useful in the treatment of osteoporosis, there is, as yet, no objective evidence of its effectiveness. On theoretic grounds one would expect that, in osteoporosis, its action would be similar to that of other agents which suppress bone resorption, such as estrogen and high calcium intakes, and that its prolonged use would be followed by a secondary decrease in bone formation.

Rickets and Osteomalacia

Definition and Histopathology

In osteomalacia, which means softening of bone, the basic abnormality is defective mineralization of osteoid tissue. During periods of growth, the mineralization defect also involves epiphyseal cartilage, and the term "rickets" is then applied.

Histologically, rickets and osteomalacia are characterized by an increase in the total amount of uncalcified osteoid tissue in the skeleton. In normal adult bone, nearly all of the bone matrix is calcified, but scattered, discrete, thin (4–12 μ) fragments of uncalcified osteoid, osteoid borders, or "seams" may be found along the margins of the bone trabeculae and in haversian systems where new bone is being laid down. In early osteomalacia and rickets, the fragments of osteoid may not be appreciably thicker than normal, but their number and the percentage of total bone surface covered by them is increased. When the disorder is more severe, the osteoid borders become distinctly thicker and involve a large proportion of the total bone surfaces (Fig. 6-9).

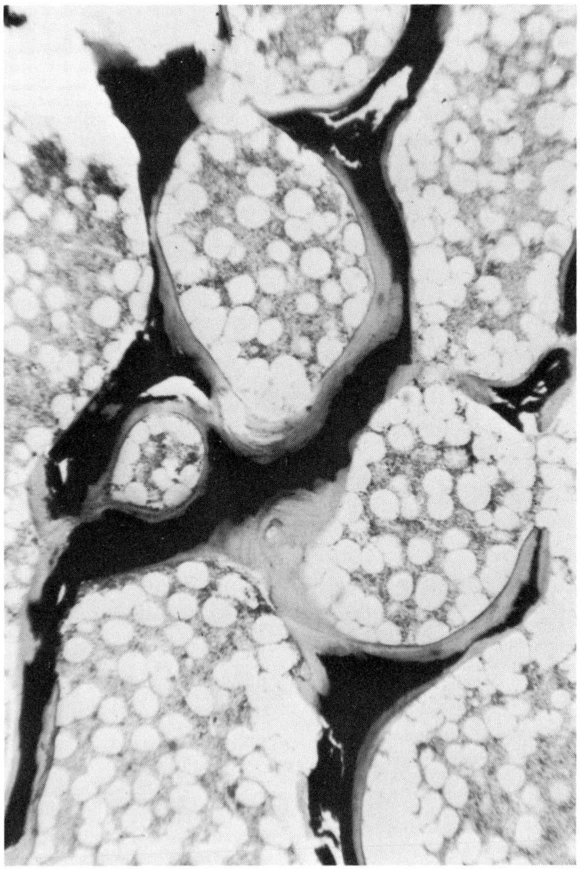

Fig. 6-9. Histopathology of undecalcified bone in osteomalacia. Mineralized areas of bone stain dark brown. There are wide borders of undecalcified osteoid along the margins of trabeculae, but the latter are normal in thickness and number. Von Kossa stain.

In rickets, the *enchondral* growth of bone is also defective; normal mineralization does not occur in the intercellular matrix between the hypertrophic cartilage cells at the base of the epiphyseal plates. After calcification, this area is normally invaded by vascular connective tissue from the metaphysis and ultimately becomes converted to trabecular bone. In rickets, this normal conversion of cartilage to bone does not take place, and the hypertrophic cartilage cells accumulate and produce the widening of the epiphyseal cartilage so characteristic of this disorder.

Secondary hyperparathyroidism frequently complicates rickets and osteomalacia due to vitamin D deficiency. In some cases, there is evidence of increased osteoclastic resorption of bone and more recently increased circulatory levels of immunoassayable parathyroid hormone have been found.[25] The most likely explanation for the secondary hyperparathyroidism is that the bone (and gut) of the D-deficient animal becomes unresponsive to parathyroid hormone with resultant hypocalcemia and parathyroid stimulation.

Pathogenesis of Rickets and Osteomalacia

The causes of rickets and osteomalacia are listed in Table 6-5. Classically, rickets and osteomalacia have been attributed to a reduction in the Ca × P product of the extracellular fluids below the critical level required for nucleation and growth of hydroxyapatite crystals in epiphyseal cartilage and bone matrix. The Ca × P product is nearly always reduced in rickets and osteomalacia except in renal failure, and elevation of this product, by whatever means, cures the disease.[30]

In certain disorders, however, osteomalacia cannot be explained in terms of this classic concept. For example, in renal osteodystrophy, osteomalacia is common even when the Ca × P product is normal or elevated, and pharmacologic doses of vitamin D may heal the lesion without any measurable change in Ca × P product. In renal tubular acidosis, histologic evidence of osteomalacia has been observed in patients with normal serum calcium and phosphorus, and in the absence of renal insufficiency. These discrepancies in the classic explanation are not surprising in view of the recent finding that the ionic composition of the fluid at the surface of bone differs considerably from that of the extracellular fluid. In addition, the process of mineralization is also affected by factors such as pH and the presence of calcification inhibitors such as pyrophosphate or other unidentified substances.[49]

Table 6-5. Causes of Rickets and Osteomalacia

Vitamin D deficiency
Dietary
Intestinal malabsorption
Postgastrectomy
Anticonvulsant drugs
Hereditary rickets simulating dietary deficiency of vitamin D
Hypophosphatemia
Simple hypophosphatemic (vitamin D refractory) rickets and osteomalacia (phosphate diabetes)
Resistant rickets (hypophosphatemic) responding to vitamin D
Hypophosphatemic rickets and osteomalacia associated with glycosuria *or* aminoaciduria
Fanconi syndrome (hypophosphatemia associated with *both* glycosuria and aminoaciduria)
Excessive intake of aluminum gels
Acidosis
Renal tubular acidosis
Ureterosigmoidostomy
Renal osteodystrophy

Rickets and Osteomalacia Due to Vitamin D Deficiency

Etiology and Incidence

Most normal (unsupplemented) diets are relatively deficient in vitamin D, which is present in significant quantities only in fish, animal liver, egg yolk, and milk and milk products.

Rickets due to dietary deficiency of vitamin D has been eliminated as a major medical problem in many countries of the world, particularly the U.S.A., where fresh and evaporated milk and almost all commercial infant formulas have long been fortified with vitamin D. In Canada and Great Britain, where fresh milk is usually not fortified with vitamin D, the incidence of this disorder is considerably higher. The minimum daily requirement needed to prevent rickets in infants and growing children lies between 100 and 400 I.U. daily, and, in adults, probably does not exceed 100 I.U. Nonetheless adult vitamin D deficiency, due to inadequate dietary intake and insufficient exposure to ultraviolet irradiation, is still encountered in Great Britain and Europe, particularly in dark-skinned immigrants and elderly females and, on rare occasions, it is found even in North America.

In adults, vitamin D deficiency is usually secondary to intestinal malabsorption due to idiopathic steatorrhea, disease of the small intestine such as regional enteritis, or prolonged biliary obstruction. Osteomalacia secondary to pancreatic insufficiency without biliary obstruction, though unusual, does occur. Patients with occult steatorrhea may have severe osteomalacia, even though their history and the appearance of their stools does not suggest abnormal gastrointestinal function. Osteomalacia has also been reported in a patient with gluten-sensitive enteropathy with impaired D-xylose excretion but without steatorrhea. Absorption of tritiated vitamin D_3 is impaired in all of these conditions, and the degree of malabsorption of the vitamin is related to the fecal fat excretion.

Osteomalacia may complicate partial gastrectomy, particularly after the Polya or the Billroth II procedure, even in the absence of steatorrhea. It is clearly due to vitamin D deficiency because the patients have no detectable vitamin D-like activity in plasma and they respond to physiological doses of this vitamin. In some of these patients, dietary intake of vitamin D or exposure to sunlight did not differ significantly from the normal, suggesting that impaired intestinal absorption was responsible for the deficiency. Some of these patients have had mild impairment of tritiated vitamin D_3 absorption.

In children, vitamin D deficiency and rickets may develop when bile fails to reach the intestinal tract, as in congenital atresia of the bile duct, infectious hepatitis in the neonatal period, or congenital cirrhosis, celiac disease, or pancreatic steatorrhea. Osteoporosis probably occurs more frequently than osteomalacia in malabsorption, but the two disorders often coexist in the latter.

Osteomalacia has recently been reported as a complication of treatment with anticonvulsant drugs. It appears to be due to vitamin D deficiency and responds to vitamin D administration. Anticonvulsant drugs seem to induce liver enzymes that accelerate the breakdown of vitamin D.

Clinical Manifestations

Vitamin D-deficient rickets rarely declares itself clinically or radiologically until the third or fourth month of life, although a study of autopsy material indicates that it frequently begins within the first 2 months.[12] Rapid growth predisposes to this type of rickets, and consequently it is more common in premature infants and is more likely to develop in healthy infants than in sick ones. In the temperate zones, it is more common among children born during the fall and early winter months when they have a limited exposure to sunlight. The infant reared in a large industrial city is at greater risk because much of the beneficial ultraviolet irradiation is filtered out by the soot and dust in the atmosphere, even in summer.

For a complete description of the clinical features of rickets, the reader is referred to Harrison's excellent account.[18] The early signs of the disorder are difficult to recognize. In mild cases, abnormalities are evident only in the skull and costochondral junctions (the classic craniotabes and enlargement of costochondral junctions), and beading of the ribs (the "rachitic rosary"). Enlargement and thickening of the ends of long bones, most readily detected at the wrists and ankles, occurs later. The rachitic infant also tends to be irritable, listless, and apathetic and sleeps poorly. Bone tenderness is much less marked than in scurvy. If the disease persists, the infant develops slowly, standing and walking are delayed, and growth is retarded. The muscles are hypotonic, and the child becomes potbellied. Clinically evident skeletal deformities such as abnormalities of the skull, delayed and abnormal dentition, thoracic deformity (pigeon breast), and bowing of the long bones do not develop until vitamin D deficiency has been present for many months. Hypocalcemic tetany is especially apt to occur when healing is initiated by very small doses of vitamin D or exposure to sunlight, or when a rise in serum phosphate levels is induced by increased phosphate intake or by phosphate liberation from tissue, as a consequence of fasting or the catabolic response to acute febrile illness.

Adults with mild degrees of osteomalacia on bone biopsy frequently have no symptoms. The earliest symptoms are usually vague aches and muscular weakness. Muscular weakness, which may also be prominent in refractory rickets and Fanconi's syndrome, may be extremely severe and may be confused with primary myopathies. This weakness is probably related to intracellular phosphate depletion and invariably responds to treatment of the underlying disorder. Gradually pain becomes the prominent feature in osteomalacia. Characteristically, it begins in the lumbosacral region and hips and later spreads to involve the spine and ribs; it is aggravated by walking or attempting to rise from the sitting position and is sometimes wrongly attributed to arthritis or neurosis. In severe disease, the patient has widespread tenderness and aching of the bones, a waddling gait, and softening of the skeleton, which lead to deformities and fractures after trivial trauma. Eventually he is confined to the wheelchair or even to bed. Hypocalcemic tetany may occur.

Radiologic Features

The earliest changes of rickets occur in the skull and costochondral junctions where they are difficult to detect radiologically, and as a result, such signs as the rachitic rosary may antedate radiologic changes. Radiographs of the wrist are usually taken for diagnostic purposes because the earliest changes are best seen at the cartilage-shaft junctions at the lower ends of the radius and ulna. There is widening of the epiphyseal cartilage, and the zone of provisional calcification, normally seen as a regular dense line adjacent to the metaphysis, becomes frayed and cupped. There are no changes in the diaphysis early in the disease, but later the cortex becomes thin and less dense and the trabecular pattern loses its sharp definition and takes on a hazy, blurred, coarse appearance. Other changes include greenstick fractures, callus formation, curvatures, and displacement of epiphyses or metaphyses.

The early stages of osteomalacia cannot be detected radiologically so that the radiographs may appear relatively normal when the patient has histological and clinical evidence of the disorder. One radiologic feature which, when present, is virtually diagnostic of osteomalacia is the pseudofracture. Pseudofractures, sometimes referred to as Looser's zones, after Looser who first described them, are sometimes the only radiologic abnormality. They are linear translucencies, which usually occur at right angles to the surface of the bone, and are seen most commonly in the ribs, the axillary borders of the scapulae just below the glenoid fossa (Fig. 6-10), the pubic and ischial rami, the iliac wings, the femoral necks, and the proximal third of the ulnae.

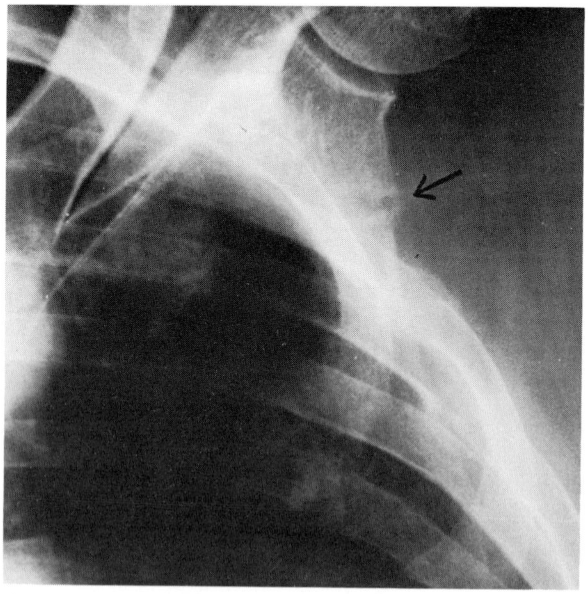

Fig. 6-10. Pseudofracture in lateral border of scapula. This lesion is pathognomonic of osteomalacia.

Laboratory Findings

The most sensitive and consistent biochemical findings in vitamin D deficiency are an elevation of the serum alkaline phosphatase and a marked diminution or absence of calcium in the urine. Hypocalcemia and/or hypophosphatemia are almost invariably present although the serum calcium and phosphorus levels may both be normal in premature or extremely young infants. Secondary hyperparathyroidism is probably responsible for the hypophosphatemia and also for the fact that serum calcium levels are often normal or only slightly depressed.

Both children and adults with vitamin D deficiency have a generalized aminoaciduria due to impaired renal tubular transport of amino acids. Recent experimental evidence suggests this abnormality is due to increased parathyroid-hormone secretion rather than a lack of vitamin D.

Diagnosis

The physician should suspect osteomalacia in patients with diffuse bone or muscle pain and muscular weakness and in those with radiologic evidence of diminished bone density. Serum alkaline phosphatase levels are usually elevated, but normal levels of this enzyme do not exclude the diagnosis. Radiologically, pseudofractures are virtually diagnostic, but in the absence of this sign, a bone biopsy prepared without decalcification is usually necessary to establish the diagnosis. A good response to small oral doses of vitamin D (1,000–2,000 I.U. daily) confirms the diagnosis of nutritional vitamin D deficiency. Rickets and osteomalacia due to malabsorption (excluding the postgastrectomy lesions), renal tubular disorders, or chronic renal insufficiency will not usually respond to 50,000 I.U. of vitamin D daily and only slowly to larger doses.

Hypophosphatasia is another rare disorder in which there is excessive uncalcified osteoid tissue. This tissue is abnormal and does not calcify in vitro, unlike epiphyseal cartilage from children with refractory rickets, which does calcify in vitro.[13] Hypophosphatasia is usually transmitted as an autosomal recessive trait but may occasionally show dominance. The clinical features are rickets, poor cranial bone formation, craniostenosis, and premature loss of teeth. This disorder may vary from the extremely severe rickets seen in infants (which is associated with a high mortality), to a relatively mild form in children or the increased fragility of long bones seen in adults. The diagnosis is based on the findings of abnormally low levels of serum alkaline phosphatase and the presence, in the serum and urine, of phosphoethanolamine, which is normally not detectable. Radiographic signs peculiar to hypophosphatasia include a ragged irregular appearance of the metaphyseal-diaphyseal junction of long bones, diaphyseal subperiosteal new-bone formation, and craniostenosis. There is no satisfactory treatment for this condition although, occasionally, corticosteroids have been beneficial and oral phosphate supplements have improved bone calcification.

Treatment of Vitamin D Deficiency

If sufficient time is allowed to elapse after treatment is initiated, any dose of vitamin D_2 (ergocalciferol) or vitamin D_3 (cholecalciferol) that would have prevented the development of the disease will cure the rickets and osteomalacia due to dietary vitamin D deficiency. In postgastrectomy osteomalacia, healing has been observed with as little as 1,000 I.U. of vitamin D per week. However, larger doses of vitamin D hasten the rate of healing and, for this reason, the recommended therapeutic dose varies from 1,000 to 10,000 I.U. daily for several months. Within 1 to 3 weeks, serum phosphorus and calcium levels rise toward normal and radiologic evidence of healing appears. Serum alkaline phosphatase levels, which temporarily may become even higher after treatment is begun, fall more slowly and may not be normal for 3 months or even longer.

Hereditary Rickets Simulating Dietary Deficiency of Vitamin D

Patients with that rare disease, hereditary rickets with autosomal dominant transmission, respond at least partially to moderate doses of vitamin D. The presence of hypocalcemia, the absence of marked hypophosphatemia, and the frequent findings of aminoaciduria all distinguish this condition from familial hypophosphatemia.

Simple Hypophosphatemic Rickets and Osteomalacia

Pathogenesis

This disorder, also called "phosphate diabetes," is now the commonest cause of juvenile rickets in many areas. The terms "vitamin D resistant" or "vitamin D refractory" are often used because the patient does not respond to physiologic doses of vitamin D, which are effective in the rickets and osteomalacia due to vitamin-D deficiency.

The fundamental biochemical defect underlying the failure of mineralization is probably hypophosphatemia which, in turn, reflects the diminished renal-tubular conservation of phosphate. In most patients, the hypophosphatemia is a familial sex-linked dominant trait. The abnormal gene is located on the X chromosome, which explains the higher incidence of the disorder in females and the increased severity of bone disease in male patients—males have no normal gene in the X chromosome to oppose the abnormal gene.

There has been disagreement as to whether the renal phosphate leak is due to a primary defect in phosphate transport or to hypersecretion of parathyroid hormone induced by failure of the intestine to absorb sufficient quantities of calcium. Although many of these patients undoubtedly have an element of secondary hyperparathyroidism, it is doubtful whether intestinal malabsorption of calcium with secondary hyperparathyroidism plays the primary pathogenetic role.[45, 46]

Clinical Manifestations and Laboratory and Radiologic Findings

The disease differs from vitamin D deficiency rickets and osteomalacia in several important respects. Patients do not have tetany because they do not have marked hypocalcemia. Dwarfism is a serious complication of cases beginning in childhood. Aminoaciduria and acidosis are not features of refractory rickets of the simple type, and urinary calcium excretion tends to be higher than in vitamin D deficiency. Alkaline phosphatase levels may be normal in patients who show clinical and biopsy evidence of osteomalacia.

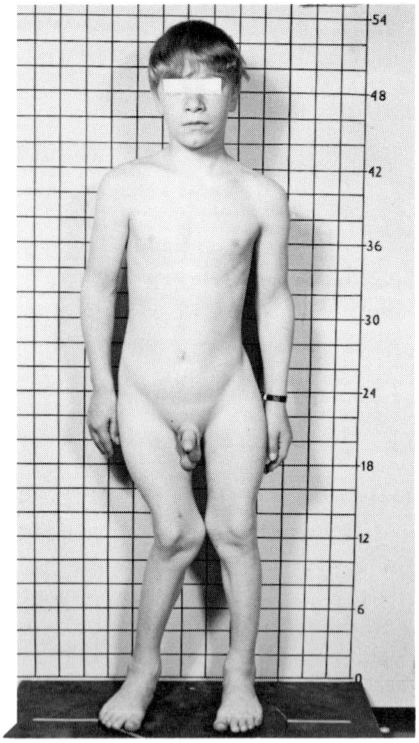

Fig. 6-11. Hypophosphatemic (vitamin D-refractory) rickets. This 12-year-old boy has marked skeletal deformity and stunted growth despite prolonged treatment with pharmacologic doses of vitamin D.

Treatment of Vitamin D Refractory Rickets

The aim of therapy is to raise serum phosphorus levels sufficiently to allow the skeleton to mineralize. For this purpose it is not necessary to restore the serum phosphorus completely to normal; indeed, it is rarely possible to do so. The classic therapy has been massive doses of vitamin D, ranging from 50,000 to 1,500,000 I.U. daily; with such doses a smaller proportion of the filtered phosphate load may be excreted in the urine and serum phosphorus levels may rise a little. Some workers attribute this effect to a direct action of vitamin D on the renal tubular handling of phosphorus, but it is probably due to parathyroid suppression brought on by the vitamin D-induced release of bone mineral into extracellular fluid.

Treatment of refractory rickets solely with large doses of vitamin D has been far from satisfactory because the response is highly variable (Fig. 6-11). Some patients respond reasonably well to 50,000–75,000 I.U./day but sometimes it is impossible to obtain healing even with much larger doses. Vitamin D therapy does not significantly improve the growth rate of these children and often does not prevent severe skeletal deformities. Frequently, serum phosphorus levels cannot be raised without at the same time promoting hypercalcemia; thus vitamin D intoxication is a common complication.

Smaller amounts of vitamin D—for example, 12,500–50,000 I.U./day—with oral phosphate supplements (sufficient to supply 1–3 gm phosphorus per day) in four divided doses appears to be superior to vitamin D alone.[45] With this combination, healing may occur more rapidly than when 4–8 times as much vitamin D is given by itself. A suitable formula for oral phosphate supplementation was given earlier in this chapter.

When surgical correction of deformities is necessary, it is imperative that the vitamin D be discontinued 4–6 weeks before operation; otherwise the patient may develop severe hypercalcemia from inactivity and immobilization in plaster during the postoperative period.

Fanconi Syndrome

Rickets or osteomalacia is a common complication of the Fanconi syndrome, and presumably it is due to the hypophosphatemia resulting from the renal phosphate leak; when present, acidosis may be a contributory factor. The serum calcium is usually normal. Serum alkaline phosphatase levels are often elevated but may be normal.[44] The bone disease is refractory to physiologic doses of vitamin D, but with pharmacologic doses, serum phosphorus levels rise and skeletal lesions heal. In addition, aminoaciduria, glucosuria, and metabolic acidosis may diminish or disappear. Acidosis, when present, should also be corrected by administering alkalis. Osteomalacia due to the Fanconi syndrome may also be successfully treated with oral phosphate supplements without vitamin D.[44]

Resistant Rickets Responding to Vitamin D

Clinically and biochemically, this disorder resembles familial hypophosphatemia but is cured by moderate doses of vitamin D ranging from 20,000 to 40,000 I.U. daily. It recurs if treatment is stopped, but doses of vitamin D required to prevent recurrence are much smaller than those required for initial treatment. This disorder is familial.

Renal Tubular Acidosis

The pathogenesis of rickets and osteomalacia in renal tubular acidosis is not clearly established although the skeletal disease is usually attributed to hypophosphatemia. Acidosis per se increases renal phosphate excretion and may contribute directly to the hypophosphatemia. Occasionally, osteomalacia has been observed in renal tubular acidosis in the presence of normal serum calcium and phosphorus concentrations; the findings suggest that chronic acidosis per se might induce osteomalacia.

In this disorder, osteomalacia responds to prolonged treatment with alkali alone. Vitamin D is probably not necessary, and pharmacologic doses of this vitamin should be avoided if at all possible because they increase the risk of nephrocalcinosis or renal stone formation—frequent complications of renal tubular acidosis.

Excessive Intake of Aluminum Gels

Huge doses of aluminum gels diminish intestinal phosphate absorption by forming insoluble aluminum phosphate and may lead to phosphate deficiency, hypophosphatemia, and eventually to osteomalacia.

Disorders of Magnesium Metabolism

Magnesium Deficiency

The range of serum magnesium values in healthy human subjects is quite narrow. With most methods in current use, the mean value for serum magnesium is between 1.6 and 2.1 mEq/liter (1.9–2.5 mg/100 ml). The normal limits deviate from the mean by less than 15%. In patients with symptomatic magnesium deficiency, serum magnesium levels usually fall below 1 mEq/liter.

The level of magnesium in the serum, however, is not always a reliable index of magnesium deficiency. Serum magnesium levels may be normal when the magnesium content of muscle is diminished; on the other hand, low serum magnesium levels do not always indicate magnesium depletion. Approximately 50% of the magnesium in the blood is normally bound to protein so that total serum magnesium levels may not accurately reflect levels of ionized magnesium. Moreover, the content of magnesium in soft tissue or in bones probably is not a reliable index of magnesium depletion because, in human magnesium deficiency, the content of magnesium in muscle is not always diminished.[43] Despite these defects, the serum magnesium level is the only guide most practicing physicians have to the state of body magnesium stores. Hence the remainder of this discussion will focus upon altered levels of magnesium in serum.[15, 23, 43]

Causes of Hypomagnesemia

Inadequate Dietary Intake of Magnesium

Normal diets contain adequate amounts of magnesium, about 25 mEq/day. When dietary magnesium is restricted, both fecal and urinary excretion of magnesium is markedly reduced within 7 days so that it is difficult to produce significant magnesium depletion in humans by this means alone. However, despite efficient conservation mechanisms, magnesium deficiency sometimes develops with marked restriction of dietary magnesium such as occurs in protein-calorie malnutrition (kwashiorkor), starvation, or prolonged intravenous feeding.

Impaired Intestinal Absorption of Magnesium

There is a high incidence (approximately 40%) of hypomagnesemia in such malabsorptive states as nontropical sprue, other small-bowel disorders associated with steatorrhea, and massive resection of the small intestine. In steatorrhea, the increased fecal excretion of magnesium may greatly exceed the dietary intake, presumably through the formation of magnesium soaps. In massive intestinal resection, the restriction of dietary fat corrects the hypomagnesemia and diminishes fecal loss of magnesium. Dietary protein deprivation or increased calcium intake diminishes the intestinal absorption of magnesium and may contribute to magnesium deficiency.

Prolonged or Severe Loss of Body Fluids

Fluid obtained from nasogastric suction contains approximately 1 mEq of magnesium per liter. Thus, prolonged loss of large quantities of intestinal secretion may significantly deplete magnesium stores, especially when associated with prolonged intravenous feeding, as in the postoperative period. Significant magnesium deficits may also develop with intestinal or biliary fistulas, or the severe diarrhea of ulcerative colitis and infantile gastroenteritis.

Excessive Urinary Loss of Magnesium

The normal urinary excretion of magnesium in adult humans is 8–13 mEq/day, but within 7 days of severe dietary restriction or in magnesium deficiency secondary to malabsorption, urinary excretion falls to less than 1 mEq/day.

Mercurial and thiazide diuretics and ammonium chloride increase urinary excretion of magnesium. In the vast majority of patients receiving diuretics, hypomagnesemia is mild and produces no symptoms, but symptomatic hypomagnesemia requiring treatment has occasionally been reported in such patients. Even mild hypomagnesemia may be significant in patients receiving digitalis because, in magnesium-deficient animals, there is an increased incidence of arrhythmias following the administration of cardiac glycosides.

In primary aldosteronism, hypomagnesemia is probably due to the effect of aldosterone in increasing both the urinary and fecal excretion of magnesium.

Increased urinary loss of magnesium leading to hypomagnesemia and occasionally to tetany has been described in diabetic acidosis. Hypomagnesemia is also a frequent finding in nonketotic diabetics; glycosuria produces an almost threefold increase in urinary magnesium.

Hypomagnesemia may develop in hypercalcemic states such as hyperparathyroidism, vitamin D intoxication, and cancer. Hypercalcemia is usually associated with augmented urinary calcium and magnesium excretion independent of the effect of parathyroid hormone, but the hypomagnesemia may be due also to a redistribution of magnesium from the extracellular compartment to some other depot such as bone.

Patients with hyperthyroidism tend to have low plasma magnesium levels and increased urinary excretion of magnesium. These abnormalities do not appear to produce symptoms and signs and are corrected by treatment with propylthiouracil.

Hypomagnesemia in Alcoholism

Hypomagnesemia develops frequently in alcoholism and may contribute to the neuromuscular excitability of alcohol withdrawal. These patients exhibit photomyoclonus, which appears to correlate with the concentration of magnesium in serum. The various factors contributing to such deficiency include inadequate dietary intake and increased urinary excretion due to a direct effect of alcohol on the kidney.

Hypomagnesemia in Parathyroid Disorders

Hypomagnesemia may be found in both primary hypo- and hyperparathyroidism, and in neither case is the exact cause clear. The lowest serum magnesium levels have been encountered in untreated patients with severe hypocalcemia; in these patients, the serum magnesium rises to normal or almost normal during treatment with vitamin D and calcium supplements without extra magnesium.

Miscellaneous Causes of Hypomagnesemia

A depressed serum magnesium concentration is frequently observed as a transient phenomenon on the day after an operation of any type. This appears to be part of the general metabolic response to surgical trauma and should not be taken to indicate magnesium deficiency.

Clinical Manifestations of Magnesium Deficiency

The clinical manifestations of magnesium deficiency have been difficult to define because the depletion of this cation is frequently associated with other electrolyte abnormalities such as hypocalcemia and hypokalemia. The symptoms and signs most frequently associated with magnesium deficiency are: weakness, muscle fasciculations, gross tremors, personality changes (especially extreme irritability and aggressiveness), choreoathetoid movements, vertigo, and convulsions. Convulsive seizures have been a cardinal feature of most severe cases of magnesium deficiency and are potentially fatal.

Other Laboratory Manifestations of Hypomagnesemia

In man, magnesium deficiency leads to increased urinary excretion of potassium, diminished total exchangeable potassium, and hypokalemia. The frequent association of hypocalcemia with magnesium deficiency was noted earlier.

Treatment of Magnesium Deficiency

Severe magnesium deficiency (serum Mg, 0.8 mEq/liter or less), particularly when associated with convulsions, should be corrected by the intravenous administration of magnesium, either as magnesium chloride or magnesium sulfate; under these circumstances, 2 mEq/kg body weight may safely be given intravenously over a 4-hour period. Magnesium sulfate is available in ampules in 10, 25, or 50% concentrations; the dosage of this preparation is expressed in terms of the official U.S.P. hydrated salt ($MgSO_4 \cdot 7H_2O$), 1 gm of which is equivalent to 8.12 mEq of magnesium. Less severe magnesium deficiency can be corrected gradually by administering 0.25–0.5 mEq of magnesium per kilogram of body weight per day until the plasma magnesium is normal. Under these circumstances, magnesium sulfate may be administered intramuscularly at 6-hour intervals in the form of a 50% solution; as much as 10 ml of such a solution can safely be given intramuscularly at 6-hour intervals, but with the larger doses, add 1% procaine because the injections are painful.

Oral magnesium supplements—magnesium hydroxide (milk of magnesia), magnesium chloride, or magnesium citrate may be used to prevent magnesium depletion when excessive losses are continuous as in steatorrhea. A convenient solution of magnesium chloride and magnesium citrate, which provides approximately 0.8 mEq of magnesium per milliliter can be prepared as follows: magnesium chloride ($MgCl_2 \cdot 6H_2O$), 4.0 gm, magnesium citrate ($MgHC_6H_5O_7 \cdot 5H_2O$), 6 gm, water to 100 ml.

References

1. Albright, F., and Reifenstein, E. C., Jr. *The Parathyroid Glands and Metabolic Bone Disease.* Baltimore, Williams & Wilkins, 1948, pp. 40–45.
2. Aurbach, G. D., Potts, J. T., Chase, L. R., and Melson, G. L. Polypeptide hormones and calcium metabolism. *Ann Intern Med 70:*1234, 1969.
3. Avioli, L. V. "Current Concepts of Vitamin D_3 Metabolism in Man." In *The Fat Soluble Vitamins,* DeLuca, H. F., and Suttie, J. W., eds. Madison, Univ. Wisconsin Press, 1970, pp. 159–172.
4. Berson, S. A., and Yalow, R. S. Parathyroid hormone in plasma in adenomatous hyperparathyroidism, uremia and bronchogenic carcinoma. *Science 154:*907–909, 1966.
5. Cope, O. The story of hyperparathyroidism at the Massachusetts General Hospital. *N Engl J Med 274:*1174–1182, 1966.
6. Copp, D. H. Hormonal control of hypercalcemia. *Am J Med 43:*648–655, 1967.
7. DeLuca, H. F. "Metabolism and Function of Vitamin D." In *The Fat Soluble Vitamins,* DeLuca, H. F., and Suttie, J. W., eds. Madison, Univ. Wisconsin Press, 1970, pp. 3–20.
8. DeLuca, H. F. "Vitamin D; Part 1." In *International Encyclopedia of Pharmacology and Therapeutics:* Sect. 51, *Pharmacology of the Endocrine System and Related Drugs;* Vol. on *Parathyroid Hormone, Thyrocalcitonin and Related Drugs,* Rasmussen, H., ed. Oxford, Pergamon, 1970, pp. 101–137.
9. Dent, C. E., and Watson, L. The hydrocortisone test in primary and tertiary hyperparathyroidism. *Lancet 2:*662–664, 1968.
10. Epstein, F. H. Calcium and the kidney. *Am J Med 45:*700–714, 1968.
11. Farquharson, R. F. Unpublished observations.
12. Follis, R. H., Jackson, D., Eliot, M. M., and Park, E. H. Prevalence of rickets in children between two and fourteen years of age. *Am J Dis Child 66:*1–11, 1943.
13. Fraser, D., Jaco, N. T., Yendt, E. R., Munn, J. D., and Liu, E. The induction of in vitro and in vivo calcification in bones of chicken suffering from vitamin D-resistant rickets without recourse to large doses of vitamin D. *Am J Dis Child 93:*84–85, 1957.
14. Garn, S. M., Rohmann, C. G., and Wagner, B. Bone loss as a general phenomenon in man. *Fed Proc 26:*1729–1736, 1967.
15. Gitelman, H. J., and Welt, L. G. Magnesium deficiency. *Ann Rev Med 20:*233–242, 1969.
16. Halmos, V., Kendall J. M., and Ogryzlo, M. A. Idiopathic hypoparathyroidism with impaired vitamin B_{12} absorption. *Can Med Assoc J 87:*173–178, 1962.
17. Harris, W. H., and Heaney, R. P. Skeletal renewal and bone disease. *N Engl J Med 280:*193–202, 253–259, 303–311, 1969.
18. Harrison, H. E. "Rickets." In *Practice of Pediatrics,* Brenneman, J., ed. Hagerstown, Md., Prior, 1963, pp. 1–63.
19. Howard, J. E. Reflections on calcium habits in man. *Can Med Assoc J 99:*41–48, 1968.
20. Howard, J. E., and Thomas, W. C. The biological mechanisms of transport and storage of calcium. *Can Med Assoc J 104:*699–703, 1971.
21. Howard, J. E., and Thomas, W. C. Clinical disorders of calcium homeostasis. *Medicine (Balt) 42:*25–45, 1963.
22. Jowsey, J., Schenk, R. K., and Reutter, F. W. Some results of the effect of fluoride on bone tissue in osteoporosis. *J Clin Endocrinol Metab 28:*869–874, 1968.
23. Martin, H. E. Clinical magnesium deficiency. *Ann NY Acad Sci 162:*891–900, 1969.
24. Meema, H. E., and Meema, S. Prevention of postmenopausal osteoporosis by hormone treatment of the menopause. *Can Med Assoc J 99:*248–251, 1968.
25. Melick, R. A., and Martin, T. J. "Immunoassay of Parathyroid Hormone in Human Plasma." In *Parathyroid Hormone and Thyrocalcitonin (Calcitonin),* Talmage, R. V., and Bélanger, L. F., eds. New York, Excerpta Medica, 1968, p. 440–441.
26. Meroney, W. H., Rubini, M. E., Rosch, P. J., Austen, F. K., Herndon, E. G., and Blythe, W. B. Decreased density of bone: An etiological approach to diagnosis. *Metabolism 8:*293–375, 1959.
27. Myers, W. P. L. Studies of serum calcium regulation. *Adv Intern Med 11:*162–213, 1962.
28. Nicolaysen, R. The absorption of calcium as a function of the body saturation with calcium. *Acta Physiol Scand 5:*200–211, 1943.
29. Nordin, B. E. C. Effects of malabsorption syndrome on calcium metabolism. *Proc R Soc Med 54:*497–500, 1961.
30. Nordin, B. E. C., and Smith, D. A. "Pathogenesis and Treatment of Osteomalacia." In *L'Ostéomalacie,* Hioci, D., ed. Paris, Masson, 1967, p. 379–399.
31. Parfitt, A. M. Delayed recognition of postoperative hypoparathyroidism. *Med J Aust 1:*702–708, 1967.
32. Posner, A. S., Eanes, E. D., Harper, R. A., and Zipkin, I. X-ray diffraction analysis of the effect of fluoride on human bone apatite. *Arch Oral Biol 8:* 549–570, 1963.
33. Arnaud, C. D., and Tenenhouse, A. "Parathyroid Hormone." In *International Encyclopedia of Pharmacology and Therapeutics:* Sect. 51, *Pharmacology of the Endocrine System, and Related Drugs;* Vol.

on *Parathyroid Hormone, Thyrocalcitonin and Related Drugs,* Rasmussen, H., ed. Oxford, Pergamon, 1970, p. 197–235.

34. Raisz, L. G. "Calcium, Phosphate, Magnesium and Trace Elements." In *Clinical Disorders of Fluid and Electrolyte Metabolism* (2d ed.), Maxwell, M. H., and Kleeman, C. R., eds. New York, McGraw-Hill. In press.
35. Rasmussen, H. "Basic Aspects of Bone Function and Calcium Metabolism." In *International Encyclopedia of Pharmacology and Therapeutics:* Sect. 51, *Pharmacology of the Endocrine System and Related Drugs;* Vol. on *Parathyroid Hormone, Thyrocalcitonin and Related Drugs,* Rasmussen, H., ed. Oxford, Pergamon, 1979, p. 1–18.
36. Rasmussen, H. Cell communication, calcium ion and cyclic adenosine monophosphate. *Science 170:* 404–412, 1970.
37. Rasmussen, H., and Pechet, M. "Calcitonin and Thyrocalcitonin." In *International Encyclopedia of Pharmacology and Therapeutics:* Sect. 51, *Pharmacology of the Endocrine System and Related Drugs;* Vol. on *Parathyroid Hormone, Thyrocalcitonin and Related Drugs,* Rasmussen, H., ed. Oxford, Pergamon, 1970, p. 237–260.
38. Reiss E., and Canterbury, J. M. Primary hyperparathyroidism. Application of radioimmunoassay to differentiation of adenoma and hyperplasia and to preoperative localization of hyperfunctioning parathyroid glands. *N Engl J Med 280:*1381–1385, 1969.
39. Rose, G. A. A critique of modern methods of diagnosis and treatment of osteoporosis. *Clin Orthop 55:* 17–41, 1967.
40. Sissons, H. A. "Osteoporosis of Cushing's Syndrome." In *Bone as a Tissue,* Rodahl, K., Nicholson, J. T., and Brown, E. M., eds. New York, McGraw-Hill, 1960, p. 3–17.
41. Smith, R. W., and Rizek, J. Epidemiologic studies of osteoporosis in women of Puerto Rico and Southeastern Michigan with special reference to age, race, national origin and to other related or associated findings. *Clin Orthop 45:*31–48, 1966.
42. Steiner, A. L., Goodman, A. D., and Powers, S. R. Study of a kindred with pheochromocytoma, medullary thyroid carcinoma, hyperparathyroidism and Cushing's disease: Multiple endocrine neoplasia, Type 2. *Medicine (Balt) 47:*371–409, 1968.
43. Walser, M. *Magnesium Metabolism. Reviews of Physiology, Biochemistry and Experimental Physiology.* New York, Springer, 1967.
44. Wilson, D. R., and Yendt, E. R. Treatment of the adult Fanconi syndrome with oral phosphate supplements and alkali. *Am J Med 35:*487–511, 1963.
45. Wilson, D. R., York, S. E., Jaworski, Z. F., and Yendt, E. R. Studies in hypophosphatemic vitamin D-refractory osteomalacia in adults. *Medicine (Balt) 44:*99–134, 1965.
46. Yendt, E. R. "Disorders of Calcium, Phosphorus and Magnesium Metabolism." In *Clinical Disorders of Fluid and Electrolyte Metabolism* (2d ed.), Maxwell, M. H., and Kleeman, C. R. eds. New York, McGraw-Hill. In press.
47. Yendt, E. R. Renal calculi. *Can Med Assoc J 102:* 479–486, 1970.
48. Yendt, E. R. "Vitamin D; Part 2." In *International Encyclopedia of Pharmacology and Therapeutics:* Sect. 51, *Pharmacology of the Endocrine System and Related Drugs;* Vol. on *Parathyroid Hormone, Thyrocalcitonin and Related Drugs,* Rasmussen, H., ed. Oxford, Pergamon, 1970, p. 139–195.
49. Yendt, E. R., Connor, T. B., and Howard, J. E. In vitro calcification of rachitic rat cartilage in normal and pathological human sera with some observations on the pathogenesis of renal rickets. *Bull Johns Hopkins Hosp 96:*1–19, 1955.
50. Yendt, E. R., DeLuca, H. F., Garcia, D. A., and Cohanim, M. "Clinical Aspects of Vitamin D." In *Fat Soluble Vitamins,* DeLuca, H. F., and Suttie, J. W., eds. Madison, Univ. Wisconsin Press, 1970, p. 125–158.
51. Yendt, E. R., and Gagné, R. J. A. Detection of primary hyperparathyroidism with special reference to its occurrence in hypercalciuric females with "normal" or borderline serum calcium. *Can Med Assoc J 98:*331–336, 1968.
52. Yendt, E. R., Guay, G. F., and Garcia, D. A. The use of thiazides in the prevention of renal calculi. *Can Med Assoc J 102:*614–620, 1970.

7

The Adrenals

Charles E. Bird and Albert F. Clark

Historical Background

The development of our knowledge of the adrenal illustrates the debt physiology and biochemistry owe to clinical medicine for providing a steady stimulus to further investigation. The adrenal did not attract much attention until 1849, when Thomas Addison published his paper "On the Constitutional and Local Effects of Disease of the Supra-renal Capsules" in which he described a number of patients with fatal asthenia associated with cutaneous pigmentation.[1] Subsequently the low blood pressure in Addison's disease was attributed to a deficiency of the pressor material demonstrated in the adrenal medulla by Schafer and Oliver in 1894. This substance, adrenaline or epinephrine, was the first hormone to be chemically isolated, analyzed, and synthesized in 1904. However, treatment of Addison's disease with adrenaline was ineffective and at times seemed to harm the patient.

In a series of studies published in the next two decades, W. B. Cannon *et al.* showed that secretion of adrenaline by the adrenal medulla was important in the normal response to fear, anger, pain and physical exertion.[4, 5] In 1927, C. H. Mayo described spontaneous excessive adrenaline secretion in a patient with paroxysmal hypertension and adrenal medullary tumor (pheochromocytoma); the hypertension was relieved by surgery.

Stewart and Rogoff engaged Cannon in an interesting verbal duel, which ran for several years in the physiological literature of the 1920's, to counteract what they believed was an unwarranted emphasis on the importance of adrenaline and the adrenal medulla.[26] They maintained that the medulla did not discharge any function essential for life. Their researches, which provided the first solid evidence concerning the vital importance of the cortex, ultimately led in 1948 to the demonstration that the recently synthesized adrenal steroid, cortisone, restored patients with Addison's disease to full vigor and safety.

Early in this century, Bullock and Sequira and others proposed that the adrenal cortex also produced sex hormones after they observed virilism in patients with adrenal tumors.

In 1932, Cushing drew the world's attention to "pituitary basophilism." This condition, a result of adrenal cortical overactivity, was characterized by hypertension, purplish striae, diabetes mellitus, osteoporosis, and truncal obesity. He emphasized the relationship between the pituitary and the adrenal cortex that had been suggested by Simmonds in 1914 and was later verified when Collip isolated the potent pituitary adrenocorticotropic hormone in 1935.

The most recent major discovery in adrenal physiology was the isolation and characterization of aldosterone in the early 1950's by Simpson and Tait. This hormone has powerful sodium-retaining and potassium-excreting properties. In 1954, Conn first recognized that aldosterone-secreting adenoma was an important cause of remediable hypertension.

Thus the debt that physiology and biochemistry owed to clinical medicine for initiating investigation of the adrenal glands has been amply repaid by basic research which has provided greatly improved methods of diagnosis and treatment of adrenal disorders.[28]

Embryology and Anatomy of the Adrenal

The fetal adrenal cortex, derived from celomic mesoderm on the posterior abdominal wall, appears during the fourth to sixth week of gestation. Clusters of cells develop at the periphery of the fetal cortex at about 10 weeks of gestation and eventually become the permanent adrenal cortex. During the seventh to eighth week of gestation, cells from the neural crest invade the cortex; these are the precursors of the adrenal medulla. The adrenals grow rapidly and at midgestation are larger than the kidney. The growth rate then decreases so that, at term, the normal ratio of kidney to adrenal size results.

Accessory adrenal glands containing both cortex and medulla are rarely found. However, isolated clumps of medullary tissue occasionally develop, particularly in the paraganglionic masses along the aorta, and in the organ of Zuckerkandl at the lower end of the aorta. "Cortical rests" are occasionally found in the ovary, testes, or close to the diaphragm above the normal site of the adrenal.

The adrenals, flat triangular structures, lie at the upper pole of either kidney. The normal adrenal weighs between 3 and 6 gm and is slightly heavier in the male than in the female. The outer cortex is golden-yellow while the medulla is reddish brown.

The adrenals are supplied by many small arteries from the renal artery, the inferior phrenic artery, and even directly from the aorta. The arterioles break up into sinusoids and drain medially into the medulla. There are usually only two or three adrenal veins; these drain from the right side into the vena cava and from the left side into the left renal vein.[25]

In the adult the adrenal cortex is composed of three distinct layers. The outermost, called the zona glomerulosa, is a thin layer of cuboidal cells arranged irregularly just beneath the capsule. Deep to this is the wide zona fasciculata in which strands of cuboidal cells run in a radial fashion towards the periphery. These strands are separated by the sinusoids. In the inactive state the cells of the zona fasciculata are filled with vacuoles, but in the active state they are much more compact. The innermost layer, the zona reticularis, is composed of irregularly shaped, deeply staining cells.

The adrenal medulla is composed of sheets of irregular cells with small nuclei. In their staining, these cells are much paler than those of the zona reticularis.

Adrenal Steroid Biosynthesis

The adrenal cortex, a complex organ, manufactures several steroid hormones, only a few of which seem to have clinical importance. The negative feedback control exerted between ACTH and cortisol explains much of the physiology, disorders of function, and tests used to assess adrenal and pituitary function (Figs. 7-1 and 7-2). A clinical model of adrenal function, with minor modifications, can explain the results of inborn errors of metabolism such as those in congenital virilizing adrenal hyperplasia.[26] As an aid to learning, the student can use this model (see Fig. 7-3) to rehearse the important relationships within the adrenal and, beyond it, with the pituitary and hypothalamus.

Classification of Steroid Hormones

On the basis of their major biological activity, the steroid hormones, which the adrenal cortex manufactures, can be divided into three groups: the glucocorticoids, the mineralocorticoids, and

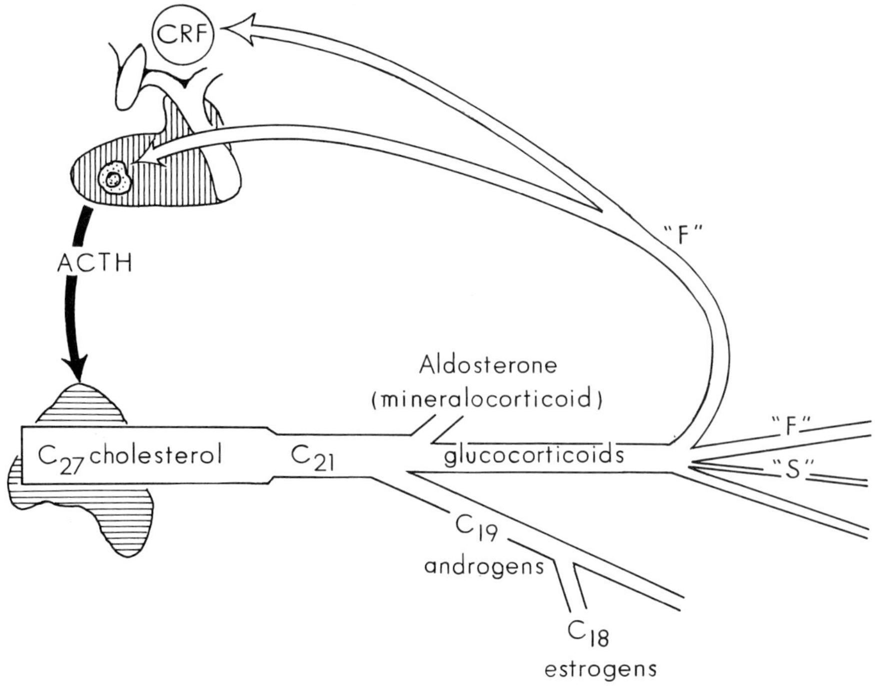

Fig. 7-1. Control of adrenal steroid biosynthesis by ACTH. Steroid hormones are designated by a combination of 4 types of nomenclature: (1) *biological action*—mineralocorticoid, glucocorticoid, sex steroids (androgens and estrogens); (2) *the number of carbon atoms* in the molecule (C_{21}, C_{19}, C_{18}); (3) *trivial name*—such as aldosterone; and (4) *alphabetical terminology*—"F" (cortisol or hydrocortisone), "S" (11-deoxyhydrocortisone). Under influence of ACTH, the adrenal produces a series of steroid hormones from cholesterol (C_{27}). Negative feedback inhibition of ACTH secretion is exerted solely by cortisol (compound F), which also inhibits the secretion of CRF (corticotropin-releasing factor).

Fig. 7-2. Measurement of adrenal metabolites in urine. The series of steroid hormones that the adrenal produced from cholesterol (C_{27}) are degraded along several pathways (see text) to produce two major groups of urinary metabolites: 17-hydroxycorticoids (17-OHS) and 17-ketosteroids (17-KS). The 17-OHS are derived from breakdown of glucocorticoid hormones ("F" and "S"). Note that the contribution of "S" metabolites is normally much less than those derived from "F." During a normal response to Metopirone test, the proportion of "S" to "F" metabolites increases considerably. The 17-KS are derived in part from breakdown of glucocorticoids, but mainly from metabolism of androgens. Normal range depicted (5–15 mg) is for the adult female; for adult males it is 8–25 mg. Measurement of metabolites of aldosterone and estrogens requires separate specialized techniques (see text).

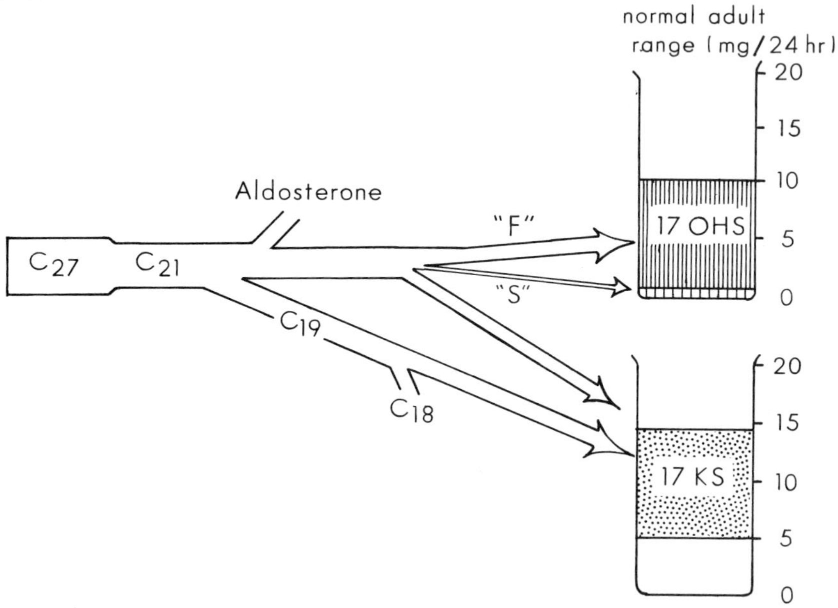

the sex steroids. Another classification based on the number of carbon atoms in the molecule describes these hormones as C_{21} steroids (hydrocortisone and aldosterone); C_{19} steroids (androgen); and C_{18} steroids (estrogens). In the initial steps of steroid hormone biosynthesis, the adrenal tissues convert acetate to cholesterol, a C_{27} compound. Thereafter cholesterol, by a series of transformations involving a loss of carbon atoms, is converted to C_{21} steroids, C_{19} steroids and C_{18} steroids. A limited alphabetical designation of the steroid hormones has also survived from an earlier nomenclature and is still useful as a kind of clinical shorthand. In this system, Compound E stands for cortisone, Compound F for hydrocortisone or cortisol (as it is commonly designated), and Compound S for 11-desoxyhydrocortisone.[13]

Control of Synthesis and Secretion

The synthesis and secretion of the glucocorticoid hormones and the "sex steroids" is largely under the control of ACTH. By the negative feedback mechanism described in Chapter 4, The Adenohypophysis, the adrenal secretion of cortisol is related to the pituitary output of ACTH. This inhibition is mediated also through the hypothalamus, which produces corticotropin-releasing factor (CRF) in response to the various stimuli that call for increased ACTH. The production of aldosterone, the principal mineralocorticoid, is mainly under the control of the renin-angiotensin system and is little affected by changes in ACTH secretion.

Transport and Metabolism

The steroid hormones and the excretory products that appear in the urine are the basis of some of the most important tests of adrenal function. After secretion, the steroid hormones are transported in the blood to the tissues, where they exert their biological effects, and eventually, after being converted mainly to water-soluble compounds, appear in the urine. In the urine, the principal excretory product of cortisol is measured as 17-hydroxycorticoid.

The major excretory products of most C_{19} steroids are measured as 17-ketosteroids, which are also, in part, derived from C_{21} steroids. However, urinary 17-ketosteroid excretion cannot be used as a direct measure of androgen production because testosterone, by far the most potent androgen, is not itself appreciably excreted as ketosteroid. The urinary 17-ketogenic steroids are derived from the metabolism of glucocorticoids; the 17-ketogenic steroid determination is sometimes confused with 17-ketosteroids, which however measures products of C_{19} steroid metabolism.

Urinary 17-ketogenic steroids give essentially the same information as urinary 17-hydroxycorticoids. In the normal individual, the plasma cortisol level shows a diurnal variation that reflects the rhythm in pituitary ACTH secretion under hypothalamic control. It suddenly rises to about 25 $\mu g/100$ ml shortly before the individual awakes in the morning and slowly falls to a minimum of less than one-half this amount some time after 6 P.M. Diurnal rhythm is abolished in Cushing's syndrome and is lost early when the hypothalamus and pituitary are affected by destructive processes.

Congenital Virilizing Adrenal Hyperplasia

We know of at least six inborn errors of metabolism involving specific enzyme deficiencies that lead to disordered hormone production in the adrenal cortex. The most common, a deficiency of C_{21} hydroxylase, interferes with the final step in the synthesis of hydrocortisone (Fig. 7-3). Through the resulting failure of negative-feedback inhibition, the pituitary ACTH output increases, producing adrenal hyperplasia and hypersecretion. The consequent overproduction of adrenal androgen produces masculinization of the female infant (female pseudohermaphroditism). In the male, pseudosexual precocious puberty describes the condition in which the androgen is derived from the adrenal and the testes remain small (in isosexual precocious puberty, the androgen is derived from the testes, which are larger than appropriate for the prepubertal boy). In these patients, depending on the degree of C_{21} hydroxylase deficiency, the production of mineralocorticoids may

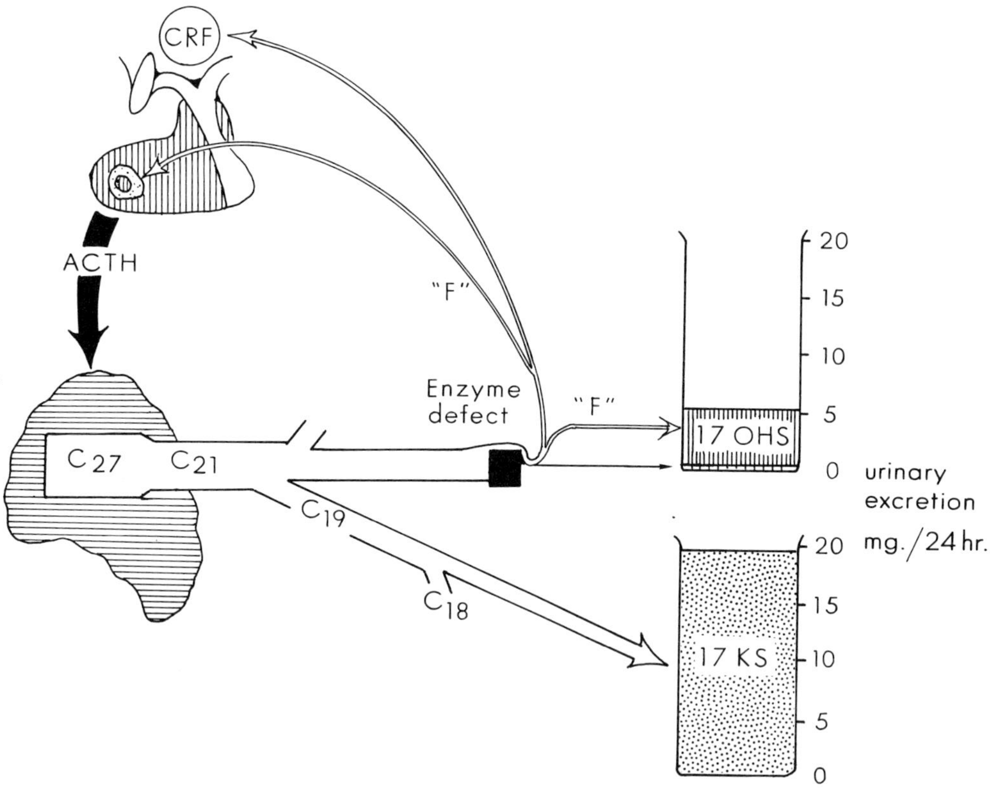

Fig. 7-3. Virilizing adrenal hyperplasia due to enzyme defect. Figures 7-1 and 7-2 show normal control of steroid hormone biosynthesis and breakdown of principal steroid hormones to their major urinary metabolites. In virilizing adrenal hyperplasia due to enzyme defect, there is compensatory response of the hypothalamic-pituitary-adrenal axis to a block in the synthesis of cortisol. If production of cortisol is impaired either because of congenital enzyme defect or drug treatment (i.e., Metopirone), subsequent overproduction of ACTH (*broad arrow*) will drive adrenal steroid biosynthesis along alternate pathways. This overproduction is reflected in high levels of urinary 17-KS (*lower right*) which, in turn, reflect increased stimulation of adrenal growth and secretion. Adrenal hyperplasia usually overcomes the block to cortisol production sufficiently to keep the patient from dying in adrenal insufficiency (*"F," upper right*). Excess androgen production, upon which major clinical features depend, continues but can be inhibited readily by small doses of cortisol or its analogues (e.g., prednisone).

be inadequate. Sodium loss and hypotension are also sometimes seen because of lack of salt-retaining hormone. The urinary 17-ketosteroids are usually increased because these are major breakdown products of the androgens produced in such excess.[29]

Since the basic defect in *all* forms of virilizing adrenal hyperplasia is impaired cortisol production, such patients are treated by providing daily cortisol maintenance in tablet form. Administration of 20–30 mg hydrocortisone or its equivalent as prednisone (5.0–7.5 mg) daily will lower ACTH production and reduce adrenal steroid secretion, thus controlling but not curing the disease. Patients with the "salt-losing" form of C_{21} deficiency also require mineralocorticoid therapy —9α-fluorohydrocortisone, 0.1 mg daily.

Because the drug metyrapone (Metopirone) produces a temporary C_{11} hydroxylase deficiency and impaired cortisol production, it is now used to test the ability of the pituitary to increase ACTH output by inducing a temporary failure of negative feedback associated with a transient hydrocortisone deficiency.[18] Metopirone does not impair the production of another C_{12} steroid, compound S; this latter compound, like cortisol (Compound F), is measured in the urine as 17-hydroxycorticoid. Therefore, a rising level of urinary 17-hydroxycorticoid on the day of Metopirone administration, or on the day after, indicates that the pituitary, as is normal, has increased its secretion of ACTH (see Fig. 7-7).

Control of adrenal steroid biosynthesis, some of the major metabolic pathways to excretion, and the diagnostic tests used to assess adrenal function have been illustrated in Figures 7-1 and 7-2. With this introduction, based on a consideration of enzyme defects, the student can now organize the more detailed presentation that follows: the metabolic effects of the steroid hormones, their clinical testing, and the diagnosis and treatment of adrenal disorders.

The Adrenal Cortex

The Steroid Hormones

The biological activity of steroid hormones depends upon specific structural features of the molecule. With respect to steroid nomenclature, the student will encounter at least three labels for most steroids; in brief, these are (1) the chemical name, (2) the trivial name(s), and (3) the alphabetic designation. The trivial name of the principal glucocorticoid is hydrocortisone (cortisol) and its chemical name is Δ^4-pregnene-11β, 17α,21-triol-3,20-dione and it still may be referred to as compound F. As in Table 7-1, the label used in this chapter is the trivial name or as close to this as possible.

The relatively flat steroid molecule is composed of four rings denoted A, B, C, and D. Figure 7-4 indicates the ring lettering and carbon numbering for 21-carbon steroids (C_{21} steroid) such as hydrocortisone. Details concerning the stereochemistry of important functional groups will be introduced where they can be applied to the interpretation of laboratory data. A C_{19}-steroid (i.e., 19 carbon atoms) would not have carbon atoms 20 and 21; testosterone and other related compounds have this basic 19-carbon nucleus. Estrogens lack carbon 19 and so are C_{18} steroids.

Although the adrenal cortex secretes a number of steroids, those of biological importance are the glucocorticoids (hydrocortisone and corticosterone) and the mineralocorticoid (aldosterone). Specific steroids are considered to be secretory products of the adrenal cortex when their concentration is higher in the blood of the adrenal vein than in peripheral blood. In the normal person, the other steroids (Table 7-1) secreted by the adrenal have minimal biological significance but, in disease, may be produced in large amounts and give rise to significant symptoms and signs.

Table 7-1. Steroids Secreted by Adrenal Cortex

Biologically active steroids
Normally secreted in amounts of physiologic significance
Hydrocortisone
Aldosterone
Normally secreted at levels not physiologically significant
Corticosterone
Deoxycorticosterone
Progesterone
Testosterone
Estrogens
Biologically "inactive" steroids
Pregnenolone
17α-Hydroxypregnenolone
17α-Hydroxyprogesterone
18-Hydroxycorticosterone
Dehydroisoandrosterone (free and sulfate)
Δ^4-Androstenedione
11β-Hydroxy-Δ^4-androstenedione

Principles of Steroid Biosynthesis and Metabolism

The following principles are basic to an understanding of steroid hormone biosynthesis and metabolism:

1. Cholesterol, a 27-carbon compound, is the basic precursor of steroid hormones.
2. During metabolic alterations, the number of

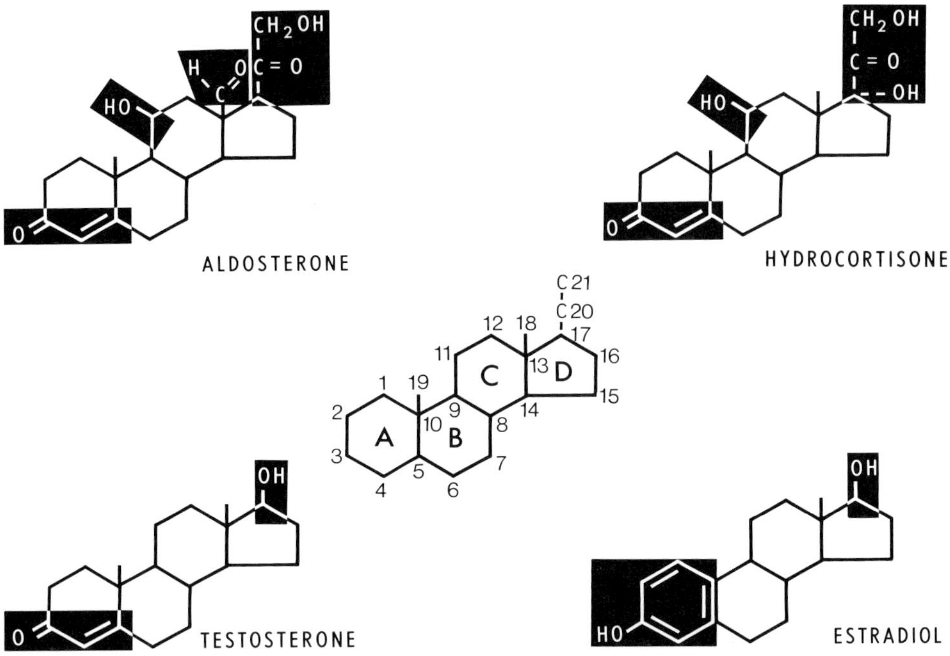

Fig. 7-4. Most important steroids in the four major classes. Note ring lettering and carbon numbering of steroid molecule—cyclopentenophenanthrene nucleus plus appropriate side chains (*center;* see also Fig. 9-11). The most important steroids in the four major classes of adrenal cortical hormones, according to predominant biological activity: (1) mineralocorticoid—aldosterone; (2) glucocorticoid—hydrocortisone; (3) androgen—testosterone; and (4) estrogen—estradiol.

carbon atoms in cholesterol or any other steroid molecule can be reduced but never increased.

3. All steroid hormones are formed and metabolized by (*a*) removing carbon atoms from cholesterol side chain, (*b*) oxidation or reduction of the basic cyclopentanophenanthrene nucleus and/or its side chain, (*c*) conjugation of the molecule with glucuronic or sulfuric acid.

4. Oxidation and reductions may occur at specific sites on the steroid molecule and can take the form of: (*a*) cleavage of a side chain, (*b*) hydroxylation (adding OH group), (*c*) oxidizing hydroxyl groups into ketones ($-OH \rightarrow =O$), (*d*) reducing ketone groups to hydroxyl groups, (*e*) dehydrogenation by removing hydrogen and creating double bonds.

5. The first step in the production of steroid hormones converts cholesterol to pregnenolone and the related compound, progesterone. This reduces the number of carbon atoms from 27 to 21.

6. The human ovary and testis are steroid-forming tissues that have no 11-hydroxylase activity. Therefore, these tissues cannot form hydrocortisone.

7. Androgenic hormones are produced from pregnenolone and progesterone first by 17-hydroxylation followed by removal ("side-chain cleavage") of two more carbon atoms, reducing the number of carbon atoms from 21 to 19. (See C_{17} Hydroxylase Deficiency in the section on Adrenogenital Syndrome later in this chapter.)

8. Estrogenic molecules (18 carbon atoms) are produced only from androgens (19 carbon atoms). Androgens can be converted to estrogens by removing hydrogen from the first ring (A) of the steroid nucleus and producing a benzene configuration. This irreversible process is called "aromatization."

Biosynthesis. The elucidation of the steroid biosynthetic pathways in the normal adrenal gland has led to a better understanding of the abnormal steroid patterns found in the blood and urine in disease states—e.g., congenital adrenal hyperplasia. The initial steps of steroid hormone biosynthesis, which will

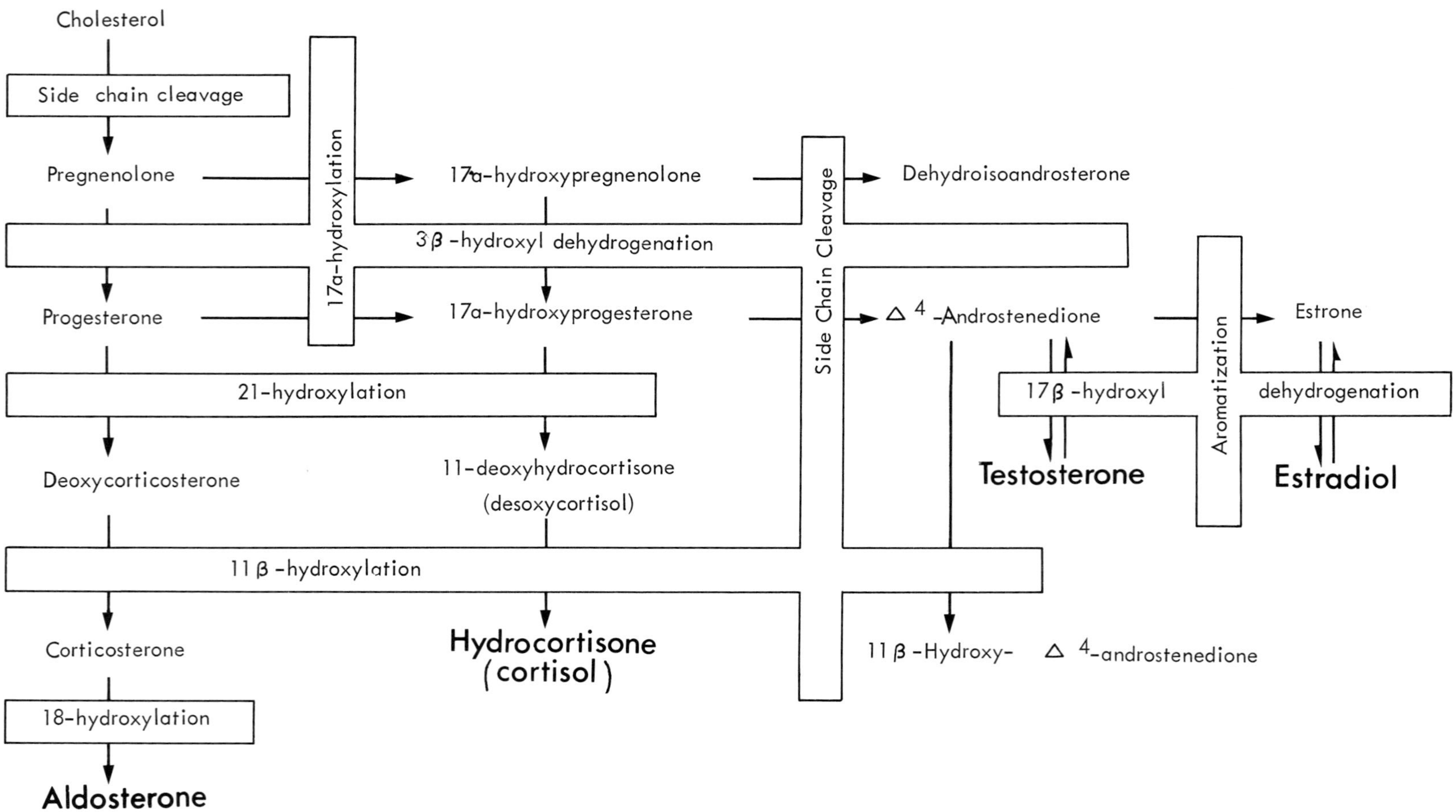

Figs. 7-5 and 7-6. Global view of adrenal steroid biosynthesis. This series depicts the principal pathways of such biosynthesis. **Fig. 7-5.** Overall view of related steps in production of the four important steroids, previously presented in their modified ring structures in Figure 7-4. **Fig. 7-6, A–D.** Divisions of the diagram in Figure 7-5 to focus attention on the biosynthetic pathways of each one of these major steroids, in turn. For easier understanding, they should be read with repeated reference to Figure 7-5.

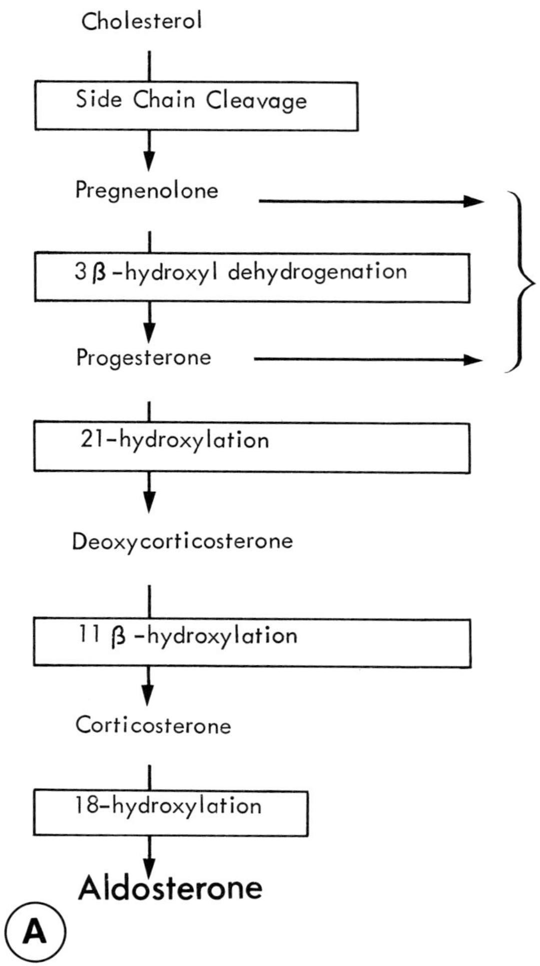
Cholesterol
Side Chain Cleavage
Pregnenolone
3 β -hydroxyl dehydrogenation
Progesterone
21-hydroxylation
Deoxycorticosterone
11 β -hydroxylation
Corticosterone
18-hydroxylation
Aldosterone
A

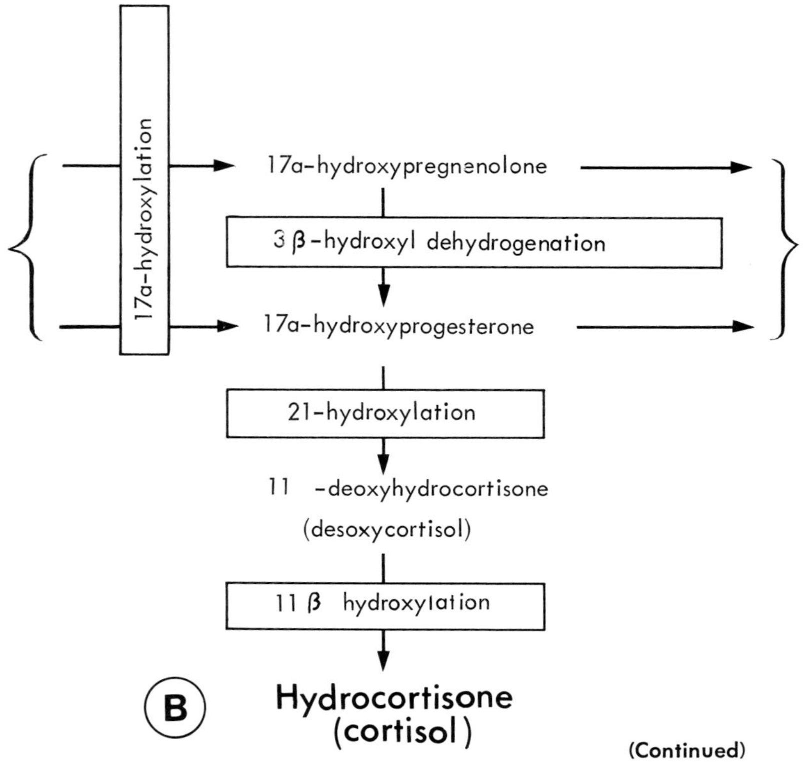
17a-hydroxylation
17a-hydroxypregnenolone
3 β -hydroxyl dehydrogenation
17a-hydroxyprogesterone
21-hydroxylation
11 -deoxyhydrocortisone
(desoxycortisol)
11 β hydroxylation
Hydrocortisone
(cortisol)
B

(Continued)

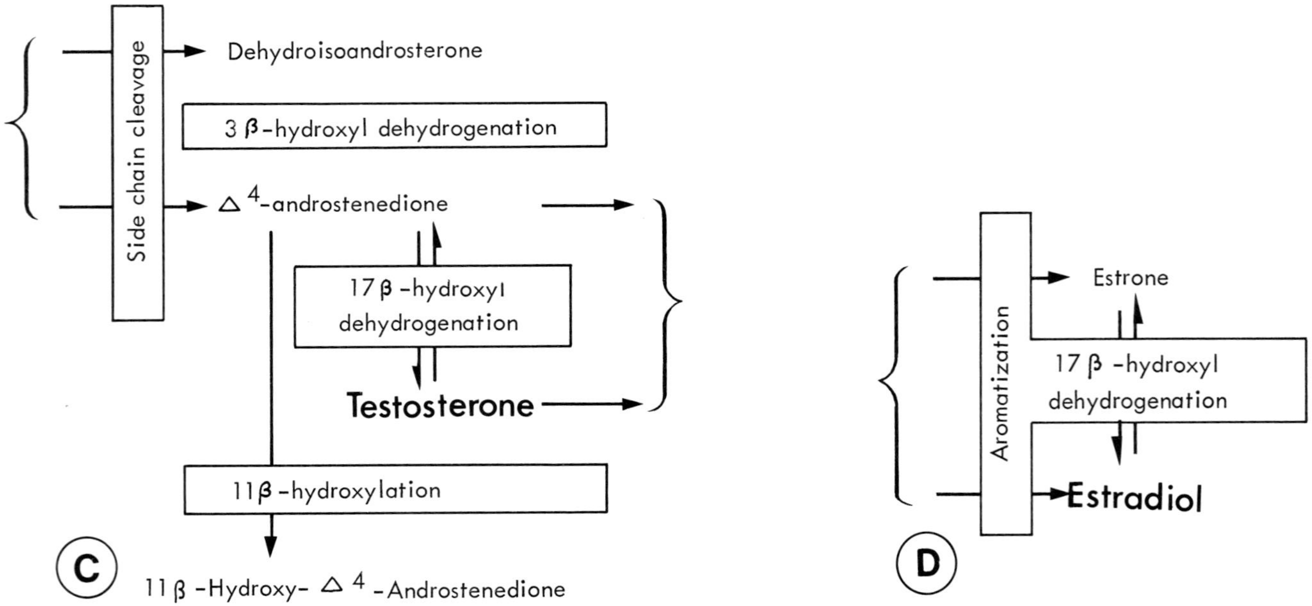
Side chain cleavage
Dehydroisoandrosterone
3 β-hydroxyl dehydrogenation
△ 4-androstenedione
17 β -hydroxyl dehydrogenation
Testosterone
11β -hydroxylation
11β -Hydroxy- △ 4 -Androstenedione
C
Aromatization
Estrone
17 β -hydroxyl dehydrogenation
Estradiol
D

(Continued)

not be discussed here, require the conversion of acetate to cholesterol. Both the adrenals and the gonads can synthesize cholesterol from acetate. In the adrenal, approximately 80% of the cholesterol used for steroid biosynthesis is derived from that in the circulation.

Cholesterol undergoes a series of transformations (Figs. 7–5 and 7–6) in its conversion to its various products: C_{21} steroids (hydrocortisone and aldosterone), C_{19} steroids (testosterone and dehydroisoandrosterone), and C_{18} steroids (the estrogens). In these transformations, progesterone is the important intermediate through which the glucocorticoids, mineralocorticoids, and the sex steroids all pass. In three steps, cholesterol (a 27-carbon sterol) loses 6 carbons to yield the 21-carbon steroid pregnenolone. The conversion of pregnenolone to hydrocortisone involves a dehydrogenation and a series of hydroxylations (at the 17α, 21, and 11β positions in this order); one of the pathways to hydrocortisone goes through progesterone which, alternatively, can be transformed via deoxycorticosterone and corticosterone to aldosterone. The formation of C_{19} steroids requires the oxidative cleavage of the two carbons of the side chain of C_{21} steroids. The conversion of testosterone and other C_{19} steroids to estrogens will be discussed in Chapter 10, The Ovary. Some steroids are secreted by the adrenal cortex as sulfate conjugates; the role of the sulfate conjugates in steroid biosynthesis is at present not clear.

Control of Biosynthesis and Secretion

Hydrocortisone

In large part, the pituitary hormone ACTH controls the rate of hydrocortisone biosynthesis and secretion by the adrenal cortex. The adrenal secretion of hydrocortisone and the pituitary secretion of ACTH are mediated through the hypothalamus via corticotropin releasing factor (CRF). That is, as the hydrocortisone level increases in plasma, the release of CRF by the hypothalamus is inhibited and the secretion of ACTH by the pituitary decreases—"negative feedback" inhibition (Fig. 7-1). Other factors such as stress, trauma, and toxic substances (chemical or bacterial) appear to act directly on the hypothalamus or pituitary to stimulate the production of ACTH (see Fig. 2-2). For further information on ACTH and CRF see Chapters 2 and 4.

The precise mode of action of ACTH is, as yet, unknown. However, one current explanation is that ACTH works by activating adenyl cyclase which produces increased amounts of cyclic 3′, 5′-AMP. ACTH is needed to maintain the normal size and function of the adrenal cortex; it stimulates adrenal growth by increasing the rate of protein synthesis. ACTH also stimulates the rate of hydrocortisone biosynthesis.

Aldosterone

The renin-angiotensin system, which plays the major part in the control of aldosterone production, responds to changes in blood volume such as those caused by blood loss, salt loss, reductions in sodium intake, and changes in posture. When the juxtaglomerular cells of the kidney are stimulated by a reduction in blood volume or a decrease in sodium concentration, they produce renin, which acts on angiotensinogen to form angiotensin I (a decapeptide). A converting enzyme cleaves angiotensin I to yield the octapeptide, angiotensin II, which stimulates the adrenal to secrete aldosterone. ACTH appears to be of some importance in aldosterone secretion, but it is not the primary controlling factor; in pituitary insufficiency, mineralocorticoid replacement is not generally required. The plasma potassium level, which exerts a minor controlling influence, acts directly on the adrenal cortex. When a woman is pregnant or is taking oral contraceptives, renin and aldosterone production increases.

Other Steroids

In the adrenal cortex, the rate of synthesis of other steroid hormones, in general, parallels that of hydrocortisone, although changes in ACTH levels may not have as great an influence on these as on hydrocortisone. In clinical conditions characterized by excess hydrocortisone production, there is usually an excess of C_{19} steroids; the most important exception is Cushing's syndrome due to adrenal adenoma, in which there is often pure hydrocortisone overproduction.

Transport of Steroid Hormones

After they are secreted into the bloodstream, steroids must be transported to the tissues to exert their biological activities. In transit, they are bound to certain proteins. This binding controls biological activity during transport; if they were not bound, they would be inactivated or, conversely, might exert undesirable or inappropriate effects (e.g., some women with hirsutism seem to have abnormally high levels of unbound testosterone). The binding of the steroid to its proteins, which can be visualized as

Steroid + binding protein $\rightleftarrows$ steroid-binding protein complex,

obeys the law of mass action. The protein-steroid complex exists in equilibrium with free steroid and free protein; as free steroid is removed from circulation, more is released by the binding protein. The complex acts as a reservoir.

Hydrocortisone

Hydrocortisone makes up about 80% of the 17-hydroxycorticoids in blood. Under normal circumstances, the hydrocortisone in blood is bound in part to a specific binding protein—an α-globulin called corticosteroid-binding globulin (CBG) or transcortin. Each molecule of protein firmly binds one molecule of hydrocortisone. CBG binds hydrocortisone most effectively, but it is only present in small amounts. Usually, CBG binds approximately one-third to one-half of the plasma hydrocortisone.

Plasma CBG levels have been measured in several physiological and pathological conditions. They are normal in most common endocrinopathies, including both Addison's disease and Cushing's syndrome. CBG levels are increased in pregnancy and after estrogen administration. In pregnancy, the levels of CBG start to rise during the second and third month and continue to rise gradually thereafter.

Albumin also binds hydrocortisone, but its affinity for the hormone is much less than that of CBG. The term "affinity" refers to the *strength* of the binding and does not indicate the protein's capacity. However, because there is so much albumin in plasma, this protein binds almost one-third of the hydrocortisone. As noted above, the binding of hydrocortisone to CBG and albumin keeps it inactive during transport. So far as we know, bound hydrocortisone is biologically inactive. Binding, especially to CBG, impedes its rate of transfer into some cells and also decreases its rate of metabolism. The excretion of hydrocortisone in the urine is more closely related to the levels of unbound hydrocortisone in the plasma than to the total levels.

Aldosterone

Aldosterone is bound to a smaller extent (approximately 40%) than is hydrocortisone and this binding does not increase during pregnancy. The principal protein involved is albumin; aldosterone is bound very weakly to CBG.

Other Steroids

Although CBG has a strong affinity for progesterone, this steroid does not interfere greatly with hydrocortisone binding because it is present in such low concentrations except in pregnancy. In pregnancy, the liver produces more CBG; thus, the *increase in capacity is great enough to bind the increased amounts of both hormones.* Another binding protein (β-globulin) with strong affinity for testosterone has recently been described, but normally there is very little of it. This protein, which has a considerable affinity for estradiol, increases during pregnancy and after estrogen administration. Other steroids, such as dehydroisoandrosterone, do not appear to be bound strongly to any protein.

Metabolism of Steroid Hormones

After secretion, steroid hormones are transported in the blood to the tissues where they exert their biological effects and subsequently are converted into water-soluble compounds, which are excreted. Such conversions alter the steroid molecule, resulting in a loss of biological activity.

Hydrocortisone

Of the biologically active steroids, the adrenal secretes more hydrocortisone than any other hormone.[23] Hydrocortisone and cortisone are interconvertible, and many tissues contain the enzyme required for this transformation.

$$\text{Hydrocortisone} \rightleftarrows \text{cortisone}$$

Hydrocortisone has a greater glucocorticoid activity than cortisone, which appears to be active only when converted to hydrocortisone.

Hydrocortisone and cortisone undergo identical transformations before excretion. Both are reduced to the "tetrahydro" metabolites. Quantitatively, the most important of these metabolites in the urine are tetrahydrohydrocortisone (THF) and tetrahydrocortisone (THE). Figure 7-7 shows the principal metabolic pathways in these transformations.

Minor Pathways

One minor pathway of hydrocortisone metabolism is side-chain cleavage not only of the hydrocortisone molecule itself, but also of the reduced metabolites. The final products of such side-chain removal are 17-ketosteroids, principally 11-oxygenated etiocholanolone derivatives (Fig. 7-8).

A second minor pathway is by further hydroxylations of hydrocortisone—e.g., 6β-hydroxylation. This metabolic pathway is of considerable importance in the newborn but is insignificant after the first few weeks of life.

Most of the steroid metabolites are excreted in the urine as conjugates of glucosiduronic and sulfuric acids which are much more soluble in water.

Half-Life

Using isotopically labeled hydrocortisone, it has been possible to study the rate at which this steroid disappears from the circulation. These disappearance times are expressed in terms of "half-life"—e.g., the time during which the hydrocortisone in the circulation falls to one-half its initial value. In humans, the half-life of hydrocortisone is 80–110 minutes. Some of its synthetic analogues, such as dexamethasone, have longer half-lives; this perhaps explains their greater biological potency—that is, they stay in circulation longer.

Aldosterone

The metabolism of aldosterone is similar to that of hydrocortisone; the main metabolite is tetrahydroaldosterone.

Other Steroids

Other C_{21} steroids have patterns of metabolism similar to those for hydrocortisone, cortisone, and aldosterone: Ring A is reduced and the 20 ketone can also be reduced. Accordingly, the principal metabolite of progesterone is pregnanediol; that of 17α-hydroxyprogesterone is pregnanetriol; and those of corticosterone and deoxycorticosterone are the corresponding "tetrahydro" compounds. The C_{19} steroids are metabolized in a similar manner.

Biological Effects

Under normal conditions, the steroids secreted by the adrenal cortex have two principal effects: (1) glucocorticoid, and (2) mineralocorticoid. These effects overlap to a considerable extent. In general, when the adrenal steroids are over- or underproduced, the patient develops clinical symptoms. The normal individual does not secrete enough adrenal androgens to produce discernible physiological effects except that, in the normal female, growth of pubic and axillary hair is partly attributed to these substances. In this section, glucocorticoid and mineralocorticoid effects are discussed as though these steroids are present in excessive amounts or their actions are not opposed by normal controlling factors.

Glucocorticoids

Metabolic Effects

The glucocorticoids, principally hydrocortisone, play an important role in the control of carbohydrate, protein, and lipid metabolism. Their overall action is catabolic; they increase protein breakdown and nitrogen excretion. However, in the liver their influence is primarily anabolic. These steroids probably exert their primary effect in the liver, causing increased gluconeogenesis, increased amino-acid uptake, and increased RNA and protein synthesis. The fact that increased RNA synthesis precedes the increase in protein synthesis indicates that hydrocortisone has its primary action on RNA synthesis. Thus, more of the enzymes involved in liver metabolism are produced. In contrast, protein in other tissues breaks

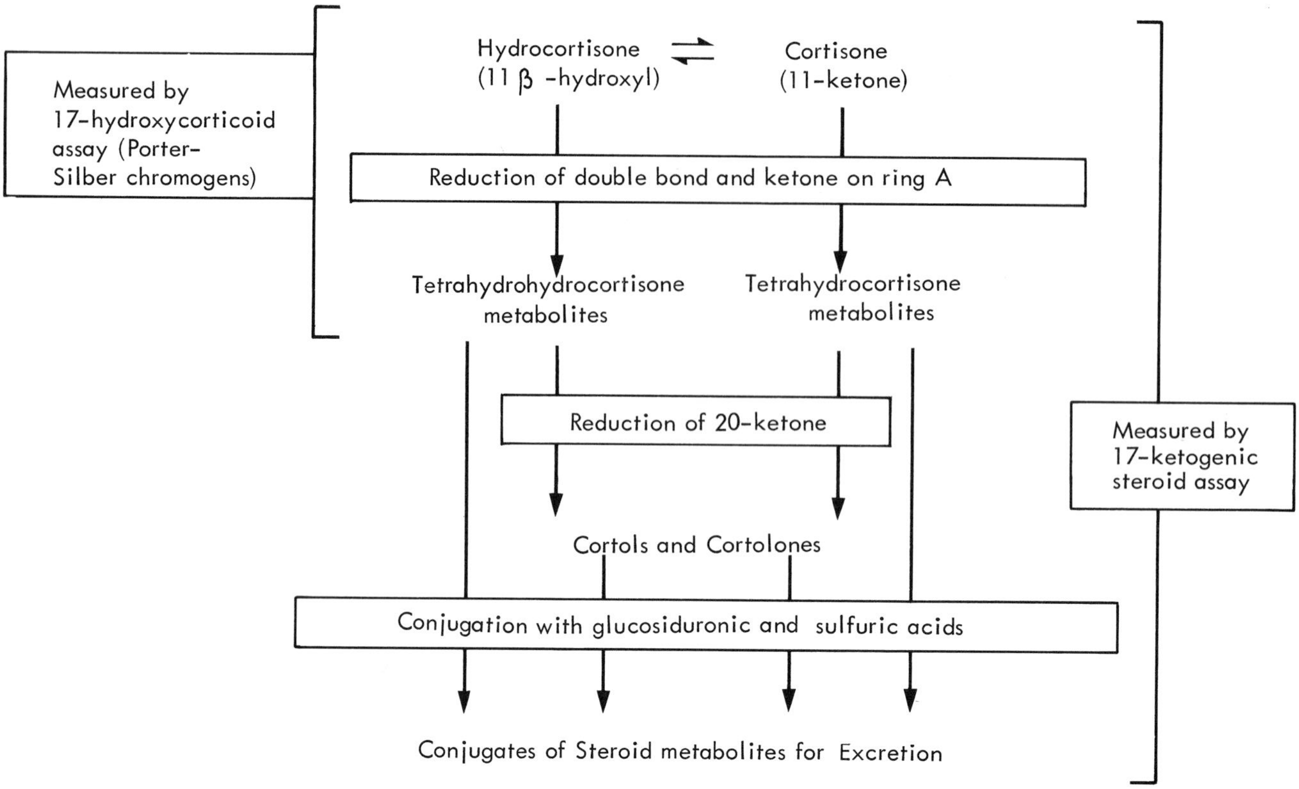

Fig. 7-7. Metabolism and excretion of the principal glucocorticoid hormones. This figure depicts the principal metabolic pathways involved in degradation and excretion of *hydrocortisone* and *cortisone*. Unlike the 17-hydroxycorticoid assay (*far left*), the 17-ketogenic steroid assay (*far right*) measures all the steroids shown in the diagram and also measures others—e.g., pregnanetriol (not shown). Thus it is easy to see why the normal range of 17-ketogenic steroids is twice that of 17-hydroxycorticoids.

down to such an extent that total body protein decreases and muscle mass decreases. Appropriately, urea and ketone production also increases.

Glucocorticoids decrease glucose utilization in muscle, adipose and lymphatic tissues and stimulate the release of free fatty acids from adipose tissues. Hence, more compounds are made available for gluconeogenesis in the liver, and blood-glucose levels increase. The glucocorticoid hormones increase the activities of a number of liver enzymes involved in amino-acid metabolism and glucose synthesis.

Hematologic and Other Effects

These effects of the glucocorticoids include:

1. Suppression of inflammatory reaction and the body's resistance to infection. Because of this anti-inflammatory action, this steroid is widely used in medicine
2. Lymphopenia through interference with DNA synthesis in lymphoid tissue
3. Eosinopenia by increasing the rate of destruction of eosinophils, an effect widely used to assay glucocorticoid activity
4. Decrease in basophils
5. Increase the neutrophils, giving a total leukocyte count of between 12,000 and 20,000/mm^3
6. Increase in erythrocytes, leading to polycythemia
7. Inhibition of the hypersensitivity reaction to antigen-antibody complexes, and intracellular synthesis of histamine
8. Stabilization of lysosomal membranes, thereby inhibiting the release of proteolytic en-

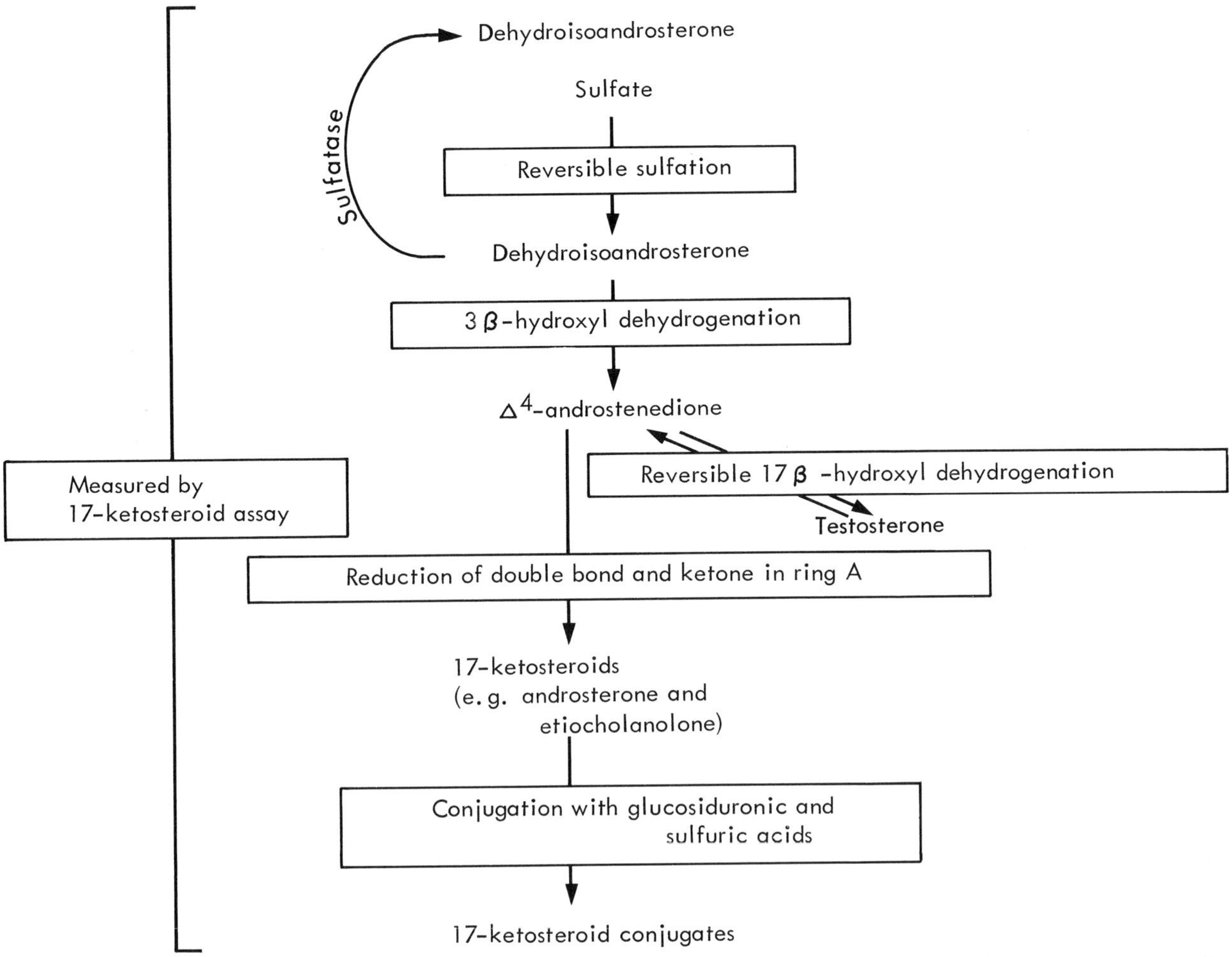

Fig. 7-8. Other pathways of excretion of glucocorticoid and androgenic hormones. This figure shows the source of most of the 17-ketosteroids in the urine. However, the 17-ketosteroid assay (*far left*) also measures other metabolites not shown on the diagram—e.g., those derived from 11β-hydroxyandrostenedione. Hydrocortisone and cortisone also may be metabolized and excreted, in part, as 17-ketosteroids.

zymes that cause cellular damage

9. Decrease in serum calcium levels, probably by inhibiting the absorption of calcium from the gastrointestinal tract

Some of the actions of the glucocorticoids depend on their relationships with other hormones. They retard growth probably by suppressing growth-hormone secretion and interfering with its action on skeletal muscle. Hydrocortisone controls ACTH release via the negative feedback mechanism. The most important action of glucocorticoids on the circulation is "permissive"; they sensitize the arterioles to the pressor effect of norepinephrine and similar drugs. Hydrocortisone and cortisone enhance water diuresis by preventing the movement of water into the cells. They may also directly inhibit the action of antidiuretic hormone (ADH).

Mineralocorticoids

Aldosterone causes sodium retention and simultaneous loss of potassium in the urine. As

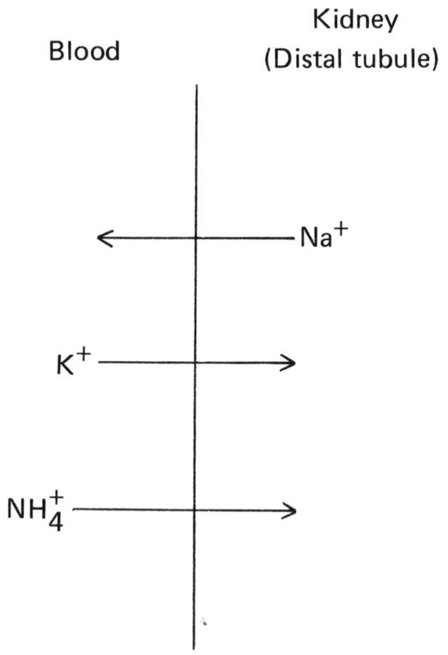

Fig. 7-9. Effects of aldosterone on kidney. Aldosterone causes sodium to be exchanged for hydrogen and potassium ions.

shown in Figure 7-9 it acts on the distal tubule, causing sodium to be exchanged for hydrogen and potassium ions. The same exchange takes place in the sweat glands, salivary glands, intestinal mucosa, and between intracellular and extracellular water. Aldosterone exerts its primary effect on sodium levels by increasing the ATP available to the "sodium pump"—the mechanism whereby the extracellular levels of sodium increase while potassium and hydrogen ion levels fall. The other important mineralocorticoid in humans, deoxycorticosterone (DOC), has approximately one-thirtieth the biological potency of aldosterone in terms of sodium retention. Compared to aldosterone, it may cause relatively greater potassium loss than sodium retention.

Other Hormones

The metabolic and physiological effects of the other steroid hormones, in particular the androgens and estrogens, will be discussed in Chapter 9, The Testis, and Chapter 10, The Ovary, respectively.

Testing Adrenal Cortical Function

To understand the rationale behind the various tests of adrenal function, the student must clearly distinguish between secretion, production, and excretion. In assessing adrenal function, we may measure one or several of the following:

1. Secretion of a compound by the adrenal, normally expressed as rate: weight per unit time
2. Production by the whole body. This includes secretion by the glands plus conversion of a suitable precursor to the compound in peripheral tissues—i.e., liver. This production is also expressed as rate: weight per unit time
3. Excretion of the compound or its specific metabolites in the urine (also expressed as rate: weight per unit time)

Tests of adrenal cortical function measure the steroid hormone or its metabolites in either blood or urine. Under normal conditions, the adrenal cortical activity is dynamic; it is continually changing. The physician must remember this circadian rhythm (regular changes from one part of the day to another) when interpreting certain of the tests. The rate of secretion of ACTH and, hence, hydrocortisone is much higher in the morning than at night. Also, some pathological states are characterized by large unexplained fluctuations in adrenal activity from one day to another, which are not due to circadian rhythm.

In general, most tests which measure steroid hormones and their metabolites in blood and urine reflect the sum of a group of chemically similar compounds. Because of this, some assays measure metabolites of compounds that have no biological significance. In general, methods that measure only one compound are longer, more intricate, and are therefore less suited to routine determination.[20]

Because urine is available in larger volumes than blood and, hence, provides larger amounts of the steroids for quantitation, most routine determinations are based on the measurement of steroids in urine. It must be remembered, however, that these methods measure metabolites excreted over a period of time and give no indication of variations (if any) during this period. Also, kidney function and other factors which influence the rate of steroid metabolism and excretion will not be indicated by determinations from urine. Consequently, these methods may not give a true measurement of adrenal secretion or activity in certain circumstances. The methods used from laboratory to laboratory vary a good deal; hence the "normal" ranges differ from hospital to hospital. In the sections which follow, these assays are discussed briefly in terms of what they measure and their possible significance. The principal metabolites derived from the products of adrenal cortical secretion appear in the urine chiefly as conjugates of glucosiduronic and sulfuric acids (Figs. 7-7 and 7-8). The normal ranges for the various urine tests are given in Table 7-2 (see also Fig. 7-2).

Table 7-2. Normal Ranges* for Steroid Assays

Assay	*Male*		*Female*
Urine (excretion per 24 hr)			
17-Hydroxycorticoids (mg)		1–10	
17-Ketogenic steroids (mg)	9–17		7–12
17-Ketosteroids (mg)	8–25		5–15
Estrogens, total (μg)	4–25		4–60
Pregnanetriol (mg)		0–4	
Pregnanediol (mg)	0–1.5		
Follicular phase			0.5–1.5
Luteal phase			2–7
Postmenopausal			0.2–1.0
Aldosterone (μg)		4–17	
Plasma (μg/100 ml)			
Hydrocortisone (μg)		5–20	
17-Hydroxycorticoids (μg)	0–1.5	1–10	0.2–1.0

* Normal ranges vary slightly from one laboratory to another, depending on the method used.

Tests for adrenal cortical function may be divided into two groups:

1. *Static:* measurements made in a baseline situation at a single time or for a stated period of time. The static tests, in particular, measure adrenocortical activity at the time of the test only or represent mean activity for a period of time. They do not indicate the total reserve of the gland.
2. *Dynamic:* measurements of changes in function over a period or periods during and after a specific stimulus or suppression.

Static Tests

Urine Determinations

Urinary 17-Hydroxycorticoids

This established method, often called the Porter-Silber chromogen assay, measures the metabolites of hydrocortisone and 11-desoxyhydrocortisone. A color reaction, it detects steroids containing a dihydroxyacetone

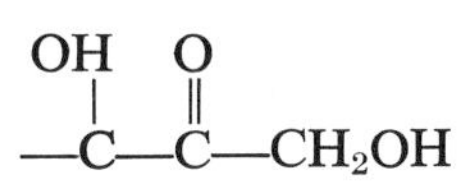

side chain and measures hydrocortisone, cortisone, 11-desoxyhydrocortisone (Compound S), and any of their metabolites containing an unaltered side chain. Cortols and cortolones will not be measured. This assay is inaccurate in low ranges because several nonsteroids give a positive reaction, and hence it is not reliable in assessing patients with suspected adrenocortical hypofunction (see Fig. 7-7 far left).

Urinary 17-Ketogenic Steroids

This assay measures any steroid that contains oxygen (OH or =O) on carbons 17 and 20, that is, hydrocortisone, cortisone, 11-desoxyhydrocortisone (Compound S), 17α-hydroxyprogesterone, 17α-hydroxypregnenolone, and all their metabolites which have an intact side chain (Fig. 7-7, far right). Thus, this assay measures a larger group of compounds than the 17α-hydroxycorticosteroid method and, by so doing, gives a more complete assessment of adrenocortical secretion and function. The name of this assay reflects the fact that it measures steroids that can be converted to 17-ketosteroids; in most of the methods, the assay does not measure 17-ketosteroids already present in the urine.

Urinary 17-Ketosteroids

By a colorimetric method this assay measures C_{19} steroids that contain a 17-ketone portion. Normally, dehydroisoandrosterone and its metabolites, principally androsterone and etiocholanolone, make up about 60% of the daily excretion (6–10 mg) in this group. This assay also measures the same metabolites formed from testosterone and Δ^4-androstenedione; approximately 1 mg/day in normal females and 3 mg in normal males. This test is not a good measure of the amount of biologically active androgen produced because (1) testosterone itself is not measured, and (2) large amounts of biologically inactive 17-ketosteroid precursors are normally secreted by both adrenals and gonads and are detected as 17-ketosteroids in this test (see Fig. 7-8).

Other Urinary Methods

Pregnanediol. This steroid is used as an index of progesterone secretion but is inaccurate because it is also produced peripherally from other steroids. For this reason, it is not reliable.

Pregnanetriol. This steroid is a metabolite of 17α-hydroxyprogesterone and 17α-hydroxypregnenolone. In some forms of congenital adrenal hyperplasia (i.e., 21-hydroxylase defect), the concentration of urinary pregnanetriol gives a good indication of the extent of the enzymatic block that characterizes this disorder.

Aldosterone. Measurement of this steroid in urine is complicated because it is present in such small amounts. This steroid has been measured by both colorimetric and double isotope procedures. In the current state of our knowledge, aldosterone production is best estimated by measuring the aldosterone secretion rate. If this technique is not available, the aldosterone excretion rate is still worth doing in patients with suspected hyperaldosteronism.

Fractionation of 17-Ketosteroids. Urinary 17-ketosteroids can be separated into individual components or groups by several chromatographic procedures. This fractionation may aid the physician in differentiating adrenal from gonadal disorders—i.e., 11-oxy compounds are increased in many adrenal disorders, in particular, adrenocortical hyperplasia. In many patients with adrenocortical carcinoma, dehydroisoandrosterone excretion is very high.

Testosterone. During the last few years, numerous assays for this steroid have been developed and its determination may soon become routine. Such an assay is the best urine method for assessing testosterone production (secretion plus conversion). Normally, the adrenal cortex secretes very little testosterone.

Estrogens. In only a few tumors does the adrenal gland produce significant quantities of estrogen. Total estrogens or individual ones (estradiol, estrone, and estriol) can be measured in urine.

11-Hydroxy and 11-Deoxy Corticoids. By extraction with specific solvents, the corticosteroids can be separated and measured as total 11-hydroxycorticoids and total 11-deoxycorticoids—i.e., Compound F metabolites and Compound S metabolites. These assays will be described in more detail in the section on the Metopirone inhibition test.

Free Hydrocortisone [Cortisol]. In the last few years, the concentration of free or unconjugated hydrocortisone in urine has been recognized as a good indicator of adrenal hydrocortisone production. These levels increase in Cushing's syndrome.

Plasma Determinations

Because the concentration of steroid metabolites is much lower in blood than in urine, only a few methods using blood have been adopted for routine laboratory use. Ideally, plasma concentrations should reflect hormone production (secretion by the gland, plus production by peripheral tissues). However, fluctuations in metabolite formation and protein binding make this direct correlation unreliable. Therefore, rather than using plasma concentrations to reflect production, most physicians now use these concentrations to record changes in diurnal or circadian rhythm.

Plasma 17-Hydroxycorticoids (17-OHCS)

This method is the only one widely used to measure steroid concentrations in blood. In many instances the method measures total 17-hydroxycorticoids, of which hydrocortisone comprises 80%. Plasma 17-OHCS levels undergo a circadian rhythm that is related to a similar rhythm in ACTH secretion. The concentration of 17-OHCS peaks (at 12–30 μg/100 ml) at 6 A.M. and then falls to its minimum (2–12 μg/100 ml) between 6 P.M. and midnight, a rhythm that is usually lost in Cushing's syndrome. Because corticosteroid-binding globulin increases during pregnancy and estrogen therapy, the plasma 17-OHCS also rises and, in these situations, is not a reliable measure of adrenal secretion.

Other Plasma Determinations

Dehydroisoandrosterone sulfate, the steroid found in highest concentration in the circulation (up to 200 μg/100 ml in normal males) has no known physiologic role; hence, it is not assayed routinely. Methods are now available for assaying plasma progesterone, testosterone, and, more recently, estrogen, but they are complex and in most hospitals are done only in research laboratories.

Dynamic Tests

During all dynamic tests of adrenal-pituitary activity, we manipulate the "axis" and, by doing serial measurements, record the effects of the manipulation. We perform three major manipulations:

1. ACTH stimulation test
2. Dexamethasone suppression test
3. Metopirone inhibition test

In the ACTH test, exogenous ACTH is given to stimulate the adrenal output of steroid hormones.

In the dexamethasone suppression test, the administration of biologically active glucocorticoid inhibits ACTH secretion and thereby decreases adrenal activity.

In the Metopirone test, the administration of this drug, by inhibiting 11β-hydroxylation of the steroid molecule, decreases hydrocortisone secretion. As a result of the reduction in hydrocortisone levels, pituitary ACTH release is increased and the adrenal is stimulated to increase 11-deoxyhydrocortisone (Compound S) secretion.

In the assessment of adrenocortical function we measure one or more of the urine 17-hydroxycorticoids, urine 17-ketogenic steroids, urine 17-ketosteroids or plasma 17-hydroxycorticoids before and during administration of compounds that stimulate or suppress adrenocortical activity.

ACTH Stimulation Test

This test measures the changes in adrenal cortical function produced by the administration of ACTH and is reported in one or more of the following parameters: 24-hour urinary excretion levels of 17-ketogenic, 17-hydroxy, and 17-ketosteroids, and plasma 17-hydroxycorticoids, depending upon which assays are available. For any of the assays, control levels must be determined before the ACTH is given. Of the various methods used to administer the ACTH, two common ones are: (1) intravenously over an 8-hour period, and (2) intramuscularly as ACTH gel. In some cases, the ACTH administration is repeated for several days. In the 8-hour intravenous ACTH test in adults, 0.25 mg of synthetic (B1-24)

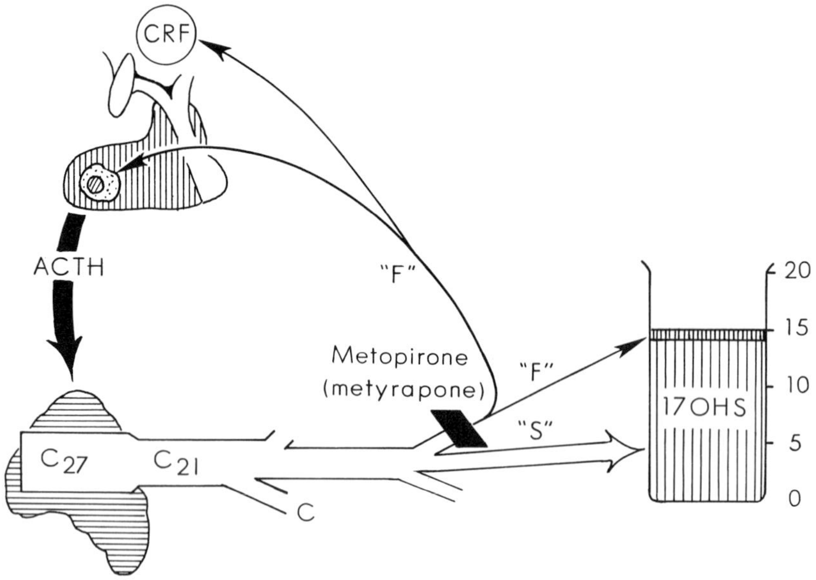

Fig. 7-10. Mechanism of the Metopirone test. Negative feedback inhibition induced by an increased plasma level of cortisol (Compound F) normally keeps the corticotroph from secreting excessive ACTH. Metopirone inhibits 11β-hydroxylation of the steroid molecule and thus decreases cortisol production. ACTH secretion increases if the hypothalamic structures associated with CRF and the pituitary corticotroph are normal. The adrenal is then stimulated to increase secretion of 11-dehydrocortisone (Compound S), the metabolite of which is measured in urine as 17-hydroxycorticoid. Thus a normal response to the Metopirone test is indicated by a rise of 17-hydroxycorticoid excretion on the day of or following Metopirone to twice the control value. When routine separation of the tetrahydro metabolites of Compounds F and S becomes possible, these changes can be followed with greater precision.

C_{27} refers to the number of carbon atoms in the cholesterol molecule, and C_{21} to the number of atoms in glucocorticoid hormones (e.g., Compounds F and S).

ACTH is added to 500 ml of physiologic saline and infused for exactly 8 hours, starting at 8 A.M. Twenty-four-hour urine collections begin at 8 A.M. at least 1 day before the test and preferably 2 days before. If adrenocortical function is normal, there should be a three- to fivefold increase in these values. If the 17-hydroxycorticoids increase less than 100% and 17-ketogenic steroids less than 200% over the individual's "baseline" values on Day 2 of ACTH administration, the patient probably has adrenocortical insufficiency. ACTH administration usually, but not always, increases the levels of urine 17-ketosteroids.

This test is most useful in differentiating primary and secondary adrenocortical hypofunction (see Chapter 4, section on Corticotropin). The response to ACTH will be very low in the primary form. In the secondary form, in which the hypofunction is due to the lack of ACTH, there will be a response although in some patients it will take more than one day of ACTH administration to elicit it. Normal subjects will show a good response on the first day.

Dexamethasone Suppression Test

This test is based on the principle that exogenous glucocorticoids suppress the secretion of ACTH and, in so doing, suppress the secretion of steroids by the adrenal cortex. The urinary excretion of steroids and plasma 17-hydroxycorticoids decreases below control levels. The very small amounts of steroids given do not contribute significantly to the products measured in the urine. With dexamethasone, two schedules are used: (1) 2 mg/24 hours (4 doses of 0.5 mg daily) for 2 days; (2) 8 mg/24 hours (4 doses of 2 mg daily) for 2 days. The low dose suppresses normally functioning adrenals so that the urine levels of 17-hydroxycorticoids decrease to less than 3 mg/24 hours on the second day. The levels of 17-ketogenic steroids decrease by more than 50%.

The higher dose is usually required to suppress the activity of the hyperplastic adrenals of Cushing's syndrome. Adrenocortical tumors are usually not suppressed by any dose of dexamethasone, however high. The "overnight" suppression test is performed by giving 1 ml of dexamethasone at 11 P.M. and taking blood for 17-hydroxycorticoids at 8 A.M. the next morning. Normally, the plasma level will be reduced to 6 μg/100 ml. In patients with adrenal cortical hyperplasia, the level will remain above 10 μg/100 ml. This test is most often used as an outpatient screening procedure.

Metopirone Test of Pituitary Function

Metyrapone (Metopirone*) inhibits the adrenocortical 11β-hydroxylase enzyme system. When administered to a human, it inhibits this enzyme in the adrenal and thus decreases the secretion of hydrocortisone, which, via the negative-feedback-inhibition control system, increases ACTH secretion. The production of the immediate precursor of hydrocortisone, 11-desoxyhydrocortisone, increases greatly (Fig. 7-10).

In this test, various doses have been administered, but in general, 500–750 mg is given orally every 4 hours for 24 hours. Twenty-four-hour urines are collected for 2 days before, during, and 1 day after the administration of Metopirone. The highest urinary steroid levels are usually found 24 hours after administration. In subjects with normal adrenal-pituitary function, levels of 17-hydroxycorticoids and 17-ketogenic steroids increase 100%. If the steroid metabolites are separated into 11-deoxy and 11-oxy compounds (Group G of other urine steroid assays), the reliability of the test can be greatly increased. By this separation we can accurately determine whether 11β-hydroxylation has been inhibited.

Before concluding that failure to respond to Metopirone is due to pituitary disease, the physician should determine whether the adrenal can respond to ACTH; this can be done by carrying out the ACTH test. The Metopirone test assesses the pituitary "reserve"—i.e., it determines whether the gland can produce more ACTH when needed. In patients with pituitary deficiency, the concentration of urine steroids does not increase.

* 2-Methyl-1,2-bis-(3-pyridil)-1-propanone, also designated SU-4885.

Steroid "Production Rates"

For these specialized determinations, we must administer the specific steroid tagged with a radioactive label (carbon-14 or tritium). A metabolite with the label is isolated from the urine and purified, and its specific activity (counts per minute per unit of weight) must be determined. However, if the method is to be valid, the metabolite must be derived only from the steroid being investigated. This procedure makes the assumption that administered steroid and the naturally

Table 7-3. Tests of Adrenal Cortical and Pituitary ACTH Responsiveness

Test	*Method of Administration*	*Response*
ACTH	0.25 mg over 8 hr	Change in urinary excretion of 17-KGS* or 17-OHCS† —three to fivefold increase over baseline value on second day of ACTH administration
Metopirone	750 mg p.o. every 4 hr for 6 doses	Twofold increase in urinary 17-KGS or 17-OHCS over baseline the day after administration
Dexamethasone		Normals show fall to below 4 mg of 17-KGS or 17-OHCS excretion per day
Low dose	0.5 mg every 6 hr for 8 doses	
High dose	2.0 mg every 6 hr for 8 doses	Hyperplasia—50% decrease from baseline urinary steroids on second day
		Tumors—no change

* 17-Ketogenic steroid.
† 17-Hydroxycorticosteroid.

Table 7-4. Normal Values in Investigation of Adrenal Cortex

Hormones and steroids	*Normal range*	*Hormones and steroids*	*Normal range*
Production rates of major hormones		Urine excretion	
Hydrocortisone (mg/day)	10–20	17-Ketogenic steroids (mg/day)	
Aldosterone (μg/day)	60–200	Males	9–17
Testosterone (mg/day)		Females	7–12
Males	5–8	17-Hydroxycorticosteroids (mg/day)	1–10
Females	0.3–0.8	17-Ketosteroids (mg/day)	
Dehydroisoandrosterone	25–30	Males	8–20
Plasma levels (μg/100 ml)		Females	5–15
Hydrocortisone	5–20 (at 8:00 A.M.)	Estrogens, total (μg/day)	
Aldosterone	0.002–0.01	Males	4–25
Testosterone		Females	4–60
Males	0.5–1.0	Pregnanetriol (mg/day)	0–4
Females	0.03–0.06	Pregnanediol (mg/day)	
Protein binding (%)		Males	0–1.5
Hydrocortisone	80	Females	
Aldosterone	70	Follicular	0.5–1.5
Testosterone		Luteal	2–7
Males	90	Postmenopausal	0.2–1.0
Females	95	Aldosterone (μg/day)	4–17
		Free hydrocortistone (μg/day)	0–200

secreted steroid mix rapidly and are metabolized in exactly the same manner. The urine must be collected until all radioactivity from the metabolite being measured is excreted. The weight of the administered (labeled) steroid is negligible; therefore any reduction in the specific activity of the metabolite excreted in the urine is due to (endogenous) unlabeled hormone production. In this way, the production rate of steroid (weight of steroid produced per 24 hours) can be calculated. For example, the production rate of hydrocortisone can be determined by administering tritium or carbon-14-labeled hydrocortisone and measuring the specific activity of urinary tetrahydrohydrocortisone. Such determinations give a much better assessment of adrenocortical production than direct measures of urinary steroids or metabolites.

Disorders of the Adrenal Cortex

Cushing's Syndrome

Cushing's syndrome is due to sustained overproduction or excessive administration of the glucocorticoid, hydrocortisone or its analogues. In 1932 Harvey Cushing, a neurosurgeon, described a group of patients who had this disorder and a basophilic tumor of the pituitary gland—an association designated Cushing's *disease*.[10] Over the years other causes of hydrocortisone excess have been recognized and the common clinical picture resulting from these many causes is referred to as Cushing's *syndrome*.[14]

Pathogenesis

Disease in the hypothalamus or pituitary may lead to overproduction of ACTH with subsequent overactivity of the adrenal. Benign basophilic or chromophobic adenomas of the anterior pituitary may produce Cushing's syndrome, and rarely, the tumor may be malignant. More frequently, however, no pituitary tumor can be demonstrated. In these instances, some as-yet-undefined hypothalamic disturbance presumably leads to overproduction of corticotropin-releasing factor (CRF) and subsequent excessive secretion of ACTH from the pituitary.

In recent years many workers have demonstrated that nonendocrine neoplasms can produce ACTH or an ACTH-like material and give rise to bilateral adrenal hyperplasia and Cushing's syndrome. The "ectopic ACTH syndrome" is encountered most frequently in patients with oat-cell carcinoma of the lung. Carcinoma of the thymus and pancreas may also produce excess ACTH. This syndrome has been reported less commonly with carcinoma of the ovary, testis, gallbladder, kidney, prostate, thyroid, breast, colon, and salivary glands, as well as bronchial adenoma. The material isolated from the tumor is, by all current techniques, identical with pituitary ACTH. This abnormal production of ACTH leads to bilateral adrenal hyperplasia and usually very high urinary steroid levels. However, because of the short course of many of these cancers, the usual clinical features of Cushing's syndrome may not develop.

A functioning adrenal neoplasm can cause Cushing's syndrome by producing excessive amounts of hydrocortisone. The tumor is independent of pituitary control, and pituitary ACTH is suppressed. The tumor may be a benign adenoma or a functioning carcinoma.

Incidence

Cushing's syndrome may be seen at any age but is most common in the third to sixth decade and affects women more often than men. The disease frequently appears during or just after pregnancy.

The commonest cause of Cushing's syndrome is a pituitary-hypothalamic disorder overproducing ACTH. The "ectopic ACTH syndrome" is more common in later life and affects men more often than women. Adrenal adenomas are more common in the left than in the right adrenal. Functioning adrenal carcinomas, which are seen chiefly in children, give rise to palpable abdominal masses and distant bony secondaries.

Symptoms and Signs

Although the classic features of this condition —truncal obesity, rounding of the face, and purple striae—are due to hydrocortisone excess (Fig. 7-11), the clinical picture may be complicated by adrenal androgen excess causing hirsutism, mineralocorticoid excess, resulting in hypokalemia with weakness, or in some adrenal tumors, estrogen excess, producing gynecomastia in males.

Overproduction of hydrocortisone affects most metabolic processes with the biologic results shown in Table 7-5.

In women with Cushing's syndrome, androgen overproduction by the adrenal leads to hirsutism and acne. Oligomenorrhea and infertility may be prominent features. The anabolic effects of the androgens occasionally produce increased body weight and muscle mass.

Mineralocorticoid excess may contribute to sodium retention, hypertension, and potassium loss. This is rarely due to aldosterone overproduction, but under excessive ACTH stimulation, deoxycorticosterone secretion may increase.

Table 7-5. Biological Effects of Hydrocortisone Overproduction

Protein metabolism
Thinning of skin
Reddish striae
Loss of bone matrix and demineralization
Poor wound healing
Muscle wasting and weakness
Capillary fragility and bruising
Impaired growth (children)
Carbohydrate metabolism
Abnormal glucose tolerance curve
Overt diabetes mellitus
Lipid metabolism
Centripetal fat distribution
Moon facies
Electrolyte balance
Sodium retention, potassium loss
Hypertension
Hypervolemia
Hematopoietic effects
Eosinopenia, lymphopenia
Polymorphonuclear leukocytosis
Erythrocytosis
General effects
Hypercalciuria and renal calculi
Gastric ulceration
Psychosis
Impaired immunological tolerance

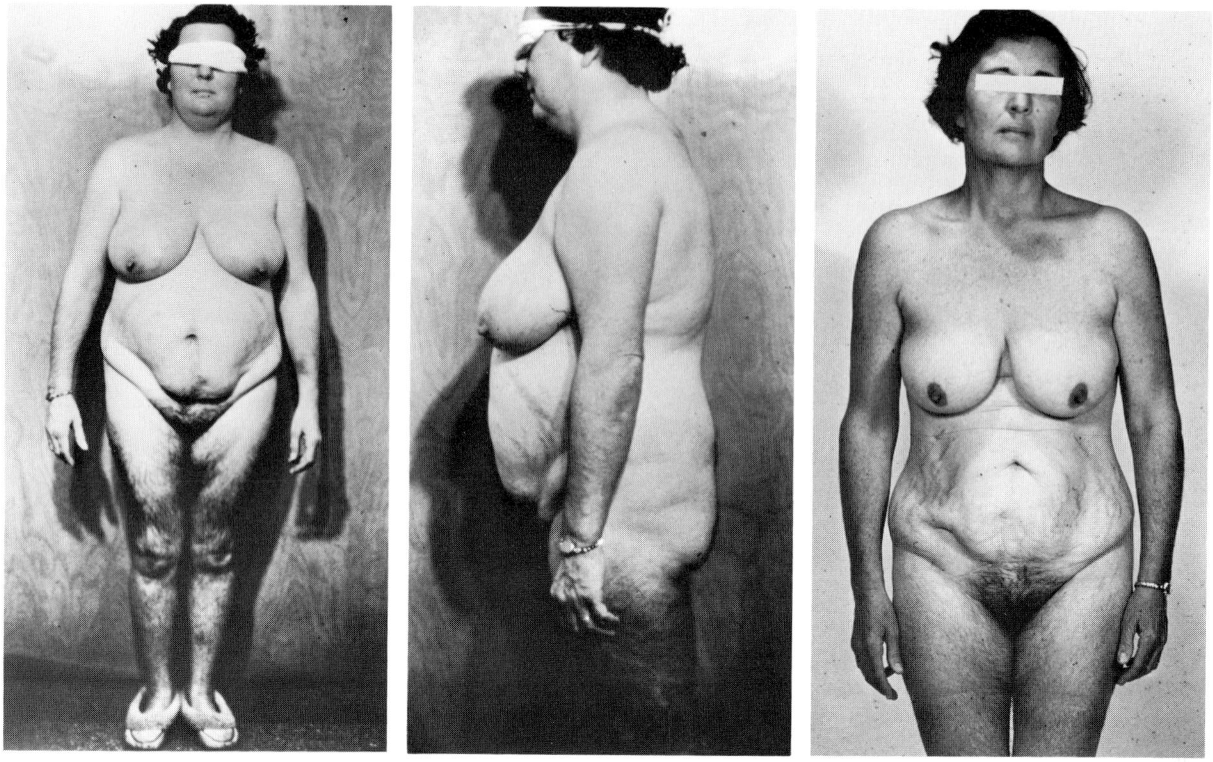

Fig. 7-11. Cushing's syndrome. A. Truncal obesity, striae, moon face, and hirsutism. **B.** Lateral view of same patient shows obvious buffalo hump and lateral abdominal striae are more clearly seen than in front view. **C.** Same patient is shown following cure of Cushing's syndrome by removal of both adrenals, which were hyperplastic. Note regression of obesity and moon face and increase in pigmentation, particularly of the areolae. This pigmentation is probably due to a pituitary oversecretion of ACTH.

In addition to the effects of the hormones, there may be clinical symptoms related to the causal disorder: Pituitary tumors may cause local pressure effects; nonendocrine tumors may cause cachexia; and large adrenal carcinomas may produce intraabdominal symptoms.

Laboratory Diagnosis

Routine Investigations and Common Positive Results

Hematologic. There is relative lymphopenia, leukocytosis, and erythrocytosis. Platelet count is normal.

Chemistry. Tests will show:

1. Abnormal glucose tolerance curve
2. Hypokalemia, hypochloremia, alkalosis
3. Hypercalciuria
4. Decreased gamma globulin

X-Ray. X-ray films reveal:

1. Demineralization and compression fractures of the spine
2. Codfish vertebrae
3. Displacement of a kidney on IVP by an adrenal neoplasm; renal calculi
4. Enlargement of the sella turcica; rarely, signs of increased intracranial pressure
5. Peptic ulcer demonstrated by a barium meal

Demonstration of Hydrocortisone Overproduction

Urine Excretion of Steriod Metabolites. In Cushing's syndrome, the outupt of 17-ketogenic steroids and 17-hydroxycorticoids is commonly elevated. The excretion of urinary 17-ketosteroids in Cushing's syndrome depends upon the cause. The level is normal in adrenal adenoma, high in adrenal carcinoma, and variable in adrenal hyperplasia.

Plasma 17-Hydroxycorticoids. The normal 8 A.M. fasting plasma 17-hydroxycorticoid level in adults is between 8 and 30 μg/100 ml. This single determination, however, cannot be used to confirm or exclude the diagnosis of Cushing's syndrome because many such patients have values within or slightly above the normal range. In Cushing's syndrome, however, the normal diurnal rhythm of plasma hydroxycorticoid secretion disappears. When this loss of diurnal rhythm is demonstrated, preferably using 4-hour samples over a 24-hour period, the diagnosis of Cushing's syndrome can be strongly suspected.

Urinary Free Hydrocortisone. Normal subjects excrete approximately 30–60 μg of unconjugated hydrocortisone in their urine in a 24-hour period. This unconjugated form is thought to directly reflect the amount of hydrocortisone produced by the adrenal. In Cushing's syndrome, the 24-hour excretion of free hydrocortisone in the urine may increase to 200 μg or more.

Chief Causes of Cushing's Syndrome

In most cases the diagnosis of Cushing's syndrome is suspected on clinical grounds and proved by laboratory evidence of hydrocortisone overproduction. The management of the syndrome, however, depends upon finding the cause. One must differentiate among adrenal (cortical) neoplasia, hypothalamic-pituitary overproduction of ACTH, and "the ectopic ACTH syndrome." The dynamic tests are used to make this differentiation, and for clarity, the results of such tests are described for each of the possible causes of Cushing's syndrome and summarized in Table 7-6.

Adrenal Adenoma

This tumor is usually autonomous and produces excess hydrocortisone with complete suppression of ACTH and hypothalamic-pituitary control. The administration of exogenous dexamethasone cannot further decrease ACTH release, nor can it directly inhibit the adrenal tumor. The autonomous adrenal overproduction of

Table 7-6. Dexamethasone Suppression, Diurnal Variation of Plasma Cortisol and Response to Metopirone in Various Types of Cushing's Syndrome

Type	*Suppression by dexamethasone*		*Diurnal variation of plasma cortisol*	*Normal or hyperactive response to Metopirone*
	2 mg	*8 mg*		
I. Bilateral adrenal cortical hyperplasia:				
Without demonstrable pituitary tumor	No	Yes	Absent	Yes
With benign pituitary tumor	No	Variable	Absent	Yes
With malignant pituitary tumor	No	No	Absent	No
From ectopic malignant ACTH-producing tumor (e.g., lung cancer)	No	No	Absent	No
From benign lung tumor (bronchial adenoma) producing ACTH-like substance	No	Variable	Absent	Variable
II. Adrenal adenoma	No	No	Absent	No
III. Adrenal carcinoma	No	No	Absent	No
IV. Secondary to obesity	Yes	Yes	Present	Yes

hydrocortisone continues and, as a result, the urinary excretion of hydrocortisone metabolites is unchanged during the administration of dexamethasone.[17]

Since the tumor is autonomous, it will not respond readily to exogenous ACTH administration. There are exceptions, however, and in some patients with adrenal adenomas, the urinary 17-hydroxy or 17-ketogenic steroids increase after ACTH administration. It is not clear whether the increase in steroid output comes from the adenoma or from the relatively atrophic adrenal tissue around the adenoma and in the opposite atrophic gland.

As mentioned earlier, Metopirone interferes with 11β-hydroxylation in the adrenal. The biosynthesis of hydrocortisone is decreased, and according to the principle of negative feedback control, the pituitary output of ACTH will undergo a compensatory increase. This in turn will increase the adrenal production of steroids. However, in patients with Cushing's syndrome due to an adrenal adenoma, there is no increase in steroid production by the adrenal. There are two possible explanations for this: Long-standing hydrocortisone excess has depressed the pituitary's response to hydrocortisone deficiency, or the autonomous adenoma does not increase its steroid output when endogenous ACTH production increases.

Adrenal Carcinoma

Very high urinary steroids, hypokalemia, and a palpable abdominal mass suggest this diagnosis. The carcinoma is completely autonomous so that urinary steroid excretion will not change when dexamethasone, ACTH, or Metopirone is given.

Adrenal Hyperplasia from ACTH Overproduction

Hypothalamic-Pituitary Dysfunction. As described in Chapter 4, the "set point" of ACTH release is elevated, and probably the output of corticotropin-releasing factor increases, causing increased ACTH secretion.

The altered "set point" results in continuous ACTH output during the "small dose" dexamethasone suppression test (2 mg/day). However, the "large dose" dexamethasone suppression test (8 mg/day) does suppress the pituitary release of ACTH and the adrenal steroid production falls, so that the urinary 17-ketogenic steroid and 17-hydroxycorticoid levels are reduced to less than 50% of control values.[17]

If the adrenals can respond, the administration of ACTH usually increases urinary steroid levels further. The increase may not develop if the hyperplastic adrenals are already stimulated to their maximum.

Similarly, the administration of Metopirone and the subsequent reduction of hydrocortisone production usually causes the pituitary to release more ACTH and the urinary steroids will rise further. If the pituitary ACTH production is already maximal, this increase in urinary steroids may not occur.

Pituitary Adenomas. Often these lesions are not demonstrated before the sella is explored. In these patients, dynamic tests give results similar to those found in nonneoplastic hypothalamic-pituitary disorders.

Pituitary Carcinomas. Because these rare tumors are autonomous, one cannot alter ACTH production by giving dexamethasone or Metopirone. Carcinomas are usually recognized when they erode the sella or compress the optic chiasma.

Ectopic ACTH Syndrome. ACTH overproduction from the "ectopic site" is autonomous and hence is not suppressed by the increased hydrocortisone production.[19] After dexamethasone administration, there is no change in urinary steroid levels. Similarly, the tumor's secretion of ACTH-like material cannot be increased by Metopirone. Because these tumors can produce enough ACTH to induce maximal adrenal response, there may be no further rise when ACTH is administered. This syndrome is characterized by very high urinary steroid levels, hypokalemia, few clinical manifestations of Cushing's syndrome, and finally the specific symptoms of the tumor. The occasionally associated bronchial adenoma is unusual because it may respond to dynamic tests; the ACTH-like material can then be suppressed or stimulated by dexamethasone and Metopirone. The results of such stimulation resemble those obtained when hypothalamic-pituitary dysfunction causes adrenal hyperplasia.

Differential Diagnosis of Types of Cushing's Syndrome

Three tests usually enable the physician to determine the type of Cushing's syndrome present in a given patient (see Table 7-4).

1. Dexamethasone suppression. The patient takes 2 mg for 2 days (0.5 mg q.i.d.) and 8 mg for 2 days (2 mg q.i.d.). The total amount of urinary 17-hydroxycorticoids on 24-hour urine collections on the second and fourth day of the test is measured to demonstrate that 17-hydroxycorticoid excretion has been suppressed, compared with the control value.
2. Diurnal rhythm of plasma cortisol levels (reflecting diurnal change in ACTH secretion). Plasma cortisol is measured at 8 A.M. and 8 P.M. In normal subjects and those with Cushing's syndrome secondary to obesity, the 8 A.M. value (8–30 μg/100 ml) will be at least twice that measured at 8 P.M.
3. Metopirone test. This test can differentiate those cases due to pituitary hyperplasia or to ACTH tumors, which usually respond, from those due to adrenal tumors or to the ectopic ACTH syndrome, which do not.

After a 24-hour control urine is obtained, 750 mg Metopirone is administered by mouth every 4 hours for 6 doses. A 24-hour urine is obtained on the day of Metopirone administration and the day after as well. Patients with normal or hyperplastic adrenals will approximately double their 17-hydroxycorticoid excretion. However, in patients with an adrenal tumor or the ectopic ACTH syndrome, the pituitary corticotrophs are inhibited, and there is no increase in ACTH output during the Metopirone test.

Management of Cushing's Syndrome

The proper treatment of this syndrome depends upon knowing the specific cause.

Adrenal Neoplasms

Adrenal Adenoma. The treatment of choice is surgical removal, after radiological demonstration of its location. However, because precise localization of the tumor may not be possible even with arteriography or venography (which is hazardous because of the risk of hemorrhage), it may be necessary to explore both adrenals. Following unilateral adrenalectomy for an adenoma, the patient requires careful management; the other adrenal, although anatomically intact, will be atrophic because pituitary ACTH secretion was suppressed. The patient is maintained with steroid supplements for several weeks and, as these are gradually reduced, normal ACTH secretion is restored. The repeated administration of exogenous ACTH in time will stimulate the atrophic adrenal but will not hasten the recovery of normal hypothalamic and pituitary regulation of the production and release of ACTH. After either unilateral adrenalectomy for Cushing's syndrome or the withdrawal of glucocorticoids after a prolonged course of treatment, ACTH output returns to normal some time before adrenal cortical secretion. Thus the adrenal appears to be inhibited directly by the effect of glucocorticoid excess as well as indirectly through decreased ACTH secretion.

Adrenal Carcinoma. The adrenal and its tumor are excised, and because of atrophy of the contralateral gland, the patient is managed with great care in the weeks that follow surgery. The prognosis in patients with adrenal carcinoma is roughly as follows: If the tumor is still encapsulated, the prognosis is fair. However, if metastases are demonstrated, survival is always short. Metastases may appear relatively late and usually develop in liver, lungs, and bone. Treatment of adrenal cancer with o, p′-DDD[2,2-bis(2-chlorophenyl-4-chlorophenyl)-1, 1 dichloroethane] has met only limited success.[27]

Bilateral Adrenal Hyperplasia

There is still considerable controvery concerning the correct therapy for these patients, and no single approach covers them all. If a pituitary adenoma is demonstrated, specific therapy must be directed against the pituitary. Methods include hypophysectomy, high-voltage radiation, implantation of radioactive isotopes, and cryohypophysectomy. (The results obtained with any one form of therapy depend, in large measure, on the experience of the local team.)

Patients with nonendocrine tumors that produce excessive amounts of ACTH are treated by attacking the neoplasm directly. In patients with an oat-cell carcinoma, considerable remission has been induced by pneumonectomy. In these tumors the prognosis is that of primary neoplasm and is not greatly influenced by the effects of hydrocortisone excess.

Therapy is particularly difficult in patients who have bilateral adrenal hyperplasia but have no evidence of extraendocrine tumors or any demonstrable pituitary tumor. Bilateral total adrenalectomy removes the source of hydrocortisone and induces a clinical remission (Fig. 7-11**C**). However, a number of these patients have developed a chromophobe adenoma of the pituitary in the first few years after operation.[22] Because adrenalectomy removes negative feedback control of pituitary ACTH production, ACTH secretion usually increases in spite of replacement therapy. In time, the high level of ACTH production leads to generalized pigmentation because of the similarity in chemical structure between a portion of the ACTH molecule and melanocyte-stimulating hormone. Later, the pituitary adenoma may cause local pressure effects.

To avoid these complications, subtotal adrenalectomy is sometimes performed, removing one adrenal and approximately two-thirds of the other. The remnant produces enough hydrocortisone to control pituitary ACTH production. However, the symptoms and signs of Cushing's syndrome may recur if the remnant undergoes further hyperplasia. Subsequent reoperation for removal of the remnant is technically difficult. On the other hand, the remnant may not provide enough hydrocortisone to control ACTH production; then the end result is similar to total adrenalectomy.

Other workers suggest that patients with bilateral adrenal hyperplasia can be treated by removing one adrenal and radiating the pituitary. When adrenalectomy is followed by a tissue dose of 4,000–5,000 R to the pituitary, 70% of patients go into remission. Pituitary radiation alone, using cobalt-60 to give a tissue dose of 4,000–5,000 R, brings remission in approximately 50–60% of patients. If after 3 or 4 months there is no remission, the patient must have further therapy. However, irradiation often makes pituitary surgery technically difficult and second courses of pituitary irradiation often induce such complications as hemorrhagic necrosis and complete anterior pituitary insufficiency.

Management of Adrenalectomy

Patients with Cushing's syndrome must be brought to operation in optimal medical condition—the attending physician must correct any hypokalemia and any plasma deficit associated with the relative polycythemia. Steroid therapy is usually not required before operation.

The adrenal can be approached through a loin incision, transabdominally or transthoracically. The transabdominal approach usually allows the best exposure of both adrenals. On the day of operation, the patient is given 100 mg of hydrocortisone sodium succinate in an intravenous infusion over 8 hours; this is repeated every 8 hours to a total of 300 mg on the operative day. The day after operation, intravenous therapy should be continued with 100 mg every 12 hours. In addition, on the evening of the second day, 100 mg of cortisone acetate is given intramuscularly. This will take effect by the third day when intravenous therapy can be discontinued. Intramuscular cortisone acetate is given every 12 hours in decreasing doses until the patient is able to take oral medication. In approximately 1 week, the patient should be on a maintenance schedule of 37.5 mg of cortisone daily—25 mg at 8 A.M. and 12.5 mg at 6 P.M. to mimic the normal diurnal variation. Sometimes additional mineralocorticoid effect is needed to correct hyperkalemia; this may be given as 9α-fluorohydrocortisone, 0.05–0.1 mg daily.

Adrenal Insufficiency

Acute Adrenal Insufficiency

The clinical picture reflects an absolute or relative lack of adrenocortical hormones. Although it may be due to pituitary insufficiency (resulting from surgical removal, trauma, hemorrhage, infarction) and a subsequent lack of ACTH, acute insufficiency is more commonly due to primary adrenal disease such as hemorrhage, infection, and infarction. Surgical removal of both adrenals can be considered a cause of acute adrenal insufficiency.

Although this is a rare disorder, it should be looked for in ill patients who are hypotensive and have the appropriate clinical settings. Some patients being treated with anticoagulants have been known to develop intraadrenal hemorrhage resulting in acute destruction of the adrenal. As well, arterial thrombosis with infarction of the adrenal presents with severe abdominal pain localized to the upper abdomen and is followed by vascular collapse. Severe systemic infection by meningococcus (the Waterhouse-Friderichsen syndrome) is characterized by high fever, meningeal irritation, petechial hemorrhages in the skin and mucosa, and vascular collapse. In patients who have no adrenal reserve, acute insufficiency can be precipitated by stress or by withdrawing glucocorticoid substitution therapy. The vascular collapse typical of this syndrome is associated with anorexia, nausea, and vomiting.

The diagnosis is confirmed after the crisis has been treated, using the same parameters as in chronic adrenal insufficiency.

Management of Adrenal Crisis

Intravenous hydrocortisone, the mainstay of therapy, starts with 100 mg of hydrocortisone sodium succinate given over 30 seconds; this is followed by 100 mg given in 1,000 ml of 5% glucose in normal saline over 8 hours. This amount of hydrocortisone should induce adequate sodium retention, but if the blood pressure does not rise, a vasopressor such as neosynephrine may be used. Fluid replacement of up to 3,000–4,000 ml on the first day is usually required because of the severe fluid and electrolyte loss from nausea and vomiting. Appropriate antibiotic coverage should also be given. Hydrocortisone is gradually reduced to maintenance level after the crisis is over.

Chronic Adrenal Insufficiency

Primary Insufficiency—Addison's Disease

Idiopathic atrophy, which is responsible for more than one-half of all primary adrenal insufficiency, has been attributed to an autoimmune disorder and, indeed, adrenal antibodies can be demonstrated in many patients. The next most common cause is tuberculosis involving the cortex and medulla, causing necrosis followed by calcification in the adrenal. Almost 95% of the gland must be destroyed to produce symptoms and signs. Two-thirds of these patients will have no history of tuberculosis, but careful investigation will show evidence of old inactive tuberculosis, most commonly in the lung.

Rarely Addison's disease may be produced by histoplasmosis, coccidioidomycosis, and blastomycosis, or by infiltration of the gland by sarcoidosis, secondary malignant tumor, or leukemia.

The clinical picture of chronic adrenal insufficiency results from the lack of hydrocortisone plus the increased pituitary secretion of ACTH and MSH. The symptoms and signs develop slowly and insidiously. The common clinical findings are:

1. Weakness
2. Weight loss
3. Hyperpigmentation
4. Hypotension
5. Anorexia
6. Vomiting
7. Nausea
8. Hypoglycemic symptoms
9. Abdominal pain

Severe fatigue or asthenia is a common and major symptom of this disease. Nearly all these patients have a dusky-brown hyperpigmentation, although some do not. The deepened color is most marked about scars, nipples, and pressure points, such as knuckles and elbows (Fig. 7-12). In addition they may have excessive pigmentation of palmar creases and often gray-blue coloring of the mucosal surfaces, such as the buccal area or vagina. These patients have black freckles or moles, especially over the upper trunk. A normal summer tan which persists well into the winter

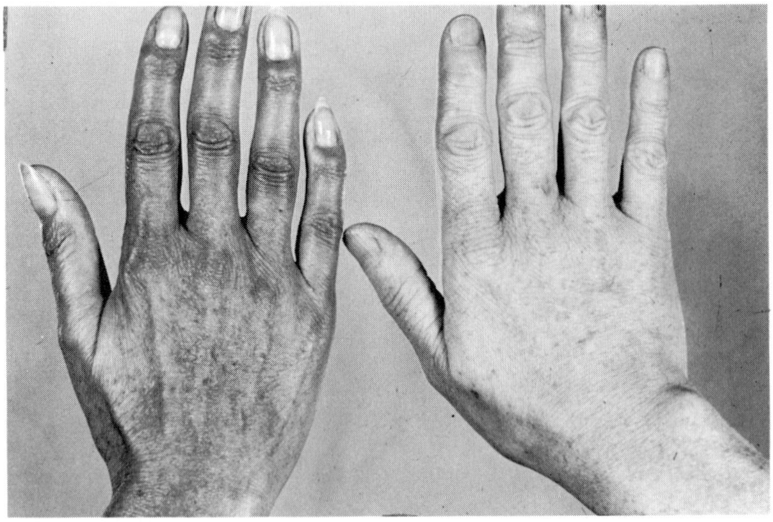

Fig. 7-12. Idiopathic Addison's disease. The pigmentation of the hand on the left is contrasted with that of a normal hand.

months should arouse suspicion, especially if it is associated with hypotension and weight loss. Changes in pigmentation are less definite in those who are naturally dark because of racial origin, but even here distinct changes in degrees of pigmentation can be detected. Areas of vitiligo may be found in 10–15% of patients with Addison's disease. These are usually irregular white patches scattered most commonly in exposed parts in the skin of the body.

Characteristically, patients with Addison's disease have low blood pressure with a narrow pulse pressure and are prone to postural giddiness.

Most of these patients will have some gastrointestinal symptoms such as anorexia accompanied by nausea and vomiting and, occasionally, diarrhea. The vomiting and diarrhea lead to further electrolyte imbalance which complicates the clinical picture.

Episodes of hunger associated with sweating and weakness suggest intermittent hypoglycemia. The Addisonian patient appears to have a reduced threshold to hypoglycemia and may have these symptoms with blood sugar levels between 40 and 50 mg/100 ml.

Gonadal function is disturbed; the patient loses libido and develops impotence or oligomenorrhea. Infertility is common but not invariable.[16] In women axillary and pubic hair may be reduced because of the lack of adrenal androgens.

Some patients may describe episodes of muscular weakness that progress to actual paralysis, or severe muscular cramping progressing to actual flexion contractures, particularly of the legs. These muscle disorders have been attributed to a disturbance in sodium and potassium balance at the neuromuscular end-plate.

Laboratory Findings. Just as the clinical signs and symptoms can be related to deficient glucocorticoid or mineralocorticoid production by the adrenal, so, too, may the laboratory findings.

Although many patients have a normal hemoglobin at the time of diagnosis, treatment and rehydration uncover an iron-deficiency anemia. The plasma volume is returned to normal and the hemoglobin falls to 10 or 11 gm/100 ml. These patients, whose iron deficiency is primarily due to poor absorption of iron, may also show eosinophilia and leukocytosis.

The untreated patient usually has a reduced serum sodium and normal or elevated serum potassium levels. With progressive dehydration, glomerular filtration falls and azotemia develops. Impaired renal perfusion causes a further rise in serum potassium. In the untreated disease, renal tubular function is altered, the tubule may not reabsorb sodium from the glomerular filtrate or exchange sodium for potassium distally. Because of impaired renal concentrating ability progressive dehydration develops.

Hypochlorhydria and gastric mucosal atrophy

are also common. There may be associated malabsorption.

The cardiovascular changes relate primarily to decreased blood volume and electrolyte disturbances. The various electrocardiographic changes are secondary to the electrolyte disturbances.

In many cases, the electroencephalogram shows a decrease in the predominant frequency and an increase in the number of short bursts of low-frequency waves.

Radiographic studies may show a small heart, evidence of pulmonary tuberculosis, abdominal calcification in the region of the adrenal, and occasionally, calcification of the pinnas of the ears, which cannot, as yet, be explained.

Although the clinical picture and the laboratory evidence discussed above may strongly suggest adrenocortical insufficiency, the specific diagnosis depends on laboratory tests designed to assess adrenal function. Indirect evidence such as impaired response to water loading, eosinophilia, and disturbed salivary sodium-potassium ratio only serve as rough screening procedures, and often give false-negative or false-positive results.[9]

For direct assessment of adrenocortical function, the physician must measure the basal activity and repeat the measurements after appropriate stimulation of the adrenal gland.[15]

1. Basal excretion of adrenocortical hormones. At least two 24-hour collections of urine are analyzed for 17-ketosteroids and 17-hydroxy- or 17-ketogenic steroids. In most patients with untreated Addison's disease, the 24-hour excretion will be low. However, it is important to note that these steroid levels may also be low in nonspecific chronic illness. Furthermore, in borderline Addison's disease, basal excretion levels may be normal—that is, the adrenal is responding at its maximal level to high levels of ACTH. The gland produces enough steroid for day-to-day function but cannot increase production in times of stress. Plasma hydrocortisone levels, which reflect the amount in the circulation at the time of sampling, may vary, depending on the time of day of sampling and on the rates of secretion or disappearance of hydrocortisone. For this reason, single plasma determinations are of little value in diagnosis. Drugs containing estrogen will give rise to erroneously high values for plasma hydrocortisone because they increase the level of protein binding and slow the disappearance rate.

2. ACTH stimulation. This method is the one most commonly used to assess the adrenal's capacity to respond to stress. After such stimulation, the amount of 17-hydroxy- or 17-ketogenic steroids and 17-ketosteroids are measured in 24-hour urine collections. The response of the adrenal is reflected by the increase in urinary steroids on the first and second day of the test, as compared to the mean control levels. If adrenal function is normal, the second day's increment will be greater than 200% of the control value.

Acute adrenal insufficiency can be precipitated in patients with Addison's disease who are undergoing ACTH testing. Under ACTH stimulation, adrenal reserve may be completely exhausted and steroid production may actually decrease below control values on the second day of the test. For this reason, if adrenal insufficiency is strongly suspected, the patient should be given dexamethasone (1 mg) or fluorohydrocortisone (0.1 mg) before the test. These doses will protect the patient and will not suppress the adrenal's response to ACTH, nor will they interfere with the determination of urinary steroids.

Secondary Adrenal Insufficiency

Deficiency of ACTH results in adrenal atrophy and impaired steroid production either as part of complete anterior pituitary failure or, rarely, as a selective deficiency of ACTH. The etiology of pituitary insufficiency has been discussed in Chapter 4.

In many ways, adrenal insufficiency due to pituitary disease mimics primary adrenal insufficiency. However, because ACTH is lacking, most such patients, rather than showing increased pigmentation, are pale and fail to tan. They may complain of the usual effects of glucocorticoid lack such as weakness, fatigue, gastrointestinal complaints, and muscle cramps.

Secondary adrenal insufficiency may eventually lead to reduced aldosterone production due not to ACTH deficiency, but to general atrophy of the gland. This is a late stage, however, and initially serum electrolytes, blood volume, and blood pressure remain close to normal.

The diagnosis of adrenal insufficiency secondary to pituitary disease can again be confirmed only after the combined assessment of pituitary and adrenal function. Thus, as in Addison's disease, the basal excretion of urinary 17-hydroxy- or 17-ketogenic steroids may be low, but these levels will increase considerably after ACTH is administered intravenously. The impaired endogenous ACTH production can be demonstrated by the Metopirone test.

Treatment of Adrenal Insufficiency

The treatment of the acute adrenal crisis has been discussed earlier in this chapter. Adequate steroid and electrolyte replacement plus specific measures directed at the complications are the cornerstones of therapy.

Chronic

In general, the patient with Addison's disease given proper steroid replacement can look forward to a full and active life. He should be carefully instructed about his disease, the need for continuous therapy, and his conduct during acute illness or stress. Nausea is usually the first symptom of relative adrenal insufficiency; in this event, the patient should double the dose of glucocorticoids for a day or two until he can consult a physician.

Glucocorticoid replacement should provide the patient with the equivalent of 20–30 mg of hydrocortisone per day.[11] For this replacement, many synthetic glucocorticoid hormones with a great range of potency are available. One and one-half tablets of any of the commercially available glucocorticoids are adequate for usual maintenance. In general, it is advisable to mimic the normal diurnal rhythm in normal subjects so that two-thirds of the glucocorticoid is given in the morning and one-third in the afternoon. Side effects from normal maintenance therapy are rare, although occasionally a patient will complain of weight gain due to fluid retention, or postprandial distress due to gastric irritation. Prednisone, being the least expensive glucocorticoid, is usually the drug of choice; the dose is 7.5 mg daily (5 mg at 8 A.M. and 2.5 mg at 6 P.M.).

Fluorohydrocortisone in a dose of approximately 0.1 mg/day further increases the patient's sense of well-being. The actual dose, which must be adjusted to the individual, may range from 0.05 mg to as high as 0.3 mg/day. The dose is selected to maintain the patient's body weight and blood pressure within normal limits. Mineralocorticoids may not be needed in secondary adrenal insufficiency if aldosterone production continues to be adequate.

Primary Aldosteronism—Conn's Syndrome

In the original description of this syndrome, primary aldosteronism was defined as "excessive production of aldosterone from a benign adrenal cortical adenoma"; this tumor may be called an "aldosteronoma" (analogous to insulinoma). Its principal features are arterial hypertension and potassium loss in the urine.[6, 7] Because aldosterone controls tissue and plasma electrolyte concentrations, these changes will alter aldosterone production. The electrolyte disturbances probably produce the hypertension which characteristically is mild and does not produce cardiomegaly or retinal vascular changes. Other symptoms in primary aldosteronism are due to hypokalemia. Impaired renal concentrating ability leads to polyuria, nocturia, and then polydipsia. Hypokalemia

Table 7-7. Causes of Hypertension and Hypokalemia

Type of disorder	*Cause*
Medicinal	Potassium-losing diuretics in hypertensives
	Licorice
Renal	Renal tubular acidosis
	Liddle's syndrome
Adrenal cortical	Increased aldosterone secretion
	Increased cortisol production (Cushing's syndrome)
	Increased DOC (11β-hydroxylase deficiency)
	Increased B,DOC (17α-hydroxylase deficiency)
	Increased 18-hydroxy DOC

(and perhaps hypomagnesemia) may result in paresthesia, muscle weakness, and even paralysis. For reasons as yet unexplained, true tetany occasionally develops in these patients.

Although the diagnosis of primary aldosteronism is difficult, it should be considered in any hypertensive patient with hypokalemia. Before diagnostic studies are made, however, certain conditions must be satisfied:

1. The patient has been off all drugs for 3 months, particularly thiazides and oral contraceptives.
2. Secondary causes of hypertension, including pheochromocytoma and coarctation of the aorta, must be eliminated.
3. The urine excretion of 17-ketosteroid and 17-ketogenic steroids must be normal. (Remember that patients with nonendocrine neoplasms causing Cushing's syndrome may be hypertensive and hypokalemic.)

In the absence of some edematous state, hyperaldosteronism is most commonly due to an autonomous adrenal adenoma or to overproduction of angiotensin II. The renin-angiotensin mechanism is activated by kidney disease. The diagnosis of primary aldosteronism is made by clearly demonstrating excessive aldosterone production and by proving that the renin-angiotensin system is not the cause of the overproduction of aldosterone. Since aldosterone production is influenced by electrolyte and water balance, it is best to carry out the diagnostic tests in a metabolic ward under conditions of controlled diet.

Indirect evidence of aldosterone overproduction includes hypokalemia, hypernatremia, and excessive loss of potassium in the urine. Patients will have alkaline urine and systemic alkalosis. Hypokalemia may result in impaired carbohydrate tolerance and diabetes mellitus.

We can measure the secretion rate of aldosterone using isotopic methods. The normal range, 50–160 μg/day, can be measured quite accurately.

Hypokalemia, hypernatremia, and excessive renal loss of potassium may also be found in patients with malignant hypertension, those with pregnancy and toxemia, and those with renal artery stenosis.

The major differential diagnosis centers on patients with primary aldosteronism and those with renal artery stenosis and presumably activation of the renin-angiotensin system and subsequent aldosterone overproduction.

Intravenous pyelography followed by retrograde femoral arteriograms and then bilateral urethral catheterization will demonstrate renal artery stenosis and decreased function of the kidney with the stenosed artery. Renin activity or, more recently, angiotensin levels may be measured in plasma from peripheral or renal veins. Because the renin-angiotensin system is not suppressible by increased levels of aldosterone in patients with renal artery stenosis, these levels will be elevated. However, in patients with autonomous adrenal tumors producing excessive aldosterone, which inhibits a normally suppressible renin-angiotensin system, renin and angiotensin levels will be low or undetectable.[8] Thus when aldosterone production is shown to be excessive and the renin-angiotensin system suppressed, the existence of primary hyperaldosteronism must then be assumed.[24] A rare type of primary hyperaldosteronism may be controlled by glucocorticoid therapy, which acts presumably by inhibiting ACTH output. Therefore, a trial of prednisone, 7.5 mg daily for 1 month, should precede surgical treatment in these patients.

Management

Removal of the adrenal adenoma is the major goal of therapy. Because the tumors may be very small (0.5 cm in diameter), careful exploration is required, usually starting with the left adrenal. If no tumor is found on the left side, the right is examined. If possible, the tumor is shelled out, leaving the rest of the gland. If the surgeon cannot palpate a tumor, he removes the left adrenal gland and one-half of the right. This tissue is then sectioned, in a search for the tumor.

During adrenalectomy the patient is managed just as one undergoing operation for Cushing's syndrome. He is given 100 mg of hydrocortisone sodium succinate in intravenous fluids every 8 hours for the first 2 postoperative days and then the dose is quickly reduced to maintenance levels. If a discrete adenoma was found and removed, the steroid supplement can be stopped. If a subtotal adrenalectomy was done, the patient may require maintenance therapy for the rest of his life.

The headaches, muscular weakness, low serum potassium, and impaired renal function all disappear or return to normal levels in the first few weeks after operation, but the blood pressure often remains elevated for months before it starts to fall. Eventually, 80% of these patients become normotensive.

Adrenogenital Syndrome

In normal subjects the adrenal produces small amounts of androgens. In men, testosterone is secreted directly into the adrenal vein and general circulation; in women, androstenedione is secreted and converted to testosterone, primarily in the liver. If immature males produce excessive amounts of testosterone, their sexual development will be precocious; in females, hirsutism and, later, virilization appear. Testosterone overproduction by the adrenal occurs in most of the congenital and acquired virilizing disorders.[3]

Other less potent androgens may contribute to the virilism produced by adrenal overactivity. Because testosterone is so potent, relatively small amounts are needed to produce virilism, hence urinary 17-ketosteroids are not increased significantly, even though testosterone is excreted, in part, by this pathway. On the other hand, the less potent androgens (dehydroepiandrosterone, androstenedione, etc.) produce definite increases in urinary 17-ketosteroids when they are associated with virilism.[12]

The adrenogenital syndrome (the adrenal overproduction of androgen) embraces both tumors and various hyperplasias. This heterogeneous group can be best understood by considering, first, the six varieties of congenital adrenal hyperplasia (see Fig. 7-3); the acquired forms of the syndrome, including neoplasms; and finally, the largest group, approximately 95% of the total, consisting of the adult type of virilizing adrenal hyperplasia. The latter disorder can be thought of as a "congenital" hyperplasia that does not express itself until adolescence and early adult life.

Congenital Adrenal Hyperplasia

The basic fault in congenital adrenal hyperplasia is the deficiency, but not complete absence, of one or more specific enzymes required for normal steroid biosynthesis.[2] In five of the six documented defects, the enzyme deficiency results in impaired biosynthesis of hydrocortisone. As a result, the adrenal secretes less hydrocortisone than normal and thus activates the negative feedback system. As discussed in Chapter 2, the hypothalamus sends more corticotropin-releasing factor to the pituitary via the portal system, and this in turn releases more ACTH and stimulates adrenal steroid biosynthesis. Under this strong stimulus, the adrenal can usually produce enough hydrocortisone to maintain life despite the enzyme deficiency.

Because enzymes in other adrenal pathways are not deficient, certain hormones may be produced in excess under this strong ACTH stimulation; most commonly testosterone. These enzyme deficiencies are congenital, and excess androgen is produced in utero. As a result, newborn boys show evidence of precocious sexual development and girls have masculinized external genitalia. Depending on the site of the enzyme deficiency, mineralocorticoid hormones may be produced in excess and give rise to hypertension with hypokalemia.

The following variants of congenital adrenal hyperplasia have been observed:

Congenital Lipoid Hyperplasia

In this rare disorder, little is known about the defect(s) in steroid biosynthesis. The adrenals are hyperplastic and the cells are filled with lipid material. These infants present with diarrhea, anorexia, vomiting, weight loss, and marked skin pigmentation. This disorder, which has been reported in both sexes, has been uniformly fatal.

3β-Hydroxysteroid Dehydrogenase Deficiency

In this disorder, the adrenal cannot convert pregnenolone to progesterone; hence no steroid is produced in adequate amounts. Male infants have ambiguous external genitalia, suggesting that enzyme defect also affects the testes, resulting in a deficiency in testicular androgens. Some of the infant girls have mild degrees of virilization, suggesting that some androgens can be produced by either the adrenals or the gonads. To date all such infants have died in adrenal crisis.

C_{21} *Hydroxylase Deficiency*

In this, the commonest deficiency, the clinical picture results from the lack of hydrocortisone production. Through the negative feedback, pituitary ACTH secretion increases and adrenal hyperplasia develops. In the female, adrenal androgen excess causes masculinization, and in the male, precocious pseudosexual development. (The latter is pseudosexual because the androgens arise from the adrenal and not the testes, which are actually small and inactive.) Depending on the degree of enzyme deficiency, mineralocorticoid production may or may not be adequate. In one-third of these patients, deoxycorticosterone and aldosterone are deficient and the clinical picture is aggravated by salt loss and hypotension. Other patients with this deficiency produce adequate amounts of mineralocorticoids and hence do not suffer from sodium depletion.

C_{11} *Hydroxylase Deficiency*

Because not enough hydrocortisone is produced, ACTH production increases and leads to an excess of the 11-deoxy precursors—e.g., 11-desoxyhydrocortisone. 11-Desoxycorticosterone overproduction leads to salt retention and hypertension. In the female, androgen excess produces virilization and, in the male infant, precocious pseudosexual development.

C_{18} *Hydroxylase Deficiency*

In this rare syndrome, aldosterone production is deficient.

C_{17} *Hydroxylase Deficiency*

To date, this recently reported deficiency has been recognized only in the female. Hydrocortisone production is impaired and excess corticosterone and 11-deoxycorticosterone are produced. Aldosterone secretion is low. Because C_{17} hydroxylation is essential to side-chain cleavage and androgen and estrogen formation, sex hormones are produced only in small amounts. The enzyme defect appears to affect the ovary also. Because of the absence of estrogen, the patient cannot mature and has primary amenorrhea. However, the patient is phenotypically female, without masculinization. She has pubic and axillary hair, but it is scanty. Deoxycorticosterone excess produces sodium retention, hypokalemia, and hypertension.

All forms of congenital adrenal hyperplasia result in impaired hydrocortisone production. The specific clinical picture and urinary steroid content depend on the site and completeness of the enzyme deficiency. Therapy aims first at replacing the deficient hydrocortisone—giving 20–30 mg of hydrocortisone (or its equivalent) per day. This dose depresses ACTH production and thus reduces adrenal steroid secretion, controlling though not curing the disorder. Patients with the salt-losing form of the disease require mineralocorticoid replacement—0.1 mg of fluorohydrocortisone per day.

Acquired Abnormalities of Adrenal Androgen Production

Adrenal hyperplasia or tumors can lead to overproduction of potent androgens without glucocorticoid or mineralocorticoid excess. In men, since the testis is the main source of testosterone, adrenal androgen excess rarely produces increased virilism that can be recognized clinically. In women with adrenal hyperplasia, testosterone production is much lower than in normal men. The ovary will secrete small amounts of testosterone and the adrenal will secrete androstenedione that is converted to testosterone in the peripheral tissues. Excessive testosterone production by either endocrine organ produces progressive hirsutism and eventually virilization.

Hirsutism in women can be defined as hair growth in unusual sites such as the chin, moustache, inner aspects of the thighs, the lumbar area, about the nipples, and in a male distribution of pubic hair. This excessive or unusual hair growth may be associated with irregular menstrual function and infertility. Virilization is defined as the above symptoms and signs plus masculinization—that is, recession of the temporal hairline, acne, increase in the prominence of the thyroid cartilage with associated voice changes, increase in muscle mass, and a redistribution of body fat to the typical male pattern. The clitoris may enlarge, sexual drive may increase, and normal feminine secondary characteristics may regress.

Mild degrees of hirsutism, though common, require careful investigation. In all such patients, it is important to evaluate the family history regarding hirsutism, the racial background of the patient and relatives, and to ask about any drugs that may lead to hirsutism. A careful gynecologic assessment is also necessary to rule out benign or malignant ovarian lesions that produce androgens and hence hirsutism or virilism.

Non-Neoplastic Adrenal Hyperplasia

The cause of excessive adrenal androgen production is unknown. As measured in the plasma, ACTH is not increased and there is no evidence of glucocorticoid or mineralocorticoid excess. When the adrenal produces enough androgen to give rise to biologic effects, the urinary ketosteroid excretion increases, reflecting excessive androstenedione production by the adrenal. Part of this excess is converted to testosterone in peripheral tissues. Testosterone and androstenedione in turn give rise to the urinary 17-ketosteroids, androsterone and etiocholanolone. In contrast, patients with ovarian disorders that produce hirsutism usually have a normal urinary ketosteroid output. Because testosterone is so potent, slight increases in its production that are not reflected in increased ketosteroid excretion can produce biologic effects.

With respect to differential diagnosis, if during the small-dose dexamethasone test (2 mg/day), urinary 17-ketosteroids fall to less than 4 mg, the excess 17-ketosteroids come from the adrenals. Dexamethasone suppression, which reduces ACTH output, will not influence ovarian androgen production, and in patients with functioning ovarian tissue producing excessive androgen, the urinary 17-ketosteroids frequently do not fall below 4 mg/day.

Because few patients with adrenal hyperplasia whose symptoms begin at puberty excrete increased amounts of urinary pregnanetriol, some investigators have suggested that they suffer from an incomplete or partial 21-hydroxylase deficiency. Presumably, this deficiency is mild enough to allow normal genital development during fetal life and normal growth up to adolescence. However, at puberty, steroid production increases, and because of the underlying enzyme deficiency, androgen production also increases, causing hirsutism and acne.

Excess adrenal androgen production can be controlled by suppressing the hyperplastic gland with prednisone in a dose of 5–7.5 mg/day.

Adrenal Neoplasia with Androgen Overproduction

Adrenal adenomas or carcinomas that do not produce excess glucocorticoids may secrete excess androgens and cause progressive virilism. In these patients, the urinary 17-ketosteroids are very high and cannot be suppressed with dexamethasone or increased by intravenous ACTH. (In virilizing ovarian neoplasms, which are very rare, the urinary 17-ketosteroids are usually normal.) As the first step in therapy, these adrenal tumors must be removed. The patient is prepared as for adrenalectomy in Cushing's syndrome, but after operation, the steroid supplement can be withdrawn because the opposite adrenal is not atrophic and will produce adequate glucocorticoid.

Occasionally, some patients will have mild degrees of hirsutism but no evidence of ovarian or adrenal dysfunction. This disorder, which does not seem to be racial or familial or related to drug treatment, is common in females of all ages. The urinary 17-ketosteroids are normal, although the testosterone excretion may be elevated. Some of these patients are helped by prednisone suppression, others with estrogen, and some with neither. As they grow older, the rate of hair growth decreases and hair becomes lighter, but the hair follicles do not cease their activity. For cosmetic reasons, these women often need local therapy by electrolysis or depilatory agents.

Feminizing Adrenocortical Tumors

These rare neoplasms, which are nearly always malignant, occur chiefly in men between the ages of 25 and 45 years. The tumor secretes excessive quantities of estrogen and, as a result, produces feminization, gynecomastia, decreased libido, atrophy of the testis, and changes in body configuration. In the few instances in which this tumor has been reported in young women, they present with precocious pseudopuberty, which may be accompanied by signs of Cushing's syndrome because of parallel hydrocortisone excess.

In such patients the excretion of estrogen metabolites and 17-ketosteroids is increased, and the adrenal cannot be suppressed with dexamethasone or stimulated with ACTH. In men with gynecomastia, this tumor must be differentiated from Klinefelter's syndrome and in prepubertal females from estrogen-secreting tumors of the ovary. Removal of the tumor may produce remission, but if the clinical signs progress and estrogen excretion increases further, the patient has functioning metastases. These secondaries, which are common, can be treated by irradiation, but the prognosis is poor.

Table 7-8. Drugs Commonly Used in Adrenal Cortical Disorders

Agent	*Form supplied*
Hydrocortisone	20 mg tablet
Cortisone	30 mg tablet
Hydrocortisone sodium succinate	100 mg/ml
Prednisone	5 mg tablet
Prednisolone	5 mg tablet
Dexamethasone	0.5 or 0.75 mg tablet
Betamethasone	0.5 mg tablet
Florinef (9α-fluorohydrocortisone)	0.1 mg tablet
Deoxycorticosterone	5 mg/ml
ACTH (Synthetic β1-24)	0.25 mg
Metopirone	250 mg capsule
Testosterone propionate	100 mg/ml
Ethinyl estradiol	0.05 or 0.1 mg tablet
Triamcinolone	1 or 2 mg tablet
Spironolactone	25 mg tablet

Adrenal Medulla

The hormones produced and secreted into the circulation by the adrenal medulla are the catecholamines—norepinephrine and epinephrine. The brain, sympathetic nerve endings, and other chromaffin cells of peripheral tissue synthesize these two hormones and dopamine.

The catecholamines are compounds with catechol as the basic nucleus and an amine group ($-NH_2$) attached to it.

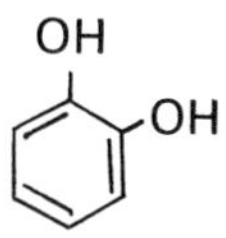

Catechol nucleus

Biosynthesis of Medullary Hormones

Tyrosine serves as the basic precursor for norepinephrine and epinephrine synthesis (Fig. 7-13). The concentration of this amino acid in plasma is 1–1.5 mg/100 ml, whereas in brain and probably other tissues it is accumulated in higher concentrations by means of an active transport system. By hydroxylation, tyrosine forms 1,2-dihydroxyphenylalanine (dopa) and, after decarboxylation, yields 1,2-dihydroxyphenylethylamine (dopamine). Hydroxylation of the β-carbon of the side chain yields norepinephrine. Methylation of norepinephrine to yield epinephrine is catalyzed by a methyl transferase. Using in vitro methods, it has been shown that the tyrosine hydroxylase reaction is the slowest of all the enzymatic conversions and is probably the step that controls the rate of production of the catecholamines.

Catecholamine Storage

In most tissues, norepinephrine and epinephrine are held in high concentration in special subcellular particles called "granules." These particles, which can be seen with the electron microscope, can be isolated by ultracentrifugation. Acetylcholine may stimulate the passage of calcium into the cell where it acts on the storage granules to liberate catecholamines.

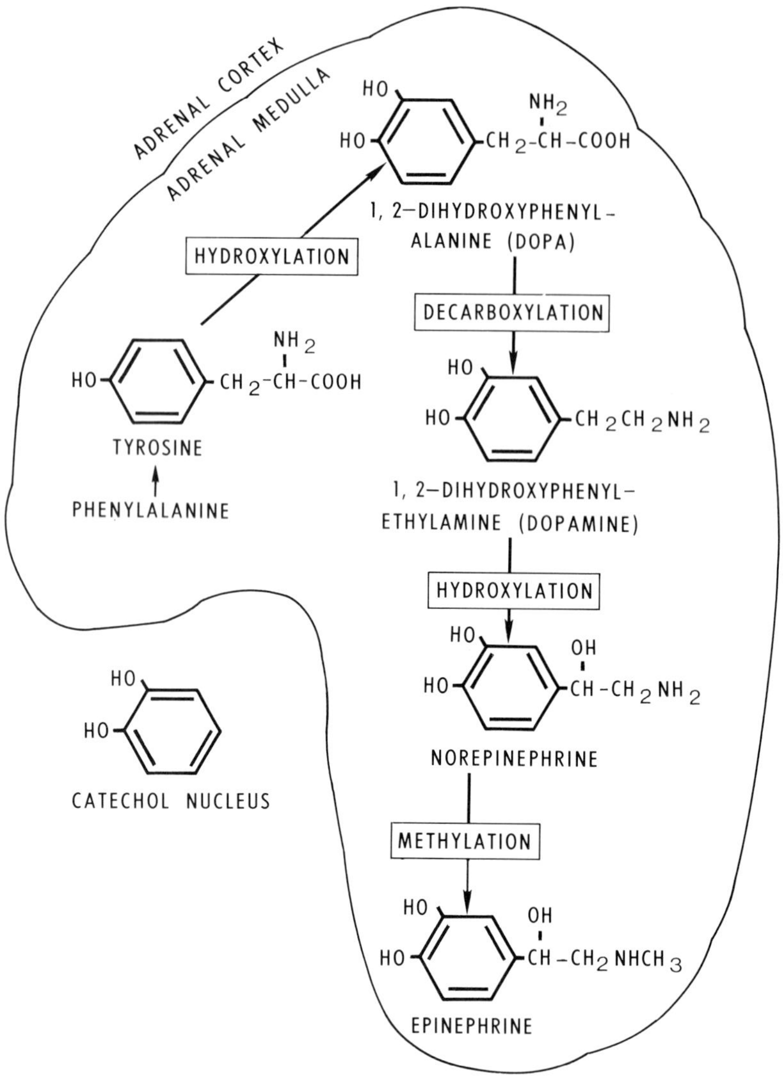

Fig. 7-13. Biosynthetic pathways of the catecholamines. See Chapter 2 for details.

Catecholamine Secretion

Small amounts of catecholamine may be secreted continuously by the adrenal medulla, but the major portion is probably secreted after stimulation of the preganglionic cholinergic fibers or under the influence of other hormones such as insulin and histamine. Almost all the epinephrine in the circulation comes from the adrenal, which also produces appreciable amounts of norepinephrine so that, after bilateral adrenalectomy, the urine epinephrine falls more than 80%, while the norepinephrine falls only slightly because, besides the norepinephrine produced by the adrenal, large amounts are produced by sympathetic ganglion cells.

Catecholamine Metabolism

Catecholamines are removed from the circulation and inactivated by four mechanisms (Fig. 7-14):

1. Re-uptake by the storage granules in adrenergic nerve endings. They are thus removed from circulation and are stored for later release.

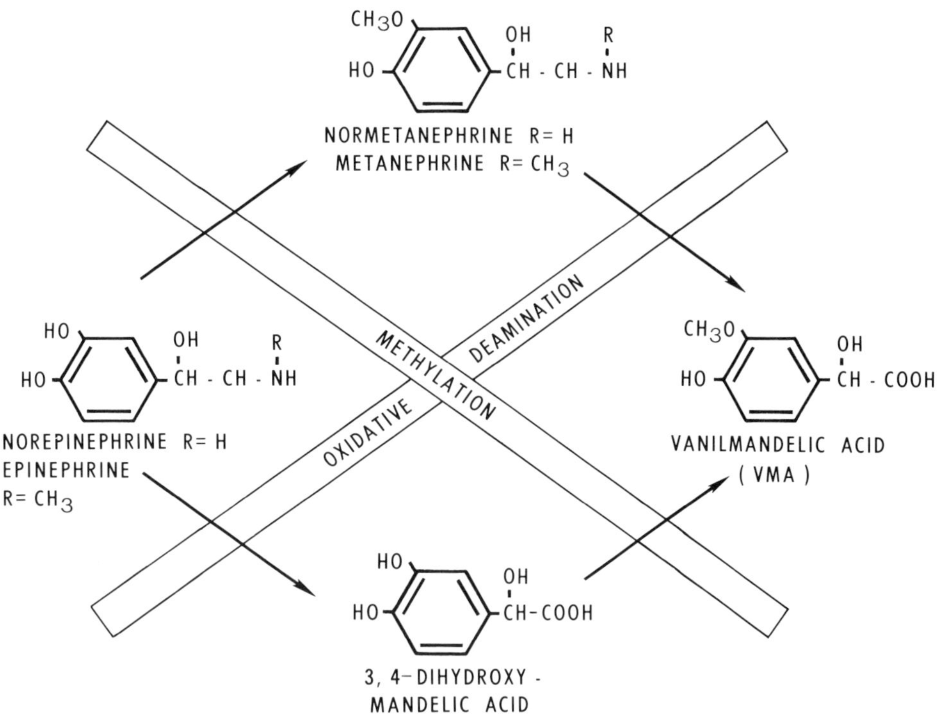

Fig. 7-14. Catecholamine metabolism. Note (*at left*) conversion of norepinephrine-epinephrine to normetanephrine and metanephrine (*top, center*) by methylation, the principal means of inactivating *circulating* catecholamines. Oxidative deamination of free or methylated catecholamines gives rise to mandelic acid derivatives (*at right* and *bottom*).

2. Methylation by catechol-0-methyl transferase, which is found in plasma, liver, and kidneys. This conversion plays the major role in the destruction of circulating catecholamines. The product of this methylation is normetanephrine or metanephrine, depending on the starting compound (i.e, norepinephrine or epinephrine).

3. Oxidative deamination by monoamine oxidase. This enzyme can act either on the free or on the methylated catecholamine. If it acts on the free compound, the resulting product is then methylated to give the principal metabolite, vanillmandelic acid (VMA). Monoamine oxidase plays a minor role in the metabolism of circulating catecholamines; its major function is in the rapid inactivation of catecholamines after their release from the storage granules into the nerve endings.

4. Excretion of unchanged norepinephrine and epinephrine.

Biological Effects

Norepinephrine constricts arterioles and venules by acting at the alpha adrenergic receptors to cause increased peripheral vascular resistance and venous tone. The net effects are changes of unpredictable magnitude in systolic and diastolic blood pressure levels. Epinephrine, by producing overall vasodilation, decreases peripheral resistance and increases cardiac output and heart rate. The end result is an increase in systolic blood pressure but either no change or a decrease in diastolic blood pressure.

Both epinephrine and norepinephrine exert metabolic effects, but the former is usually more potent than the latter. Epinephrine causes an increase in oxygen consumption and elevation of body temperature. Breakdown of liver and muscle glycogen increases because phosphorylase levels are increased after epinephrine administration.

Biochemical Tests

Although daily catecholamine production can be assessed by several methods, the routine hospital laboratory commonly uses urine assays. Blood catecholamines are most difficult to measure because of the small quantities present (<1 μg/liter). The measurements done on urine are:

1. Vanillmandelic acid (VMA) (normal range 1.8–9.0 mg/24 hours)
2. Normetanephrine and metanephrine (normal range <1.3 mg/24 hours)
3. Catecholamines: norepinephrine (normal range 10–70 μg/24 hours), and epinephrine (normal range 0–20 μg/24 hours

These tests are normally done on 24-hour urines collected in dark bottles containing hydrochloric acid. A number of drugs and/or their metabolites interfere with these assays, and so false results will be obtained if collections are made while the patient is on these medications—e.g., tetracyclines and/or certain antihypertensive drugs. The patient should not ingest coffee, vanilla, or certain vegetables and fruits during the collections.

Any of these three urine assays will detect tumors that produce excessive amounts of catecholamines. The first two, VMA and normetanephrine-metanephrine, are easier to perform and are more economical because these metabolites are present in much higher quantities than epinephrine and norepinephrine.

Once the physician knows that the patient has a catecholamine-producing tumor, the urinary norepinephrine-epinephrine ratio may help him locate it. The enzyme that methylates norepinephrine to epinephrine is found only in the adrenal medulla and the organ of Zuckerkandl; if more than 20% of the total catecholamines are epinephrine the tumor is almost certainly in one of these two sites. If only norepinephrine is increased, the tumor may be found in sites other than the adrenal although an adrenal source is still the most common in this group.

The pattern of urine metabolites depends in part on the size of the tumor. If the ratio of norepinephrine plus epinephrine to VMA is high, the tumor is usually small because the catecholamines are not stored. If the ratio is low, the tumor is large because catecholamines are being stored and metabolized in the tumor.

Table 7-9. Biochemical (Urinary Excretion) Tests Used in Disorders of the Adrenal Medulla

Compound	*Unit of measure*	*Normal range*
Catecholamines		
Noradrenaline	μg/day	10–70
Adrenaline	μg/day	0–20
Vanillmandelic acid	mg/day	1.8–9.0
Metanephrines	mg/day	<1.3

Pheochromocytoma

Although this a a relatively rare tumor, it is responsible for 1% of all arterial hypertension. Since the hypertension can usually be cured by removing the tumor, pheochromocytoma should be sought in all hypertensives. In 95% of patients, the tumor is in the adrenal medulla, although functioning chromaffin tumors have been found in the chest, neck, urinary bladder, and at other sites. The tumor is usually benign, but 5% are malignant and metastasize to bone and liver. In 20–40% of familial and 8% of sporadic cases, the tumor is bilateral.[21]

The production of norepinephrine and epinephrine may be sustained or intermittent. The clinical picture, which varies, depends on the physiologic effects of the excessive catecholamines.

These amines produce diastolic hypertension, which may be sustained or intermittent and which may range from mild to malignant. The patient may develop cardiomegaly, left ventricular hypertrophy, and an unusual cardiomyopathy leading to congestive heart failure. Retinal arterial spasm can progress to hemorrhages and exudates in the severe forms of hypertension. The metabolic effects of catecholamines may manifest as tremor, anxiety, weakness, and weight loss. Tachycardia, hyperventilation, and flushing are common. Headaches, excessive perspiration, and postural hypotension are also frequently found.

The incidence of neuroectodermal disease (neurofibromatosis) in association with pheochromocytoma is increased because of a common embryologic defect. Other associated disorders include medullary carcinoma of the thyroid gland, true erythrocytosis, and an increased incidence of cholelithiasis.

Except for hypertension with retinopathy and cardiomegaly, there are few specific findings. Café-au-lait spots may be seen with neurofibromatosis. In 30% of these patients blood pressure increases when the abdomen is carefully examined to produce pressure on the tumor. The pheochromocytoma itself may be palpable in 10%. In patients with bladder pheochromocytomas, the blood pressure may rise when the patient voids.

Diagnosis

Routine Procedures

Hemoglobin and hematocrit may be high normal, but there are no specific changes in the leukocytes or platelets. The plasma volume may be reduced. The urinalysis is unremarkable, except for occasional glycosuria. Plasma glucose and fatty acid levels may be elevated. Serum electrolytes are normal.

X-Ray Examinations

A tumor may rarely be detected on the chest film. An intravenous pyelogram may show displacement of the kidney, and in malignant tumor, bone X-rays may show metastases. Over the adrenal on the affected side, selective retrograde femoral arteriography may show increased vascularization.

Definitive

Excretion of Catecholamines or Their Metabolic Products Vanillmandelic Acid or Normetanephrine. In 90–95% of patients, the excretion is increased either constantly or intermittently. If the latter, increased excretion is detected only on days of physiologic stimulation of the tumor using histamine, glucagon, or tyramine.

Pharmacologic Testing. In patients who have a pheochromocytoma and hypertension, 1–5 mg of phentolamine (Regitine, Ciba; an alpha-blocking agent) intravenously may cause the blood pressure to fall. However, some patients with pheochromocytoma are extremely sensitive to this drug and may have prolonged hypotension. If the diagnosis is strongly suspected, start with 1 mg and then increase to 5 mg if the test is negative with the smaller dose. In a positive test, the fall in blood pressure greater than 35/25 mm Hg is sustained for at least 4 minutes.

In patients with pheochromocytoma and intermittent hypertension, it may be necessary to stimulate the tumor's production or release of catecholamines. Histamine releases catecholamines and raises blood pressure by causing a reflex sympathetic discharge. Under the usual procedure, with the patient at rest, ingesting no drugs, an intravenous infusion of 5% glucose in water is started and allowed to run freely. The blood pressure is measured at intervals until stable and then 25–50 μg of histamine base is injected intravenously and the pressure recorded at 30-second intervals for 5 minutes. In all patients there is an initial fall in pressure, but a positive test requires an ultimate increase greater than 60/30 mm Hg. Side effects occur in all patients and include tachycardia, anxiety, and a pounding headache. The sudden rise in blood pressure can induce cerebral vascular hemorrhage. Regitine should be available in a syringe for injection to counteract any massive rise in blood pressure. This test has few false negatives, but the side effects make it upsetting to patients. Because patients have died as a result of this test, it should be done only by those with much experience and, even then, this type of test is rarely indicated.

Tyramine also causes a release of catecholamines from the nerve endings; 500–1,000 μg intravenously is given under the same controlled conditions as for histamine. This test is positive in only 75% of patients with pheochromocytoma, but it causes no appreciable side effects. For no obvious reason, most of the false negatives have been in individuals with the familial form of the disease.

Glucagon (0.5–1.0 mg) given intravenously can also be used to stimulate catecholamine output; it elevates the blood pressure significantly in patients with pheochromocytoma but has no effect on normal subjects.

Table 7-10. Pharmacological Tests Commonly Used in Disorders of the Adrenal Medulla

*Agent**	*Method of administration*	*Response*
Phentolamine (Regitine)†	2 mg IV (increase to 5 mg if no response)	Fall in blood pressure of 35/25 mm Hg or more for at least 2 minutes
Glucagon	1 mg IV	Rise in blood pressure of 60/30 mm Hg or more
Tyramine	1 mg IV	Rise in systolic pressure of 30 mm Hg or more

* Histamine should not be used because of danger of excessive response.
† A short-acting alpha blocker.

Treatment of Pheochromocytoma

The tumor should be removed if possible. However, before operation, the patient must be carefully managed. In very ill patients or those with maligant pheochromocytoma and secondaries, only medical treatment is feasible and is really only an extension of the preoperative program.

The patient is prepared for operation with an alpha adrenergic blocker. This is given orally in a dose of 40–100 mg/day to control the blood pressure. In addition, a beta blocker such as propranolol can be used to control the blood pressure and heart rate. Regitine has also been used, but this agent has a much shorter action and must be administered every 4 hours. Recently catecholamine excess has been controlled with agents that block the synthesis of catecholamines (for example, alpha methyl paratyrosine). In time, this type of drug will become the pharmacologic agent of choice.*

Once the symptoms and signs of catecholamine excess are under good control, exploration can be considered. The anesthetic agent must be selected with care: the preferred agents are thiopental with nitrous oxide, although some groups find halothane [bromochlorotrifluoroethane (2-bromo-2-chloro-1,1,1-trifluoroethane)] to be very efficient. These agents are chosen because they are least likely to produce cardiac arrhythmia. During the operation, it is important to monitor the electrocardiogram, central venous pressure, and arterial blood pressure so that alterations can be detected and treated appropriately. For hypertensive crisis, phentolamine is given in a dose of 1–5 mg and for hypotension, Neo-Synephrine. If an arrhythmia develops, give propranolol intravenously in a dose of 2–5 mg.

The gland is usually approached anteriorly. With the blood pressure and cardiac rhythm under good pharmacologic control, the risks of operation are greatly reduced, but occasionally hypertensive crises during or after operation may threaten the life of the patient.

After the tumor has been removed, the patient usually makes an uneventful recovery although, on occasion, the blood pressure may drop and vasopressors must be given for the first few days to maintain adequate circulation.[30]

* 1. *Phenoxybenzamine* (Dibenzyline), a long-acting alpha-blocker, 10 mg 4 times daily, is preferred over phentolamine for the control of blood pressure during operation. It should be started 3 days before operation. To prevent postural hypotension the patient should be kept in bed for 2 days until intravascular volume expands under the influence of alpha blockade.

2. *Propranolol,* used in the management of arrhythmias, 10 mg 4 times daily by mouth, given only after Dibenzyline. Otherwise, blood pressure will rise because norepinephrine has both alpha and beta effects. During operation, propranolol can be given intravenously in a dose of 2–5 mg to control arrhythmias.

3. Ortho methyl tyrosine, an investigational drug, is available to treat hypertension due to metastatic pheochromocytoma; it blocks the synthesis of norepinephrine.

References

1. Addison, T. Anaemia—disease of the supra-renal capsules. *London Med Gaz 43:*517–518, 1849.
2. Bongiovanni, A. M., and Root, A. W. The adrenogenital syndrome. *N Engl J Med 268:*1283–1289, 1342–1351, 1391–1399, 1963.
3. Camacho, A. M., and Migeon, C. J. Testosterone

excretion and production rate in normal adults and in patients with congenital adrenal hyperplasia. *J Clin Endocrinol Metab 26:*893–896, 1966.
4. Cannon, W. B., Britton, S. W., Lewis, J. T., and Groeneveld, A. Studies on the conditions of activity in endocrine glands. XX. The influence of motion and emotion on medulliadrenal secretion. *Am J Physiol 79:*433–465, 1927.
5. Cannon, W. B., Querido, A., Britton, S. W., and Bright, E. M. Studies on the conditions of activity in endocrine glands. XXI. The role of adrenal secretion in the chemical control of body temperature. *Am J Physiol 79:*466–507, 1927.
6. Conn, J. W. Aldosteronism in man: Some clinical and climatological aspects, part II. *JAMA 183:*871–878, 1963.
7. Conn, J. W. Presidential address: I. Painting background. II. Primary aldosteronism, a new clinical syndrome. *J Lab Clin Med 45:*3–17, 1955.
8. Conn, J. W., Cohen, E. L., and Rovner, D. R. Suppression of plasma renin activity in primary aldosteronism; distinguishing primary from secondary aldosteronism in hypertensive disease. *JAMA 190:* 213–221, 1964.
9. Cope, C. L. and Black, E. G. The reliability of some adrenal function tests. *Br Med J 2:*1117–1122, 1959.
10. Cushing, H. The basophil adenomas of the pituitary body and their clinical manifestations. *Bull Johns Hopkins Hosp 50:*137–195, 1932.
11. DiRaimondo, V. C., and Forsham, P. H. Pharmacophysiologic principles in the use of corticoids and adrenocorticotropin. *Metabolism 7:*5–24, 1958.
12. Dorfman, R. I., Forchielli, E., and Gut, M. Androgen biosynthesis and related studies. *Recent Progr Horm Res 19:*251–273, 1963.
13. Eisenstein, A. B. *The Adrenal Cortex.* Boston, Little, 1967.
14. *The Human Adrenal Cortex: Proceedings of a Conference.* Conference on the Human Adrenal Cortex, University of Glasgow, 1960. Edinburgh, Livingstone, 1962.
15. Jenkins, D., Forsham, P. H., Reddy, W. J., and Thorn, G. W. Use of ACTH in the diagnosis of adrenal cortical insufficiency. *Am J Med 18:*3–14, 1955.
16. Knowlton, A. I., Mudge, G. H., and Jailer, J. W. Pregnancy in Addison's disease. *J Clin Endocrinol Metab 9:*514–528, 1949.
17. Liddle, G. W. Tests of pituitary-adrenal suppressibility in the diagnosis of Cushing's syndrome. *J Clin Endocrinol Metab 20:*1539–1560, 1960.
18. Liddle, G. W., Estep, H. L., Kendall, J. W., Williams, W. C., and Townes, A. W. Clinical application of a new test of pituitary reserve. *J Clin Endocrinol Metab 19:*875–894, 1959.
19. Liddle, G. W., Givens, J. R., Nicholson, W. E., and Island, D. P. The ectopic ACTH syndrome. *Cancer Res 25:*1057–1061, 1965.
20. Loraine, J. A. *Hormone Assays and Their Clinical Application,* ed. 2. Edinburgh, Livingstone, 1966.
21. Manger, W. M. *Hormones and Hypertension.* Springfield, Ill., Thomas, 1966.
22. Nelson, D. H., Meakin, J. W., Dealy, J. B., Jr., Matson, D. D., Emerson, K., and Thorn, G. W. ACTH-producing tumor of the pituitary gland. *N Engl J Med 259:*161–164, 1958.
23. Peterson, R. E., Wyngaarden, J. B., Guerra, S. L., Brodie, B. B., and Bunim, J. J. The physiological disposition and metabolic fate of hydrocortisone in man. *J Clin Invest 34:*1779–1794, 1955.
24. Slaton, P. E., Schambelan, M., and Biglieri, E. G. Stimulation and suppression of aldosterone secretion in patients with an aldosterone-producing adenoma. *J Clin Endocrinol Metab 29:*239–250, 1969.
25. Soffer, L. J. *The Human Adrenal Gland.* Philadelphia, Lea & Febiger, 1961.
26. Stewart, G. N. The adrenal glands. *Arch Intern Med 43:*1929.
27. Temple, T. E., Jones, D. J., Liddle, G. W., and Dexter, R. M. Treatment of Cushing's disease. *N Engl J Med 281:*801–805, 1969.
28. Thorn, G. W. The adrenal cortex. I. Historical aspects. II. Clinical considerations. *Johns Hopkins Med J 123:*49–77, 1968.
29. Wilkins, L. *The Diagnosis and Treatment of Endocrine Disorders in Childhood and Adolescence,* 3d ed. Springfield, Ill., Thomas, 1965.
30. Williams, R. H. *Textbook of Endocrinology,* 4th ed. Philadelphia, Saunders, 1968.

8

Hypertension and Hypokalemia

John C. Laidlaw

The finding of hypokalemia in a patient with diastolic hypertension may be of considerable diagnostic significance in that it may lead to the detection of a number of types of hypertension which are potentially curable. The major types of hypertension are as follows:

Primary
- Essential hypertension*

Secondary
- Renal
  - Glomerulonephritis
  - Pyelonephritis
  - Renal artery stenosis*
  - Coarctation of aorta
  - Polycystic disease
  - Collagen disease
  - Eclampsia
  - Rare renal diseases*
- Neurologic
  - Psychogenic
  - Brain tumor
  - Poliomyelitis
- Endocrine
  - Acromegaly
  - Primary hypothyroidism
  - Pheochromocytoma
  - Adrenal cortical hyperfunction*
  - Oral contraceptive medication*

The types associated with hypokalemia, indicated by an asterisk, include hypertension associated with the administration of oral contraceptive medication, a variety of forms of adrenocortical hyperfunction associated with the increased secretion of one or more steroids possessing mineralocorticoid activity, renal artery stenosis, and certain rare renal diseases. An asterisk has been placed opposite essential hypertension because a number of patients who were believed to have essential hypertension were found to have hypokalemia and increased production of a newly recognized mineralocorticoid, 18-hydroxydeoxycorticosterone (18-hydroxy DOC). To appreciate the mechanisms involved in the production of hypertension and hypokalemia, the physician requires an understanding of such matters as the function of adrenal mineralocorticoids in the human, the control of aldosterone secretion, the causes of hypokalemia and the manifestations of potassium deficiency.

A mineralocorticoid may be defined as an adrenal steroid which, when administered to the human subject, produces renal sodium and water retention and potassium loss. Natural mineralocorticoids in the human are:

High glucocorticoid-mineralocorticoid ratio
- Cortisol (F)

Corticosterone (B)
High mineralocorticoid-glucocorticoid ratio
Aldosterone
Deoxycorticosterone (DOC)
18-hydroxy DOC
18-hydroxy B

The glucocorticoids, cortisol and corticosterone, both possess mineralocorticoid activity, particularly when given in large doses intravenously. The "pure" mineralocorticoids are those listed as having a high mineralocorticoid-glucocorticoid ratio. These compounds also possess some glucocorticoid activity because they may produce potassium deficiency and thereby lead to impaired glucose tolerance. Of these mineralocorticoids, aldosterone is the most potent. While 18-hydroxy DOC and 18-hydroxy B have been shown to possess mineralocorticoid activity in animals, their precise activity in this regard in humans is presently unknown.

A number of syndromes characterized by hypertension and hypokalemia are associated with increased secretion of one or more of all of the hormones listed, but no hypertensive condition has been described in which there is only an excess of 18-hydroxy B. In hypertensive disorders associated with increased aldosterone secretion, however, production of 18-hydroxy B is always increased. Hypertension associated with increased 18-hydroxy DOC is discussed briefly later in this section.

The principal control of the secretion of cortisol, corticosterone, desoxycorticosterone, and 18-hydroxy DOC is ACTH.

The chief controlling mechanism of aldosterone and 18-hydroxy B secretion is the renin-angiotensin system, which is illustrated in Figure 8-1. Renin, an enzyme produced by the juxtaglomerular cells in the kidney, acts on an alpha 2 globulin, angiotensinogen which is produced in the liver, to give rise to a 10 aminoacid peptide angiotensin I. Through the action of converting enzyme, which is present in plasma and a number of tissues, particularly the lung, angiotensin I is converted to angiotensin II by the removal of a further two amino acids. Angiotensin II is a highly potent hypertensive agent and, in addition, its presence in excess increases aldosterone secretion. In renovascular hypertension, there is increased renin production, which leads to a rise in both angiotensin II and aldosterone.

In the presence of an autonomous increase in aldosterone secretion, such as occurs in primary aldosteronism due to adrenocortical tumor, renin production is suppressed. In clinical situations, renin is ordinarily measured indirectly by determining the ability of the patient's plasma, when incubated, to generate angiotensin II. This so-

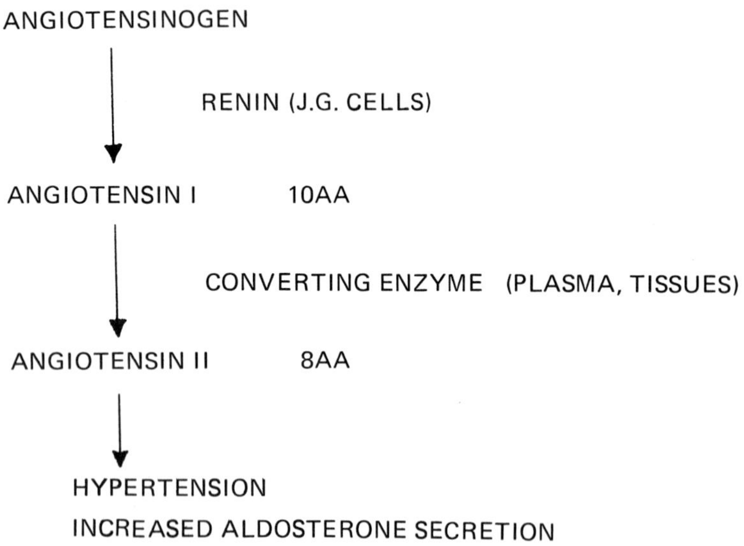

Fig. 8-1. Renin-angiotensin system.

called "plasma renin activity" determination is performed on blood obtained when the patient has been on a low sodium intake (10–15 mEq/day) for 3 days and has been upright for at least 2 hours. The low sodium intake and the upright posture both stimulate renin secretion.

The following list gives a number of factors that control aldosterone production via the renin-angiotensin system, and other factors that affect aldosterone secretion more directly.

- Renin-angiotensin system
  - Sodium
  - Intravascular volume
  - Progesterone
- Potassium
- Sodium
- ACTH

The renin-angiotensin system, and hence aldosterone, may be stimulated by a low sodium diet, by a fall in intravascular volume, and by progesterone or spironolactone (Aldactone). Progesterone and Aldactone interfere with the renal action of aldosterone, thereby inducing a sodium and water diuresis that stimulates both renin and aldosterone production. High potassium intake stimulates the production of aldosterone by direct action on the adrenal cortex. Sodium deficiency may also increase aldosterone production by direct action on the adrenal cortex as well as by stimulating the renin-angiotensin system.

ACTH appears to be less important in controlling aldosterone secretion as demonstrated by the fact that most patients with panhypopituitarism have a normal or low-normal aldosterone production. When ACTH is given to normal human subjects, aldosterone secretion rises for the first 24 hours or so, but subsequently returns to or towards control levels while ACTH is continued. The mechanism for this biphasic effect of ACTH on aldosterone is unknown.

The normal range of serum potassium levels in the human is 3.6 to 5.0 mEq/liter. Although hypokalemia is defined as any value below 3.6 mEq/liter, normal subjects rarely have serum potassium levels which are consistently below 4.0 mEq/liter. Hence any patient who has serum potassium values consistently between 3.6 and 4.0 mEq/liter may well have potassium deficiency.

To obtain a valid measurement of serum potassium concentration, certain precautions have to be taken. For example, placing a patient with hypokalemia on a low sodium intake may return the serum potassium levels to normal. Secondly, contracting the muscles in the forearm, with the tourniquet applied, may elevate the serum potassium level of blood removed under these conditions by as much as 1 mEq/liter. Thirdly, appreciable hemolysis may artificially increase serum potassium levels. The causes of hypokalemia are as follows:

- Gastrointestinal
  - Impaired intake
  - Vomiting
  - Diarrhea
- Renal
  - Primary renal disease—renal tubular acidosis, Liddle's syndrome
  - Drugs and hormones—potassium-losing diuretics, mineralocorticoids
- Passage into cells
  - Hypokalemic periodic paralysis

The causes relevant to the syndrome of hypertension and hypokalemia result in renal loss of potassium and include certain types of primary renal disease, the administration of certain drugs, and the increased production of mineralocorticoids.

The manifestations of renal loss of potassium are:

- Clinical
  - Muscle weakness
  - Paresthesia, tetany
  - Polydypsia, polyuria
- Biochemical
  - Hypokalemia
  - Metabolic acidosis
  - Hyposthenuria
  - Alkaline urine
  - Normal or high urine potassium
- Pathological
  - Vacuolar nephrosis

In all types of potassium deficiency, there may be muscle weakness, paresthesias and tetany due to the alkalosis associated with potassium deficiency, and polydypsia and polyuria due to resistance to the effect of endogenous antidiuretic hormone. Urine potassium is normal or high when there is renal potassium loss but low when the potassium is being lost from the gastrointestinal tract. In severe potassium deficiency, there may be vacuolar changes in the proximal and distal convoluted tubular cells and in the cells of the collecting tubules.

The causes of hypertension and hypokalemia are given in Table 7-7. It should be stressed that, in all of these states, although serum potassium levels are often depressed, this is not always so. Any hypertensive patient on long-term treatment with a potassium-losing diuretic may, of course, develop hypokalemia. When hypokalemia in such patients is severe, that is below 3.0 mEq/liter, the physician should suspect an underlying condition which might contribute to the hypokalemia. Excessive intake of licorice, either by itself or as a flavoring in certain drinks, may produce hypertension and hypokalemia because the flavoring contains a chemical substance that mimics the action of aldosterone.

Patients with renal tubular acidosis rarely develop hypertension until late in the course of their disease. Systemic acidosis, rather than the alkalosis ordinarily found in potassium deficiency, is a hallmark of this condition. Liddle's syndrome is a rare familial condition in which there is a primary disturbance in the exchange of sodium for potassium at the level of the renal tubule. Patients with this syndrome exhibit a primary renal loss of potassium, and as a result aldosterone production is suppressed.

With regard to the adrenocortical causes of hypertension and hypokalemia, those associated with increased aldosterone will be described below. Increased cortisol production may produce this syndrome, particularly when it is due to increased ACTH secretion from a carcinoma arising in a tissue other than the anterior pituitary gland—the so-called ectopic ACTH syndrome. Increased deoxycorticosterone levels are found in the type of congenital adrenal hyperplasia known as 11β-hydroxylase deficiency. This enzyme deficiency leads to impaired cortisol production and a secondary androgen and mineralocorticoid excess.

There is increased secretion of both corticosterone and deoxycorticosterone in a type of congenital adrenal hyperplasia known as 17α-hydroxylase deficiency. This deficiency leads to an impaired production of cortisol, androgen, and estrogen. Most of the patients with the deficiency have been female, and have presented with hypertension, hypokalemia, and primary amenorrhea. Finally, a number of patients who were thought to have essential hypertension but who had hypokalemia, low plasma renin activity, and normal or low aldosterone levels showed increased production of 18-hydroxydeoxycorticosterone (18-hydroxy DOC). In some of these patients, the hypertension and mineralocorticoid excess were relieved by small doses of glucocorticoid (dexamethasone). The proportion of patients with presumed essential hypertension but with increased 18-hydroxy DOC secretion remains to be determined.

Among the causes of hypertension and hypokalemia associated with increased aldosterone production, those types associated with elevated plasma renin activity include oral contraceptive medication, renal artery stenosis, and malignant hypertension. "The pill" is believed to produce hypertension by the following steps: The estrogen in this medication induces a rise in renin substrate; this leads to increased formation of angiotension II which then stimulates aldosterone production. In patients who are found to be hypertensive while taking oral contraceptives, the medication should be discontinued and the patient's blood pressure measured over several months before extensive investigation is undertaken.

When renal artery stenosis is detected on renal arteriography, it is important to determine whether the stenosis is playing a part in the hypertension. This is best achieved by determining the plasma-renin activity in blood removed from the renal vein from both kidneys. When the plasma renin activity in blood obtained from the affected kidney is two or more times greater than that from the opposite renal vein and peripheral venous plasma-renin activity is increased, the hypertension can often be ameliorated by correction of the renal artery stenosis or by nephrectomy.

When hypertension, hypokalemia, and increased aldosterone secretion are associated with suppressed plasma renin activity, the condition may be due to one of three causes: an adrenocortical tumor (Conn's syndrome) or one of two types of adrenocortical hyperplasia. In the first type of hyperplasia, the hypertension and hypokalemia are relieved by small doses of glucorticoid (glucocorticoid-remediable aldosteronism); in the latter, they are not. The incidence of Conn's syndrome in patients thought to have essential hypertension now appears to be approximately 1–2%.

Glucocorticoid-remediable aldosteronism is probably very rare, only eight cases having been reported since 1966. This condition may be detected by studying the response of the patient's blood pressure and serum potassium levels to a 2-week course of dexamethasone, 2 mg by mouth daily. The type of adrenocortical hyperplasia which is associated with aldosterone excess but is not relieved by glucocorticoid is probably as common as Conn's syndrome. The differentiation of these two conditions *before operation* is usually difficult. In this type of adrenal hyperplasia, subtotal or total adrenalectomy usually relieves the hypokalemia but rarely produces marked improvement in the hypertension.

In summary, hypertension may be associated with hypokalemia in a number of clinical states. This syndrome most commonly occurs in hypertensive patients who are receiving potassium-losing diuretics. In any such patient when serum potassium levels are very low, i.e., below 3.0 mEq/liter, there may well be an underlying condition which is contributing to the potassium deficiency.

The second most common cause of hypertension and hypokalemia is oral contraceptive medication. The third most common is renal artery stenosis. Finally, a number of primary adrenal cortical disturbances are associated with an increased secretion of one or more mineralocorticoids.

Investigation of a patient with hypertension and hypokalemia may require admission to hospital for 2 weeks or so during which, among other tests, the physician determines plasma renin activity on constant normal and low sodium diets, and aldosterone secretion or excretion on a constant normal sodium intake. One must use particular care in the selection of patients for such an investigation. It seems reasonable to submit to such a study any patient who is under the age of 30 and who has hypertension and serum potassium levels below 3.0 mEq/liter.

With respect to the use of spironolactone (Aldactone) in the differential diagnosis of patients with hypertension and hypokalemia, it should be stressed that Aldactone may relieve hypokalemia without affecting the hypertension in a patient with signs of mineralocorticoid excess, irrespective of the type of mineralocorticoid or the source of the primary lesion (renal or adrenal). Furthermore, Aldactone may relieve both hypertension and hypokalemia in all three conditions associated with hypertension, increased aldosterone secretion, and suppressed plasma renin activity.

A discussion of the conditions which cause hypertension and hypokalemia belongs in a textbook of endocrinology because application of the principles of endocrine function has helped to unravel the complex relationships between potassium, renin, and the adrenal mineralocorticoids, and thus has assisted in the diagnosis and treatment of "curable" hypertension.

References

1. Conn, J. W. The evolution of primary aldosteronism: 1954–67. *Harvey Lect 62*:275–291, 1966–67.
2. Salti, I. S., Stiefel, M., Ruse, J. L., and Laidlaw, J. C. Non-tumorous "primary" aldosteronism: I. Type relieved by glucocorticoid (glucocorticoid-remediable aldosteronism). *Can Med Assoc J 101*: 1–10, 1969.
3. Ferriss, J. B., Brown, J. J., Fraser, R., Kay, A. W., Neville, A. M., O'Muircheartaigh, I. G., Robertson, J. I. S., Symington, T., and Lever, A. F. Hypertension with aldosterone excess and low plasma-renin: preoperative distinction between patients with and without adrenocortical tumor. *Lancet 2*:995–1000, 1970.
4. Melby, J. C., Dale, S. L., and Wilson, T. E. 18-Hydroxydeoxycorticosterone in human hypertension. *Circ Res Suppl 2*:28–29, 143–153, 1971.

9

The Testis

Charles E. Bird

Embryology

The primitive gonad appears during the fifth week of gestation as a thickening of celomic epithelium on the medial surface of the urogenital ridge. In the sixth week of gestation, the ridge is invaded by primitive germ cells from the entodermal yolk sac cells. The gonad now consists of a cortex, which is the forerunner of the ovary, and the medulla, the forerunner of the testis. During the seventh and eighth weeks of gestation, the testis becomes recognizable, as epithelial cords become defined. The interstitial cells of Leydig appear during the fourth month and actually decrease in number about the eighth month of pregnancy. The seminiferous tubules develop a central lumen in the seventh month.

Embryology of the Genital Ducts

As the gonad differentiates in the male, the wolffian (mesonephric) duct becomes dominant. This structure will form the duct of the epididymis, the vas deferens, the common ejaculatory duct, and the seminal vesicle. As well, it forms the trigone of the bladder on both sexes. The müllerian (paramesonephric) duct regresses in the male, leaving only two structures, the hydatid and prostatic sinuses.

Descent of the Testis

The testis initially develops in the retroperitoneal tissues at the level of the lumbar spine. Because the gubernaculum testis grows more slowly than the lumbar and pelvic regions of the trunk, the testis is pulled caudally by the gubernaculum. The testis reaches the inguinal ring by the fifth month and enters the inguinal canal during the seventh month, reaching the scrotum in the eighth month. The inguinal canal usually closes before birth, but if it does not, the testis may be retracted into the inguinal canal or even into the abdominal cavity.

Anatomy

In the adult male, the testes are located in the scrotum; the left is usually lower than the right. They are firm, ovoid organs measuring 4–6 cm in length. The grayish-white testes are covered by a visceral layer of the tunica vaginalis propria. The tunica albuginea forms the thick dense capsule. Connective tissue septums from the tunica albuginea divide the testes into lubules. Each lobule contains two or three seminiferous tubules which are 30–70 cm in length and 150–200 μ in diameter. The tubules converge on the posterior surface of the testis to form the tubuli recti which anastomose in the rete testes. The ducti efferente join the rete testes to the ductus epididymis. The epididymis is convoluted on the posterior surface of the testes and leads into the ductus deferens.

Blood and Nerve Supply

The main arterial supply from the internal spermatic artery enters the testes in the posterior surface and divides into branches along the septums between the lobules. The venous drainage follows the arterial supply to form the pampiniform plexus on the posterior surface. This in turn forms the spermatic vein which, on the left, drains into the left renal vein and, on the right, into the vena cava. The sympathetic nerve supply is from the hypogastric plexus.

Histology

In the seminiferous tubules, the Sertoli or sustentacular cells, considered to be nutrient cells, are found close to the basement membrane. They have large oval nuclei with large nucleoli.

The spermatogenetic cells undergo repeated mitosis to produce the mature spermatids from the immature spermatogonia. The spermatogonia are located at the periphery of the tubule and, as maturation and division proceed, the germ cells move toward the lumen.

Recent work by Heller and Clermont has shown that the complete process of spermatogenesis requires about 74 days. This is a relatively constant period and the induction of spermatogenesis may take 2 months or more.

Interstitial tissue is composed of supporting tissue for the tubule plus the Leydig cells. The Leydig cell has a large round nucleus with a nucleolus and a coarse chromatin network.

Physiology of the Testis

In normal man, the major functions of the testes are hormone production and spermiogenesis.

Hormone Production

The Leydig cell and possibly the Sertoli cell produce hormones. Biologically, testosterone is the most important hormone secreted by the testis, although it also produces androstenedione, dehydroisoandrosterone, and 17β-estradiol. Interstitial-cell stimulating hormone from the pituitary directs the production of testosterone in the testis by a "negative feedback" mechanism. The circulating level of testosterone in the plasma acts on the hypothalamus to inhibit the secretion of a "releasing factor." This factor stimulates the pituitary to release stored interstitial-cell stimulating hormone and probably also increases its production. The details of this control at the level of the hypothalamus and pituitary have been discussed earlier in Chapters 2 and 4.

In the testis, steroid biosynthesis follows the same metabolic pathway described for the adrenal cortex (Chapter 7).

The testis does not possess the 11β-hydroxylase enzyme, however, so that cortisol and other 11-oxy compounds are not formed. Testosterone is transported in plasma bound to protein. Seventy per cent of the circulating testosterone is bound to albumin, which has a low affinity and high binding capacity for testosterone. Twenty per cent of the circulating testosterone is bound to a specific beta globulin which has a high affinity and low binding capacity. The remaining 10% is unbound. The bound form exists in dynamic equilibrium with the free and biologically active form. (In females, over 95% of the circulating testosterone is bound to proteins. The percentage bound increases during pregnancy and exogenous estrogen therapy.)

Normal men produce between 4 and 8 mg of testosterone per day. The testis secretes most of this, but some is secreted by the adrenal gland or formed from androstenedione in nonendocrine tissues (such as the liver or even whole blood). The plasma level in men ranges between 0.5 and 1.0 μg/100 ml of whole blood. The half-disappearance time is approximately 30–40 minutes. Most of the testosterone is converted to etiocholanolone or androsterone in the liver but, in normal men, approximately 30–130 μg appears unchanged in the urine each day.

Before the secretion of interstitial cell-stimulating hormone increases at puberty, the plasma level and secretion rate of testosterone are very low. At the other end of life, the secretion rate and plasma level of testosterone drop off past the age of 70 in normal men.

Biologic Effects of Testosterone

Morphologic

When secondary sexual characteristics develop in the male at puberty, the beard grows, pubic hair develops, the voice deepens, the thyroid cartilage enlarges, the temporal hairline recedes, muscle mass increases, the penis, prostate, and seminal vesicles enlarge, testicles increase in size, the rugal folds of the scrotum become pigmented and develop, and after a sudden growth spurt, the epiphyses close.

Metabolic

Increase in protein anabolism causes a sudden growth spurt and an increase in muscle mass and strength that is reflected in a positive nitrogen balance and a rapid gain in weight.

Psychic

The rise in testosterone production at puberty increases physical and emotional drive, induces libido, and awakens sexual potentia.

When testosterone production falls after castration or when the pituitary-testicular axis is disrupted by disease, all these manifestations regress —i.e., sexual drive is reduced, secondary sexual characteristics regress, and protein anabolism decreases.

Spermiogenesis

In the normal adult male, the germ cells develop and mature in an orderly fashion. The pituitary gonadotropin (FSH) acting on the tubules stimulates the spermatogonia to mature through the spermatocyte and spermatid phases to the mature spermatozoa. Testosterone is also required because it stimulates the growth of the seminiferous tubule and, with estrogen, may contribute directly to spermatogenesis.

Hypogonadism

This general term means diminished or absent gonadal function. In primary disease of the testis, one or both specific functions of the testis will be lost. In secondary hypogonadism, a patient with pituitary disease loses both gonadotropins and does not produce hormone or sperm (Table 9-1).

Diagnosis of Hypogonadism

Clinical Examination

The major determinant of the clinical picture is the age of onset. Prepubertal hypogonadism is characterized by a failure of sexual maturation. The patient usually has a eunuchoidal habitus. His span is more than 2 inches greater than his height. The distance from the soles of his feet to the symphysis pubis is 2 inches greater than the distance from the symphysis to the top of his head. His voice remains high-pitched, facial and pubic hair growth never starts, and the genitalia remain infantile.

Postpubertal hypogonadism leads to a gradual regression in secondary sexual characteristics and an associated decrease in libido; eventually impotence develops.

There may be associated symptoms of the disease causing the hypogonadism: a history of local pain or inflammation in the testes, or symptoms suggestive of pituitary disease such as headache or changes in visual fields.

Laboratory Evaluation

Seminal Fluid Examination

The patient masturbates into a clean glass container and submits the fresh specimen for examination within 1 hour. The normal volume of the ejaculate ranges from 2.5 to over 6 cc. Sixty per cent or more of the sperm should be motile. The total count ranges from 50 to 100 million sperm per cubic centimeter. However, it cannot be concluded that fertility is impaired until the count drops below 20 million per cubic centimeter.

Table 9-1. Classification of Hypogonadism

Primary
Deficiency of Leydig cell and seminiferous tubule function
Functional prepubertal castrate syndrome
Deficiency of seminiferous tubule function alone
Klinefelter's syndrome
Adult seminiferous tubule failure
Orchitis (mumps, gonorrhea, leprosy)
Irradiation
Myotonia dystrophica
Deficiency of Leydig cell function
Adult Leydig cell failure (male climacteric)
Secondary
Hypogonadotropic hypogonadism
Complete form
Incomplete form
Delayed puberty
Prepubertal pituitary failure
Selective pituitary failure
Severe anterior pituitary insufficiency

Hormone Assays

Gonadotropins in Postpubertal Patients. Pituitary function is assessed by measuring the level of gonadotropins in the urine or, more recently, in plasma. As determined by a bioassay in mice, normal men and women excrete 5–30 mouse units per 24 hours. In postmenopausal women, the level increases over a range of 30–8,000 mouse units per 24 hours. With pituitary disease, the excretion of gonadotropins falls. With primary gonadal disease, testosterone no longer inhibits hypothalamic-pituitary function and, hence, urinary gonadotropins increase.

The level of the urinary 17-ketosteroids reflects both adrenal and testicular steroid production. Thus the significance of the level of ketosteroid excretion must be interpreted with care. 17-Ketosteroid assay does not measure testosterone although it does measure the testosterone metabolites—androsterone and eticocholanolone. Because of its high biologic potency, a slight increase in testosterone production induces major clinical changes without changing the quantity of ketosteroid excretion. Thus the urinary 17-ketosteroids provide a poor index of testosterone production.

Testosterone. In plasma or urine testosterone can now be measured directly. In men, there is a high correlation between the level of testosterone in plasma or urine and the clinical picture (the same does not hold true for women). Gonadal production of testosterone can be stimulated by the administration of human chorionic gonadotropin (HCG) in a dose of 3,000 I.U./day for 5 days. An increase in testosterone excretion proves that the gonad is responsive.

Testicular Biopsy

When a man has oligospermia or azoospermia but normal pituitary function, a biopsy of the testis is often necessary to determine the nature and extent of the underlying local lesion. The microscopic findings will distinguish defective spermiogenesis from obstruction to the passage of the sperm. The Leydig cells can be examined microscopically at the same time.

Chromosomal Studies

As discussed in Chapter 11, specific techniques allow us to determine the patient's genotype. The presence of the perinuclear Barr body in more than 20% of the cells from a buccal smear means that the patient has at least 2 X chromosomes in many of the cells. More complete discussion of these tests can be found in the chapter Chromosomal Studies in Endocrinology.

Clinical Syndromes of Hypogonadism

Functional Prepubertal Castrate Syndrome

In this syndrome, testosterone production and spermiogenesis fail at puberty despite the normal increase in pituitary secretion of ICSH and FSH at this time. Boys with this condition have normal external genitalia but the testes are either absent or atrophic. Since the patients have a normal male phenotype, the abnormality has arisen after 8 weeks' gestation. Most commonly, an unknown developmental fault during gestation results in testicular atrophy, leaving wolffian duct derivatives behind. Rarely, postnatal destruction of the testes by bilateral herniorrhaphy, infection, or trauma may produce the syndrome.

Because testosterone has not produced its biologic effect, these boys do not develop secondary sexual characteristics. They may have a eunuchoid habitus and gynecomastia, and in the scrotum there are only tiny remnants of testicular tissue.

Chromosomal studies show a normal male pattern. The urinary excretion of FSH will rise to abnormally high levels. The urinary 17-ketosteroid excretion may be low or normal and the urinary estrogen excretion is normal.

These patients are permanently infertile but should have long-term androgen therapy to produce normal physiologic and psychologic maturation. The safest and most efficient method is the parenteral administration of testosterone: 300 mg of testosterone cyclopentylpropionate intramuscularly every 3 or 4 weeks.

Deficient Seminiferous Tubule Function

Klinefelter's Syndrome

In this, the commonest form of male hypogonadism, the basic defect is a cytogenetic abnormality (Fig. 9-1). The patients with this disorder can be classified into one of two major groups—the true syndrome, and the variants of the syndrome.

Patients with true Klinefelter's syndrome always have a chromatin-positive buccal smear, and more than 20% of the cells will contain a darkly staining perinuclear chromatin mass—"the Barr body." These patients have at least two X chromosomes and a Y chromosome in some of their cells—thus, a total of at least 47 chromosomes. Some have suggested that this abnormality results from a nondysjunction in one of the gametes. Before puberty, these patients are phenotypic males and show no obvious abnormality. At puberty some body hair develops, but their body builds may range from normal male to eunuchoid. Frequently they have gynecomastia. The testes will be small (less than 1.5 cm in longest diameter) and firm. The urinary FSH level will be high, urinary 17-ketosteroids normal or slightly reduced, and plasma tesosterone levels will vary. On biopsy of the testes, there is hyalinization and fibrosis of the seminiferous tubules, no elastic fibers around the hyalinized tubules, and a variable degree of Leydig cell hyperplasia (Fig. 9-2).

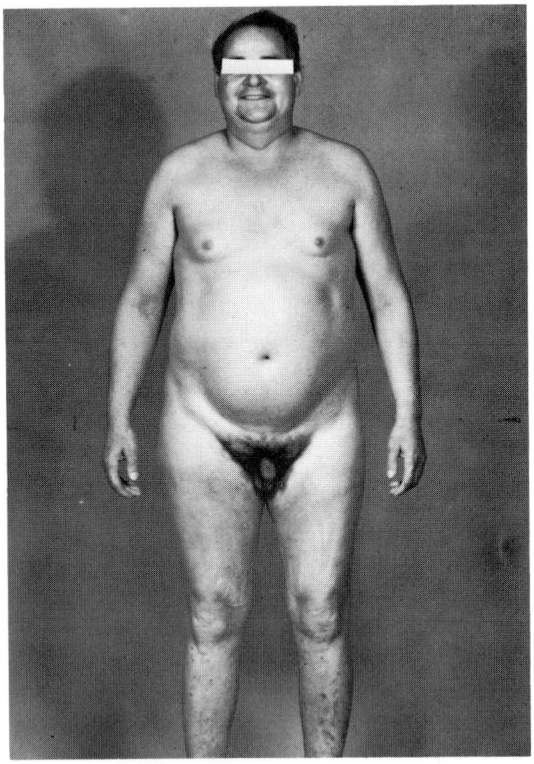

Fig. 9-1. Klinefelter's syndrome. This 34-year-old man with gynecomastia has normal potency but small testes and is sterile because of aspermia. He has normal pubic and facial hair and is balding. External genitalia are normal. He has had no androgen treatment. He has a 47,XXY karyotype characteristic of Klinefelter's syndrome, and positive sex chromatin on buccal smear.

In variants of Klinefelter's syndrome one of a number of abnormal chromosome patterns may be present, including mosaics with 48 or 49 chromosomes in some cells. Thus, these patients have at least two X's and a Y in some cells and so fit the definition of Klinefelter's syndrome. The defect may be found in only some of the cells. This mixture results in the varying clinical picture of the syndrome. Since the defect can appear in only some cells, the classification of the syndrome as chromatin-positive or chromatin-negative on the buccal smear can lead to some confusion. Clinically, the individuals range from an almost com-

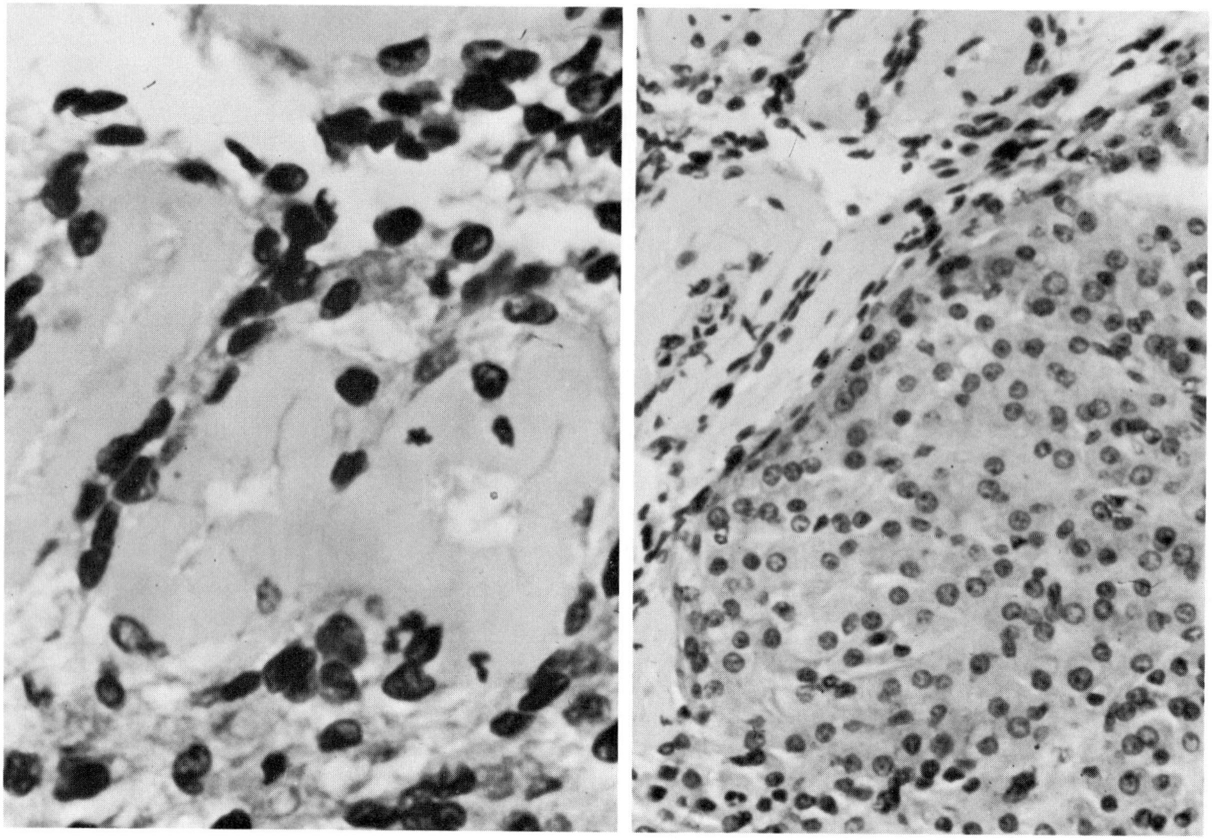

Fig. 9-2. Testis in Klinefelter's syndrome. A. The characteristic alterations in Klinefelter's syndrome are hyalinization of the seminiferous tubules and absence of spermatogenesis.

B. In this section of the same testis shown in **A**, the Leydig cells appear in large clumps, as a result of either hyperplasia or condensation of stroma (H & E × 400).

pletely normal male capable of some spermatogenesis to a typical eunuch with azoospermia. Some members of the variant group may be mentally retarded. Personality disorders are also common.

A few patients with Klinefelter's syndrome have been described who have a normal XY chromosome. This is a rare diagnosis and must be based on typical clinical and laboratory findings of Klinefelter's syndrome despite a negative buccal smear and normal chromosome pattern.

The fertility of each patient depends on the cytogenetic abnormality and the degree of azoospermia; in any event, it cannot be influenced by therapy. Some patients benefit from long-term androgen therapy in that they develop secondary sexual characteristics. However, their response to treatment may be disappointing either because the peripheral tissues may be resistant to androgen, or because there is a defect in the mechanism that converts androgen to a biologically active form.

Kallman's Syndrome

This syndrome is probably due to a lesion of the hypothalamus or its higher connections in association with agenesis of some portion of the olfactory pathway.

Germinal Cell Aplasia (Sertoli-Cell-Only Syndrome)

In this uncommon disease of unknown etiology, the patient seeks help because of infertility.

The biologic effects of testosterone are normal, and the testes are of normal consistency but slightly smaller than normal.

The urinary gonadotropins may be elevated, but the excretion of urinary 17-ketosteroids is normal. These men have azoospermia and, on testicular biopsy, there are no germinal cells in the seminiferous tubules, although the basal Sertoli cells appear normal. The interstitial tissue and Leydig cells are normal.

There is no specific treatment for the infertility, and androgen therapy is not required.

Adult Seminiferous Tubule Failure

Mumps Orchitis. This, the commonest of the few systemic infections that involve the testis, rarely occurs in prepubertal children; when it does, recovery is always complete. In the adult male, orchitis accompanies epidemic parotitis in 20% of cases. Although usually unilateral, it may be bilateral. The inflammatory response leads to local edema and severe pain. The edema may be followed by chronic progressive tubule fibrosis and hyalinization, leading to infertility. A smaller firm testis will be detected within 6 months.

Gonorrheal Orchitis. This rare complication of gonococcal urethritis is characterized by acute pain, swelling, and systemic manifestations of infection. Although antibiotics control the infection, permanent tubular destruction and fibrosis may result.

Leprosy. This disease may cause an indolent inflammation in the testis resulting in atrophy and infertility.

Irradiation. Exposure to X-rays or radioactive material can destroy the germinal cells and cause fibrosis of the tubules.

Idiopathic Failure. After puberty, progressive tubular fibrosis can occur without known cause. Males with this condition have normal Leydig cell function, elevated urinary gonadotropins, and oligospermia, but rarely azoospermia.

Myotonia Dystrophica. This disease is found only in males and is characterized by frontal baldness, lenticular opacities, and testicular atrophy. Approximately 80% of these men have significant hypogonadism. Biopsy reveals severe fibrosis and hyalinization of the tubules.

Deficiency of Leydig Cell Function

Adult Leydig Cell Failure ("Male Climacteric")

There is considerable controversy as to whether otherwise normal males have such failure. Men normally suffer a slowly progressive reduction in sexual drive with the passage of time. However, now that an adequate number of cases have been studied, a specific diagnosis of Leydig cell failure can, at times, be made.

Characteristically, these men lose libido and potency over a year or so. In addition, they complain of fatigue, depression, loss of memory, inability to concentrate, and nervous irritability. They suffer from hot flushes and excessive sweating, symptoms typical of the menopausal syndrome in the woman.

The urinary 17-ketosteroids may be normal or slightly low. The urinary gonadotropin excretion, however, is high, as is that found in the postmenopausal woman. In the normal man, increased gonadotropin excretion does not accompany aging and gradual reduction in sexual drive. Although the rates of testosterone production have not yet been reported in these men, one would anticipate that these values will be lower than in otherwise normal men in the same age group. The sperm count will be reduced. Biopsy of the testis may show histologically normal tubules and nonspecific degenerative changes in Leydig cells.

Since the etiology is unknown, the main clinical problem is to separate true Leydig cell failure from psychogenic impotence, which presents with the same vague clinical picture. Currently, urinary gonadotropin excretion is the best laboratory index for separating the two disease states; it is high in Leydig cell failure and normal in psychogenic impotence.

A trial of intramuscular testosterone has been used as a therapeutic test to support the diagnosis. The libido and potency of patients with true Leydig cell failure markedly improve and nonspecific symptoms are reduced. On the other hand, parenteral testosterone does not help psychogenic impotence.

Secondary Male Hypogonadism

Hypogonadotropic Eunuchoidism

In the male, normal puberty occurs between the ages of 12 and 19. Increased testicular secretion produces most of the physical and psychologic changes. A rise in pituitary gonadotropin stimulates the increased testicular production of testosterone. The "trigger" in the hypothalamus that produces the increased gonadotropin secretion is unknown, but if the mechanism is not activated, normal puberty does not occur. Because of the wide age range of normal puberty, the diagnosis of hypogonadotropic hypogonadism should not be made before the male is 20 years of age or older.

Complete Form

When testosterone production does not increase, secondary sexual characteristics fail to develop. The patients have a eunuchoidal habitus with disproportionately long extremities (Fig. 9-3). The external genitalia remain infantile and body and facial hair does not develop. The testes

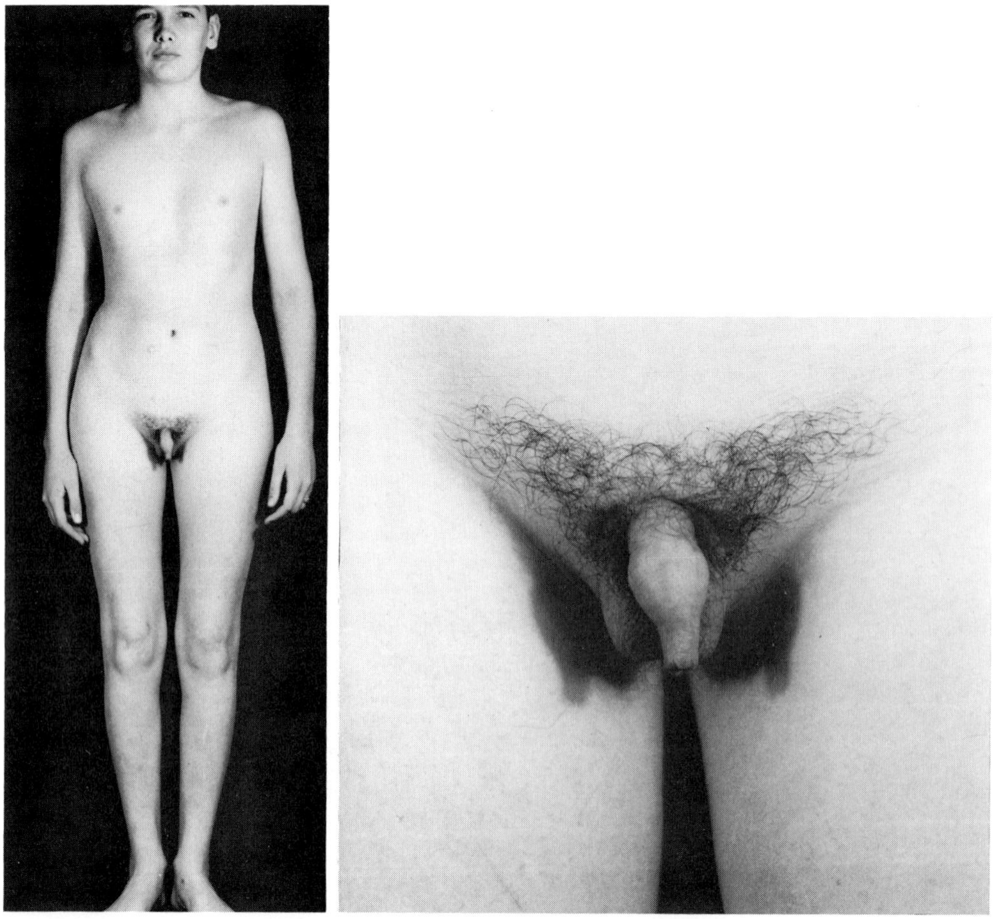

Fig. 9-3. Hypogonadotropic eunuchoidism. This 23-year-old man has features typical of eunuchoidism. He is tall (154 cm) and thin (61 kg), and has long, tapering extremities: arm span 164 cm (more than the height) and the symphysis pubis to floor measurement 82 cm (more than half the height). His musculature is poor, facial features are juvenile, skin is fine, and he has no facial or body hair. There is no temporal recession of scalp hair. However, he has sparse axillary and pubic hair. His testes are small and soft and his phallus is small. The voice is high-pitched. This patient has familiar hypogonadotropic eunuchoidism, associated with the Marie type of cerebellar ataxia. The karyotope is normal. (From Volpé, R., Metzler, W. S., and Johnston, M. W. *J Clin Endocrinol Metab 23*:107–115, 1963. Reproduced with permission.)

are very small and, on biopsy, the seminiferous tubules are immature and Leydig cells poorly differentiated (Fig. 9-4). The urinary gondadotropin excretion is low but 17-ketosteroid excretion is only slightly decreased, because adrenal function is unimpaired. Occasionally, these patients may have local disease in the hypothalamus such as a craniopharyngioma, in which case the 17-ketosteroids may be greatly reduced if ACTH secretion is also impaired.

The best initial therapy is intramuscular chorionic gonadotropin in a dose of 3,000 I.U. 3 times a week. When this is continued for 6 months, the Leydig cells are stimulated, testosterone production rises, and the secondary sexual characteristics develop. Therapy should then be withdrawn and the patient observed. In most cases, secondary sexual characteristics will gradually recede. If this occurs, the patient is started on long-term androgen therapy.

Incomplete Form

In patients with the incomplete form of hypogonadotropic eunuchoidism gonadotropin production is borderline low and testosterone production rises over prepubertal levels. The testosterone increase, however, is insufficient to bring about complete maturation. Intramuscular administration of chorionic gonadotropin increases testosterone production further and sexual maturation occurs. In some patients, after 6 months' therapy, the pituitary takes over and induces adequate gondadotropin production and spermiogenesis, the testes produce gonadotropin, and spermiogenesis and testicular hormone production continue. In others, endogenous gonadotropin production remains inadequate, and the patient, who must be treated with long-term androgen, must be considered infertile.

Delayed Puberty

Because puberty may not occur until age 20, a diagnosis of hypogonadotropic hypogonadism should not be made before this age. Until 20, the maturation of boys can be accelerated by the administration of gonadotropins but many will mature spontaneously (see Fig. 4-12). If these boys are treated and do not develop sexually, they then should be called "hypogonadotropic eunuchs."

Prepubertal Severe Anterior Pituitary Insufficiency (Pituitary Dwarfism)

More complete discussion of panhypopituitarism will be found in Chapters 2 and 4. The failure to develop gonadal function is partially masked by

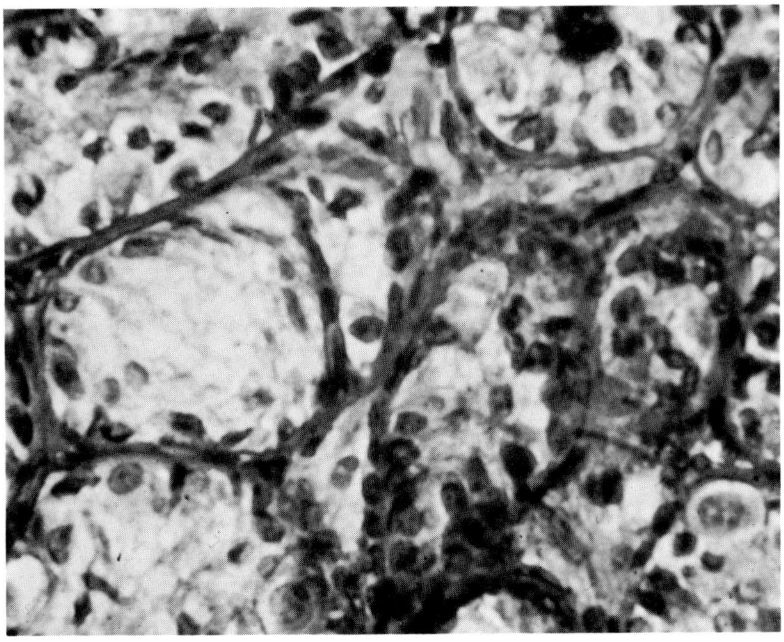

Fig. 9-4. Testis in hypogonadotropic eunuchoidism. Section from testis of patient in Figure 9-3 shows small seminiferous tubules without lumens and without Sertoli cells. Interstitial tissue was composed of only undifferentiated mesenchymal cells and contained no Leydig cells (H & E × 400). This infantile picture persists because there was no gonadotropic stimulation. (From Volpé, R., Metzler, W. S., and Johnston, M. W. *J Clin Endocrinol Metab 23*:107–115, 1963. Reproduced with permission.)

other endocrine deficiencies, but in the testes, both hormone production and spermiogenesis fail. The urine excretion of gonadotropin is low, and, histologically, the testis is characteristically immature. Androgen is only one part of the general endocrine replacement treatment required by these patients.

Postpubertal Pituitary Failure

In these patients the symptoms of clinically more important adrenal and thyroid deficiency predominate. The patient may complain bitterly of decreased libido and impotence. He has oligospermia and infertility, but these are not recognized because of the other major clinical problems.

Androgen replacement therapy is of major importance, especially in younger men. Intramuscular testosterone will stop regression of secondary sexual characteristics and increase libido. Usually, however, the patient remains oligospermic and infertile, although in a few patients fertility has returned after adequate testosterone therapy combined with thyroid and adrenal replacement.

A specific deficiency of gonadotropins may develop in the adult male. Most commonly, however, this is the first clinical evidence of progressive pituitary failure. As time passes, thyroid and finally adrenal function are also impaired because the pituitary is not producing specific tropic hormones. The predominant clinical features result from a decrease in testosterone production and regression of secondary sexual characteristics, loss of libido, and development of impotence. Oligospermia and infertility may be the presenting complaints.

Male Sexual Precocity

Isosexual Precocious Puberty

Boys who develop testicular spermiogenesis and hormone production before age 9 have isosexual precocious puberty. Testicular stimulation by premature activation of the hypothalamic-pituitary control of gonadotropin release results in a true early puberty. Most commonly, no focal lesion can be identified in the hypthalamus or pituitary. Less frequently, tumors or congenital lesions may be detected. Other evidence of hypothalamic-pituitary dysfunction such as diabetes insipidus, obesity, or somnolence may accompany isosexual precocity.

There is no satisfactory therapy for isosexual precocious puberty, although long-acting medroxyprogesterone (Provera) induces a fall in gonadotropin production and a subsequent fall in testosterone production. This, however, only slows down the process.

Other Forms of Sexual Precocity

Excessive Testosterone Production

This disorder occurs in patients with congenital adrenal hyperplasia in whom the defect is in 21-hydroxylation or 11-hydroxylation. A more complete discussion of this disorder is found in Chapter 7, The Adrenals. In males the excessive testosterone production leads to precocious sexual development without spermiogenesis. The testes remain small and soft. Biopsy reveals immature tubules and Leydig cells. Standard replacement therapy with glucocorticoids reduces the adrenal testosterone production. This treatment allows normal growth patterns but does not cure this disorder.

Functioning Interstitial Cell Tumors

These tumors of the testis produce excessive amounts of testosterone. If this occurs before age 9, precocious sexual development will ensue. Again, spermiogenesis does not occur and the other testis remains small and immature. When the tumor is removed, the rate of development of sexual characteristics slows.

Other Testicular Disorders and Related Abnormalities

Gynecomastia

Gynecomastia is benign glandular enlargement of the male breast. It is important to separate gynecomastia from breast enlargement due to tumors such as lipoma or carcinoma, and from enlargement due to an increase in adipose tissue. The tumors will be unilateral, firm, infiltrating, and nontender. Adipose tissue is diffuse, bilateral, and not localized just in the region of the areolae.

Gynecomastia, although most common at puberty, may be found at any age. It may be unilateral but is most frequently bilateral. The enlargement may vary from a small button of subareolar tissue to the full-sized breast of the normal adult female.

Once the diagnosis is made, the cause must be found. The histologic pattern of the tissue at biopsy may help to point to the hormonal basis. Predominance of interlobular tissue suggests excessive pituitary gonadotropin production, whereas ductal hyperplasia suggests excessive estrogen effect.

In Klinefelter's syndrome and in the functional prepubertal castrate syndrome, gynecomastia may be found in association with excessive pituitary gonadotropins. In the rare feminizing adrenocortical tumors and in certain testicular tumors, excessive estrogen production causes gynecomastia. Disordered liver metabolism, as in cirrhosis, leads to an increased biologic effect of estrogen and thus gynecomastia. Exogenous estrogen therapy in carcinoma of the prostate induces gynecomastia.

Gynecomastia has been observed in other endocrine disorders—hyperthyroidism, hypothyroidism, acromegaly, and Cushing's syndrome.

Certain drugs, such as digitalis and Dilantin, have been considered to cause gynecomastia. In the occasional patient, testosterone may cause gynecomastia because of the in-vivo conversion of testosterone to estrogen. Gynecomastia has been found in patients with bronchogenic carcinoma and in patients with spinal cord lesions causing paraplegia. The mechanism in these cases is unknown. Gynecomastia has been noted during the refeeding of patients suffering from severe malnutrition. Suppression of the pituitary production of gonadotropins is low during starvation, and during refeeding there is a rebound overproduction leading to gynecomastia. Management of gynecomastia at puberty centers on reassurance of the patient and his parents. The patient should be told that it may persist for even 2 or 3 years but will gradually subside without therapy. Occasionally, if the size of the breast produces a social problem, plastic surgery can be considered.

When gynecomastia is secondary to other disease states, therapy is directed at the underlying process.

Galactorrhea

Galactorrhea with milk production by the male breast is a much rarer phenomenon than gynecomastia. It may occur from a breast that is only slightly enlarged and is probably due to the same causes as gynecomastia (increasing estrogen effect) with the addition of prolactin excess.

Testicular Feminization

This condition, which may be familial, provides the most extreme example of male pseudohermaphroditism (Fig. 9-5). The patients usually have female external genitalia with abdominal or inguinal testes. They are the most feminine of creatures and their puberty is characterized by exuberant breast development and a striking absence of pubic and axillary hair. The patient presents with primary amenorrhea and has a shallow vagina ending in a blind pouch. Buccal smear is chromatin-negative and the karyotype is normal male (46,XY). On culdoscopy, the examiner finds no uterus, tubes, or ovaries. This aberrant development appears to be due to a failure of all tissues to respond to androgen from fetal life onward. Because of the threat of malignant change, the testes are usually removed and the patient maintained thereafter on female hormone replacement.

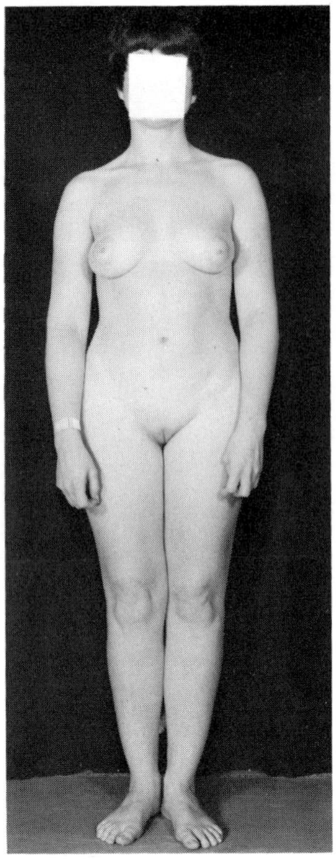

Fig. 9-5. Testicular feminization. This 26-year-old "woman" with testicular feminization presented with primary amenorrhea. She has well-developed breasts but no pubic hair. The faint bulgings in both groins are the undescended feminizing testes. When they were later removed during repair of indirect inguinal hernias, the testes contained multiple Sertoli-cell adenomas. This patient is now on low-dose sequential estrogen-progesterone substitution because she could not tolerate the usual doses of estrogen. She has two "sisters" with the same disorder.

Cryptorchidism

The incidence of this disorder is difficult to assess. Care must be taken to separate true cryptorchidism from the migratory or retractile testis, which lies in the upper scrotum and freely withdraws into the inguinal canal. Normally, the testis descends into the scrotum at about 8 months' gestation, but descent may be delayed until shortly after birth. The incidence of cryptorchidism at birth ranges from 5% to 10%. However, the testis spontaneously descends during the first year so that in man the incidence is less than 0.5%. Unilateral cryptorchidism is four times as common as bilateral cryptorchidism.

The etiology of the disorder is not clear, although on occasion it may be due to mechanical obstruction to descent. In most cases, however, it probably represents a defect in embryogenesis. For diagnosis, the patient should be repeatedly examined in the upright and supine position in a warm comfortable room. The Valsalva maneuver or lower abdominal pressure will often cause a mobile testis to descend into the scrotum.

Treatment of cryptorchidism is still controversial. The decision to attempt orchiopexy is based on at least three factors: the likelihood of spontaneous descent, the potential fertility of the undescended testis, and the possibility of detecting neoplastic change in the testis.

Current studies suggest that the production of LH by the pituitary and the increased output of testosterone by the testis precedes spermiogenesis in the testis. Thus, the signs of puberty may appear before active spermiogenesis occurs. On this basis, it is suggested that specific therapy can be delayed until the first signs of puberty are noted, thus allowing maximal times for spontaneous descent of the testis. Delay beyond puberty usually leads to degenerative changes and eventually atrophy of the testis. This degeneration has been attributed to the higher temperature to which the testis is exposed in the inguinal canal or abdomen.

Cancer is more frequent in the undescended and atrophic testis. Thus, orchiopexy makes the testis more accessible to examination to allow detection of this change.

In cryptorchidism, the first step in therapy is a course of chorionic gonadotropin, 4,000 I.U. 3 times weekly for 3 weeks. This may stimulate descent of the testis. There is still argument, however, as to whether this really causes a descent of the testis or merely speeds up descent of a testis that would come down normally. If the testis fails to descend following chorionic gonadotropin, orchiopexy is then carried out. If, at the time of operation, the undescended testis is atrophic, it should be removed.

Tumors of Testis

Although testicular neoplasms are uncommon, their concentration in the third and fourth decades makes them one of the most common malignancies in this age group. Malignant neoplasms of the testis comprise slightly more than 4% of all tumors affecting the genitourinary tract and 0.5–1.0% of all cancers in the male.

The tumors may be germinal or nongerminal. The classification and incidence of each type are shown in Table 9-2.

Tumors are more common in the right than in the left testis. They are bilateral in about 2% of cases. The most common bilateral tumors are lymphomas and seminomas. About 5% of men with testicular tumors give a history of undescended testis, the tumor being intraabdominal or in the scrotal testis.

The initial clinical symptom (a slowly increasing, nontender swelling) is usually neglected by the patient. Occasionally, he may have local pain or tenderness that leads to the mistaken diagnosis of epididymitis or orchitis. Later, the patient may complain of a dragging ache in the scrotum. The amount of local and distant spread is variable. Careful palpation of the scrotal contents is required to detect small tumors.

Germinal-cell tumors commonly have functioning chorionic elements that explain the high level of urinary chorionic gonadotropin on assay. These patients often have gynecomastia. Pituitary gonadotropins are often increased for some unexplained reason. Interstitial or Leydig cell tumors have endocrine function resulting in virilization and precocious puberty in young boys or producing feminization in men with gynecomastia, decreasing libido, and decreasing body hair growth. The first line of therapy is orchidectomy with appropriate lymph-node resection. Postoperative irradiation may be effective, depending on the radiosensitivity of tumors. Recently, chemotherapy has been used with some success in the treatment of embryonal tumors.

Table 9-2. Distribution of Tumors of the Testis

Classification	*Incidence* (%)
Primary	
Germinal seminoma	40
Embryonal (embryoma, choriocarcinoma, embryonal carcinoma, teratocarcinoma)	32
Combined seminoma and embryonal	14
Nongerminal interstitial cell (Leydig cell)	1.5
Sertoli cell	1
Stromal	1
Secondary (metastatic)	8
Uncertain	2.5

Homosexuality

Recently, Kolodny *et al.* reported low sperm counts and low testosterone levels in a group of male homosexuals. This work promises to reopen the question of the possible prepubertal influence of steroid sex hormones on human sexual behavior.

References

1. Campbell, M. F. *Urology,* ed. 3. Philadelphia, Saunders, 1970.
2. Federman, D. D. Disorders of sexual development. *N Engl J Med 277:*351–360, 1967.
3. Federman, D. D. Testicular deficiency. *Adv Intern Med 16:*81–102, 1970.
4. Heller, C. G., and Clermont, Y. Kinetics of the germinal epithelium in man. *Recent Progr Horm Res 20:*545–575, 1964.
5. Kolodny, R. C., Masters, W. H., Hendryx, J., and Toro, G. Plasma testosterone and semen analysis in a group of male homosexuals. *N Engl J Med 21:* 1170–1174, 1971.
6. Simmer, H. H., Pion, R. J., and Dignam, W. J. *Testicular Feminization; Endocrine Function of Feminizing Testes: Comparison with Normal Testes.* Springfield, Ill., Thomas, 1965.
7. Sohval, A. R. Hormonal factors in male sex development and function. *Mod Trends Endocrinol Ser. 2,* pp. 180–200, 1961.
8. Volpé, R., Metzler, W. S., and Johnston, M. W. Familial hypogonadotrophic eunuchoidism with cerebellar ataxia. *J Clin Endocrinol Metab 23:*107–115, 1963.

General Reference

The Human Testis: Proceedings of the Workshop Conference, Positano, Italy, 1970. In *Advances in Experimental Medicine and Biology,* vol. 10, Rosemberg, E., and Paulsen, C. A., eds. New York, Plenum, 1970.

10

The Ovary

Carol Ann Cowell and Richard Wilson

A healthy ovary performs the vital role in female development. Puberty and menopause, the major biological events in a woman's life, reflect profound changes in ovarian function which affect appearance, attitude, and behavior. This chapter outlines, for each life stage, normal and abnormal ovarian functions and their relationship to the female role (Fig. 10-1).

The stages of ovarian function are:

- Prereproductive
  - Fetal
  - Childhood
- Reproductive
  - Puberty
  - Adolescence
  - Maturity, including pregnancy
- Postreproductive
  - Menopause
  - Senescence

Ovaries are almond-shaped structures that, for half of a woman's life, produce hormones and eggs. Normal ovaries are also dynamic sex organs that provide the basis for a woman's sexual identity. Their normal functions assure such attributes as breasts, female body contours, menstruation and the probability of fulfilling her childbearing role.

Ovarian malfunction may distort a woman's image of herself and make it difficult to achieve a mature psychosexual sense of well-being. The physician can usually correct psychological or physical abnormalities when they occur, thereby influencing the development or preservation of a woman's self-esteem. Therefore it is important that he familiarize himself with the ovarian life cycle and its complex effects.

The influence exerted by the ovary on woman's sense of identity was not recognized until the twentieth century, yet the Egyptians understood that the ovaries were related to reproduction, and removed them for contraceptive purposes. In the second century, the king of Lydia castrated women and used these female eunuchs in sexual orgies. Shortly thereafter, in Asia Minor among the Aeramyttes and Gyges tribes, members of the royal harems were castrated to prevent conception and to keep them attractive; their masters were disappointed when beauty faded rapidly after castration produced menopausal changes.

Edgar Allan first demonstrated the ovary's endocrine function when, using the vaginal smear assay, he demonstrated the effect of an "ovarian follicular hormone" (estrogen). Subsequently, Corner and Allan, guided by the histological alterations of the endometrium, described another ovarian hormone, progesterone, which was believed to originate in the corpus luteum. In recent years, our knowledge of ovarian endocrine activity and its control has been greatly expanded. Investigators have defined the endocrine role of the gonads, isolated their hormones, and clarified the interrelationships between these and other glands that control and influence gonadal function.

The human ovary has two major physiological functions: the cyclical release of ova; the production and release of sex hormones that affect target cells in other organs. These processes are inti-

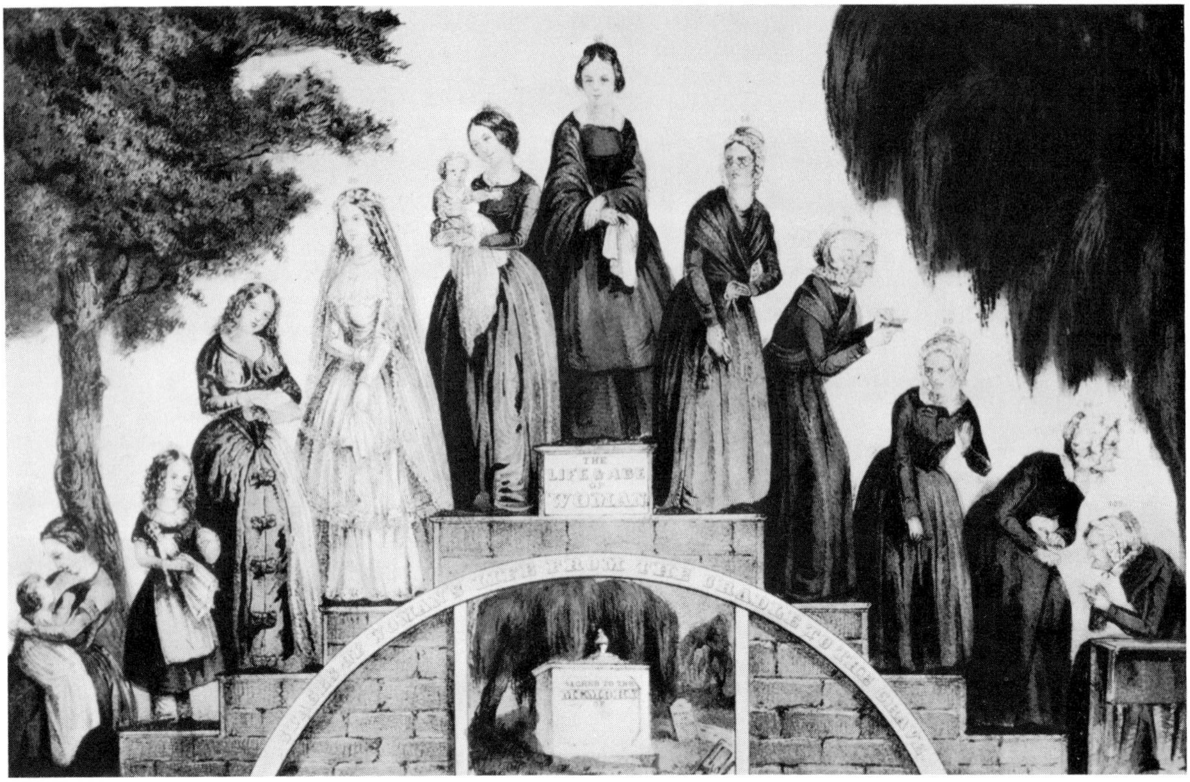

Fig. 10-1. Stages in a woman's life from cradle to grave. In this Currier and Ives print, puberty has been represented by a 16-year-old girl, whereas today puberty and the menarche occur 3 or 4 years earlier.

mately related, and malfunction of one nearly always disturbs the other.

This chapter deals chiefly with the ovary as a gland of internal secretion, producing and releasing into the bloodstream, hormones that affect the entire organism. We will consider abnormalities of ovarian development and/or function in relationship to the general homeostatic mechanisms, including genetic constitution, endocrine control, and end-organ response.

This chapter presents clinical manifestations of disturbed ovarian function and discusses the reasons for these disturbances. Complex classifications are avoided because they confuse rather than clarify. Ovarian infections and tumors, and conditions such as endometriosis, are described only as they affect reproductive and endocrine activity. The symptoms of abnormal function—menstrual disturbances, hirsutism, virilization, infertility, and unusually early or delayed sexual development—are not diseases. They indicate abnormal function; hence, the investigation of suspected ovarian malfunction is directed toward a specific cause. This break with pedagogic tradition should generate a better understanding of the ovary and its effects on the individual.

The Fetal Ovary

Genetic sex is normally determined at the time of conception by the presence or absence of the Y chromosome in the sperm that fertilizes the ovum. The sex-determining genes, either X or Y, cause the primitive gonad to develop either as an ovary or as a testis. The X and Y genes have little direct influence upon the other sexual characteristics, such as internal and external genitalia. These will always develop as female unless an active masculinizing influence acts upon the fetus during intrauterine life. The fetal testis, which functions in utero, normally exerts this influence and stimulates development of the male ductal system and external genitalia.

In the female embryo, either the maternally or paternally derived X chromosome is partially inactivated 12–18 days after fertilization and becomes the chromatin body (Barr body) in the nucleus of the cell. After this transformation, all descendants of that X chromosome are similarly inactive. Thus, each female *somatic cell* functions as if it had only one genetically active X chromosome, as the male cell does. However, the female primary *germ cells* in the embryo maintain the second X chromosome, which determines normal ovarian differentiation. The primordial gonads of chromosomal males and females are identical until the sixth week of embryonic life and can develop into either testes or ovaries. Multiple sex-determining loci on the short and long arms of the two X chromosomes in the female primary germ cells seem to determine normal ovarian development and function.

Primary germ cells have been identified in the dorsal endoderm of the yolk sac in the 24-day human embryo (Fig. 10-2). During the fourth and fifth weeks of intrauterine development, while undergoing mitosis, these cells migrate from the yolk sac and pass through the hindgut wall and the dorsal mesentery to reach the primitive gonads in the urogenital ridge. The female primary germ cells change into primary oogonia, some of which organize the stromal cells around them and become primary oocytes at a time when the primary germ cells stop producing oogonia. The two ovaries may contain as many as 6 or 7 million oogonia at the seventh month of development. Some of the priary oocytes and the surrounding stromal cells then develop further into primary follicles. The number of follicles is greatest at birth; from then on, they diminish rapidly.

Within a surviving primary follicle, ovum development is arrested at the late prophase of the first meiotic division; it remains in that state until the follicle develops and the ovum ovulates from the ovary, 12–47 years later. Just before ovulation, the first polar body is extruded from the ovum, and the haploid oocyte (i.e., that with one-half the normal complement of chromosomes) begins its second meiotic division, which is not completed (i.e., the second polar body is not extruded) until the ovum is fertilized.

Development of female internal and external genitalia does not depend upon the gonads. The male genital ducts and external genitalia, however, depend upon the fetal testis for their development and differentiation (see Chapter 9, The Testis). Thus, persons with nonfunctioning or absent gonads have female external and internal genitalia. In order to acquire male features, one must have a Y chromosome, a functioning male gonad, and normal end-organ response during intrauterine life. The female gonad has little endocrine function in utero.

Sex of rearing, assigned to the infant at birth, is based on the appearance of the external genitalia. The attendants nearly always assign the correct sex; however, if doubt exists, the physician should defer this decision until sex-chromatin pattern is determined and chromosome cultures are done. Sex of rearing can usually be altered without drastic effect until the child is 18 months old; beyond this age, it may cause serious, perhaps irreversible, psychological harm.

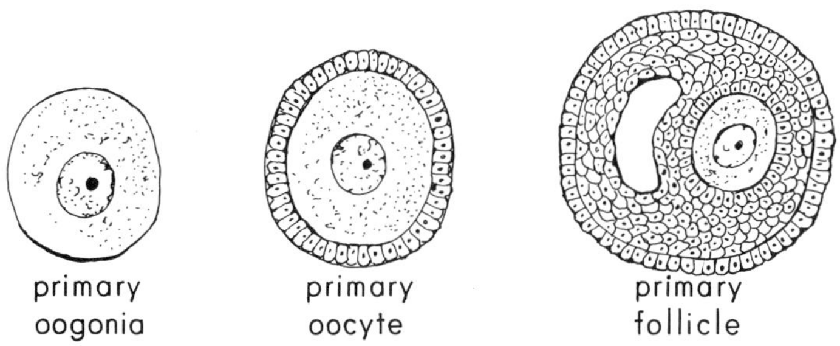

Fig. 10-2. Stages in the development of an ovum.

Ovary During Childhood

Childhood consists of two phases: infancy to age seven, and age seven to puberty. Body growth, the most obvious change during the initial phase, is accompanied by little apparent sexual development.

In the immature girl, the ovaries are small and have only an occasional tiny follicle on their surfaces. These few follicles, which grow and then atrophy, secrete enough estrogen to exert an inhibiting (negative feedback) effect upon the estrogen-sensitive hypothalamic receptor area (Figs. 10-3 and 10-4). Between seven and ten years, this sensitivity to estrogen decreases; as sexual maturation begins, the ovary is stimulated to increase its production of estrogen. Maturation of the ovarian regulatory mechanism is diagrammed and explained in Fig. 4-2. This gradual estrogen increase changes fat distribution, muscle development, and pubertal growth, making the body more recognizably female. External genitalia change little anatomically, but estrogen gives the genitalia a fuller look and causes the superficial cellular layer of the vaginal mucosa to mature; this latter effect can be quantitated on a vaginal smear (cytohormonal assessment) done in later childhood.

The sexual self-image becomes firmly established between 18 months and puberty. Femininity is asserted in many ways: choice of dress, activities, interests, and reaction to environment. Childhood is not a period of total ovarian and sexual quiescence, but rather a slow preparation for the rapid changes of puberty.

The hypothalamic-pituitary-ovarian axis can function in an adult manner in the prepubertal girl: In idiopathic precocious puberty, the pituitary, gonads, and end-organs respond as they do in an adult (Fig. 10-4). Certain hypothalamic lesions also precipitate adult functioning, probably by destroying the receptor area—the upper end of the negative feedback loop. These observations suggest that the ovary normally prevents premature puberty by a negative feedback mechanism that suppresses the hypothalamus.

The regulation of ovarian function resembles other endocrine control systems, except that the ovaries function cyclically. This demands a high degree of coordination among the hypothalamic centers, the adenohypophysis, and the ovary. Progesterone, androgens, and estrogens primarily inhibit, but sometimes stimulate, the hypothalamus to coordinate the activity of the hypothalamic-pituitary axis. Figure 10-3 shows the basic three-gland and target-cell regulatory mechanism, and Figure 10-4 shows the extra stimulatory (positive feedback) loop present in the ovary.

The reproductive control centers in the hypothalamus will be female, regardless of the individual's genetic sex, unless they are exposed to male sex hormones in utero. Hypothetically, these hypothalamic reproductive control systems may be viewed as having three areas: receptor, steady state, and cycling (Fig. 10-5).

The *receptor area* integrates the environmental, emotional, biochemical, and other neural stimuli reaching the hypothalamus, and profoundly influences the *cycling area,* which in turn initiates and maintains the female pattern of cyclic gonadal activity. In the normal male, and in females with endocrine disturbances such as congenital adrenogenital syndrome, the cycling area is blocked by androgens secreted by the testes and adrenals. In the human female, this type of hypothalamic block is usually not permanent, but in the rat and some other lower animals, hypothalamic organization can be changed permanently from female to male by injecting androgens within 5 days of birth.

The *steady state area* in the male maintains testicular activity at a relatively constant level. In the female, as long as the cycling center functions well, the steady state area remains relatively inactive. However, when cycling has been disturbed, this area will support ovarian function at a low but constant level.

Little is known about the receptor area and its influence on other areas of the hypothalamus. However, we know more about the releasing factors for FSH and LH (FSHRF and LHRF), which the cycling and steady state areas produce to effect the release of the gonadotropins from the anterior pituitary. These releasing substances are

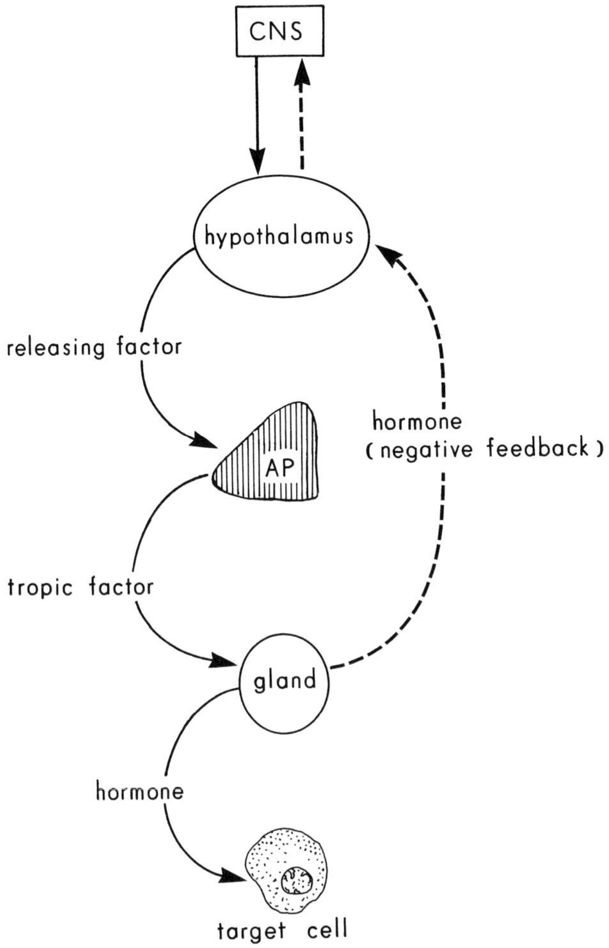

Fig. 10-3. Basic endocrine-gland target-cell regulatory system. This scheme applies more accurately to the thyroid, where the chief aim of regulation is to maintain a steady state and provide for variations in function in response to need.

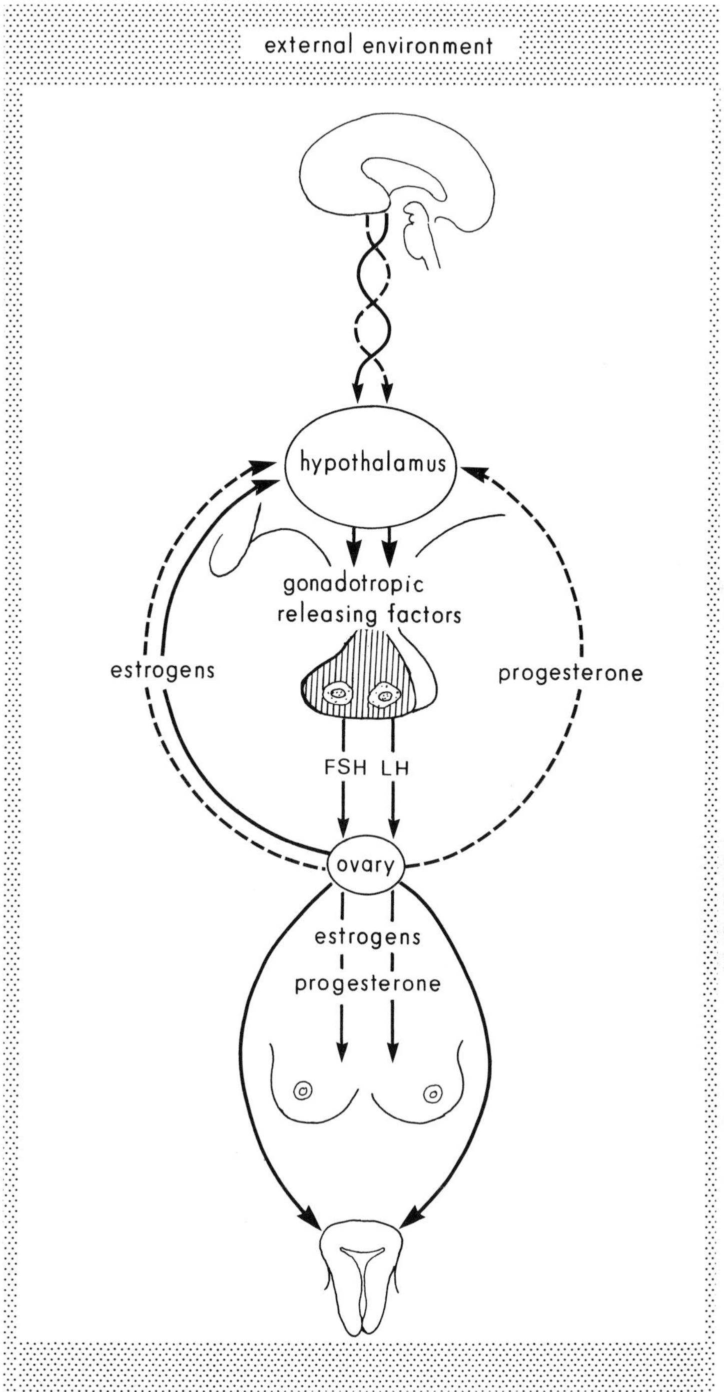

Fig. 10-4. Control of ovarian function: Solid lines represent stimulation, broken lines indicate inhibition. Regulation of ovarian function requires more complex arrangements than that shown in Figure 10-3. In positive feedback, low levels of estrogen stimulate the hypothalamus to increase its production of releasing factors. The end result of this is to increase ovarian estrogen production. When circulating estrogen rises sufficiently, hypothalamic stimulation ceases; that is, high levels inhibit—a pattern known as "negative feedback."

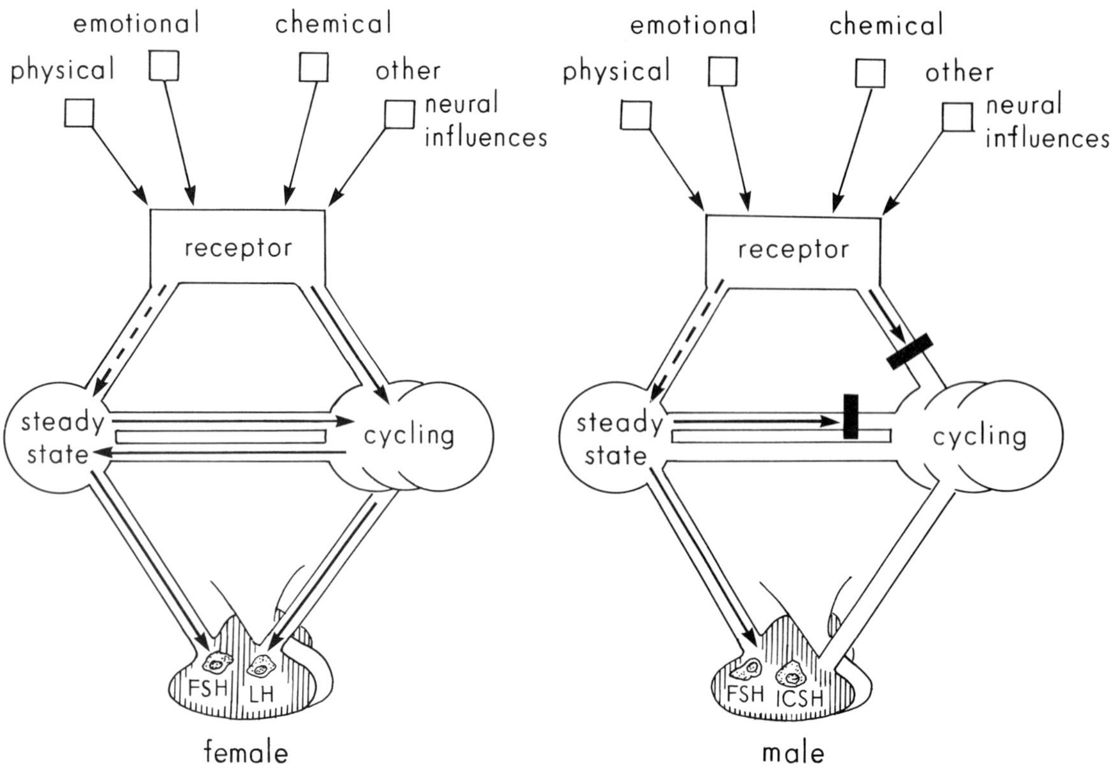

Fig. 10-5. Hypothalamic reproductive control centers. Reproduction depends on a complex integration of nervous and endocrine systems. Something is known about the endocrine structures contributing to this regulation but very little is known about comparable nervous structures. In any event, the hypothalamus is the meeting ground of these two systems. Although such centers as "the steady state area" are shown in bold outline, they are only useful as working hypotheses. The cycling center is characterized by periodicity. In the male, this center does not function because exposure to androgens before birth renders it inoperative (*black blocks*). In the female, the receptor center integrates the various stimuli and controls the periodicity of the cycling center (*solid arrow*) between these centers, but has much less influence on the steady state (*broken arrow*). The cycling area cannot function unless it is balanced by a normal steady state center. When these two centers work in harmony, they stimulate the anterior pituitary to produce and release the types and quantities of gonadotropins necessary to produce ovulation. In the male, the only gonadotropin-releasing stimuli reaching the anterior pituitary are those which come from the steady state area.

true hormones: They are secreted into the bloodstream and pass, via the hypophyseal portal system, to the pituitary gland.

The hypothalamus and the releasing factors play several roles in sexual development and the regulation of reproduction. As the female approaches puberty, the receptor area of the hypothalamus becomes less sensitive to gonadal hormones, hence less easily inhibited (see Fig. 4-2). The hypothalamus then produces more releasing factors and the pituitary releases greater amounts of gonadotropins, which stimulate production and release of increasing amounts of ovarian hormones.

In the physically mature woman, LHRF from the cycling area triggers a surge of luteinizing hormone from the anterior pituitary. This cyclic surge of LH causes ovulation. Although we do not understand the complex factors which control the ovulatory LH surge, ovulation can be induced in some animals by electrical stimuli, copulation, or light. These stimuli are not effective in the human female because of the inherent rhythmic activity of the hypothalamic cycling area. This rhythm can be disturbed, however, by alterations in the usual duration of light or darkness, and by other environmental, emotional, and chemical stimuli.

Abnormal Function

Under a microscope, immature ovaries show evidence of considerable follicular activity, but to the naked eye only an occasional small follicular cyst is visible. Infrequently, these cysts become large enough to be detected during physical examination. Occasionally, children also develop ovarian tumors. Rarely, these tumors may produce androgens or estrogens, and the hormones then exert masculinizing or feminizing influences, and may produce precocious pseudopuberty and vaginal bleeding. Any childhood or prepubertal vaginal bleeding is abnormal and its cause must be determined. In this age group, vaginal bleeding is commonly due to ingestion of estrogenic hormones (usually oral contraceptives), to a foreign body in the vagina, or to local inflammatory lesions; it is rarely due to a hormone-producing ovarian tumor.

Premature Sexual Development

In both sexes, precocious sexual development may be either isosexual (along the expected lines for that sex) or heterosexual (accompanied by symptoms and signs contradictory to the assigned sex). The physician must recognize this distinction if he is to reach a correct diagnosis.

Precocious true puberty must be distinguished from precocious pseudopuberty (Table 10-1). The former is specific, in that gonadotrophins are being produced and ovulation has occurred or is imminent—in this instance, sexual development is abnormal only because of the age. A child with precocious true puberty may show, before 8 years of age, any or all of the signs of puberty, occurring in proper sequence: breast enlargement, pubic hair, advanced bone and somatic maturation, menstruation, and ovulation.

Precocious true puberty cannot be heterosexual, but precocious pseudopuberty may be.

The most common cause of pseudopuberty in the female is congenital adrenal hyperplasia.

Table 10-1. Classification of Sexual Precocity

Isosexual
Central nervous system (true puberty)
Organic: postinflammatory, hamartoma, intracranial neoplasm, tuberous sclerosis
Congenital abnormalities: polyostotic fibrous dysplasia (McCune-Albright syndrome)
Constitutional
Ovarian (pseudopuberty)
Feminizing tumor
Teratomatous choriocarcinoma
Nonneoplastic cyst with hormonal function: theca-lutein follicle cyst
Adrenal feminizing tumors (pseudopuberty)
Other causes (pseudopuberty)
Exogenous estrogens
Hypothyroidism
Heterosexual (pseudopuberty)
Adrenal
Hyperplasia
Congenital or
acquired
Androgen-producing adrenocortical adenoma or carcinoma
Ovarian
Androgen-producing ovarian tumor

Heterosexual development occurs because the adrenals secrete excessive amounts of androgen (see Chapter 7, The Adrenals). Functioning ovarian and adrenal tumors and exogenous estrogen or androgen administration also cause precocious isosexual or heterosexual pseudopuberty.

Uterine bleeding is the most significant sign of sexual maturity. Children who exhibit breast enlargement, premature growth of pubic and axillary hair, and advanced somatic and genital development but who do not have recurrent uterine bleeding, have precocious sexual development rather than precocious puberty.

Heterosexual precocious pseudopuberty is abnormal, not only because the secondary sexual characteristics appear before the expected time, but also because these characteristics are of the opposite sex. In the female, the target tissues show masculinization. All the androgen comes from the adrenal gland during childhood, except in the case of extremely rare androgen-secreting ovarian tumors. The signs of heterosexual precocious pseudopuberty are: virilization, rapid linear growth followed by early epiphyseal fusion and ultimately short stature, excessive muscular development, clitoral hypertrophy, acne, hirsutism, premature development of pubic hair, and deepening of the voice.

It should be emphasized that heterosexual precocious pseudopuberty is a disorder of childhood, and its end-organ effects differ from the virilization occasionally seen in the newborn with ambiguous genitalia or in some females at the expected time of puberty. In all three situations, the specific cause is excessive androgens, but the effect differs in each because of the age of onset. During his investigation, the physician must determine the abnormal source of androgen in order to prescribe treatment.

Isosexual precocious puberty, which is constitutional (i.e., true puberty), is diagnosed only after excluding organic central nervous system lesions, estrogen-secreting tumors, estrogen consumption, and juvenile hypothyroidism (see Chapter 16, section on Thyroid Deficiency). The physician examines these patients according to the principles outlined in the section dealing with evaluation of the hypothalamic-pituitary-ovarian axis. The treatment of isosexual precocity, of course, depends upon the cause. In some instances of precocious true puberty, hormone therapy is useful, usually progesterone or a synthetic analogue that will not cause epiphyseal fusion. Progesterone treatment delays epiphyseal closure by inhibiting pituitary gonadotropin secretion, thus depressing ovarian function; this gives the patient a longer period of growth.

Ambiguous External Genitalia

Ambiguous external genitalia are usually recognized at birth. Unless the anomaly is pronounced, the physician may be unable to assign the correct genetic and gonadal sex, or he may assign the wrong sex. In the female infant, the ambiguity ranges from minor degrees of labial fusion, clitoral hypertrophy, and a perineal opening, to complete labial fusion and a penile urethra. When labial fusion is complete, these females often are mistaken for males.

Genital ambiguity has two principal causes: Often, the female fetus has been exposed to androgens, usually because of congenital adrenal hyperplasia; less commonly, the mother has received or is producing androgenic hormones which caused the change. In the infants, the sex chromosomes, internal genitalia, and ovaries are entirely normal.

Gonadal dysgenesis, a much rarer cause of genital ambiguity, results from chromosomal nondysjunction. Mitotic nondysjunction causes chromosomal mosaicism involving a Y chromosome; for example, XX/XY or XO/XY (see Chapter 11, section on Gonadal Development). The abnormal gonads, by producing some androgens and other substances, misdirect the embryonic development of the external and internal genitalia and produce varying degrees of sexual ambiguity.

Androgens given or produced after birth do not cause genital ambiguity but can cause clitoral hypertrophy and other signs or symptoms of masculinization.

Virilization in Childhood

Female children can become virilized at three different periods in early life (Table 10-2). Although the cause is always excessive androgen, the physical signs are different for each age group.

Virilization of the Newborn

Exposure of the fetus to androgens induces various degrees of ambiguity of the external genitalia (see section on Ambiguous Genitalia).

Postnatal Exposure to Androgens (Heterosexual Precocious Pseudopuberty)

As previously described, this syndrome is due to diseases of the adrenal or, rarely, the ovary. This disorder is nearly always due to a tumor or to disturbed metabolic activity of structurally normal glands. Exogenous androgens or the prolonged effects of androgens in unrecognized congenital adrenal hyperplasia also produce virilization in childhood. Except in congenital adrenal hyperplasia, these children have no genital ambiguity because the external genitalia differentiated along female lines before the production

Table 10-2. Effects of Excess Androgens at Various Stages of Female Development

Period	*Effect*	*Sources of androgens**
In utero	Ambiguous genitalia	Maternal adrenal hyperplasia or tumor Exogenous Fetal adrenal hyperplasia
Childhood	Heterosexual precocious pseudopuberty	Adrenal hyperplasia or tumor Ovarian tumor Exogenous
Puberty	Masculinization instead of expected feminization	Adrenal hyperplasia or tumor Ovarian tumor Exogenous
Postpuberty	Defeminization and then virilization	Adrenal hyperplasia or tumor Ovarian tumor Ovarian dysfunction (Stein-Leventhal syndrome) Exogenous

* Exogenous sources of androgen: mother or drugs.

of excess androgens. The clitoris, however, will respond to androgens at any age.

Virilization or genital ambiguity in childhood causes obvious psychological problems. Surgical, medical, and psychiatric treatment is directed toward stabilizing, restoring, or reinforcing the appropriate sexual identity.

Pubertal Virilization

If excessive androgens circulate at puberty, the girl becomes virilized rather than feminized. This condition develops when the girl has:

1. Some form of intersex or gonadal dysgenesis and unsuspected testicular tissue which begins to produce androgens at the onset of puberty
2. Virilizing ovarian or adrenal lesions beginning at puberty

Postpubertal Virilization

The normal postpubertal female can be virilized at any time by excessive androgen. This androgen excess is expressed in: initial defeminization—regression of female characteristics (breast atrophy, amenorrhea); then masculinization—the appearance of masculine features such as hirsutism, clitoral hypertrophy, deepening of the voice, etc. Again, the androgen may come from the adrenal, the ovary, or be taken as medication.

Abnormal Somatic Features

Classically, Turner's syndrome (45,XO) is associated with gonadal dysgenesis and a complex of extragenital abnormalities, which alone are almost diagnostic (see Chapter 11, Chromosomal Studies in Endocrinology for details). In the female neonate, the physician should strongly suspect this condition (especially if the birth weight is low) if he observes the following:

1. Unexplained peripheral lymphedema, especially of the lower extremities and feet
2. Webbing of the neck (see Chapter 16, Hormones and Growth)

Children with Turner's syndrome are short and, as adults, are seldom more than 5 feet tall. They frequently appear in psychiatric and cardiac clinics because of a low I.Q. and cardiovascular anomalies, particularly coarctation of the aorta. At the anticipated time of puberty, they remain sexually infantile. Other somatic peculiarities include cubitus valgus, shield-like chest, low posterior hairline, high arched palate, strabismus, inner epicanthal folds, multiple pigmented nevi, and a short fourth metacarpal. The external genitalia are female because the gonads did not function in utero. The short stature and somatic abnormalities, including gonadal dysgenesis, are due to monosomy—one gene containing several monosomic loci on the X chromosome.

Abdominal Masses

Ovarian tumors are rare in childhood but must be considered in the differential diagnosis of an abdominal mass or pain. The most common of these tumors is the dermoid cyst (benign cystic teratoma). Other, less common cystic lesions may attain enormous size—for example, follicular cysts, which sometimes develop in the newborn, perhaps as a result of maternal or placental gonadotropic stimulation. Functioning ovarian tumors are rare in the infant and child; the most common, granulosa cell tumors, are invariably accompanied by anovulatory vaginal bleeding and precocious sexual maturation—isosexual precocious pseudopuberty. Theca lutein cysts occur and may also produce signs of sexual precocity. Mucocolpos, a pseudotumor seen in infancy and childhood, has no relationship to the ovaries. Children with mucocolpos are born with an imperforate hymen, and the retained secretions gradually produce pelvic masses.

Puberty and Adolescence

Adolescence and puberty are not synonymous. During adolescence (*adolescere:* to grow), the child is transformed physically, psychologically, and socially into an adult. Puberty (*puber:* adult), the most dramatic event of adolescence, is the child's physical and sexual maturation.

The teenage girl who requires medical attention often finds herself in limbo: she is too old for the pediatrician and is thought to be too young for the gynecologist. Menstrual disorders and concern about body growth are the principal sex-related problems of teenagers, but they frequently ask doctors for information concerning sexual identity, intercourse, pregnancy, contraception, and venereal disease.

Puberty is marked by rapid physical growth and maturation of the sexual apparatus (Figs. 10-6 and 10-7). The total process has many emotional and social dimensions. The female may fear that physical changes threaten her comfortable "little-girl" role, whereby she receives love and favor without physical or psychological sexual connotations. Puberty usually has a greater impact on the adolescent female than the adolescent male. Menarche is more disturbing than a nocturnal emission.

The manifestations of puberty (pubescence) appear earlier in each generation (Fig. 10-8), so that a girl achieves biological maturity many months earlier than her mother or grandmother did. Most girls become impatient for adolescent changes if these have not started by age 13 or 14. Puberty can be a traumatic experience for the girl who, though normal, is out of phase with her peers. Often, the physician has not examined external genitalia during an annual physical examination or consciously observed body contours, and hence does not recognize that maturation is out of phase. Physicians, because they feel uncomfortable, often defer a gynecological examination despite the tremendous importance of normal development to the adolescent's emotional stability. A properly trained physician can satisfactorily examine a girl of any age. In its simplest form, the examination includes only visual inspection, digital rectal and abdominal examination, and a vaginal swab for cytohormonal assessment. Using specially designed speculums and a good light, the vagina and cervix can be examined even in the very young girl.

Normal Ovarian Function in Adolescence

Normal puberty implies not only correct timing, but also serial changes in proper sequence. Of course, individual variation is great, and the young patient and her mother should be helped to appreciate this fact. Each girl has her own biological clock that controls her growth and development, and no two girls experience precisely the same rate of physical change during adolescence (Fig. 10-9). The physician should stress this individual variation.

Puberty is an orderly process extending over several years. It is characterized in the female by linear growth, development of secondary sex characteristics, menstruation, and ovulation (Fig. 10-10).

The mechanisms which trigger puberty have never been clearly defined, but they seem to depend on maturation of the central nervous system, especially of the hypothalamus and pineal gland. In the female, pubertal somatic changes reflect increased ovarian estrogen production. Target-organ response is influenced by genetic factors, the amount of circulating estrogen, and the sensitivity of the organ. Increased numbers of ovarian follicles mature, but as a rule a girl does not ovulate for a variable period of a few months to 2 years after the menarche. Ovulation occurs when the hypothalamic receptor site matures enough to throw off the effects of ovarian suppression and begins to stimulate the cycling area.

The adrenal gland also participates in sexual maturation through increased production of androgen, which contributes to the linear growth spurt and the growth of pubic and axillary hair—the adrenarche.

Menstruation and Ovulation

The Chemistry of Sex Hormone Production

Steroid hormones are produced by the ovary in metabolic steps identical to those in the other steroid-producing glands—the adrenal cortex and the testis. The following principles govern steroid-hormone formation and metabolism:

1. Cholesterol, a 27-carbon compound, is the precursor of steroid hormones.
2. Metabolic action can reduce, but never increase, the number of carbon atoms in cholesterol or any other steroid molecule.
3. All steroid hormones are formed and metabolized by:

    Removing carbon atoms from side chains of the basic cyclopentenophenanthrene nucleus (Fig. 10-11).

    Oxidation or reduction of the nucleus or its side chains.

    Conjugation with glucuronic or sulfuric acid.

4. The first step in the production of steroid hormones—the conversion of cholesterol to pregnenolone and the related compound progesterone

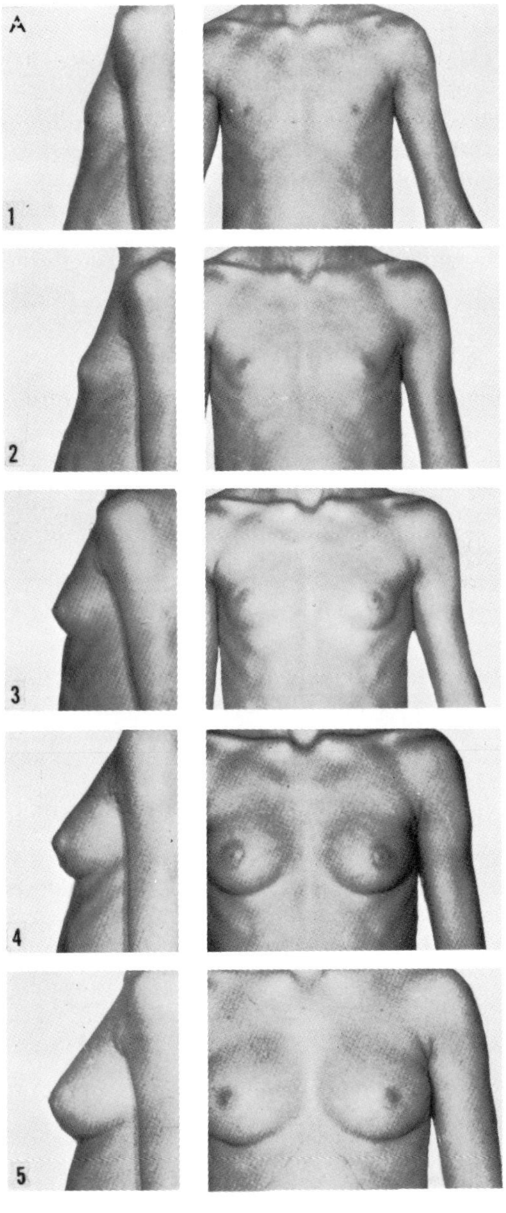

Fig. 10-6. Stages of development of the female breast. Development of the female breast is influenced by ovarian hormones, and represents an end-organ response to increasing circulation levels of estrogen. Stages are: **(1)** preadolescence, **(2)** breast bud, **(3)** elevation and enlargement of breast and areola, **(4)** areola and papilla, secondary mound, **(5)** mature breast. (Tanner, J. M. *Growth at Adolescence*, ed. 2. Oxford, Blackwell, Sci., 1962. Reproduced with permission.)

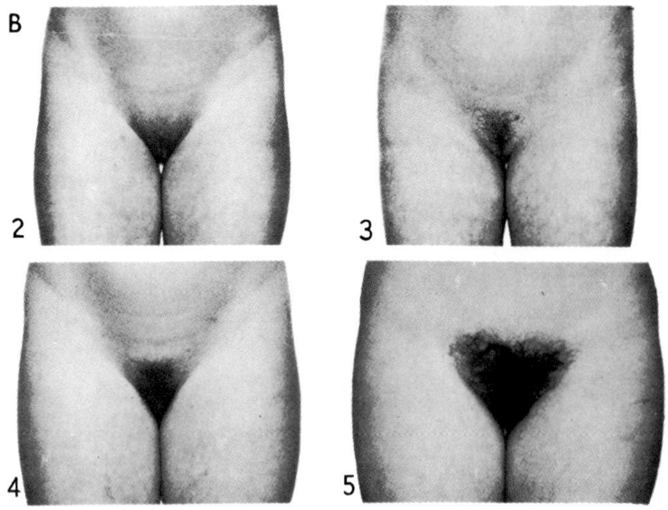

Fig. 10-7. Stages of development of female pubic hair. Pubic hair develops largely under the stimulus of increasing secretion of adrenal androgens. Little is known about the mechanisms that coordinate breast development (thelarche) and the appearance of pubic hair (adrenarche): occasionally these two events may occur at widely different times, and sometimes long before the onset of menses (menarche). Thus, in the female, puberty should be viewed as a series of biological events whose sequence, while usually coordinated, may occasionally occur inappropriately. The numbers **2**, **3**, **4**, and **5** correspond to stages shown in Figure 10-6. (Tanner, J. M. *Growth at Adolescence,* ed. 2. Oxford, Blackwell Sci., 1962. Reproduced with permission.)

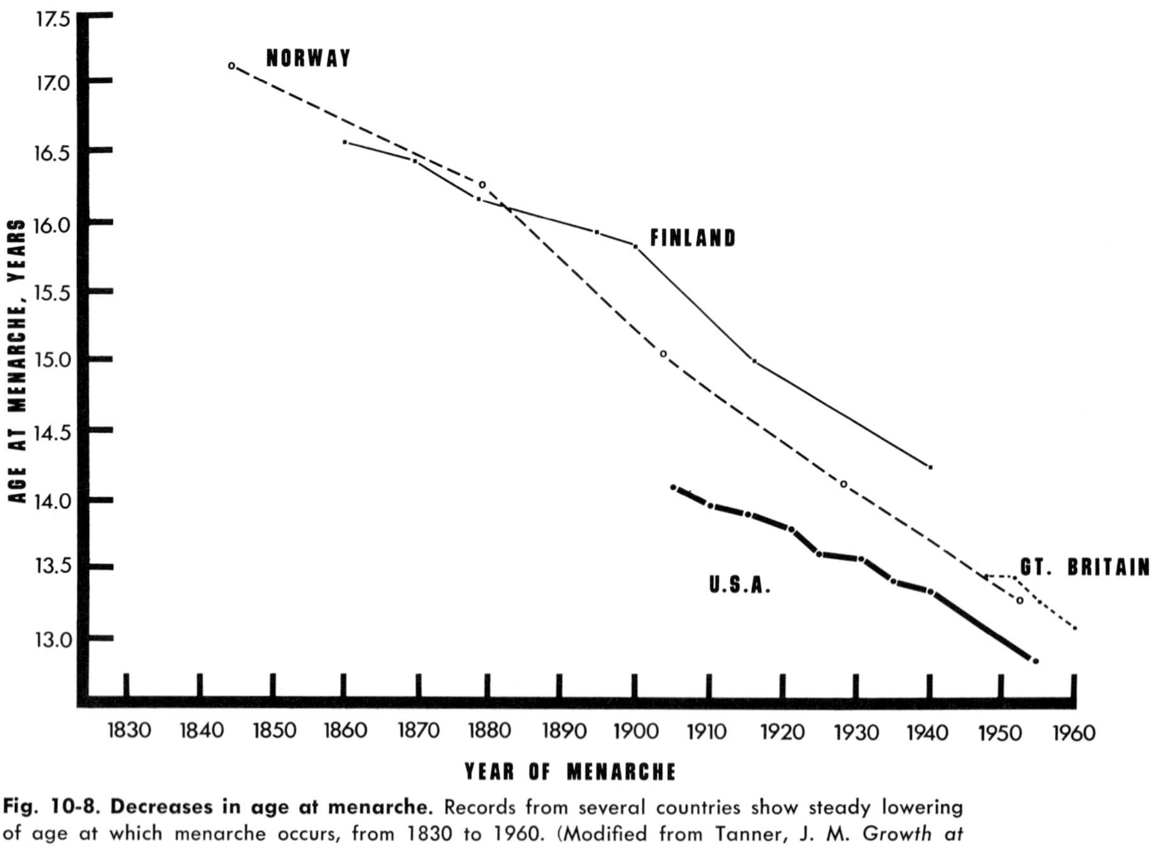

Fig. 10-8. Decreases in age at menarche. Records from several countries show steady lowering of age at which menarche occurs, from 1830 to 1960. (Modified from Tanner, J. M. *Growth at Adolescence,* ed. 2. Oxford, Blackwell Sci., 1962. Reproduced with permission.)

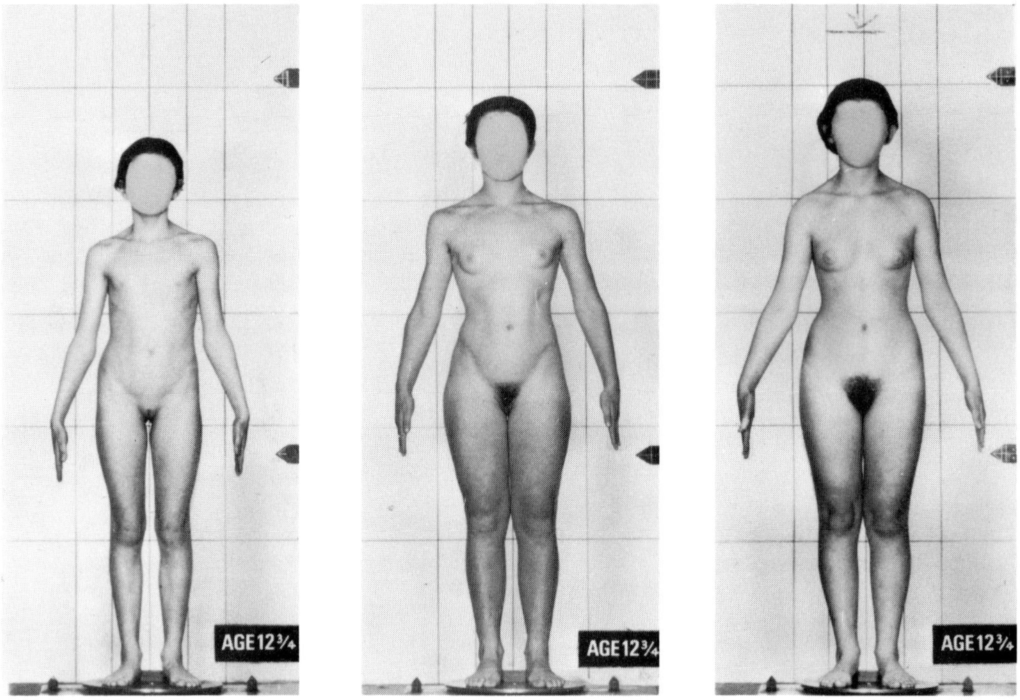

Fig. 10-9. Female sexual development. Three girls have wide physical variation at a single chronological age—12.75 years. (Tanner, J. M. *Growth at Adolescence*, ed. 2, Oxford, Blackwell Sci., 1962. Reproduced with permission.)

—reduces the number of carbon atoms from 27 to 21.

5. Oxidation and reduction of any carbon atom takes the form of:

A. Oxidation (adding =O-ketone group)

B. Hydroxylation (adding —OH group)

C. Oxidizing hydroxyl groups into ketones and the reverse reduction (—OH ⇆ =O)

D. Dehydrogenation—removing hydrogen and creating double bonds

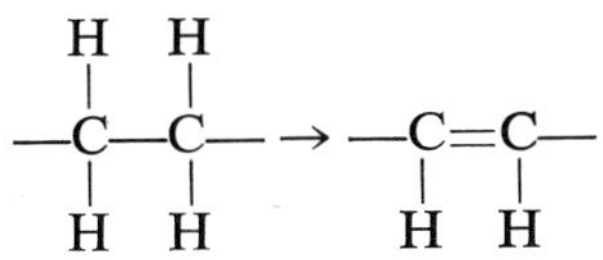

6. The human ovary and testis are steroid-forming tissues that have no 11-hydroxylase activity (Point 5*B*). Therefore, these tissues cannot form glucocorticoids.

7. Androgenic hormones are produced from pregnenolone and progesterone by removal (side-chain cleavage) of two more carbon atoms, reducing the number of carbon atoms from 21 to 19 (Fig. 10-12).

8. Estrogenic molecules (18-carbon atoms) are produced only from androgens (19-carbon atoms). Androgens are converted to estrogens by removing hydrogen (Point 5*D*) from the first ring (*A*) of the steroid nucleus and producing a benzene configuration. This irreversible process is called aromatization (Fig. 10-13).

The Menstrual Cycle

The normal menstrual cycle depends upon an intact hypothalamic-pituitary-ovarian axis. The hypothalamus is the key to ovulation and menstruation: It integrates biochemical, environmental, and emotional stimuli and produces the releasing factors that stimulate the anterior pituitary. The anterior pituitary glands of the male and female are structurally identical, but they function differently because they are exposed to different hypothalamic stimuli.

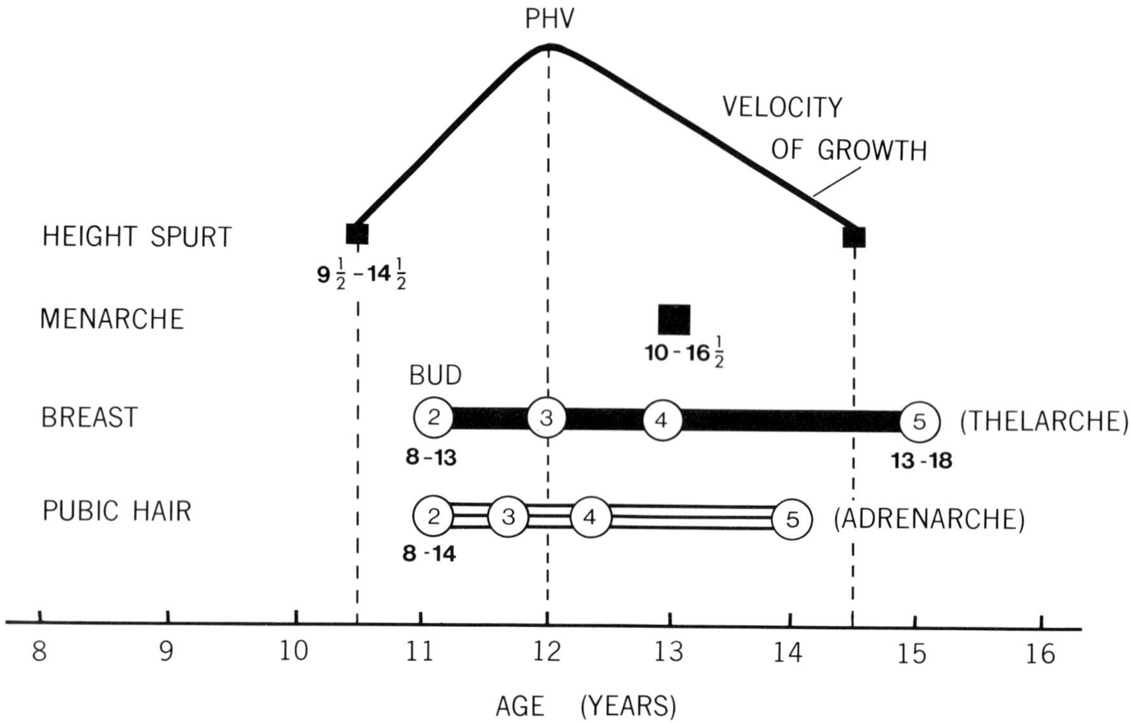

Fig. 10-10. Progress of puberty.

1. Linear growth: The sudden growth spurt, usually the first sign of pubescence, is due to sex steroids, especially androgen. Estrogens precipitate epiphyseal closure and thus terminate growth, usually 1 or 2 years after the menarche.
2. Thelarche: Breast budding, a manifestation of estrogen production, occurs 2–3 years before the menarche.
3. Pubarche (adrenarche): Growth of secondary (sex) hair reflects increased androgen production.
4. Menarche: The first menstrual period, the climax of puberty, occurs at an average age of 12.8 years. The hypothalamic cycling area responsible for the LHRF surge just before ovulation does not function until the girl produces adult amounts of estrogen. Therefore early menstrual cycles are not fertile or ovulatory but are episodes of "withdrawal bleeding" caused by a decline in estrogen level after there has been sufficient stimulation of the endometrium to permit it to bleed. (From Marshall, W. A. and Tanner, J. M. *Variations in the Pattern of Pubsental Changes in Boys. Arch Dis Child 45*:239, 1970.)

How the gonadotropins act upon ovarian cells to control steroid production is not known. Neither are the mechanisms known by which progesterone, androgen, and estrogen are produced in the ovary, although some investigators have suggested that FSH stimulates the ovary to produce androgens.

During menstruation, when circulating ovarian hormones are at their lowest, FSHRF begins to stimulate the anterior pituitary again. Concurrently, the cycling center synthesizes and stores large quantities of LHRF, which, in the LH "surge," discharges suddenly at midcycle and sweeps much of the stored LH from the anterior pituitary. The FSH-primed ovarian follicle then releases the ovum. The rising levels of ovarian hormones produced during the first half of the menstrual cycle do not shut off hypothalamic activity as in simple negative feedback. Once initiated, the activity of the cycling center proceeds inevitably to ovulation. Therefore, if a woman begins using oral contraceptives more than a week after her cycle begins, even large doses of hormone will not prevent ovulation.

During the first half of the menstrual cycle, the ovary releases androgens and estrogens, which the ovarian follicle has produced from 21-carbon-atom or progesterone-like precursors. Unquestionably, the ovary contains and releases some progesterone before ovulation. After ovulation the corpus luteum, which is independent of hypothalamic pituitary control, secretes a large amount of progesterone and some estrogen. Biochemically, ovulation produces a metabolic step backward, since the corpus luteum removes carbon atoms from the progesterone molecule less efficiently than the developing follicle. Progesterone and estrogen released after ovulation maintain the endometrium until the corpus luteum ceases to function and hormone levels fall. The endometrium then degenerates and menstruation begins.

Mechanisms of Endometrial Bleeding

The endometrium may bleed for many reasons, only a few of which are related to ovarian function. In women of reproductive age, most endometrial bleeding represents cyclic menstruation, but other causes—pregnancy, inflammatory processes, neoplasms, and trauma—must be considered whenever the bleeding pattern becomes abnormal. In this section, we will only examine endometrial bleeding related to the ovary's endocrine function.

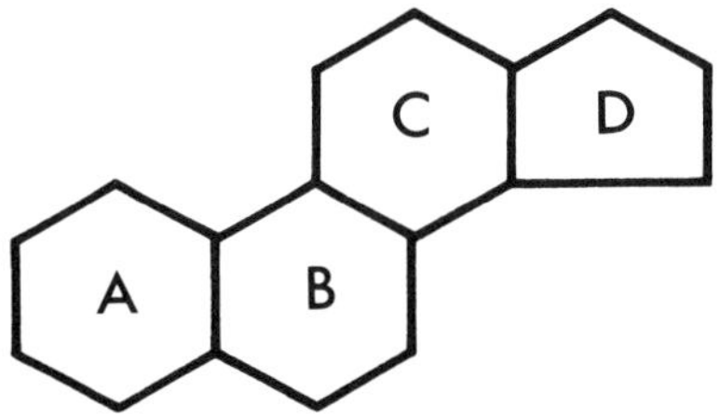

Fig. 10-11. Cyclopentenophenanthrene nucleus. This molecule forms the core of every steroid hormone. If the hormone does not have this nucleus, it cannot be called a steroid (see also Fig. 7-4).

Interaction between ovary and endometrium requires the following:

1. Endometrium that can respond to ovarian hormones
2. Sufficient ovarian stimulation so that the endometrium can develop to the point where it can bleed—the "bleeding threshold"
3. Certain specific adjustments in circulating hormone levels:

   Any drop in estrogen level from above to below the bleeding threshold causes a type of withdrawal bleeding that bears no relationship to ovulation.

   Estrogen levels constantly above the bleeding threshold will not sustain the endometrial lining indefinitely; the endometrium eventually degenerates and breakthrough bleeding occurs. Because most commercial preparations

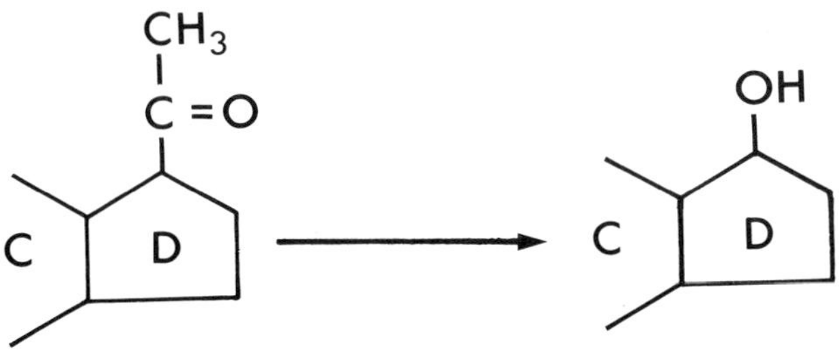

Fig. 10-12. Side-chain cleavage. Androgens are formed by the removal of two carbons from a 21-carbon steroid molecule; that is, they are 19-carbon steroids (see also Fig. 7-4).

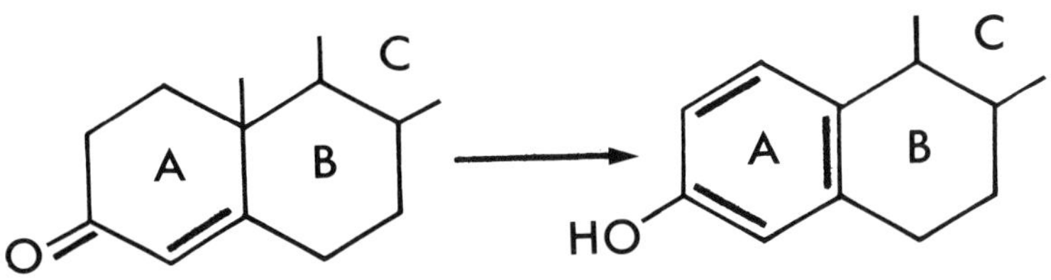

Fig. 10-13. Aromatization. To form estrogens, ring A of the cyclopentenophenanthrene nucleus is converted to a benzene configuration with three double bonds (see also Fig. 7-4).

have a constant estrogen level, they are associated with breakthrough bleeding.

After ovulation, large quantities of progesterone act upon the estrogen-prepared endometrium and stimulate the endometrial glands to secretory activity. When the corpus luteum ceases to function, and all supporting hormones are withdrawn, the endometrium degenerates and is shed—the phenomenon of menstruation.

Many types of bleeding, as well as some amenorrhea, can be explained by these simple principles. Many amenorrheic women have estrogen levels which either never quite reach the bleeding threshold or are constantly rising (as in pregnancy) and thus give the endometrium sufficient support to prevent breakthrough bleeding.

Prostaglandins

Forty years ago, Goldblatt and von Euler described this class of 20-carbon, long-chain, hydroxy fatty acids in male seminal fluid. Six primary prostaglandins, with a wide spectrum of biological activities, appear in human tissues. The exact mechanism of action remains unknown, but investigators presently believe that prostaglandins are involved in energy transfer by affecting the concentration of cyclic AMP.

Prostaglandins' contractile effect upon uterine muscles initiated the worldwide clinical trials, presently underway, to determine the value of purified prostaglandins in the induction of labor and as abortifacients. Prostaglandins also influence steroidogenesis and ovulation in primates, possibly by counteracting the effects of gonadotropins.

The role of prostaglandins in menstrual cycles, fertility and pregnancy remains far from clear, but this group of substances may well contribute to our understanding and eventual control of reproductive processes in animals and man.

Abnormal Ovarian Function in Puberty and Adolescence

Most adolescent endocrine problems are merely constitutional variations of normal physical and sexual growth and development; less than one-third represent true endocrine disease. When they occur, these diseases are usually due to abnormal function of the thyroid, adrenal cortex, or ovary.

The young patient, or her mother, perceives disturbances of the hypothalamic-ovarian axis as menstrual dysfunction or an alteration in normal development. Their anxiety is often more difficult to manage than the endocrine dysfunction itself, because failure to menstruate can produce profound emotional tensions. These, in turn, may interfere with the girl's self-image and the progressive reinforcement of her sexual identity. In this section, we will also discuss some less common complaints, such as hirsutism, which may have endocrine significance.

The investigation of gynecologic endocrine abnormalities in adolescence requires detailed pediatric, preadolescent, and medical histories and records of linear growth, breast development, and pubic-hair growth. Emotional health must be assessed, and the family history of maturation and development ascertained. Physical examination of the adolescent should include measurement of height, arm span, and assessment of general body build. If a girl is unusually short for her age, this suggests estrogen deficiency. Certain stigmas, such as webbing of the neck, may suggest ovarian dysgenesis. Abnormal amounts and male patterns of body hair may indicate excess androgen production such as that due to adrenal hyperplasia. Progressive virilization, defeminization, or failure of feminization also indicate increased androgen production.

Delayed Puberty and Menarche

In the teenage girl, the most frequent sign of abnormal ovarian function is delayed development. Here one must distinguish between delayed puberty and a simple delay in menarche in an adolescent whose sexual development is otherwise normal. Delayed puberty represents true sexual infantilism, due to malfunction of the hypothalamus, pituitary, or gonads. Ovarian failure may be acquired or, more commonly in the adolescent, may result from congenital ovarian abnormalities such as gonadal dysgenesis or agenesis.

In delayed menarche, however, the first menstrual period is merely late in a girl who has matured normally in all other respects. The age of menarche is influenced by familial tendency, type of body build, climatic conditions, and overall physical and emotional development. Because of this complex interaction, many have used the average age of menarche as an index of a civilization's living standards and well-being. Menstruation should begin before age 16, and its absence beyond this age is abnormal.

Amenorrhea

Amenorrhea is the absence of expected menstruation. In primary amenorrhea, the first period has never occurred. When menstrual flow is obstructed by congenital lesions such as cervical or vaginal atresia, or an imperforate hymen the condition is known as cryptomenorrhea, which must be distinguished from primary amenorrhea. Cryptomenorrhea distorts the internal genitalia through pressure and can usually be treated effectively. The term *secondary amenorrhea,* the abnormal cessation of menstruation, is applied after 3 months have passed with neither menstrual flow nor any signs of pregnancy. *Oligomenorrhea* (infrequent periods) is closely related to secondary amenorrhea; their causes, investigation, and treatment are identical. They differ only in degree.

In this context, amenorrhea in an otherwise normal woman must be distinguished from the amenorrhea which is one of a number of abnormal symptoms and signs. Here, therapy is aimed not at the amenorrhea itself, but at the underlying endocrine, metabolic, systemic, or psychological disease.

Amenorrhea in an Otherwise Normal Adolescent

Primary and secondary amenorrhea without apparent endocrine or systemic disease are common complaints (Fig. 10-14). The physician must decide when and to what depth investigation is warranted. Delayed menarche before age 16 is rarely cause for concern, and an otherwise normal girl should not be subjected to extensive diagnostic procedures. However, if a girl has not menstruated by age 15, and has also not matured physically (delayed puberty or sexual infantilism), a full diagnostic study should be done.

After 16, delayed menses is rarely due to slow maturation, and a normally developed adolescent with this complaint deserves fairly extensive investigation. One-half of all girls who do not menstruate by age 18 have primary ovarian failure or congenital anomalies of the reproductive system. In the older girl, "primary amenorrhea due to constitutional factors" may only be diagnosed after excluding psychic, endocrine, and/or systemic causes. Sudden cessation of menses after previously normal regular periods (secondary amenorrhea) may indicate serious disease and must be investigated. Amenorrhea in a girl with previously irregular menses is of less significance. In secondary amenorrhea, the possibility of pregnancy must always be considered.

Functional Approach

The recognition of other symptoms and signs naturally depends on the awareness of the girl and on the physician's skill in elucidating details of history and performing the physical examination. When the physician discovers other symptoms and signs (e.g., headaches, visual disturbances, virilization, hypertension, glycosuria, etc.), these must be investigated. Frequently the doctor discovers that the amenorrhea is a sign of a disease such as adrenal hyperplasia, which is only peripherally associated with ovarian function. Treatment of the primary disease cures the amenorrhea.

If the girl has menstruated previously, this proves that the hypothalamic-pituitary-ovarian axis exists and can function, that the endometrium can respond, and that the outflow tract is open. The apparently normal girl who complains of primary amenorrhea presents the most perplexing investigative problem.

Investigation of the Reproductive Axis

1. Higher centers: history and emotional assessment*

* Simple, inexpensive.

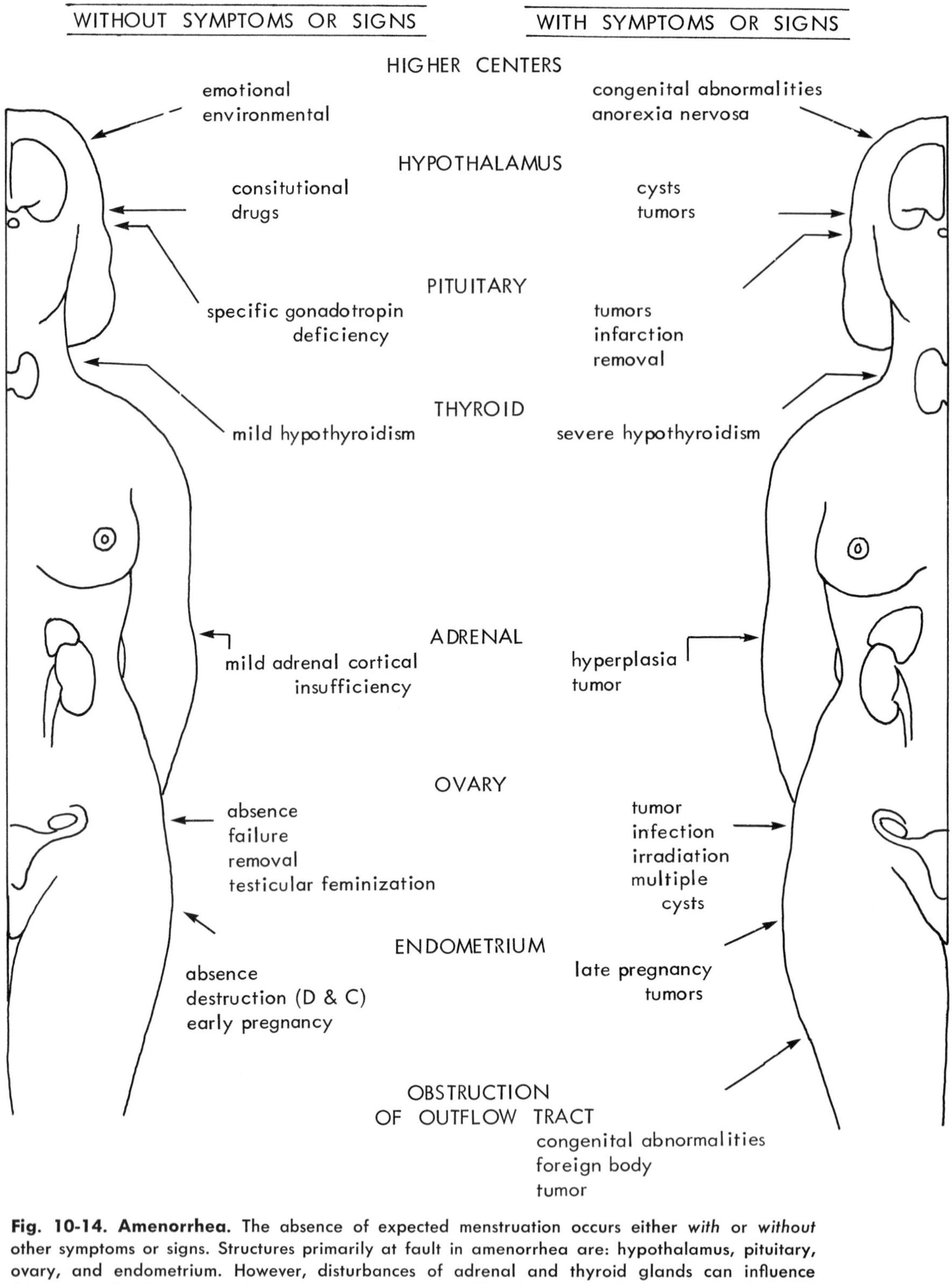

Fig. 10-14. Amenorrhea. The absence of expected menstruation occurs either *with* or *without* other symptoms or signs. Structures primarily at fault in amenorrhea are: hypothalamus, pituitary, ovary, and endometrium. However, disturbances of adrenal and thyroid glands can influence this system. Finally, emotional stress is a common cause. This figure provides a brief catalogue of the diverse causes of this *symptom*.

2. Hypothalamus: clomiphene citrate stimulation test†
3. Pituitary:
   Visual fields*
   Radiograph of pituitary fossa
   Gonadotropin assay
   ACTH and growth-hormone assessment
4. Ovary:
   Buccal smear for chromatin body*
   Vaginal smear for hormone effect*
   Progesterone withdrawal test*
   Endometrial biopsy for hormone effect (ovulation)
   Pregnanediol and estrogen assays
   Visualization and biopsy—culdoscopy; laparoscopy
5. Uterus and vagina:
   Physical examination*
   Endometrial biopsy
   Estrogen and progesterone withdrawal test*

All young women with primary or secondary amenorrhea must have complete histories and examinations, including pelvic assessment and a vaginal smear. A buccal smear should be made for sex chromatin determination. In most instances, these measures will rule out pregnancy and mechanical obstruction, and will clarify genetic sex. At this point, the physician obtains further information by determining the patient's response to an oral test dose of progesterone.

Withdrawal bleeding after five daily doses of progesterone or an analogue demonstrates the functional integrity of the reproductive tract and the pituitary-ovarian axis. The bleeding indicates that the endometrium must have been exposed to sufficient estrogen to prepare it for secretion and subsequent menstruation when the progesterone is withdrawn.

If progesterone does not produce withdrawal bleeding, further evaluation should be performed: chromosome cultures, bone-age determination, and tests to exclude pregnancy and thyroid, adrenal, and pituitary disturbances. A radiograph of the sella turcica may show erosion by a tumor; measurement of 24- or, preferably, 48-hour total urinary gonadotropins distinguishes between patients who have no estrogen because pituitary gonadotropin production or release has failed, and those who have no estrogen because of ovarian failure. Repeated high gonadotropin concentration indicates ovarian absence, dysgenesis, or failure. The patient who has consistently low urinary gonadotropins and a vaginal smear that reflects estrogen deficiency requires a thorough neurological examination because her amenorrhea may be an early symptom of an intra- or extrasellar intracranial lesion.

* Simple, inexpensive.
† Rarely done.

Chromosome cultures can provide evidence of sex chromosome abnormalities often associated with ovarian dysgenesis. More extensive investigation includes endometrial biopsy, and direct visualization and biopsy of the gonads by laparoscopy.

Before embarking upon extensive investigation, the physician should evaluate the patient's mental state and nutrition to exclude anorexia nervosa, extreme inanition, obesity, and schizophrenia.

Treatment

When amenorrhea is due to a generalized disease, the physician will treat the underlying cause. If, as in most cases, no specific cause can be found, he is left with "hypothalamic amenorrheas"—either primary (constitutional delayed menarche) or secondary.

Although it has no medical significance, late menarche may cause the young patient intense anxiety. Treatment is largely supportive and expectant: periodic reevaluation and therapeutic conservatism are essential. Both mother and daughter must be reassured that the girl is normal; if menstruation will allay anxiety, artificial periods can be induced. If the patient is producing enough estrogen, oral progesterone may be used cyclically on days 21–25 to cause withdrawal bleeding. A more reliable program is oral estrogen followed by progesterone in 21-day cycles: If the endometrium can respond, and if the outflow tract is not obstructed, this will induce regular withdrawal bleeding. Either of these programs can be continued for 3–6 months and then discontinued to determine whether spontaneous menstrual function will ensue. Again, the adolescent should not receive hormone replacement until she has completed her linear growth, or the epiphyses may close prematurely.

It is more difficult to decide whether and when hormonal therapy should be used in girls with constitutional delayed puberty. Obviously, a 16- or 17-year-old girl with the body of a child requires treatment because she may become psychologically disturbed. Replacement therapy should be started in delayed puberty that is due to an irreversible factor such as pituitary gonadotropic insufficiency or gonadal dysgenesis, as soon as the girl has reached adequate or maximum height. However, if the diagnosis of constitutional delayed puberty is made after the exclusion of all other causes, it is advisable to wait until age 15 for the spontaneous onset of puberty. After this age, the physician must choose between watchful expectancy and initiating sexual development with hormones; in any event, the choice must be individualized. The most important factors are the desires of the young patient and her height at the time of consultation.

Amenorrhea Accompanied by Systemic Symptoms and Signs

Amenorrhea can be caused by any systemic disorder that disturbs the hypothalamic-pituitary-ovarian axis: malignancies, chronic malnutrition, severe obesity, generalized infections, and so on. Of the major psychiatric disorders which produce amenorrhea, *anorexia nervosa* presents a particularly frustrating problem. In this disorder, which is not uncommon and may be overlooked rather easily in its earliest stages, up to 10 percent of patients develop irreversible, potentially fatal malnutrition. Although the primary cause is psychological, the secondary endocrine disturbance is so marked that the full-blown syndrome must be distinguished from hypopituitarism. Typically, an adolescent girl decides to go on a crash diet and, without obvious cause, slips almost imperceptibly into a life-threatening situation. She develops a total aversion to food, and her weight loss continues unchecked. The first evidence of associated endocrine dysfunction, amenorrhea, is due to hypothalamic suppression by the higher centers. Eventually, the patient becomes severely emaciated, develops muscular atrophy, hypothermia, bradycardia, and a generalized downy hirsutism in the presence of normal axillary and pubic hair. Despite these severe changes, she remains alert, active, and, because she insists that nothing is wrong, mildly hostile. Tests of endocrine activity are usually normal, apart from decreased or absent urinary gonadotropin. Anorexia nervosa can be distinguished from hypopituitarism by the patient's appearance (i.e., her vigor, lack of lethargy, persistence of sex hair) in conjunction with a typical history. The girl urgently needs psychiatric treatment, and menses will usually return spontaneously when she gains weight. As part of her treatment, the physician may induce menstruation with cyclic estrogens and progestins before their spontaneous return.

Nonendocrine Obesity. The connection between amenorrhea and nonendocrine obesity is not understood. Obese patients of all ages have more anovulatory menstrual cycles than normal females. The disturbance is probably psychological rather than organic.

Adiposogenital Dystrophy. This rare hypothalamic lesion is characterized by obesity and by the failure of the genital tract to develop beyond the infantile stage. The term should be applied only to females with a demonstrated hypothalamic lesion.

Galactorrhea. When amenorrhea is accompanied by nonpuerperal lactation, the patient usually has either an organic lesion of the central nervous system or is taking a psychotropic drug such as phenothiazine. However, some anxious patients with the "galactorrhea-amenorrhea syndrome" have not been taking any drugs to account for the disturbance. The amenorrhea and lactation are believed to reflect hypothalamic "blockade," and consequent suppression of the gonadotropin-releasing and prolactin-inhibiting factors. Pituitary gonadotropins are thus not released, and the pituitary prolactin cells are no longer inhibited. Lactation is stimulated by the prolactin produced by the independent cells of the anterior pituitary (Figs. 10-15 and 10-16).

Inguinal Hernias. Primary amenorrhea is usually the major complaint of patients with the

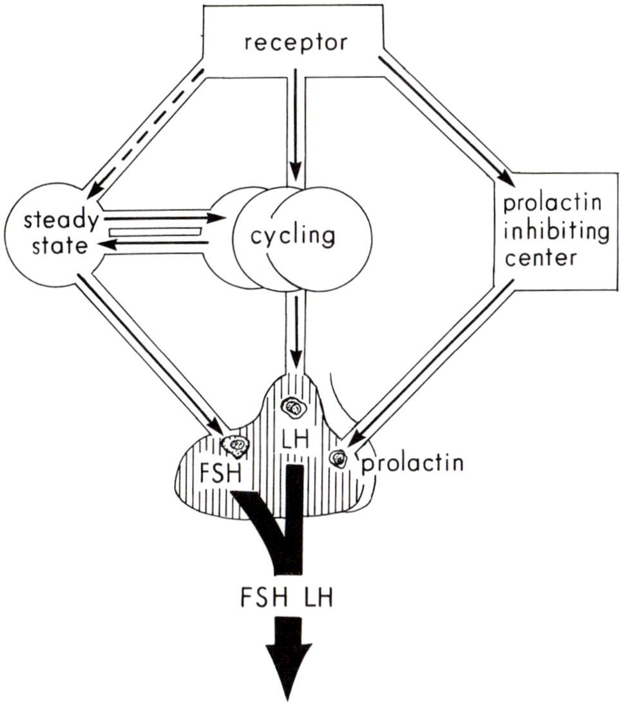

Fig. 10-15. Normal hypothalamic inhibition of pituitary lactogenic hormone. The anterior pituitary manufactures three types of gonadotropin: FSH, LH, and prolactin (luteotropic hormone—LTH, or lactogenic hormone). The higher controls for the release of FSH and LH (depicted here as "steady state⇆cycling center") are separate from those for prolactin.

A specific center exists—the prolactin-inhibiting center, whose only function is to suppress prolactin production by the pituitary. The receptor center controls this area as well as steady state and cycling centers (see Fig. 10-5).

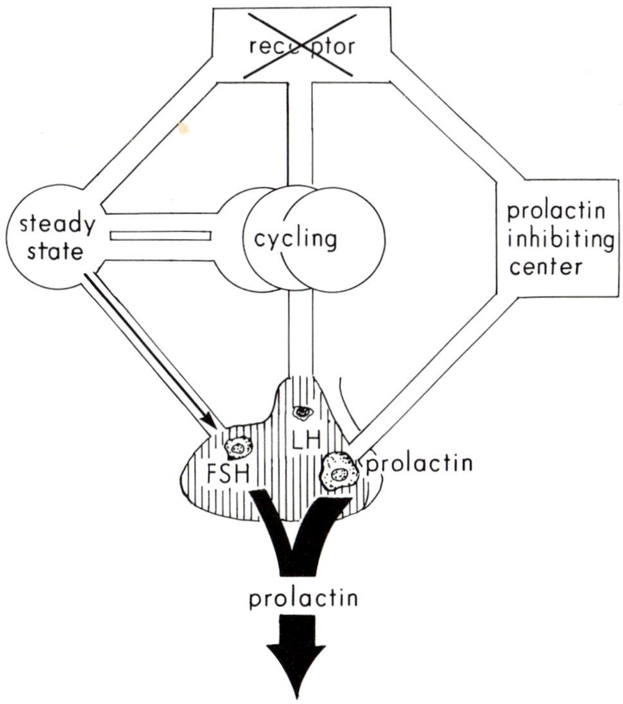

Fig. 10-16. Galactorrhea due to pituitary "escape" from hypothalamic inhibition. In a lesion that blocks or destroys the receptor area, cycling and prolactin-inhibiting centers cease to function, although the steady state may continue to operate autonomously at a low level. This receptor lesion produces amenorrhea, "escape" of the pituitary, and an outpouring of prolactin, hence galactorrhea.

testicular feminization syndrome. Sometimes these girls have inguinal hernias containing testicular tissue. This syndrome is discussed more fully in the section on testicular feminization.

Amenorrhea with Signs of Androgen Excess

Hirsutism (hypertrichosis) is an abnormal, sometimes sudden, increase in body hair. Although it may be due to androgen excess, it does not always indicate endocrine dysfunction. More often it reflects familial and racial background or enhanced end-organ sensitivity. Hirsutism is usually not accompanied by other signs of virilization, and in most cases menstrual function and body contours remain normal. When there is actual endocrine disease, the excess androgen comes from the adrenal cortex or the ovary and frequently produces other signs of defeminization or frank virilization.

When amenorrhea is accompanied by hirsutism and/or actual virilization, the woman usually has both psychological and physiological problems. The excess androgen comes from one of the following sources:

1. Ovarian
   - Stein-Leventhal (polycystic ovary) syndrome
   - Masculinizing ovarian tumors
2. Adrenal cortical
   - Congenital, postnatal, or acquired adrenogenital syndrome
   - Cushing's syndrome
   - Androgen-secreting adrenal tumors
3. Iatrogenic

Virilization denotes both defeminization (loss of female function and attributes), and masculinization, which may include any of the following changes: hirsutism, a male pattern of genital hair, temporal hairline recession (android alopecia), clitoral hypertrophy, deepening of the voice, and masculinization of body habitus. Virilization with hirsutism is always caused by excess androgen secretion, and it implies a major endocrine disorder.

Virilizing adrenal disorders are discussed elsewhere, but the reader should note that postnatal virilization can be distinguished from that which begins in utero. In the postnatal form, except for clitoral enlargement, the external genitalia appear normal; in the prenatal form, because of partial or complete labial fusion, there are varying degrees of genital ambiguity. The most common cause of prenatal virilization, or female pseudohermaphroditism, is congenital adrenocortical hyperplasia—an inborn metabolic error.

In all cases of androgen excess, amenorrhea is caused by androgenic blockade of the hypothalamus (negative feedback). The ovaries are not stimulated, no estrogen is synthesized, and the girl suffers either primary or secondary amenorrhea.

There are two causes of ovarian androgen excess: androgen-producing ovarian tumors, and disturbances of ovarian hormone formation. The latter covers a broad spectrum of poorly understood lesions, which are discussed later as "polycystic ovarian disease."

Amenorrhea with Abnormalities of Stature

Certain ovarian, pituitary, thyroid, and adrenal disorders, which occur before a child has completed her somatic development, affect her linear growth and prevent menstruation. Disordered ovarian function may be associated with either excessive height or short stature.

Excessive Height. Premenarchal ovarian failure causes excessive height because lack of estrogen delays epiphyseal closure. Such youngsters do not menstruate and have a eunuchoid, sexually infantile appearance. The underlying ovarian failure may be due to surgical castration, radiation, or destruction by disease. Certain forms of gonadal dysgenesis produce the same clinical picture.

Short Stature. Turner's syndrome (XO) and chromosomal mosaics (XOXY) involving gonadal dysgenesis are accompanied by an adult stature of less than five feet and other characteristic somatic abnormalities. Although the gonads do not produce estrogen, the dwarfing here is due to actual loss of the chromosomal material that determines growth.

Amenorrhea with Postmenarchal Metabolic Disturbances

Several endocrine disorders, such as adrenal hyperplasia and hypothyroidism, which produce secondary amenorrhea, may appear at any time during a woman's life. Basically, they reflect abnormalities of the secondary influences upon the hypothalamic-ovarian axis: the thyroid, pituitary, adrenal, and pancreas. In any case of amenorrhea, the physician must be alert to other signs and symptoms of underlying endocrine or systemic disease.

Pituitary, Thyroid, and Adrenal Disorders

Premenarchal pituitary, thyroid, and adrenal disturbances affect growth. Hypopituitarism at this time produces dwarfism, largely through lack of growth hormone, but TSH deficiency may also contribute. However, a functioning anterior-lobe tumor may stimulate *excessive* linear growth in two ways: It produces growth hormone, and through pressure causes hypogonadotropism that delays epiphyseal closure by inhibiting estrogen secretion. The amenorrhea and sexual infantilism are due primarily to insufficient gonadotropin production. Primary hypothyroidism may cause severely stunted growth (see Chapter 16).

Excessive adrenocortical androgens at first accelerate linear growth of the long bones, but later cause premature epiphyseal closure. As a result, girls with an adrenocortical tumor are taller than their peers during late childhood, but are shorter than average during adolescence and as adults.

Other Menstrual Disturbances

Other than amenorrhea and disturbed development, the major physical complaint of adolescent girls is abnormal uterine bleeding in the form of irregular anovulatory cycles, polymenorrhea, or menorrhagia. Nearly all abnormal uterine bleeding in adolescence is dysfunctional (sometimes called functional), and very rarely reflects organic disease. *Dysfunctional uterine bleeding* is a temporary, transient, and reversible symptom; it takes the form of anovulatory cycles accompanied by profuse, prolonged, or too-frequent bleeding, and by definition involves no systemic or genital tract disease.

Anovulatory cycles occur normally for a few months to a few years after the menarche; only a few adolescents develop menstrual patterns that are cause for concern. The amount of bleeding depends on several variables: amount and constancy of estrogen production; endometrial end-organ response to estrogen; and the efficiency with which the endometrium is shed in the absence of progesterone.

Some physicians suggest that the adolescent ovary is incapable of a full response to gonadotropins. It produces enough estrogen to induce endometrial proliferation, but when estrogen production falls below the level necessary to maintain the endometrium, withdrawal bleeding results. If these fluctuations in estrogen production are erratic, menstrual periods may become too frequent or prolonged.

The principal objective in treating adolescent menstrual dysfunction is to minimize symptoms by conservative measures until the endocrine and genital systems assume a normal pattern.

The severity of a menstrual disturbance is judged largely by the patient's history and by a hemoglobin determination, hematocrit, platelet count, peripheral smear, and reticulocyte count. Pregnancy is always a possibility.

Investigation should include complete physical and rectoabdominal pelvic examinations, with smears for cytohormonal assessment. Further diagnostic procedures are dictated by this baseline assessment. An adolescent rarely requires a D&C. If a girl has menstrual irregularity, but is not anemic, she needs only reassurance. If the irregularity interferes with normal activities, or if her hemoglobin falls, she should receive one of the combined cyclic estrogen-progestin preparations and an iron supplement for 5–6 months. When there is profuse bleeding, immediate treatment depends on the amount of blood lost. Transfusion may be necessary, but should be avoided if possible in all girls and young women. Uterine bleeding can be stopped within hours by intravenous estrogen (Premarin), 20–60 mg, repeated every 3–4 hours until the bleeding stops; this treatment should be followed by cyclic estrogen-progestin therapy. Less profuse bleeding can be stopped within 48 hours by oral estrogen-progestin preparations. The initial dose is three to four times that used to suppress ovulation in contraceptive therapy.

Abnormal Function and Failure of the Ovary in the Adult

Normally, the human ovary releases ova and the right kinds and quantities of hormones, at the right time. Abnormal ovarian function is a failure or disturbance of these interdependent processes and may occur at any time in the life cycle (Table 10-3). Disturbances of ovarian hormone production fall into three groups:

1. Excessive hormone production during childhood or old age

Table 10-3. Some Causes of Disordered Ovarian Function

Organ Level	*Etiologic Factors*
Hypothalamus (FSHRF and LHRF) ↓	Organic disease Tumors Infections Psychoses Functional disorders Pharmacologic blockade Secondary influences—chronic illness, etc.
Pituitary (FSH and LH) ↓	Organic disease with destruction Tumor, infarction, etc. Congenital abnormalities
Ovary (Estrogen, progesterone, androgens) ↓	Congenital absence or developmental defects Removal or loss of function due to: Castration Radiation Tumors Inflammation Menopause, etc.
Uterus and other target organs (Endometrial response—menstruation)	Congenital absence Surgical removal Destruction of the endometrium by: Inflammation Radiation Excessive curettage, etc. Secondary influences on the hypothalamic-pituitary-ovarian axis: Chronic illness Nutritional disturbances Metabolic diseases

2. Failure of hormone production during adolescence and the reproductive years

3. Hormonal imbalance, such as excess androgen production, occurring at any time

The release of ova is closely related to hormone production, and hormonal disturbances are nearly always associated with anovulation. Normal regular periods are important to a woman. She may

Table 10-4. Detailed Etiologic Classification of Abnormal Ovarian Function

- Hypothalamic-pituitary factors causing failure or abnormality of gonadotropin secretion
  - Congenital (e.g., congenital absence of gonadotropin secretion)
  - Acquired
    - Neoplastic
      - Tumors
      - Cysts
    - Physiologic
      - Constitutional delayed puberty
      - Pregnancy
      - Post partum
    - Traumatic
      - Vascular accidents
      - Infarction
      - Surgery
    - Functional
      - Chiari-Frommel syndrome
      - Stein-Leventhal syndrome or polycystic ovarian disease
    - Psychogenic
      - Anxiety or environmental disturbances
      - Anorexia nervosa
      - Psychoses
      - Pseudocyesis
  - Pharmacological blockade
    - Androgens
      - Exogenous
      - Endogenous
    - Estrogens
      - Exogenous
      - Endogenous
    - Progestins (oral contraceptives)
    - Drugs
      - Phenothiazines
      - Reserpine
- Ovarian etiologic factors
  - Congenital developmental defects (failure of the ovaries to respond to gonadotrophins)
    - Congenital absence
    - Gonadal dysgenesis
      - Turner's syndrome—XO
      - Mixed (mosaicism)—XO/XX, XO/XY
    - Male hermaphroditism
      - 46,XY with dysgenetic gonadogenesis and virilization at puberty
      - True hermaphroditism
      - Syndrome of feminizing testis
  - Acquired (due to loss of function or removal of the ovaries)
    - Surgical castration
    - Physiological—menopause
    - Pelvic radiation
    - Neoplasms of the ovary
      - Primary
      - Secondary function
    - Inflammatory destruction of the ovaries
    - Previous peritonitis, tuberculosis, mumps, chronic pelvic inflammatory disease
- Secondary influences on the hypothalamic-ovarian axis
  - Chronic illness
    - Renal disease
    - Tuberculosis
    - Cirrhosis
  - Metabolic diseases
    - Thyroid
      - Hyperthyroidism
      - Hypothyroidism
    - Adrenal
      - Cushing's syndrome
      - Congenital adrenal hyperplasia
    - Pancreas (diabetes)
  - Nutritional disturbances
    - Malnutrition and inanition
    - Exogenous obesity
- "Apparent" ovarian failure (apparent lack of uterine end-organ endometrial response)
  - Congenital obstruction of the outflow tract
    - Imperforate hymen
    - Vaginal atresia
  - Acquired obstruction to outflow tract
    - Cervical stenosis
    - Tumor
  - Absence of the uterus
    - Congenital lack of development
    - Surgical removal
  - Destruction of the endometrium
    - Inflammation
    - Neoplasm
    - Radiation
    - Excessive curettage

lament the inconvenience of menstruation, but any major departure from the established pattern provokes concern. In fact, menstrual disturbance is one of the principal reasons why women seek medical attention.

Normal female function is impossible without end-organ response to ovarian hormones and an intact hypothalamic-pituitary-ovarian axis. Ovarian failure or dysfunction can be caused by ovarian abnormalities (primary hypogonadism), or by a disturbance of the hypothalamic-pituitary-ovarian control mechanisms (secondary hypogonadism) (Table 10-4). This distinction is useful only in separating primary ovarian failure from other diseases resulting in ovarian dysfunction. Some causes of disordered ovarian function are listed in Tables 10-3 and 10-4. As the tables show, disruptions can occur anywhere within the axis and produce identical clinical results; the physician can only reach an accurate diagnosis by appropriate investigation of each component.

Polycystic Ovarian Disease (Stein-Leventhal Syndrome)

This diagnostic label was once common, but it is now recognized that the classic syndrome is rare. In 32 years, Stein found only 106 patients who fitted precisely into this category: They all had enlarged, smooth, cystic ovaries, amenorrhea, infertility, obesity, and hirsutism. The complete syndrome is an advanced stage of hypothalamic-pituitary dysfunction, characterized by excess ovarian or adrenal androgens. Greater understanding of ovarian physiology and steroid hormone formation has divided the classic syndrome into a number of ovarian and adrenal disorders, of which polycystic ovaries are the common feature.

Although the exact cause remains unknown, polycystic ovarian disease represents a disturbance of the neuroendocrine controls that regulate gondadotropin production. An older theory held that the thickened ovarian capsule mechanically prevented ovulation and interfered with the pituitary-ovarian axis. More recent evidence suggests that the basic disturbance is in the hypothalamic cycling center, which controls the production and release of pituitary LH.

If the cycling mechanism breaks down, both FSH and a small amount of LH will be released at a constant level through the steady state area, much as in the normal male. Because of this continuous, even, low-level stimulation instead of normal fluctuations, ovarian steroid synthesis (specifically, the conversion of androgens to estrogens) is not completed, excess androgen is released, and the woman does not ovulate. If the ovary is subjected to *constant* gonadotropin stimulation, it functions almost like a testis, producing mostly dehydroepiandrosterone (DHA) and some testosterone. Increased androgen release maintains a constant level of hypothalamic blockade, eventually causing ovarian cortical fibrosis and follicular cysts; amenorrhea or anovulation persists.

Normal ovarian steroid production can be restored and ovulation stimulated by treatment with drugs such as clomiphene citrate, which temporarily blocks all stimuli reaching the hypothalamic receptor area and allows the cycling area to readjust to a female pattern of activity. We have no satisfactory explanation for the success of ovarian wedge resection, but probably the trauma of the operation temporarily inactivates the ovaries, thus allowing the hypothalamic–pituitary axis to resume its female rhythm.

Clinical and Laboratory Features

The typical patient is a young woman in her late teens or twenties, who, after normal puberty and a few years of irregular, anovulatory cycles, develops either oligomenorrhea or secondary amenorrhea. These young women have increased facial and body hair, but few are actually virilized. Many have acne. Most are obese, but of normal stature and feminine appearance. Biochemically, both total gonadotropin and urinary 17-ketosteroid excretions are normal. Serum testosterone levels may be above normal, and this could account for the signs of androgen excess. Urinary 17-ketosteroids do not reflect testosterone secretion or excretion (see section on Fractionation of 17-Ketosteroids in Chapter 7). The physician bases his diagnosis primarily on the woman's history and physical examination, and does biochemical studies to rule out pituitary and adrenal disease.

Therapy

Experts increasingly recommend medical measures rather than surgery. The objectives of medical treatment are to suppress abnormal ovarian steroid formation by giving cyclic estrogens and progestins, or to correct anovulatory infertility. When the primary complaint is infertility, clomiphene citrate is of great value. The dosage must be low because the polycystic ovary is very sensitive and enlarges enormously if it is overstimulated by gonadotropins released as a result of the clomiphene therapy.

Abnormal Bleeding

In 1837, a male gynecologist named Dewees compiled the following list of causes of dysfunctional uterine bleeding:

Women most obnoxious to menorrhagia are those:
(1) who live indolently and indulge in stimuli
(2) who use little or no exercise
(3) who keep late hours
(4) who dance inordinately
(5) who are intemperate
(6) who have borne many children
(7) who have been subject to febrile affections
(8) who have much leukorrhoea
(9) who are too prodigal in the joys of wedlock
(10) who are advancing towards the non-menstrual period
(11) who yield too readily to passions or emotions

In the adult as in the adolescent, abnormal uterine bleeding (Table 10-5) should be viewed as a sign or symptom and not a disease. It is divided into two types: *dysfunctional* and *specific*. When there is no specific, demonstrable organic cause, the bleeding is dysfunctional. In most instances, dysfunctional bleeding results from subtle endocrine abnormalities that disturb the hypothalamic-pituitary-ovarian axis. Investigation must rule out a variety of diseases, such as tumors, blood dyscrasias, accidents of pregnancy, and so on, which disturb menstrual function.

Etiology and Investigation

Anovular bleeding occurs when only estrogens stimulate the endometrium. The bleeding results when estrogen levels fall below those necessary for endometrial support. Two varieties of anovular bleeding exist: estrogen withdrawal bleeding and breakthrough bleeding. The bleeding is typically irregular in frequency, amount, and duration. Since ovulation does not occur, the corpus luteum never forms, and therefore never releases the progesterone necessary to prepare the estrogen-stimulated endometrium for normal menstruation. Since the endometrium shows no progesterone-induced secretory changes in an anovulatory cycle, diagnosis can be made from either an endometrial biopsy or a D&C performed in the latter half of the cycle, when secretory changes would be expected. In the perimenopausal and postmenopausal woman with irregular bleeding, curettage is mandatory to rule out malignancy of the reproductive tract.

Therapy

Anovulatory dysfunctional bleeding results from an ovarian disturbance, which must be diagnosed before specific treatment can begin. However, severe bleeding must be controlled before the primary cause can be investigated. Treatment is therefore divided into two phases: immediate and specific.

Immediate Control

This can be accomplished by therapeutic D&C, very rarely hysterectomy, or by increasing circulating estrogens by intravenous injections. Give an initial dose of 20–60 mg of Premarin, followed by 20 mg every hour until vaginal bleeding stops.

Specific Therapy

The next goal is to establish regular, cyclic menses. Progesterone promotes the complete, even shedding of the endometrium. The founda-

Table 10-5. Descriptive Classification of Functional Menstrual Disturbances

Patient's Classification	*Clinical Designation*	*Characteristics*
"Periods have stopped"	Secondary amenorrhea	Cessation of periods—no period for 3 months or more
"Periods are coming too often"	Polymenorrhea	Cycle interval less than 21 days
"Periods are very irregular, and I often skip 1 or 2 months"	Oligomenorrhea	Cycle interval from 35 to 90 days
"Periods are too heavy or too long"	Menorrhagia Hypermenorrhea Polymenorrhagia	Clots, soak more than 6 perineal pads each 24 hr, duration longer than 7 days
"Periods are too little, too short"	Hypomenorrhea	Spotting, scanty flow, lasting less than 2 days
"Bleeding out of cycle"	Metrorrhagia Dysfunctional uterine bleeding	Abnormal bleeding of any amount which is acyclical and anovular
"Continuous bleeding"	Metrostaxis	

tion of therapy is, therefore, to supply enough progestational agent to artificially promote normal endometrial maturation and shedding.

Synthetic Progestational Agents. Progestational agents (without estrogens) can be administered for four or five cycles from day 15 or 20 until day 25. Most women will then resume normal ovarian function. These synthetic hormones include compounds containing both 19- and 21-carbon atoms. A more popular routine is the use of estrogen in combination with a progestational agent for three weeks of each four-week cycle, for several months. The physician may use combined estrogen and progestin; or he may prescribe estrogen alone for the first 14 days, followed by estrogen combined with a progestin for the next seven days.

Androgens. Although the male hormones can reduce bleeding by producing endometrial atrophy, they should not be used because of their masculinizing effect at other target organs such as hair follicles.

Stimulating Ovulation. The anovulatory cycle is obviously infertile and can be treated with clomiphene citrate, which stimulates the hypothalamic cycling mechanism and thus produces ovulatory cycles.

Surgery. After diagnostic D&C, most dysfunctional uterine bleeding can be treated with a three- or four-month course of cyclic hormone therapy. In women near the menopause the same conservative approach will usually suffice, but if this treatment fails, hysterectomy should be recommended.

As we have mentioned, D&C removes the endometrium, thus controlling bleeding for varying periods of time in 30–60 percent of women with dysfunctional uterine bleeding.

Counseling. In acyclical uterine bleeding, explanation and reassurance are often as important as hormones; by helping the woman to adjust to stress, they increase the effectiveness of hormone therapy. General treatment in all cases should include attention to diet, regulation of weight, and if blood loss has been significant, supplemental iron.

Radiation Therapy. We mention radiation only to condemn it. Occasionally, it may be considered when hormonal therapy is not advisable and when the risk of hysterectomy is inordinately high.

Absence or Cessation of Menses in the Adult

Primary and secondary amenorrhea in the mature woman have the same causes and are approached in the same way as in the adolescent. Associated signs and symptoms have the same significance. We will therefore discuss only those special syndromes ordinarily confined to the mature woman.

Primary Amenorrhea

Primary amenorrhea in the adult warrants painstaking evaluation. In most cases, some form of gonadal dysgenesis or intersex disorder exists which requires chromosomal analysis and direct visualization of the gonads.

Testicular Feminization

In hereditary testicular feminization (see Fig. 9-5), gonadal differentiation is normal (see also discussion of the same topic in Chapter 9 and section on Pseudohermaphroditism in Chapter 11). Although at birth these individuals are genetic and gonadal males (they are sex-chromatin negative and have normal male 46,XY karyotypes and testes as gonads), physical appearance is that of normal females, and they continue to develop as girls through childhood. At puberty, if the testes have not been removed, these persons become more feminine, even voluptuous. The syndrome is usually unrecognized until early adult life, when treatment is sought for primary amenorrhea and/or infertility. They look and feel like women. The external genitalia are normal, but the vagina ends in a blind pouch, and there are no internal genitalia. The testes are frequently in the inguinal canals or the peritoneal cavity. Characteristically, axillary and pubic hair is scant, and one-third of these patients have none at all.

Testicular feminization appears to be due to tissue insensitivity to androgens, perhaps because of a deficiency (at the end-organ) of the enzyme, which converts testosterone to its active form. The testes, which are normal, produce testosterone and estrogen. But while the testosterone has no effect on any of the usual target organs, the estrogen does and produces feminization. Once this diagnosis is established, the patient must be handled with great care. She regards herself as a woman, and treatment should strongly emphasize the feminine gender role. These individuals are potentially good wives and adoptive mothers. The testes are removed after puberty because of a risk of testicular cancer, and the patients then receive estrogen and progesterone supplements indefinitely. The vagina is usually large enough for intercourse; if it is not, an artificial vagina can be created.

In testicular feminization, inheritance is either sex-linked recessive or a male-limited autosomal dominant; thus in any affected family, one-half of the genotypic males will be affected and will be raised as females, and one-half the genotypic females will be carriers of the abnormal gene.

Secondary Amenorrhea

The factors that disrupt the coordination of hypothalamus, pituitary, ovary, and uterus in the adult are the same as in the adolescent. However, in the mature female, several additional causes must be kept in mind:

1. Pregnancy
2. The effects of parturition on the hypothalamus and pituitary
3. Premature menopause or early gonadal failure
4. Secondary amenorrhea seen occasionally after discontinuance of contraceptives

Pregnancy and Amenorrhea

Temporary amenorrhea up to six months after pregnancy is normal. If it persists longer, the woman must be investigated to rule out anterior pituitary failure secondary to a hypotensive episode during delivery. Because this function seems to be the most vulnerable, the first (and often the only) manifestation of mild pituitary insufficiency is reduced or absent gonadotropin secretion. If the pituitary ischemia were more severe, other pituitary (endocrine) functions would fail in order of their vulnerability—ACTH and adrenal function are usually the last to be depressed. The diagnosis of persistent postpartum amenorrhea secondary to gonadotropic deficiency (Sheehan's syndrome) is based on the history of a pregnancy complicated by hypotension and subsequent low or absent gonadotropins, with or without depressed thyroid or adrenal function. Pituitary tumors, which may produce the same picture, must be excluded by appropriate investigation.

Amenorrhea and Persistent Lactation

Postpartum amenorrhea and persistent lactation in otherwise normal women is called the Chiari-Frommel syndrome (see Fig. 10-14). Women with pituitary tumors and those who have not had a recent pregnancy may also have these symptoms—the Ahumada-del Castillo syndrome. Both groups have markedly reduced pituitary gonadotropin excretion and low or undetectable serum estrogen. The endometrium and vaginal mucosa are profoundly atrophic, and vaginal cytology shows no superficial cell maturation. Clinical examination and laboratory tests show normal thyroid and adrenal functions, indicating that pituitary dysfunction is limited to gonadotropins. The same clinical picture can also be produced by prolonged intake of phenothiazines in high doses, which presumably blocks the hypothalamus.

These disorders may be due to inhibition of the hypothalamic gonadotropin-releasing factors and prolactin-inhibiting factor, resulting in hypogonadotropism and abnormal prolactin secretion by the anterior pituitary. Treatment is often unsatisfactory, but high doses of sequential estrogen and progesterone or treatment with clomiphene citrate is occasionally successful.

Precocious Menopause (Premature Gonadal Failure)

Premature menopause refers to secondary amenorrhea and hot flashes in a woman under 40 (frequently in her late twenties or thirties), who has previously had normal ovulatory cycles. It has been suggested that an insufficient original endowment of primordial ovarian follicles is the cause of this disorder. And a sex chromosome abnormality is discovered in some cases. It may be congenital; sometimes more than one member of a family is affected. These women have no other signs or symptoms of underlying endocrine or pelvic disorders. All laboratory studies are normal except that 24-hour gonadotropin excretion is in the range appropriate to normal menopause; diagnosis is based on this finding. There is no known treatment; obviously, ovulatory stimulants will be ineffective. However, prolonged gonadal steroid replacement prevents the genital and systemic effects of long-term estrogen deprivation.

Other Functional Disorders of Menstruation

Primary (Essential) Dysmenorrhea

Sometimes, within a few years of the menarche, the menses are accompanied by incapacitating abdominal pain although there is no demonstrable organic pelvic pathology. This type of dysmenorrhea is never experienced during an anovulatory cycle because progesterone, acting on the estrogen-prepared myometrium and uterine vasculature, produces the discomfort.

The precise pathophysiology of abdominal cramps is unknown. Physicians base their diagnosis on a typical history and normal pelvic findings, and confirm it by suppressing ovulation with a synthetic combined estrogen-progestin preparation, given from day 5 to day 25. In essential dysmenorrhea, this treatment induces painless withdrawal bleeding.

Usually, young women with dysmenorrhea are treated with large doses of reassurance and small doses of simple analgesics. In instances of severe discomfort, ovulation can be suppressed for several months with a combined estrogen-progestin compound. In very rare cases, presacral neurectomy (section of the pelvic nerves) may be considered when other therapy (including the suppression of ovulation and dilatation of the cervix) fails.

Premenstrual Tension

The normal, minimal, premenstrual tension which accompanies the latter part of the secretory phase of the cycle may occasionally be greatly exaggerated, causing oppressive physical and emotional tension and irritability. The usual complaints include headaches, gastrointestinal upsets, weight gain, and occasionally overt peripheral edema. Violence and suicide in women are more common during this period than at any other time in the cycle. These symptoms seem to result from the retention of excessive sodium and fluid caused by a slight alteration in the estrogen-progesterone ratio. Estrogen promotes sodium retention, while progesterone promotes its secretion. During the premenstrual period, adrenocortical activity may increase, and a relative excess of aldosterone may contribute to the retention of sodium and fluid. This syndrome can be controlled with small amounts of supplemental progestational substances or diuretics and probably represents a relative progesterone deficiency. Although it may occur at any time during a woman's reproductive life, premenstrual tension is usually severe only in women over 30.

While explanation and reassurance are frequently adequate treatment for this disorder, two kinds of specific therapy are available:

1. Direct measures to minimize sodium and water retention:
   - Limit sodium intake and restrict fluids in the 7–10 days before menses
   - Give diuretics to facilitate salt and water excretion in the same period
2. Augmentation of ovarian progesterone production: give small doses of progesterone during the second one-half of the cycle. This is done to achieve a more favorable progesterone balance and counteract the effect of increased adrenal cortical aldosterone.

Hormones and Sexual Function in the Female

A woman's sexual identity depends on her ability to live comfortably with the various criteria of womanhood. Sexually, the female can be identified by six characteristics:

1. Chromosomal arrangement and chromatin pattern
2. Gonads that are structurally and functionally ovaries
3. Female sex-hormone production
4. Morphologically female external and internal genitalia
5. A female sex of rearing
6. Acceptance of a female role

The first four criteria are organic; the sex of rearing and gender role are psychological. *Gender role* may be defined as "all the things a person says or does to claim the status of a boy or man, girl or woman—the role an individual visualizes for himself or herself." Hence, the physician must recognize that he may do the individual great harm if he attempts to alter this gender role. In a normal female, sex is confirmed when all organic and psychological criteria agree. A conflict between psychological and morphological sexuality indicates a major psychiatric problem, such as homosexuality, transsexuality, or transvestism.

In sexual identity, we find the summation of many physical characteristics and psychological influences. We cannot yet fix the exact relationship between hormones and female sexual behavior because strong psychological factors make it difficult to isolate and evaluate the specific effects of sex hormones.

The term "sexual function" includes three factors: desire, activity, and gratification. Only recently has the sexual gratification of the woman been recognized as essential to successful sexual relationships. The late Alfred Kinsey and his coworkers and W. H. Masters and Virginia Johnson have all emphasized the similarities, not the differences, between male and female sexual behavior and response: Except for male ejaculation, there are few differences between male and female orgasm. Although women are biologically more suited to multiple orgasm than men, they achieve it less often, probably because of psychological blocks. About 95 percent of women reach orgasm at some time during their life, but only 70 percent achieve it during their first year of regular sexual activity.

Masters and Johnson described the physiological reactions of both men and women during the four phases of sexual stimulation: excitement, plateau, orgasm, and resolution. They define orgasm as the summit of physical and emotional gratification in sexual activity; it represents a sudden release from the vasocongestion and muscular tension produced by sexual stimuli. Orgasm is physiologically the same whether stimulation is heterosexual, homosexual, or achieved through masturbation; but psychologically, each woman's response is unique. Classifications such as clitoral and vaginal orgasm are artificial.

Although men and women respond much the same, their periods of greatest sexual activity differ. A man's sexual drive is usually strongest between the ages of 17 and 25; women feel sexual desire most strongly during their thirties. The decrease in the older woman's sexual activities is principally because her partner ages, not because her libido decreases. As a woman ages, other forms of sexual activity—masturbation and erotic dreams—increase.

A woman's sexual activity may increase during her late forties and early fifties: She may take a renewed interest in her husband because she no longer fears pregnancy or because she wants to get pregnant once more. This apparent increase in sexual activity represents a psychological rather than physical change. Although a woman's sexual desire remains strong in spite of the absence of sex steroids, the intensity and duration of her physiological reactions are reduced. After menopause, some women experience pain during coitus due to atrophic changes in the vagina, or painful uterine contractions both during and after orgasm as a result of hormonal imbalance. Hormone replacement cures both conditions by revitalizing the local tissues and restoring a more physiological hormonal balance.

Sustained sexual capacity depends upon regular opportunity for sexual expression. Postmenopausal women who have coitus infrequently (once a month or less) find it difficult to accommodate the penis. The problem could trigger a serious cycle of hostility to coitus in both partners.

Hormones and Sexual Identity

Sex of rearing and the corresponding gender role are determined at birth by the appearance of the external genitalia. Psychosexual identity is therefore not inherent but is acquired in infancy and is well established by 18 months of age.

Sexual identity is largely independent of chromosomal or gonadal sex, and nearly always conforms to sex of rearing. It is constantly reinforced by the attitudes of others, by clothes, and by a child's comparison of his or her genitalia with those of other children. Even if the child develops paradoxical secondary sex characteristics and heterosexual hormonal patterns, sexual identity may not be disturbed if it has been strongly fixed early in life. Total change of sex after 18 months should be undertaken only after serious consideration of all aspects, and only if the individual will be available for long-term counseling and close supervision.

After adolescence, a patient may decide independently to seek medical assistance in changing sex. These transsexual patients are genetically and physically normal, but usually have serious psychiatric disturbances and should be directed to special clinics which deal with these and similar problems. Any physician confronted with such patients, although he will soon direct them elsewhere, should show them the same consideration he shows his other patients. He should not allow his own sexual attitudes to influence his approach.

Evidence is now emerging that a hormonal abnormality may, in special circumstances, induce homosexuality and transsexuality. Recently, Kolodny *et al.** proposed a relationship between low sperm counts, low testosterone levels, and homosexuality. However, these aberrations are still generally regarded as acquired personality disorders. There have been recent suggestions that human beings are naturally, not environmentally, assigned to their gender role. This theory proposes that, in the human fetus, genetic and prenatal hormonal influences confer intrinsic sexuality, as they do in animals whose adult sexual role is determined by prenatal hormones. In the human, both physical sex differentiation and psychological development seem to be female unless the hypothalamus has been "programmed" to maleness through prenatal and perinatal exposure to androgens and other "male inducer" substances. Later castration of the male or adminis-

* Kolodny, R. C., Master, W. H., Hendryx, J., and Toro, G. Plasma testosterone and semen analysis in male homosexuals. *N Engl J Med* 285:1170–1174, 1971.

tration of androgens to the female may modify sexual behavior but will not reverse it.

Money, using female children and animals exposed to excessive prenatal androgens either through the mother or from congenital adrenal hyperplasia, showed that these androgens disturb psychosexual identity and behavior. His results indicate that the effects of these hormones are more than sexual.

Human females androgenized in utero exhibit the following characteristics:

1. Increased energy expenditure in all activities, with a preference for male sports, toys, and clothes, and a conspicuous lack of maternal instinct
2. Superior I.Q. in both verbal and nonverbal areas
3. Greater than average female sexual arousal by visual stimuli
4. A tendency toward scientific or professional careers

None of these characteristics in any way indicates a predisposition toward lesbianism.

In the female monkey, fetal androgens induce aggressive, rambunctious behavior. They also cause the female to assume the male position in sexual activities. On the other hand, if a genetically male fetus is not exposed to and affected by androgen, his sexual behavior will be female. These individuals (for example; testicular feminization, Turner's syndrome, or 46,XY gonadal agenesis) have strong maternal instincts, and they make excellent adoptive mothers. They exhibit none of the tomboyish behavior seen in girls exposed to prenatal or perinatal androgens.

Hormones and Female Libido

Whatever the mechanism, female libido depends primarily upon *adrenal* androgens: Male libido requires testicular androgens. The administration of estrogen to normal women does not significantly influence libido, but removal of the ovaries does decrease it—a loss that is restored by exogenous estrogen. The importance of the androgens to female libido is supported by clinical observations; for example, exogenous androgens stimulate libido, occasionally to a pathological degree, which may be due to increased clitoral size or sensitivity, as well as to a central hypothalamic reaction.

Before puberty, serum concentrations of gonadotropins and sex steroids are low and difficult to measure. But when adolescence begins, the gonads are activated, and the production of estrogens and androgens increases. Urinary 17-ketosteroids increase without a proportional increase in 17-hydroxycorticoids. In both sexes, the adrenal glands enlarge at puberty and produce increased amounts of androgens. The androgens from gonads and adrenals stimulate growth, muscle development, and pubic hair, and can cause acne. Adolescent changes in adrenal function are not due to an increased secretion of ACTH.

Prepubertal females with the congenital adrenogenital syndrome may have premature or exaggerated sexual desire. Adrenalectomy and hypophysectomy produce almost complete loss of female libido, which can be restored by testosterone. In such circumstances, corticosteroids alone do not restore libido, which depends on androgens. Loss of libido may provide a clue to unrecognized pituitary or adrenal deficiency.

The effects of estrogen and progesterone on libido are not as clearly definable as those of androgens. Libido varies during the menstrual cycle, and usually declines during the luteal phase. The average cycle of sex interest is shown in Figure 10-17.

A woman's sexual responsiveness is greatest during ovulation. Just before menstruation, there is a less significant rise, possibly due to an engorgement of the vessels in the vulva and pelvic organs, which is similar to that during sexual excitement. There is often another rise just after menstruation, possibly as a reaction to abstinence.

Figure 10-18 depicts the effect of pregnancy on female libido for the three trimesters and the postpartum period. During the first trimester, the expectant mother has to make many physical and psychological adjustments, and her sexual responsiveness decreases somewhat. In the mid-trimester, she usually feels well, but her sexual desire continues to diminish throughout pregnancy, and she may need reassurance that this decline is neither permanent nor harmful.

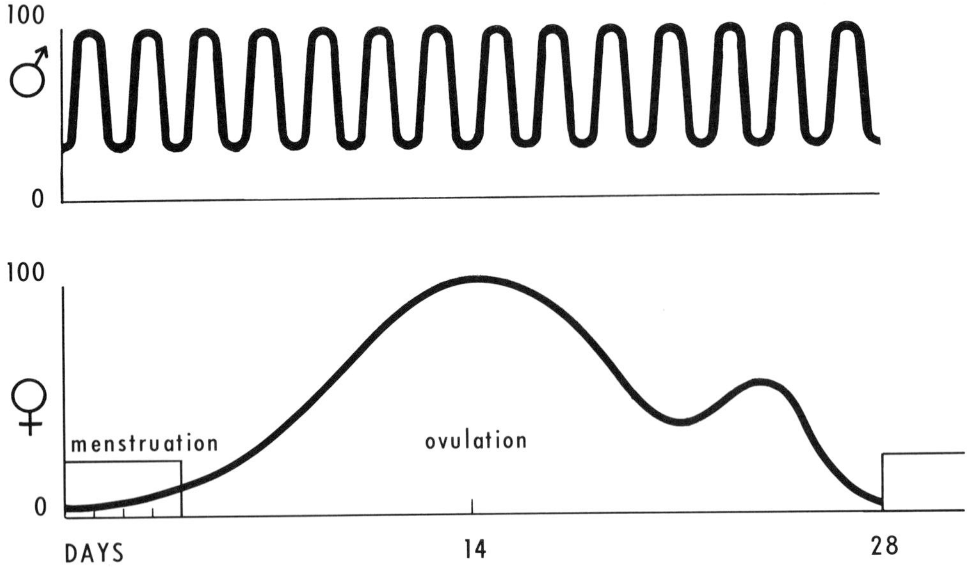

Fig. 10-17. Comparison of male and female libido. Male libido is relatively constant, fluctuating slightly in 48-hour cycles. Female libido is at its lowest during menstruation and rises to a peak at ovulation. It then declines, with a small second peak premenstrually, due to pelvic engorgement.

Female libido is strongest at a time which favors conception—namely, ovulation; and if procreation is the principal object, coitus should take place at this time.

Sperm live approximately 72 hours; the egg survives only about 12 hours after ovulation. (Adapted from *Pacific Med Surg* 73:60, 1965.)

Oral contraceptives can also reduce sexual desire. In our monogamous culture, any such reduction presents a problem: Despite the wife's loss of interest, her husband's sexual desires usually remain strong.

Frigidity is a condition in which a woman has a low or absent sex drive and cannot be sexually aroused. Its cause is psychological, usually rooted in a sense of shame, guilt, or fear. It should be noted that a woman who is sexually motivated

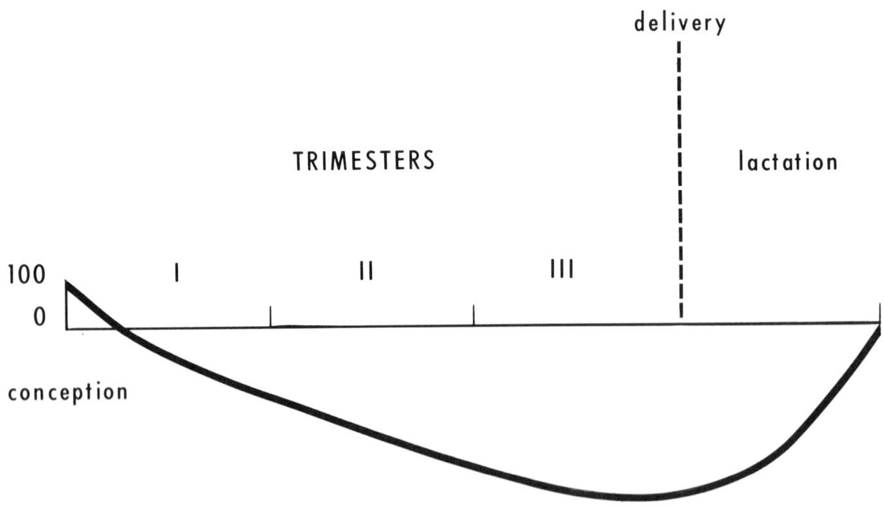

Fig. 10-18. Effect of pregnancy on libido. During pregnancy, relative to the nonpregnant state, libido declines progressively until delivery. (Adapted from *Pacific Med Surg* 73:60, 1965.)

and responsive to her mate's advances but who cannot achieve orgasm is not frigid.

Other significant aspects of sexual function are the frequency of coitus and the level of gratification achieved. Although hormones are important to sexual behavior and satisfaction, psychological factors are even more important. Sexual activity can continue unchanged in spite of hormonal deprivation, but psychological stress can distort sexual behavior, producing either frigidity or nymphomania. Such disturbances do not respond to drugs but require prolonged psychotherapy.

Reproductive Inefficiency and Excess

Since the physical test of a woman's sexuality is the ability to bear children, pregnancy demonstrates normal ovarian and sexual function. *Reproductive inefficiency* describes childlessness due to either infertility or habitual abortion. Infertility can be caused by one of many congenital or acquired conditions, but this discussion will consider only the endocrine disturbances that interfere with normal ovarian function (i.e., gametogenesis and/or steroid production, including faulty function of the corpus luteum).

To investigate fertility, the physician carries out specific endocrine studies to determine whether ovulation occurs and whether the corpus luteum functions properly. The indirect measures for detecting ovulation have been described elsewhere. Absolute confirmation of ovulation still depends upon recovering the ovum, observing its release, or confirming pregnancy. Achievement of this absolute proof of ovulation is usually impractical, and we rely on the indirect tests which indicate probable ovulation.

Apart from clinical signs and symptoms of ovulation—regular periods, dysmenorrhea, midcycle pain—the indirect methods all measure the end-organ effects of progesterone. The most practical and reliable current indicators of the effects of progesterone are: an increase in basal body temperature; glandular secretion on endometrial biopsy in the second half of the cycle; increase in urinary pregnanediol determinations; and a shift in serial vaginal cytology in both the early and late phases of the cycle. Where available, LH radioimmunoassays are used to predict ovulation. The release of progesterone from the corpus luteum can be indirectly assessed by daily estimates of pregnanediol excretion (generally impractical), by repeated postovulatory endometrial biopsies, by serial vaginal cytology, and by careful records of basal body temperature. Serum progesterone can be directly assayed by a sensitive radioimmune technique which currently is impractical for routine clinical investigation.

Anovulatory cycles are obviously infertile, regardless of whether menstruation seems normal. When menstrual dysfunction does accompany the anovulatory cycle, it is another manifestation of the hormonal imbalance found in anovulatory cycles. The cause of both the anovulation and menstrual dysfunction comes from a disturbance of the hypothalamic-pituitary-ovarian axis.

The hormonal changes that accompany anovulation are discussed in the sections dealing with amenorrhea and dysfunctional uterine bleeding. Anovulatory infertility is treated by correcting the specific disease or malfunction from which it results and hoping that ovulation will resume. Until recently, little or nothing could be done for disturbances of the hypothalamic-pituitary axis, but the availability of clomiphene citrate, and the pituitary gondadotropins themselves provide the opportunity to treat this type of anovulation.

The induction of ovulation is described in the section dealing with therapeutic agents. Oligomenorrhea and oligoovulation have been treated with progestins to induce artificial regular cycles, with the hope of an increase in fertility after cessation of progestational therapy. However, this is rarely effective.

Idiopathic Infertility

When complete investigation reveals no physical or functional abnormality in the infertile couple, the infertility is considered idiopathic. Although no specific therapy can be recommended, the couple should be assured of their normality and encouraged to persist. Correct frequency and timing of intercourse (midcycle) are stressed in counseling these and other infertile couples.

Inadequate Luteal Phase

Ovulation does not ensure that the corpus luteum will function adequately during the second half of the ovarian cycle. Luteal phase failure takes one of two forms: inadequate progesterone production and release, or premature cessation of corpus luteum function leading to premature progesterone withdrawal. In either kind of malfunction, abortion results because the fertilized ovum encounters a poorly prepared endometrial bed. This rare condition must be differentiated from anovulation, because an inadequate luteal phase can be corrected by supplemental oral progestational agents from day 16 or day 26 of the cycle. If the woman becomes pregnant, supplemental progesterone must be continued until the placenta takes over progesterone secretion from the corpus luteum, usually by the 110th day of gestation. Progestins, which would masculinize the female fetus (i.e., those structurally related to testosterone, C_{19}), should be avoided. The oral administration of C_{21} synthetic progestins will not masculinize the fetus.

Although slightly irregular menstruation may accompany inadequate luteal function, infertility is usually the only complaint. Poor corpus luteum function produces a fluctuating response of the progesterone-dependent events in the postovulatory phase: The temperature graph is low or irregular when it should be elevated; or, with premature corpus luteum failure, basal body temperature drops abruptly in 3–4 days instead of remaining elevated for 8–10 days. Repeated endometrial biopsies or several postovulatory vaginal smears show the inadequate progesterone effect resulting from corpus luteum malfunction.

Habitual Abortion

This term applies to any woman who has had three or more *consecutive* spontaneous abortions. Such abortions have many causes, but only two are related to the ovary: genetic abnormalities of the ova, and abnormal ovarian hormone production by a defective corpus luteum. Inadequate progesterone production by the corpus luteum either prevents the otherwise normal embryo from implanting or, after implantation, fails to maintain the decidua necessary to nourish the embryo.

Because of the difficulty of determining which abortions are caused by progesterone insufficiency, each clinician develops his own treatment program for habitual aborters: Either he gives none of them progestins during pregnancy, or he treats them all prophylactically. It is unwise, however, to give large doses of progestins after the abortion has become inevitable, since this treatment may only arrest expulsion of abnormal products of conception.

Thyroid Deficiency During Pregnancy

Inadequate thyroid function may cause recurrent abortion. Although thyroid hormone deficiency does not disturb ovarian activity directly, it seems to inhibit the metabolic activity of the endometrium and the implanted ovum. A thyroid supplement should be administered, preferably before conception. Thyroid tests during pregnancy are somewhat difficult to evaluate because estrogen stimulates hepatic production of thyroxine-binding globulin and thus artificially elevates protein-bound iodine and total serum thyroxine uptake values, with a fall in T_3 resin uptake.

In primary hypothyroidism complicating pregnancy, these tests will all be lower than in normal pregnancy, and the serum TSH, which may now be measured easily by radioimmunoassay, will be elevated.

Reproductive Excess

It is clear that population control cannot be achieved by copulation control, nor can the problems of overpopulation be solved simply by the availability of effective contraceptives. About 85 percent of North American women in the reproductive age group have access to methods of birth control, yet each has an average of 2.3 children; however, the rate of reproduction is inversely related to income, with the poorest families producing the most children. Population grows too rapidly, not because we lack contraceptives, but because social attitudes fix the ideal number of children at three or four, rather than at one or two. Each married woman can produce 2.2 children and still maintain the United States population at its present level of over 200 million. If each woman bears one additional child, however, the population in the year 2000 (less than 30 years away) will be more than 360 million.

In most of the world, population control still depends on the production and distribution of inexpensive, convenient, and acceptable contraceptives. Until birth rates approximate death rates, overpopulation will continue to be a threat. Although there are thousands of causes of death, there is only one life-precipitating agent. We spend millions to prevent death, but give little thought to controlling reproduction, which, in excess, might eventually destroy all life on earth.

The Endocrine Control of Fertility

Menstrual cycles can be manipulated at many stages by hormonal readjustment, and oral contraceptives represent the most successful application of this principle. The standard preparations, using estrogen and progestin either in combination or in sequence, inhibit ovulation by suppressing gonadotropin release.

We may soon be able to manipulate other steps in reproduction: the rate of gamete transport; implantation; the sperm's positive mobility and penetration of cervical mucus. Large amounts of estrogens given during the 4–5 days after fertilization can prevent the ovum from implanting securely, either by accelerating ovum transport in the tube or by making the endometrium unreceptive. Other studies suggest that some hormones may prevent implantation by destroying the egg. A single dose of such a drug at the end of each cycle would be sufficient.

Systemic long-acting progestins, such as Depo-Provera, injected at two- to four-month intervals, are contraceptive and relieve the patient of daily responsibility, thus avoiding errors in medication, especially in women of low intelligence or with language barriers. Unpredictable breakthrough bleeding episodes make this approach less than ideal, however.

At present, hormonal control of fertility is the safest, most effective, and most widely accepted method. However, nonhormonal chemicals and immunological methods may eventually replace the hormones.

The Ovary and the Menopause

Menopause means the cessation of menstruation, but this word has unfortunate connotations for many women. The physician can help dispel the impression that menopause is the onset of old age, with all its associated degenerative diseases and debility. Many women can now achieve goals that the responsibilities of childbearing and rearing had previously denied them. The physician can assist a patient with this sociological, emotional, and physical remodeling.

The North American woman expects to live at least 10 years longer than her mother did and her husband will. She spends approximately one-third of her life without the function of her ovaries—those organs which are largely responsible for her femininity. The reproductive capacity of the man declines slowly over many years, and he remains unaware of waning testicular function. The ovaries, on the other hand, cease to function suddenly; this may precipitate major problems of adaptation.

At one time or another, women in the menopausal age group attribute almost every symptom to decreasing ovarian function; their families, and frequently their physicians, may concur. As a result, North American women spend millions of dollars each year on estrogenic hormones, sedatives, and other medications for the treatment of alleged "menopausal symptoms." However, even in carefully controlled studies, it has been difficult to demonstrate that specific hormone therapy has any significant symptomatic effect. Regardless of treatment, the symptoms gradually subside, but the degenerative processes, such as osteoporosis, persist and may accelerate after the ovary fails. Within the medical profession, there are two conflicting points of view regarding the menopause and its treatment. Greenblatt's statement, "Why should any physician deny to every woman in the autumn of her life the chance to enjoy an Indian summer, rather than endure a winter of discontent?" reflects some investigators' views that the menopause is a disease resulting from a deficiency of ovarian hormones, just as Addison's disease results from deficiency of adrenal cortical hormones. Other physicians believe that the menopause is a physiological process, which may require some supportive therapy but usually not hormonal replacement.

The woman facing ovarian failure sees the menopause as an event that will affect nearly every part of her body and her entire life. The symptoms which are attributed to it include hot flashes, depression, nervousness, insomnia, lassitude, headache, backache, myalgia, dizziness, faintness, abdominal pain, constipation, diarrhea, dyspareunia, and loss of libido. Of these, only the hot flashes—a phenomenon during which a woman suddenly feels very warm and flushed, and subsequently begins to perspire—can be attributed directly to the estrogen deficiency and gonadotropin excess (Fig. 10-19).

Signs of menopause include a redistribution of fat to the lower trunk, wrinkling of the skin, loss of height, cessation or irregularity of menstruation, and atrophic vaginitis, all of which relates directly or indirectly to estrogen deficiency. These respond, to a greater or lesser degree, to estrogen therapy. We have evidence that, in women, the onset of cardiovascular degenerative disease and osteoporosis is directly related to the decline in ovarian function (Fig. 10-20).

After the menopause, all women develop osteoporosis, which gives rise to significant symptoms in 25–30 percent. Estrogen therapy delays the onset of such osteoporosis for 5–10 years, and

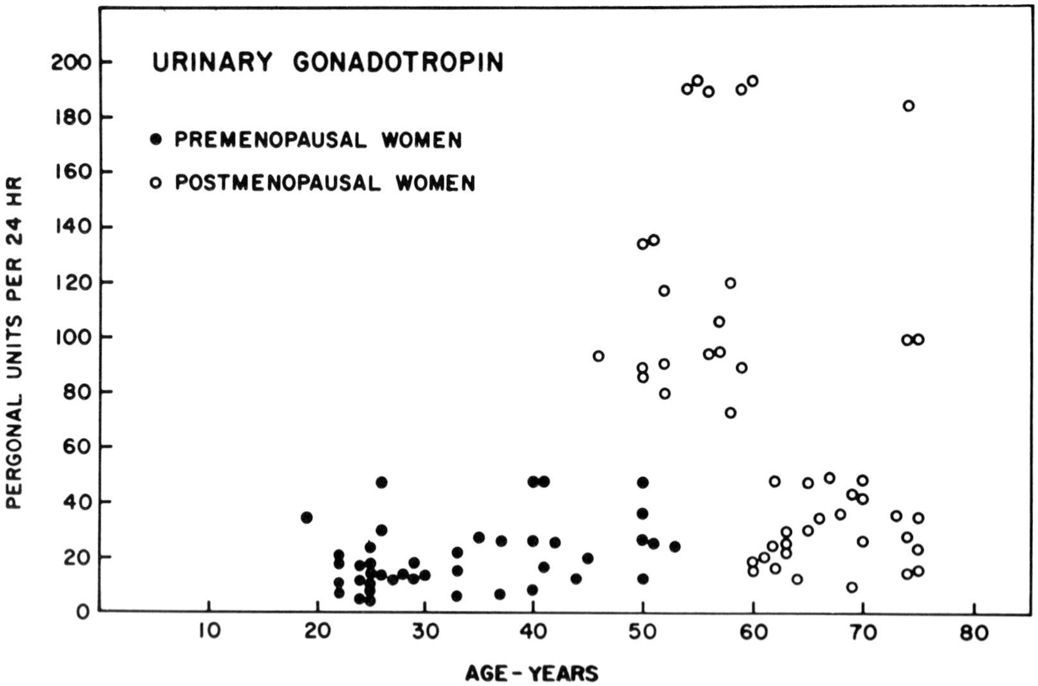

Fig. 10-19. Relation of gonadotropin level to age. Abscissa shows human urinary gonadotropin excretion (Pergonal units); ordinate, age in years. Before menopause, levels are relatively low but rise sharply with ovarian failure and decrease again some years later. (From Ryley, G. *Clin Obstet Gynecol* 7:444, 1964. Reproduced with permission.)

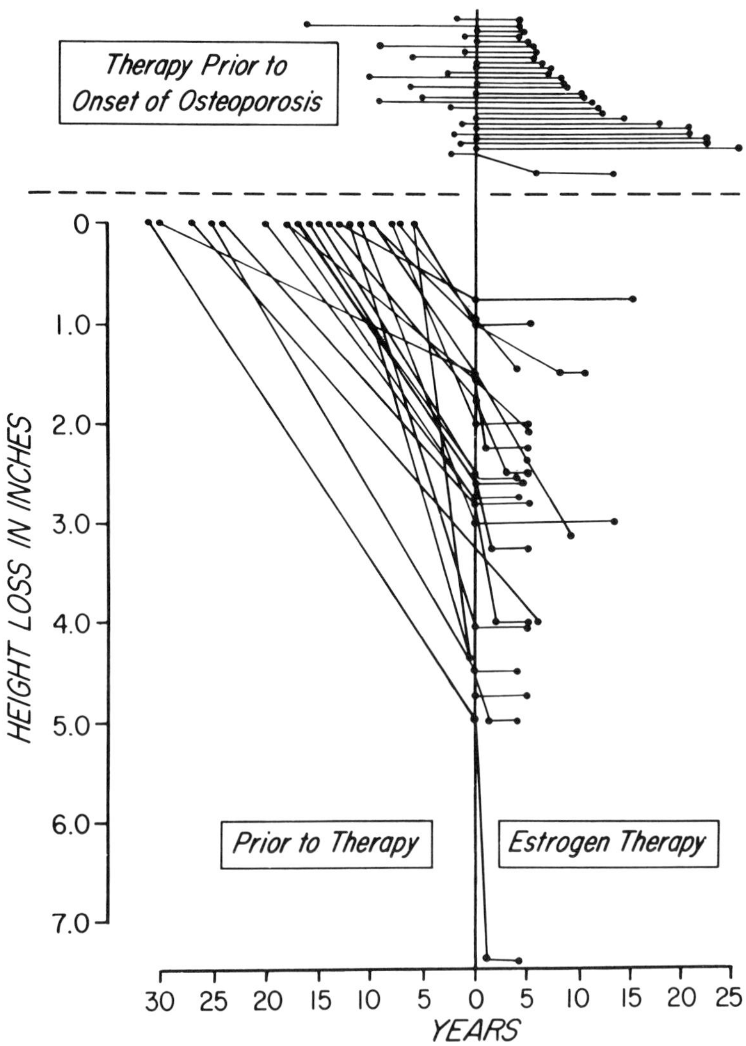

Fig. 10-20. Osteoporosis with and without estrogen treatment. The portion of the figure above dotted line shows that women who were treated before onset of osteoporosis nearly always maintain their height for many years. Below dotted line, women with osteoporosis but no treatment suffer a marked loss in height—up to 5 inches. Estrogen therapy frequently slows or halts this loss. (From Henneman, P. H. Postmenopausal Osteoporosis, *Clin Obstet Gynecol* 7:541, 1964. Reproduced with permission.)

during this interval, the women have few or no symptoms related to the bony skeleton. Then, if therapy is continued, the process advances more slowly.

Women often ask why, if we have conclusive evidence of its benefits, should not all women receive estrogen replacement after the ovaries fail. Theoretically simple therapeutic programs are often extremely difficult to implement; for example, estrogen replacement therapy may be associated with such side effects as irregular bleeding, fluid retention, and the other symptoms and signs that often plague the menstruating woman. From the point of view of symptoms only, some women find the cure (replacement therapy) worse than the disease. In addition, women receiving estrogen therapy must remain under close medical supervision, which is inconvenient and time-consuming for both the woman and her physician.

Every woman does not require the same amount of estrogen to achieve adequate substitution. The physician, if he is to regulate the dose carefully, requires considerable understanding of the effects and biochemistry of the hormones. The irregular bleeding which frequently follows estrogen therapy in the postmenopausal woman may mask an underlying endometrial cancer; therefore every case of breakthrough bleeding must be thoroughly investigated. Finally, although there is no scientific evidence that estrogens induce cancer in the postmenopausal female, many physicians still accept this relationship.

Treatment of the Menopause with Hormones

Certain menopausal women should receive replacement therapy, and these women can be selected on the basis of definite indications. These include:

1. Premenopausal surgical castration
2. Onset of menopause before 40 years of age
3. Severe symptoms and signs that can be related to estrogen lack

Contraindications to replacement therapy include a history of malignancy, such as carcinoma of the breast; uterine fibroids; hypertension; a history of thrombophlebitis; or the presence of severe liver disease.

Finally, each woman must be assessed individually before replacement therapy is begun or is refused, and the basis for the decision thoroughly explained to her.

Objectives of Therapy

Therapy may be aimed at symptomatic relief or physiological replacement. The woman herself wishes to retain or recapture her youth and to obtain relief from the many symptoms she attributes to the menopause. Sedatives or very small doses of estrogen usually relieve most of her symptoms but do not prevent osteoporosis or cardiovascular degeneration. To achieve physiological replacement, the physician must give almost as much estrogen as the woman produced during her reproductive years. Since no two women are identical, the physician must plan a replacement program for each woman individually, just as he would if she suffered from adrenal deficiency or diabetes mellitus.

Many hormonal products are available for the treatment of menopausal symptoms and signs. These include the "natural" estrogens extracted from pregnant mares' urine, and a number of synthetic products, such as the nonsteroid diethylstilbestrol and the steroid hormones ethinyl estradiol and mestranol. The progestational agents are useful in treating menopausal symptoms when estrogens themselves are contraindicated—for example, to treat a woman with a history of carcinoma of the breast. These agents are also administered for a short period to produce regular withdrawal bleeding following several weeks of estrogen therapy.

Estrogens can be administered in several patterns:

1. Continuous low-dose estrogen
2. Continuous high-dose estrogen
3. Intermittent low-dose estrogen—that is, three weeks of therapy followed by one week without therapy
4. Intermittent high-dose estrogen
5. Combined estrogen-progestational agent therapy, either in an intermittent or continuous fashion
6. Sequential estrogen/estrogen-progestogen therapy, administered either continuously or intermittently

The currently popular treatment program is intermittent low-dose estrogen therapy, such as 0.625 mg of conjugated natural estrogens (Premarin) for three weeks, followed by one week without therapy. This routine produces symptomatic relief but rarely vaginal bleeding. Sequential oral contraceptives, another popular therapy, stimulate the endometrium sufficiently to produce regular withdrawal bleeding.

If administered, therapy should be tailored to a woman's needs and contain sufficient estrogen to achieve physiological replacement with few side effects. This usually requires sequential estrogens, at a level from 40 to 80 μg for 2–3 weeks, followed by one week of the estrogen combined with a suitable progestational agent to produce regular shedding of the endometrium and withdrawal bleeding. As the menopause approaches and ovulation becomes infrequent, many women require both hormonal replacement and continued protection against conception. In these women, the physician should use one of the sequential contraceptive agents which will achieve both purposes.

The cytohormonal index described frequently as the "femininity index," while a good guide to the effect of estrogen at one end-organ (the vagina), does not give an accurate measurement of the degree of physiological replacement. Many factors, such as adrenocortical function, local bacterial flora, and other medications, affect the cytohormonal index. Changes in the index in response to estrogen therapy remain the simplest general measure of the end-organ effect, but this alone should not be used to determine the dose of estrogen needed to achieve symptomatic relief and physiological replacement.

Objective measurement of therapeutic results of estrogen replacement is almost impossible. Randomized double-blind studies indicate that psychotherapy alone may relieve such symptoms as hot flashes, while the cytohormonal index remains unchanged. Such studies also demonstrate that women receiving physiological estrogen replacement generally feel better and cope more effectively than those receiving placebo. However, many women expect therapeutic miracles, which the profession cannot yet offer.

Principles of Endocrine Diagnosis

Fundamental Principles

Diagnosis of endocrine disorders need not depend on memorizing seemingly unrelated facts and procedures. Investigation can follow the step-by-step approach used in solving a mathematical problem of several unknowns. When one unknown is identified, it is used in subsequent equations until the final solution is reached. This method applies to any endocrine dysfunction, because all such systems depend on a linear neuroendocrine axis. This concept is shown in Figure 10-13. By using data that describe the function of glands along the axis or the effects of their hormones upon target tissue, the physician can solve the unknowns in the equation and thus determine:

1. The precise level at which the axis-circuit has been affected
2. The cause of the malfunction: the endocrine gland, or impairment of axis function by extrinsic influences

The mechanisms of endocrine malfunction are fairly uncomplicated, but merely pinpointing them does not provide a diagnosis. The physician must discover the specific cause of axis-circuit disruption by testing, in sequence, the integrity of each component. Careful selection and interpretation of clinical and laboratory procedures are essential; equally important is the choice of measures to assess secondary influences on axis-circuit function. The data provided by these investigations lead eventually to final *etiologic* diagnosis. Only then can proper treatment be prescribed. Regardless of the endocrine level being investigated, tests are either direct or indirect quantitative measures, which reflect the function of a specific axis-circuit component.

The student can apply the axis-circuit concept to endocrine diagnosis more effectively if he remembers the following possibilities:

1. Sometimes the entire axis can be tested as a unit. For example, when clomiphene citrate is given, a stimulus is applied to the top of the axis (hypothalamus) and the response of the entire system evaluated at the terminal target organ (endometrium). Clomiphene works (ovarian follicle stimulation) only if the entire axis is intact. It appears to "stir up" the hypothalamus, which stimulates the pituitary to release gonadotropins. The response (ovulation) is measured in the ovary, at the opposite end of the axis by applying the indirect methods of detecting ovulation. If the axis is intact but not functioning, and if the woman does not ovulate or menstruate until she receives clomiphene, one may conclude that:

    The fault is within the hypothalamus.

    Clomiphene reverses the fault.

    The defect is functional, and probably not due to organic disease; therefore—

    The axis is intact but is not functionining normally.
2. Within a particular axis, data about an endocrine gland may be obtained by:

Direct or indirect inspection: for example, the ovary by laparoscopy; or the adrenal by specialized radiological techniques, such as retroperitoneal CO_2 injection (pneumography)

Assessing its hormone production: measurements of related biochemical, immunological, and biological assays. The assessments can often be made by stimulating or inhibiting glands, as in the dexamethasone suppression (see Chapter 7) and ACTH stimulation tests, and measuring the resulting increase or decrease in hormone output.

Assessing target-organ response: Target-organ responses to hormones produce the symptoms which cause the patient to see a doctor. The responses of the target tissues vary for different hormones, but there is a good deal of overlap: Growth hormone, adrenocortical, thyroid, and sex hormones all effect bone growth, but in each case the effect is different. Apart from the fact that target tissues produce the signs and symptoms of endocrine dysfunction, their response can provide indirect measures of hormonal activity, which is related to the functional integrity of the endocrine gland producing the hormone. The diagnostic value of target-organ evaluation will become clearer in the following section.

Evaluating the Ovarian-Endocrine System

The Ovarian Axis

The ovaries should not be investigated as isolated organs, but must be examined within the total axis-circuit. The hypothalamus, regulatory area of the reproductive system, contains a receptor site and steady state and cycling areas—the "gonadostat." The receptor site integrates the environmental, emotional, and biochemical stimuli, then relays nerve impulses to the gonadostat and regulates its response. The sexual area of the hypothalamus secretes FSH- and LH-releasing factors, which stimulate the anterior pituitary to release gonadotropin. The pituitary, the next endocrine organ in the axis, is the target for the releasing factors. Last in this series are the ovaries, which are both target organs and endocrine glands. The ovarian sex steroids complete the circuit by exerting positive and negative feedback on the hypothalamic receptors (Figs. 10-4 and 10-5). The ovarian hormones also produce recognizable peripheral target-organ changes.

Target-Tissue Response and its Evaluation

The major target-tissue effects of the sex steroids (particularly of estrogen and progesterone) occur in the reproductive tract. It must be emphasized, however, that the gonadal steroids produce general effects on calcium and lipid metabolism and electrolyte balance.

Target-tissue response is useful in assessing the ovarian endocrine axis and the output of the glands along it only if the physician is familiar with the following:

1. The target organs or tissues for each hormone
2. The effect of each particular hormone on each target tissue
3. How to use the target-tissue changes in evaluating endocrine function

Target tissues are the same in prepubertal, postpubertal, and postmenopausal women, but their responses to hormonal stimulation are different during each life stage. A response may be normal (menstruation at age 14) or pathological (menstruation at age five, or failure to menstruate by age 18).

The following endocrine disturbances can occur at any age:

1. Deficient or absent sex steroids
2. Excessive abnormal steroids, such as androgens or corticosteroids
3. Unbalanced estrogen and progesterone output
4. Continuous estrogen production and target-tissue stimulation due to failure of ovulation, i.e., progesterone production and release.

In women of any age, stimulation of the target tissues by excessive, abnormal, or deficient sex steroids can produce:

1. Feminization
2. Defeminization, hirsutism, and virilization
3. Sexual infantilism

The following target tissues can be assessed clinically for response (or lack of response) to estrogen and progesterone, and for stimulation by androgen:

1. General somatic effects
   - General growth and body habitus
   - Bone growth, epiphyseal closure, and body height
   - Pattern and texture of extragenital hair growth
   - Sebaceous and sweat-gland activity
   - Enlargement and development of larynx
2. Genital growth
   - Growth of internal genital structures
   - Ovulation
   - Growth and development of external genitalia
   - Secondary sex organs—breasts, pubic hair, and axillary hair

Target Organ Response to Estrogen

Estrogen produces most of the typical female characteristics: fat distribution, breast growth, and development of the internal and external genitalia. It stimulates selectively the growth of all tissues derived from the müllerian ducts and also has a generalized effect on body physiology, metabolism, shape, and composition, as well as emotional tone. Peak levels of estrogen are essential to induce feminization of the pubertal girl; complete lack of estrogen results in sexual infantilism.

Table 10-6. Office Assessment of Gynecologic-Endocrine Patient

- History
  - Gynecologic
    - Menstrual
      - Age at menarche
      - Cycle
        - Regularity
        - Interval
        - Duration
        - Associated pain
        - Volume of flow
      - Premenstrual symptoms
        - Breast tenderness
        - Bloating
        - Headaches
        - Irritability
      - Date of last menstrual period
    - Obstetrical
      - Number of pregnancies
      - Complications and outcome
  - Endocrine
    - Events during and after puberty
      - Breast development
      - Hair growth and distribution
    - Symptoms of other endocrine disease—e.g., heat or cold intolerance
  - Social and family background
  - Fertility
    - Health of husband
    - Frequency and technique of intercourse
    - Contraceptive methods
- Physical examination
  - Endocrine target organs
    - Body shape
    - Sex hair
      - Distribution
      - Texture
    - Skin
      - Secretions
      - Acne
    - Breast development
    - External genitalia
      - Clitoris
      - Vaginal orifice
  - Assessment of pelvic organs
    - Uterus
      - Presence
      - Size
      - Position
      - Shape
      - Mobility
    - Ovaries
      - Presence
      - Size
  - Tests
    - Sound uterus for possible obstructions
    - Quality of cervical mucus
      - Spinnbarkeit (elasticity)
      - Ferning (crystallization)
    - Vaginal cytology (maturation index)
    - Buccal smear (chromatin body)

Somatic Effects

It has long been assumed, though not adequately documented, that it is estrogen which terminates the growth of the pubertal girl by closure of the epiphyses. For reasons that are not entirely clear but probably relate to increased testosterone production, boys grow taller than girls, as a result of an adolescent spurt which begins later, is more intense, and lasts longer. Lack of estrogen production in a girl who has not lost the genetic material for growth can produce eunuchoid proportions (i.e., excessive height due to continued increase in leg length). If there is little estrogen effect, androgens induce sebaceous gland activity, which causes acne. Because estrogen is anabolic, its decline after the menopause may contribute to the osteoporosis seen in this period.

Gynecologic Investigation of Endocrine Disorders

We have discussed in detail information providing a unified concept of the reproductive tract as a

Table 10-7. Protocol for In-Hospital Assessment of Hypothalamic-Pituitary-Ovarian Interactions†

Day 1*
- Medical photography (if not carried out previously)
- Buccal smear plus chromosome cultures
- X-rays
  - Pituitary fossa
  - Routine chest
  - IVP (where indicated)
  - Hysterosalpingogram (in selected cases)
- O.T. test (1:2000)
- Blood tests
  - Routine hematology
  - Electrolytes
  - BUN, FBS (2-hr p.c.)
  - Thyroid function
    - Serum T_4, T_3 uptake
    - PBI
    - TSH
- Urine for routine analysis and culture
- Daily pelvic examination
  - Serial vaginal smear for cytohormonal assessment
  - Cervical mucus assessment
    - Quantity
    - Ferning effect
    - Spinnbarkeit
- Assessment of patient by social services and behavioral sciences

Day 2
- Commence 24-hr urine collections for baseline determination of:
  - Total gonadotropin excretion (bioassay)
  - 17-OHCS and 17-KS
- Capsule for ^{131}I uptake
- Daily pelvic for smears
  - Cytohormonal
  - Cervical mucus assessment
- Immunoassay for gonadotropins

Day 3
- Continue urine collections
- ^{131}I scan
- Read O.T. test
- Daily pelvic for smears
- Serum estrogens and androgens (including testosterone) × 3

Day 4
- Commence progesterone withdrawal test—medroxyprogesterone acetate 10 mg orally × 5
- Operating room for
  - Examination under anesthesia
  - D&C (if indicated)
  - Laparoscopy for
    - Direct visualization of gonads and internal genitalia
    - Ovarian biopsy (if indicated)
    - Photographs of laparoscopic findings
- Review of nurses' notes, discussion of patient's behavior, attitudes, and adjustment with nursing staff

Day 5
- Remove Michel clip from laparoscopy procedure
- 17-KS and 17-OHCS results
  - Dexamethasone suppression if indicated (low and high dose)
- Arginine and insulin infusion tests (growth hormone)

Day 5 +
- Review of findings with patient, and instruction regarding treatment if any is instituted:
  - Ovarian suppression
  - Reproductive tract priming or development
  - Adrenal suppression (prednisone)
- Follow-up appointment in 6 weeks
- Discharge home

Days 8–12
- Contact patient regarding results of progesterone withdrawal test

* The following regimen should be observed throughout the patient's hospital stay: (1) regular diet; (2) no medication; (3) full ambulatory ward activity; (4) daily weight-taking.

† See also Pituitary Investigation Protocol—Addendum, Chapter 4.

specific endocrine system. Such a concept, particularly with regard to investigation and diagnosis, can lead to a flexible approach to all gynecologic endocrine problems.

Baseline Office Assessment

Investigation begins with a comprehensive medical history and a thorough physical examination, of particular importance since gynecologic complaints are frequently the first signs of serious systemic disease. The patient's age may also affect diagnostic procedures and treatment. Table 10-6 provides for collecting the essential information.

Specific Assessment

The history and physical examination will define the patient's specific problem reasonably well. If additional laboratory, radiologic, or surgical procedures are necessary for a precise diagnosis, they should be done in the hospital, preferably in a metabolic unit. Infertility studies are an exception to this rule; they should be begun on an outpatient basis, and include charting of basal body temperature, serial evaluation of cervical mucus (Table 10-6) and the maturation index. Postcoital tests, tubal insufflation, and endometrial biopsies at the beginning and end of the cycle complete the outpatient investigation.

In the hospital, the tests listed in Table 10-7 are usually ordered for assessment of hypothalamic-pituitary-ovarian axis function and of other endocrine function such as thyroid, adrenal cortex, and islets of Langerhans. Further laboratory tests and surgical procedures are selected according to the results of these investigations.*

Summary

While the ovary is responsible for many female characteristics, women live long after the menopause. Ovarian hormones are partially responsible for this longevity, and thus contribute to the increasing proportion of elderly women in our communities. Postmenopausal life can still be sexually and socially fulfilling, if the environment provides the necessary resources and support. Continued replacement of ovarian hormones may further reinforce the natural difference between aging in men and in women and accentuate the problems of our older female population.

Aging is inevitable, despite our youth orientation and our refusal to face resolutely its psychic-emotional problems. The physician can, by the use of hormones and other drugs, radically alter the biochemical environment of the woman, but he cannot compensate for the loss of her husband or the gradual withdrawal of her children into their own lives. Loneliness and a sense of uselessness contribute heavily to the high incidence of reactive depression in older women.

The health professional must deal with these social and psychological consequences of variations in ovarian function throughout a woman's life. His objective is to recognize and understand her problems, and to optimize physical and emotional health at each of the stages depicted in the Currier and Ives print (Fig. 10-1).

* See Appendix: Addendum to Chapter 10.

References

Neuroendocrinology

1. Martini, L., and Ganong, W. F., eds. *Neuroendocrinology,* Vol. I and II. New York, Acad. Press, 1966.
2. Nalbandov, A. V., ed. *Advances in Neuroendocrinology.* Chicago, Univ. Illinois Press, 1963.
3. Martini, L., Fraschini, F., and Motta, M. Neural control of anterior pituitary function. *Recent Progr Horm Res 24:*439, 1968.
4. Chally, A. V., Arimura, A., Bowers, C. Y., Kastin, A. J., Sawano, S., and Redding, T. W. Hypothalamic neurohormones regulating anterior pituitary function. *Recent Progr Horm Res 24:*497, 1968.

Gonadotropins

5. Armstrong, D. T. Gonadotropins, ovarian metabolism and steroid biosynthesis. *Recent Progr Horm Res 24:*255, 1968.
6. Butt, W. R. *The Chemistry of the Gonadotropins.* Springfield, Ill., Thomas, 1967.
7. Rosenberg, E., ed. *Gonadotropins 1968: Proceedings of the Workshop Conference, Vista Hermosa, Mexico, June 24–26, 1968.* Los Altos, Calif., Geron-X, Inc., 1968.
8. Swyer, G. I. M., ed. Control of human fertility. *Brit Med Bull 26:*1–97, 1970.
9. Immunoassay of gonadotrophins. 1st Symposium, Karolinska symposia on research methods in reproductive endocrinology, Stockholm, 1969. Ed. E. Diczfalusy. *Acta Endocrinol (Suppl) 142:*1–382, 1969.

Pediatric and Adolescent Gynecology

10. Dewhurst, C. J. *Gynaecologic Disorders of Infants and Children.* London, Cassell, 1963.
11. Gardner, L. I., ed. *Endocrine and Genetic Diseases of Childhood.* Philadelphia, Saunders, 1969.
12. Heald, F. P., ed. *Adolescent Gynaecology.* Baltimore, Williams & Wilkins, 1966.
13. Huffman, J. W. *The Gynaecology of Childhood and Adolescence.* Philadelphia, Saunders, 1968.
14. Jones, H. W., Jr., and Heller, R. H. *Paediatric and Adolescent Gynaecology.* Baltimore, Williams & Wilkins, 1966.
15. Lang, W. R., consulting ed. Paediatric and adolescent gynaecology. *Ann NY Acad Sci 142:*547–834, 1967.
16. Marshall, W. A. Sex differences at puberty. *J Biosoc Sci Suppl 2:*31–41, 1970.
17. Marshall, W. A., and Tanner, J. M. Variations in pattern of pubertal changes in girls. *Arch Dis Child 44:*291–303, 1969.

Steroid Biochemistry

18. Dorfman, R. I., and Ungar, F., eds. *Metabolism of Steroid Hormones.* New York, Acad. Press, 1965.
19. Gorski, J., Toft, D., Shyamala, G., Smith, D., and Notides, A. Hormone receptors: studies on the interaction of estrogen with the uterus. *Recent Progr Horm Res 24:*45, 1968.
20. Martini, L., and Pecile, A., eds. *Hormonal Steroids I.* New York, Acad. Press, 1964.
21. Fieser, L. F., and Fieser, M. *Steroids.* New York, Reinhold, 1959.

See also Reference 4.

General Endocrinology

22. Gold, J. J., ed. *Textbook of Gynaecologic Endocrinology.* New York, Hoeber, 1968.
23. Gual, C., and Ebling, F. J. G., eds. *Progress in Endocrinology: Proceedings of the III International Congress of Endocrinology.* Amsterdam, Excerpta Medica, 1969.
24. Lloyd, C. W., ed. *Human Reproduction and Sexual Behaviour.* Philadelphia, Lea & Febiger, 1964.
25. Paschkis, K. E., Rakoff, A. E., Cantarow, A., and Rupp, J. J., eds. *Clinical Endocrinology,* ed. 3. New York, Hoeber, 1967.
26. Williams, R. H., ed. *Textbook of Endocrinology,* ed. 4. Philadelphia, Saunders, 1968.
27. Simmer, H. H., Pion, R. J., and Dignam, W. J. *Testicular Feminization.* Springfield, Ill., Thomas, 1965.

11

Chromosomal Studies in Endocrinology*

Patrick Edward Conen

This review will attempt to show the close association and interdependence of knowledge between genetics and endocrinology.

The student will strengthen and extend his knowledge of genetics by carefully studying patients with interesting endocrine problems, particularly those with gonadal abnormalities.

Although man is the most closely studied animal we know, we can only learn more about him by careful observations of chance experiments of nature and simulation of these in the laboratory.

In this chapter, some methods and the significance of chromosomal analyses will be presented that will help in diagnosis and further understanding of endocrine disorders. Studies of sex chromatin and dermatoglyphics (skin ridge patterns) will also be described to help in interpretation of chromosome findings. The following glossary of terms used may prove helpful:

Autosome: A chromosome other than a sex (X or Y) chromosome

Crossing-over: An exchange during cell division of corresponding parts of the maternal and paternal homologous chromosomes

Deletion: Loss of a portion of a chromosome

Diploid: Containing a set of maternal and a set of paternal chromosomes (total 46); see *Haploid*

Gene: The smallest unit of inheritance of a single characteristic

Haploid: Containing a single set of chromosomes (total 23); normal in gametes

Homologous chromosomes: Chromosomes of the same type, one derived from the mother and one from the father, which form a pair in the diploid cell

Karyotype: The number, size, and morphology of an individual's chromosomes

Meiosis: Cell division in germ cells resulting in the production of haploid cells (23 chromosomes) from diploid cells (46 chromosomes)

Mitosis: Cell division in somatic cells, resulting in the preservation of the chromosome number (46)

Monosomy: Presence of only one of a given pair of chromosomes in a diploid cell

Mosaicism: Occurrence in a single individual of more than one genotype derived from one zygote

Nondisjunction: Failure of a pair of newly divided chromosomes to separate during cell division; one daughter cell receives both chromosomes and the other daughter cell receives neither

X chromatin: Chromatin mass (Barr body) visible in most female nuclei; generally the number of

* This work was supported by the Ontario Cancer Research and Treatment Foundation.

Barr bodies is one less than the number of X chromosomes

Y chromatin: An X or Y chromosome

Translocation: Transfer of a chromosome segment to an abnormal site, either on another chromosome or the wrong position on the same chromosome

Morphologic Sex

Sex determination of an individual occurs at conception when an X-bearing sperm fertilizes an egg to form an XX female or a Y-bearing sperm and egg form an XY male zygote. The presence or absence of the sex chromatin mass determines cellular or *cytological sex*. During *sex differentiation* in early fetal life, the gonads (testes or ovaries) form and the *primary sexual characteristics*—the internal and external genitalia—develop, and at puberty the *secondary sexual characteristics* develop.

Sexual Identity (Gender)

The *sexual role* (gender), a psychosocial phenomenon, is determined by the *sex of rearing*. This role and the individual's complex relationships with other members of the family and society, begin when the infant is identified as male or female. If, at maturity, the adult is to play the role appropriate to his gender, he must, as an infant, have close contact with and receive affection from parents and others. Monkeys reared with a warm sack containing a milk and food supply and totally deprived of any contact, sound, or sight of other animals grow and develop secondary sex characteristics normally. However, of monkeys so reared, all males and many females are sexually ineffective when later put with other animals and, although they are anatomically normal, are thus "sterile."

The parents are so anxious that the child be confirmed at once in his or her gender that they may be disproportionately concerned with sexual identity, even when, for example, the child has a life-threatening heart defect as well as an abnormality of the genitalia. According to psychologists and sociologists, interest and curiosity about sexual matters reflects the instinctive drive to preserve the species, a goal only slightly less important than preservation of self.

After the baby has been born, friends' and relatives' inquiries about the infant's sex and name understandably increase the parents' acute anxiety if the doctors cannot tell them unequivocally that the baby is a boy or girl. Several sex chromosome disorders and many conditions with normal chromosomes may result in changes in the external genitalia that make it difficult to determine whether the infant is male or female.

The decision is vital in these "intersex" conditions because the many medical and social problems which these children may face in adult life will be compounded if the child is reared in the wrong sex. The physician must make a correct and early diagnosis of intersex, discuss the treatment proposed, and help the parents and their relatives understand the eventual outlook for the child.

Until recently, the sex of rearing of a child with abnormal genital organs was determined only by the anatomy and possible function of these underdeveloped organs. That these decisions were sometimes wrong or incompletely managed became apparent when a "boy" would menstruate and develop breasts, or when a "girl" would develop a deep voice and facial hair. If the sex of rearing was altered after early childhood, the psychological effects were usually disastrous.

With recent improvements in technique and knowledge to be described in this chapter, sex diagnosis should become more accurate. However, because these investigations are complex, several weeks may pass before a definite decision can be made on the sex of the child. In the interval, the physician should carefully explain the purpose and progress of these tests to the parents so that they can understand. They may be told that a girl had incompletely formed internal genital organs and will require treatment at puberty if she is to develop as a normal woman, or that she will probably not have children of her own but can marry, adopt children, and live a normal life. The parents should also be helped to prepare their explanations for relatives and friends.

Thus at any age, intersex poses a difficult challenge during diagnosis and treatment. In addition, the physician must spend considerable time counseling the parents, following the child, and giving further treatment as he or she grows to adulthood.

Chromosomal Analysis in Clinical Investigation

In the past decade, chromosomal analyses have established normal patterns (Fig. 11-1), and abnormal chromosomal patterns have become important in the diagnosis of endocrine disorders, particularly abnormalities of sex development. These analyses are often supported by the results of nuclear sex tests (X and Y chromatin) and dermal patterns (skin-ridges) described later in this chapter. All these tests are used in conjunction with the clinical findings and family history. Some of the important points that should be considered for any disorder when dealing with such patients are:

1. Incidence in the general population
2. Effect on development of gonads, ducts, and genitalia
3. Whether all affected individuals seek medical attention
4. Important diagnostic features, clinical and laboratory
5. Age of onset and likely medical problems
6. Which problems can be treated
7. Explanations to the patient concerning the condition
8. Residual limitations after treatment
9. Tests which may increase scientific knowledge

In the clinical investigation of some disorders, chromosomal analyses are used directly as a diagnostic test. Patients with sex chromosome disorders (abnormalities of X or Y chromosome), although they frequently have abnormal gonads and genitalia, usually survive until adult life when defective sexual development and infertility become obvious. In autosomal disorders (all chromosomes except X and Y), the patients have severe physical defects and often die in infancy; for this reason, compared with sex chromosome abnormalities, such disorders contribute little to our knowledge of endocrine disease. Correlation of the chromosome abnormality and features of clinical disorders has given us insight into genetic

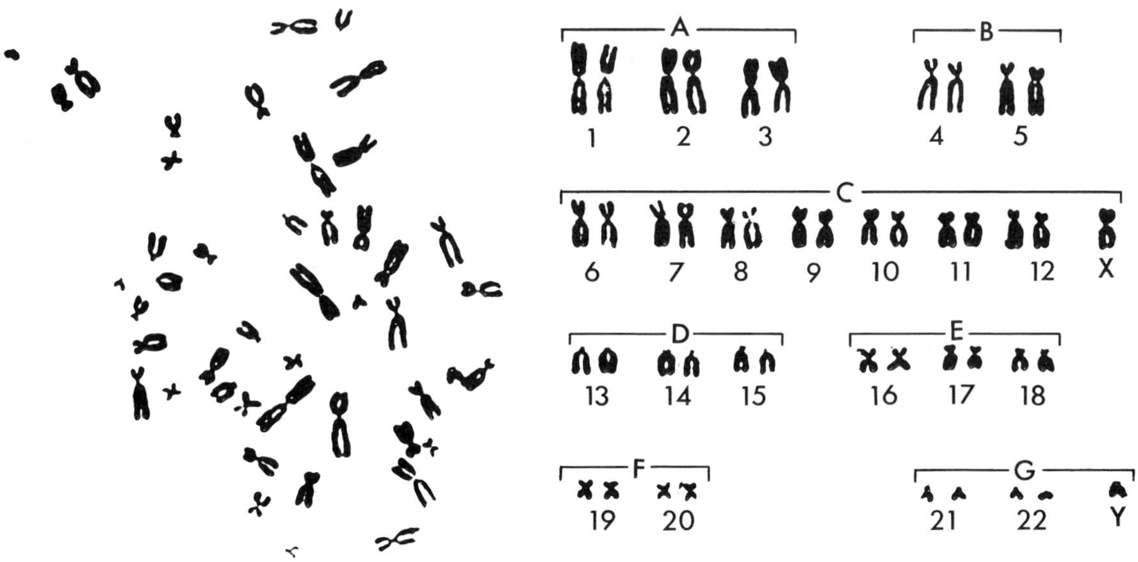

Fig. 11-1. Normal metaphase cell and karyotype. The left half of the figure is a photomicrograph of the chromosomes in a dividing cell at the metaphase stage of mitosis. In the right half of the figure, the chromosomes have been cut from the photomicrograph and arranged according to size and shape to form groups A–G.

With improved techniques, particularly quinacrine fluorescence and modified Giemsa staining, all chromosome pairs of the human set can now be identified.

effects that are due to abnormalities of parts of chromosomes ("chromosome mapping").

The way in which chromosome analyses have clarified our understanding of basic abnormalities is illustrated by the rapid expansion of our knowledge concerning two relatively common intersex conditions, Turner's syndrome and Klinefelter's syndrome.

Turner's Syndrome. Patients with this disorder are infertile, short females, with gonadal dysgenesis, absence of secondary sex characteristics and many other anomalies, particularly webbing of the neck (Fig. 11-2). Turner's syndrome was originally believed due to pituitary hypofunction and later to a primary ovarian defect. However, because patients are sex-chromatin negative, it was then thought that they represented male pseudohermaphrodites or individuals with almost "complete" sex reversal. In Turner's syndrome, the incidence of color blindness resembles that of males (1:10) rather than females (1:100). For this reason, some workers suggested correctly that this syndrome might represent an XO chromosome complex. (Color blindness is due to an X-linked abnormal gene and, hence, females would not be color-blind unless such a gene was present on both X chromosomes.) Subsequently, the discovery of the abnormal 45,XO karyotype confirmed that this syndrome was indeed a chromosomal disorder rather than male pseudohermaphroditism. The disturbances of pituitary and gonadal function are secondary.

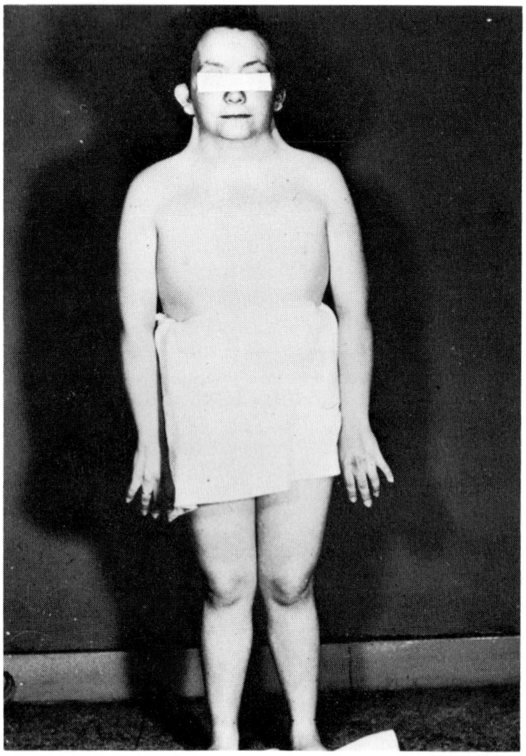

Fig. 11-2. Turner's syndrome. At the time this photograph was taken, Miss B.R. was 26 years of age and 4 feet 7 inches tall (121 cm). She had never menstruated and had developed no secondary sex characteristics. She has low-set ears, webbed neck, and broad shield-like chest, and cubitus valgus (not visible in photo). She also had coarctation of the aorta and agenesis of the right kidney. Her cells were X chromatin negative. Chromosome analysis showed 45,XO karyotype.

Klinefelter's Syndrome. Patients with this disorder are infertile eunuchoid males with small testes. (See also Chapter 9, section on Clinical Syndromes of Hypogonadism.) This syndrome was previously difficult to distinguish from other forms of eunuchoidism. When patients with Klinefelter's syndrome were found to be chromatin-positive (like the pattern in normal females), complete sex reversal was postulated. It is now known that they have 47 chromosomes with an XXY pattern, which explains the X chromatin mass (inactive second X) and the development of testes (due to the Y chromosome).

Once the exact chromosomal status was determined in Turner's and Klinefelter's syndromes (usually 45,XO and 47,XXY, respectively), these and other intersex conditions could be explained and classified. These diagnoses can now be made at all ages (important in newborn surveys for incidence of these conditions). The X chromatin mass can be studied, and in addition, the effect of the Y chromosome and supernumerary X chromosomes can be explained.

General Considerations of Genetically Determined Diseases

In this chapter the emphasis will be placed on chromosomal and sex chromatin defects because they are common in disorders of sex differentia-

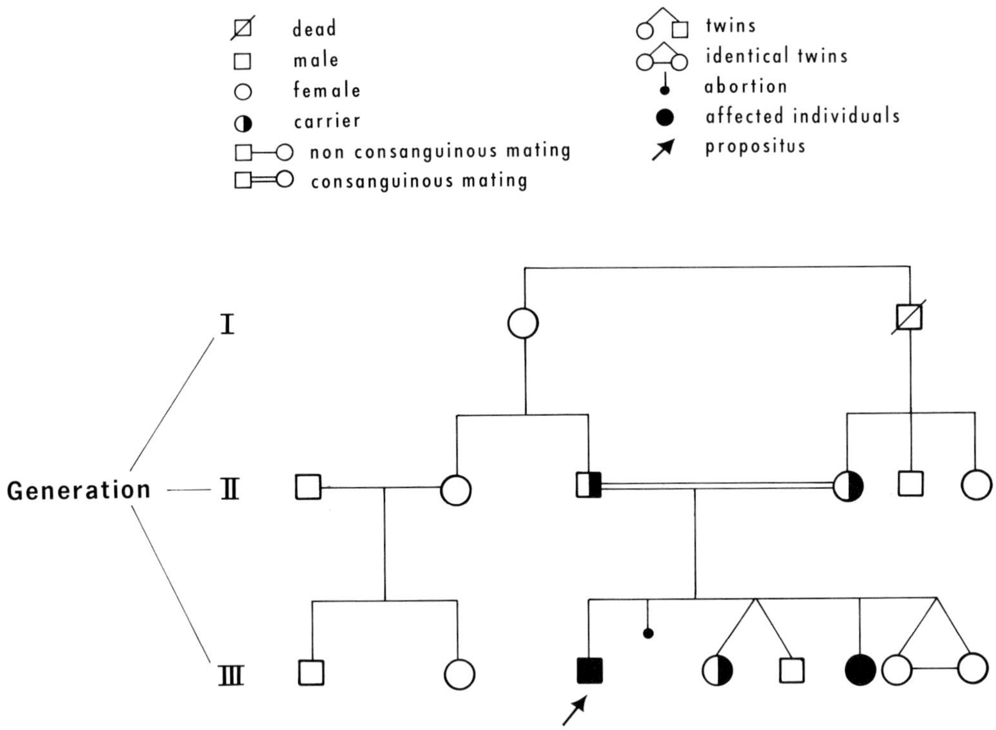

Fig. 11-3. Schematic pedigree. This "map" shows the relationship between individuals of three generations of one family and the results of all pregnancies. The arrow shows the first affected individual that comes to the investigator's attention (propositus). These pedigrees must record all "individuals" including abortuses, must indicate whether each individual has the disorder under study or make plain whether they have survived long enough to manifest it. (Ages on birth year should be included.) Only from such complete pedigrees can we determine the mode of inheritance and predict risk of transmission of the defect.

tion, but the reader should remember that, in general, chromosomal disorders make up only a small fraction of genetic diseases. If he wishes to elucidate the pattern of inheritance of single-gene (dominant/recessive: autosomal/X-linked) and multifactorial disorders, the investigator must obtain a detailed family history and construct a pedigree chart (Fig. 11-3). In such charts, he must record the outcome of all pregnancies so that he can estimate the true fetal wastage and the proportion of males and females affected. The fetal-wastage data will help in estimating the frequency of an abnormal condition in the family, and sex ratios will identify X-linked disorders, particularly if only males are affected or if many males fail to survive to birth. Such pedigree charts help the physician to recognize or exclude disorders that have a known pattern of inheritance and, in genetic counseling, to advise family members of the risks of abnormal offspring.

Chromosomes

These particles of nuclear material are most clearly visible at cell division (mitosis, Fig. 11-4), particularly in metaphase. Between cell divisions (interphase), chromosomes are so long and closely intertwined that individual chromosomes cannot be identified although they are present at all stages of the cell cycle (Fig. 11-5). During part of interphase, the DNA replicates to provide

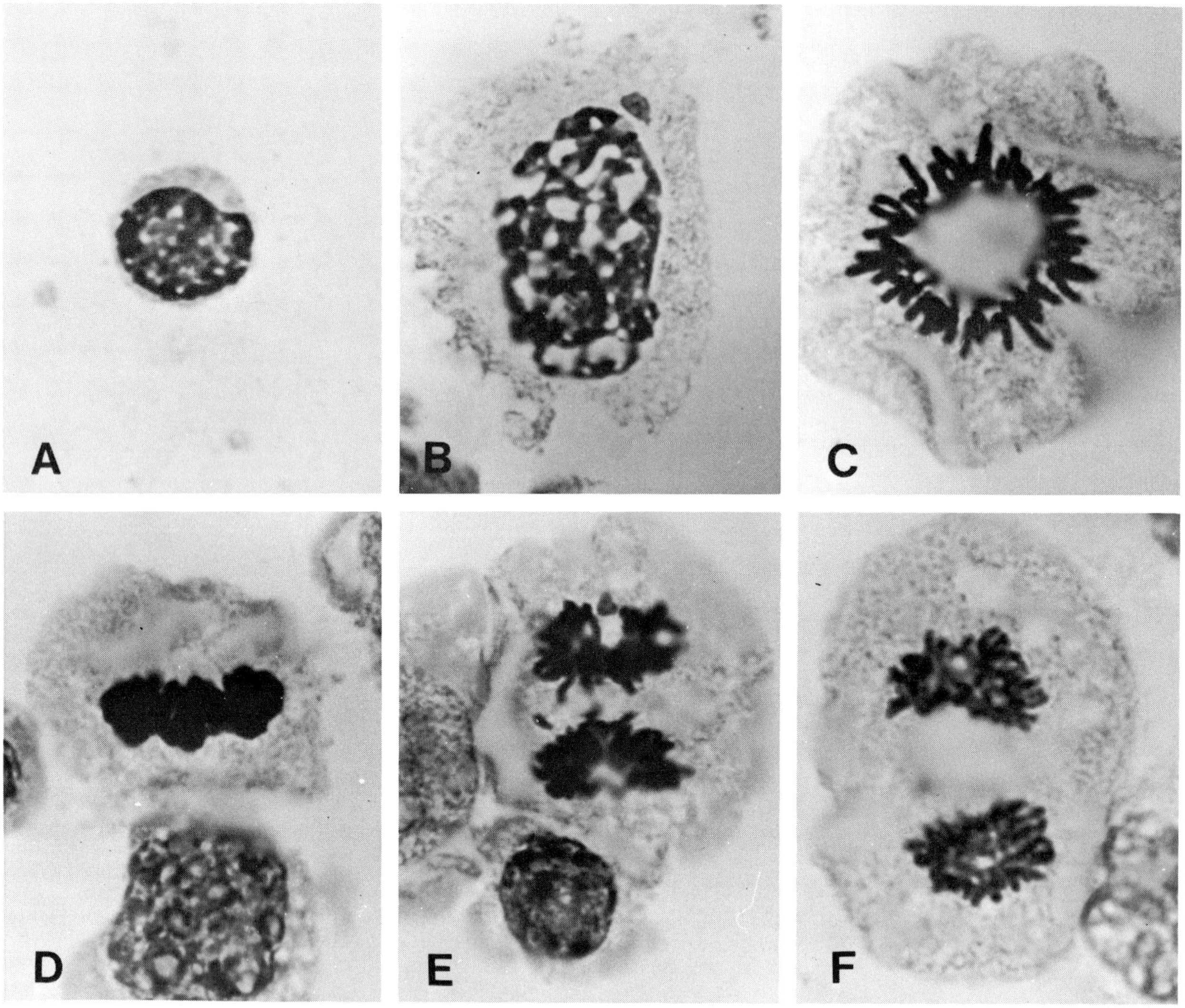

Fig. 11-4. Stages in mitosis. A. Lymphocyte in interphase. **B.** After transformation by phytohemagglutinin. **C.** Face view of the mitotic plate with attached peripherally arranged chromosomes. **D.** Side view of similar mitotic plate. **E.** At anaphase, there is almost complete separation of the paired chromosomes to form daughter nuclei. **F.** At telophase separation is complete and cytoplasmic division is beginning.

genetic material to be shared between two daughter cells at the next cell division. Thus, at the end of interphase, the cell contains exactly double the amount of DNA arranged in two strands (chromatids), compared with the original amount in one chromatid at the beginning (Figs. 11-5 and 11-6). The centromere joins the two arms of a chromatid, holds the two chromatids together after replication (Fig. 11-6), and, in mitosis, attaches to a spindle fiber to permit chromatid movement to daughter cells. In all tissues, through the complex process of mitosis, the amount and individual parts of DNA molecules are equally distributed to the two daughter nuclei. In the more complex reduction-division (meiosis) in germ cells, independent assortment of maternal

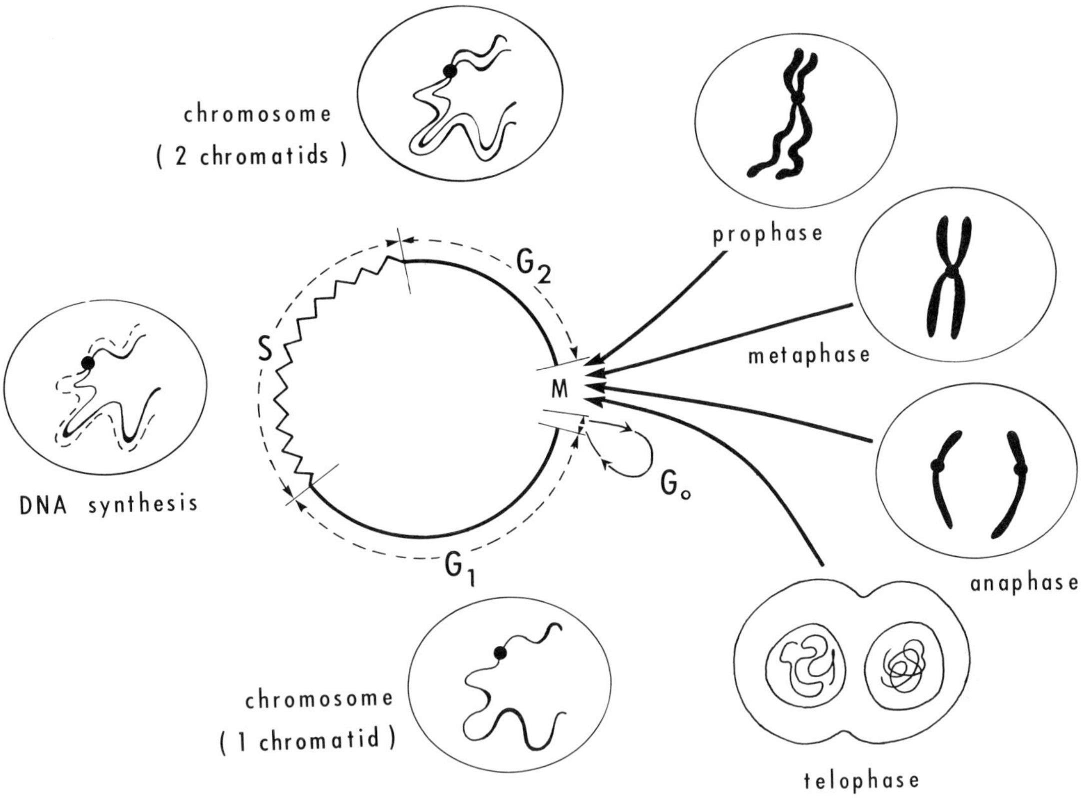

Fig. 11-5. Stages of cell cycle. *Center.* Stages of cell cycle from mitosis (M) through interphase —Gap 1 (G_1), DNA synthesis (S), and Gap 2 (G_2)—to the next mitosis. *Periphery.* Nuclei (with only one chromosome depicted for simplicity) corresponding to each stage.

Some cells enter Gap 0 (G_0) stage until their activity is needed. In G_1, the chromosome has a single chromatid that replicates during S to form two chromatids by G_2. At these stages the chromosomes cannot be seen until they contract and can be separately recognized in mitosis.

Gap 1 is the first period of protein synthesis between mitosis and synthesis. Gap 2 is the second period of protein synthesis between S and mitosis. A second chromatid (shown partially formed in diagram) is formed during period of DNA synthesis. Gap 0 is the resting stage with no protein or DNA synthesis (e.g., small lymphocyte).

Fig. 11-6. Chromosome structure. The G_1 chromosome has one chromatid (*crosshatched*). A second chromatid (*open line*) is formed by DNA replication in *S* period and is complete by G_2. The *centromere* separates DNA material of the chromosome into a short and a long arm. Chromosomes are classified by their length, relative to other chromosomes, and the centromere position, which may be central (metacentric), off center (submetacentric, as in this figure), or near the end of the chromosome (acrocentric).

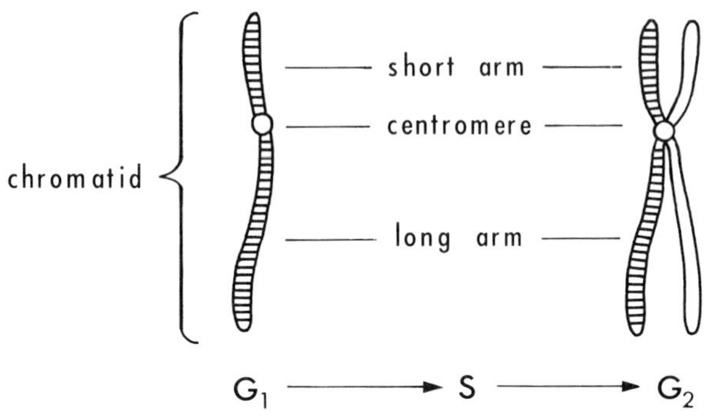

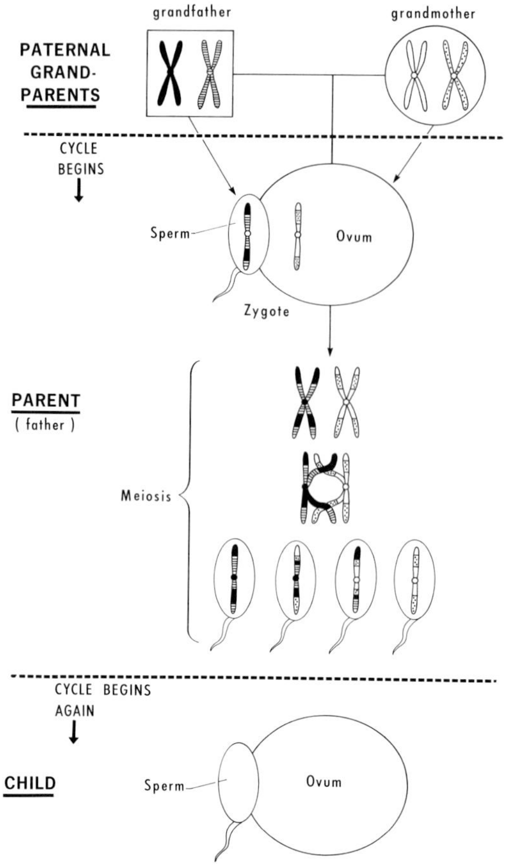

Fig. 11-7. Meiosis and mixing of genes. This diagram illustrates mixing of genetic material in the No. 3 chromosome in a male. Relationship to preceding and succeeding generations are shown above *dotted line* (*grandparents*) and below the line (*child*).

Genetic mixing occurs at meiosis in spermatogenesis and many crossovers (chiasmas) occur between chromosome pairs, only one of which is shown in the diagram. The genetic contents of this pair of chromosomes is represented by combinations of crosshatching, etc.

Note that the chromosome inherited via sperm from paternal grandfather is a mixture of the pair in the grandfather's cells and similarly for the chromosome inherited via ovum (oocyte) from paternal grandmother.

In meiosis in the father, one crossover between upper arms and one in lower arms of a chromatid are shown. This results in four different patterns of genetic material in the four sperm. For simplicity, crossovers in only two chromatids are shown.

An infinite number of combinations can occur, thus ensuring mixture of genetic material and considerable variety and differences in each generation.

and paternal chromosomes provides different combinations of genes within the chromosome; thus the genetic contributions of mother and father are mixed and the genetic endowment of the offspring varies (Fig. 11-7). However, functionally useful genes are grouped in close apposition on the chromosome, which limits the chance of their separation during crossing-over. It should be stressed that the exact arrangement of DNA in a chromosome is still unknown.

Improvements in Chromosome Preparation and Related Tests

For many decades, because of inadequate techniques of examination, the chromosome number was erroneously believed to be 48 (Table 11-1). In 1956, when techniques had improved, the normal human chromosome number was set correctly at 46, and since 1959, using this standard, several hundred different chromosome abnormalities have been described. The technical improvements that set the stage for these advances were relatively

Table 11-1. Improvements in Techniques and Knowledge

1949	**X chromatin (Barr body) in females***
Pre-1956	Erroneous belief: 48 human chromosomes
1956	46 human chromosomes proved
1959	Mongolism, Klinefelter's and Turner's syndromes, etc., identified
1960	Phytohemagglutinin (PHA) used
1961	Autoradiography used
1963	Chromosome culture kits developed
1963	Microtechniques (fingerprick) developed
1964	XYY syndrome identified (? tall, aggressive)
1965	Prenatal tests (amniocentesis) developed
1965+	Newborn surveys
1970	**Fluorescence tests of Y chromosome in males***
1970	Identification of all chromosomes now possible

* The two convenient nuclear sex tests are shown in bold face for emphasis.

simple: *mitosis-arresting agents* were introduced to increase the number of mitotic figures available for study; individual cells were swollen by *hypotonic fluids* to disperse the chromosomes in the cytoplasm; and the cells were *"squashed" or air-dried flat* (Fig. 11-8) to present the chromosomes in one plane, making them easier to count and photograph. The following list gives details of the procedure.

1. Culture cells until enough cells in mitosis are present.
   Blood lymphocytes 72–96 hours
   Skin fibroblasts 2–6 weeks
2. Arrest dividing cells at metaphase stage of mitosis by colchicine.
3. Swell in hypotonic fluid to separate chromosomes.
4. Fix in Carnoy's fluid.
5. Flatten by air-drying or "squashing" to provide chromosomes in one plane of focus (Fig. 11-8).
6. Stain and make permanent slides.

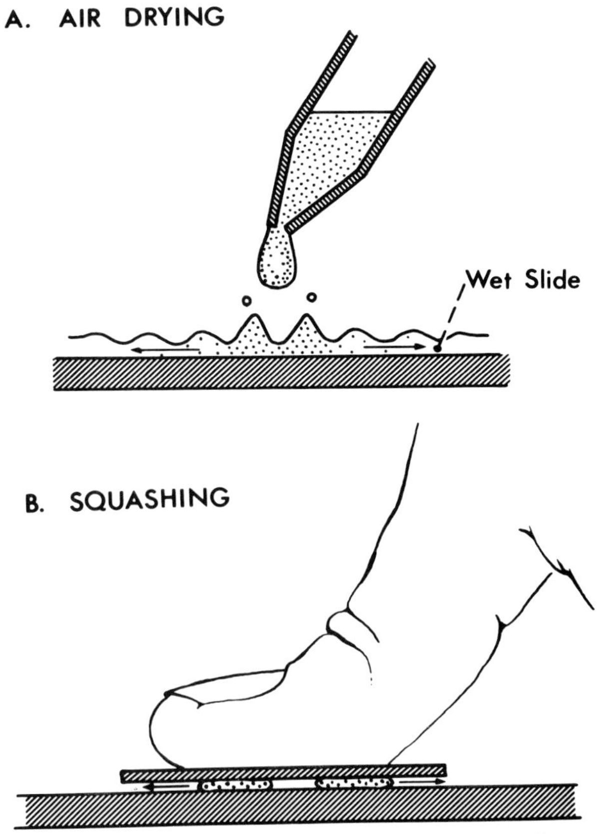

Fig. 11-8. 'Air-dry squash.' Two methods, air-drying and squashing, are used to flatten the cells, separate the chromosomes from each other and put them in one plane of focus. Cells in acetic acid–alcohol suspension (represented by dots in the diagram) may be flattened (A) by rapid air drying on a glass slide or (B) by squashing the cells flat beneath a coverslip by even pressure with the thumb.

Many tissues can be used for chromosome studies (Table 11-2). Originally, for analysis, tissues with a high mitotic rate, such as marrow, were needed, but now marrow cells are needed only to investigate leukemias. With phytohemagglutinin, lymphocytes can be cultured from peripheral blood for chromosomal analysis, and, with microcultures of whole blood, chromosomal analyses can be made from fingerprick samples. When unusual chromosomal abnormalities are being studied, fibroblasts grown from skin samples may confirm the findings from lymphocyte culture or may reveal additional patterns. In the differential diagnosis of individuals with infertility or with a suspected chromosomal abnormality that cannot be detected on mitotic preparation, the meiotic cells in tissue obtained at testicular biopsy can be studied.

Table 11-2. Tissues Used in Chromosome Studies

Source	*Cells*	*Purpose*
Cultured blood	Lymphocytes	Autopsy
Cultured spleen	Lymphocytes	Special cases or autopsy
Cultured spleen and other tissues	Fibroblasts	Leukemias
Direct marrow		Very special cases only (meiosis)
Direct adult testis	Germ cells	
Direct fetal ovary	Germ cells	Routine

Chromosomal Analysis

In chromosomal analysis, a technician counts the number of chromosomes in each of several

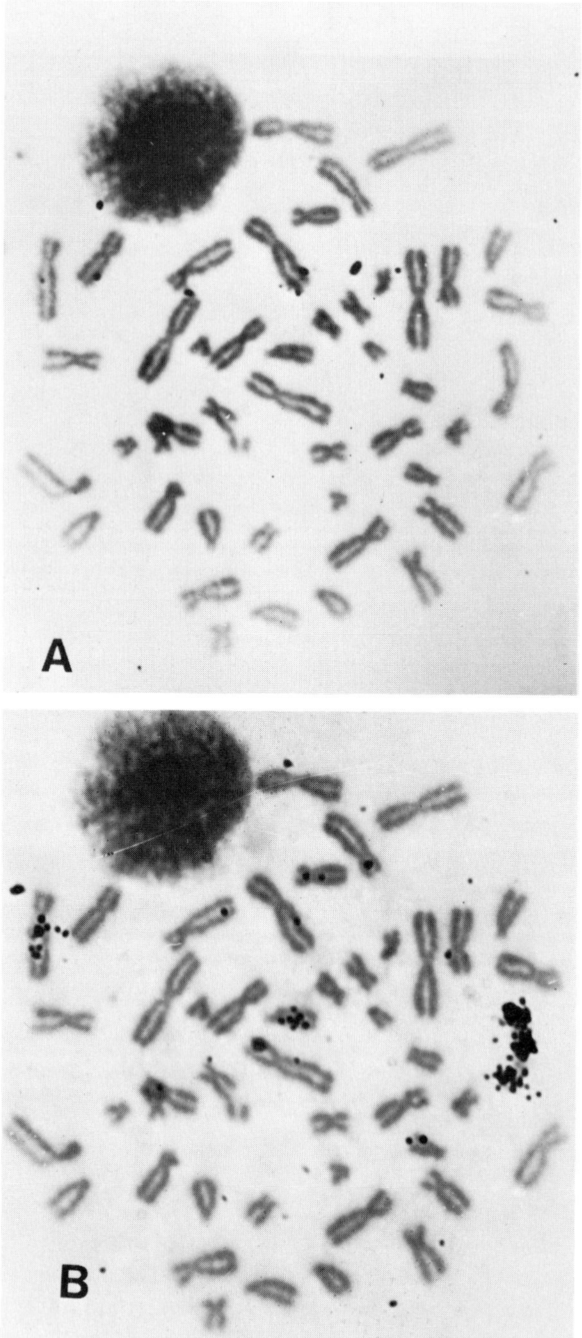

Fig. 11-9. Metaphase cell (A) before and (B) after autoradiography. An interphase nucleus is at the upper left of these photographs. The late-labeling X (*arrow*) is clearly demarcated by heavy concentration of silver grains over it. One of the D and one of the B group chromosomes are lightly labeled. The dots in the photomicrograph (A) are dirt and not silver grains.

cells, and establishes a basic chromosome number. The general procedure is as follows:

1. Select cells with well-spread, clear chromosomes.
2. Analyze chromosomes from many cells, into groups and pairs.
3. Cut, from prints, chromosomes from some cells (left half of Fig. 11-1).
4. Arrange in pairs to form a karyotype (chromosomal pattern): The pairs are arranged and numbered in descending order of size (longest is No. 1; smallest is No. 22). The sex chromosomes are omitted from this sequence (right half of Fig. 11-1).
5. On the basis of size and centromere position, the chromosomes are sorted into seven groups: A (1–3), B (4–5), C (6–12,X), D (13–15), E (16–18), F (19–20), G (21–22,Y). Only certain pairs (1, 2, 3, 16, 17, 18) and the Y chromosome can be separately identified.

Additional chromosomes can be identified by their characteristic "labeling pattern" by autoradiography, fluorescent staining, and a modified Giemsa technic. In autoradiography, radioactive thymidine added to the culture becomes incorporated into some chromosomes during stages of DNA synthesis (replication).[27] This radioactivity can be detected because it produces silver grains in a photographic emulsion left in close contact with the cell for some weeks. Figure 11-9 shows the same cell (A) before autoradiography and (B) with the exposed, developed emulsion lying over the chromosomes. The significance of late replicating chromosomes, which replicate their DNA later in the cell cycle than other chromosomes, is as follows:

1. They are involved in chromosomal disorders.
2. They have relatively terminal centromeres.
3. They are associated together in the cell.
4. They are involved in translocations.
5. They probably contain some less genetically active or important regions.

An exciting new technique for chromosome identification is fluorescence microscopy of

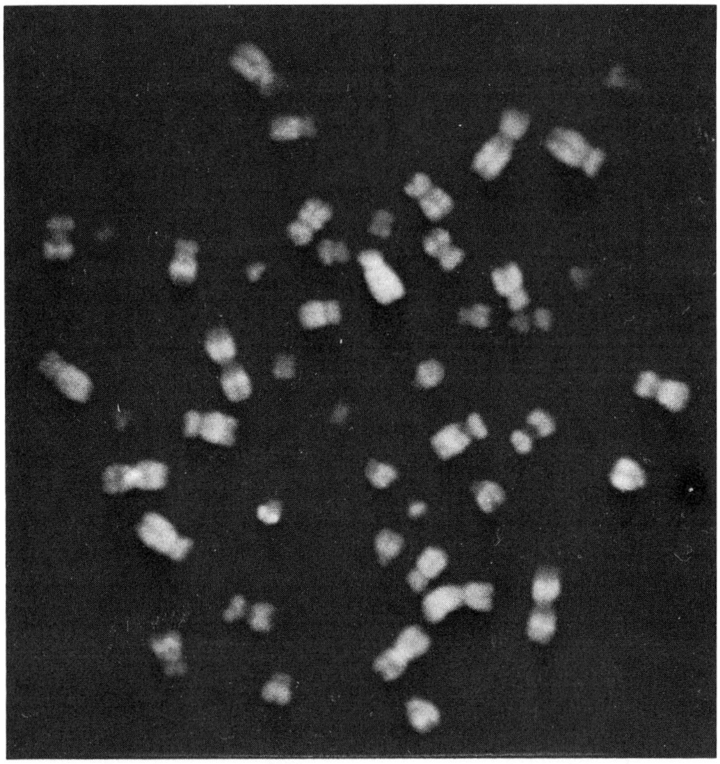

Fig. 11-10. Fluorescence photomicrograph of chromosomes. The chromosomes in this cell have been 'stained' with quinacrine dihydrochloride and examined with transmitted dark-field blue-violet light. There are areas of bright and dull fluorescence along the lengths of the chromatids that enable most chromosome pairs to be identified (not just the groups as by conventional staining). New DNA-denaturation-Giemsa stain techniques appear also to characterize individual chromosomes with the advantage that such preparations can be viewed by ordinary microscopes and the preparations are permanent.

quinacrine-stained metaphase cells. The method reveals a characteristic banding pattern along with length of the chromosomes (Fig. 11-10).[5,17,25,45] Another new technique, which produces a characteristic banding pattern along chromosomes, is Giemsa stain after DNA denaturation–renaturation or enzyme pretreatment.[8,9,15,31,37,38,43]

Such techniques will eventually replace tritiated thymidine autoradiography because all human chromosomes can be identified in minutes, whereas autoradiography takes many weeks and only identifies about one-half of the number of chromosomes present (Table 11-3). The additional accuracy and information they provide will enable "computer karyotyping" to be feasible. These techniques are also discussed later in this

Table 11-3. Comparison of Methods for Chromosome Analysis

	Standard microscopy	*Fluorescence microscopy*
Advantages	Well-known standard methods and results	All chromosomes identifiable by characteristic patterns of fluorescence
Disadvantages	Only 1–3; 16–18 and Y chromosomes identifiable Autoradiography (laborious) is required for additional identification of B 4–5; D 13–15, and a second X	Expensive equipment Method new

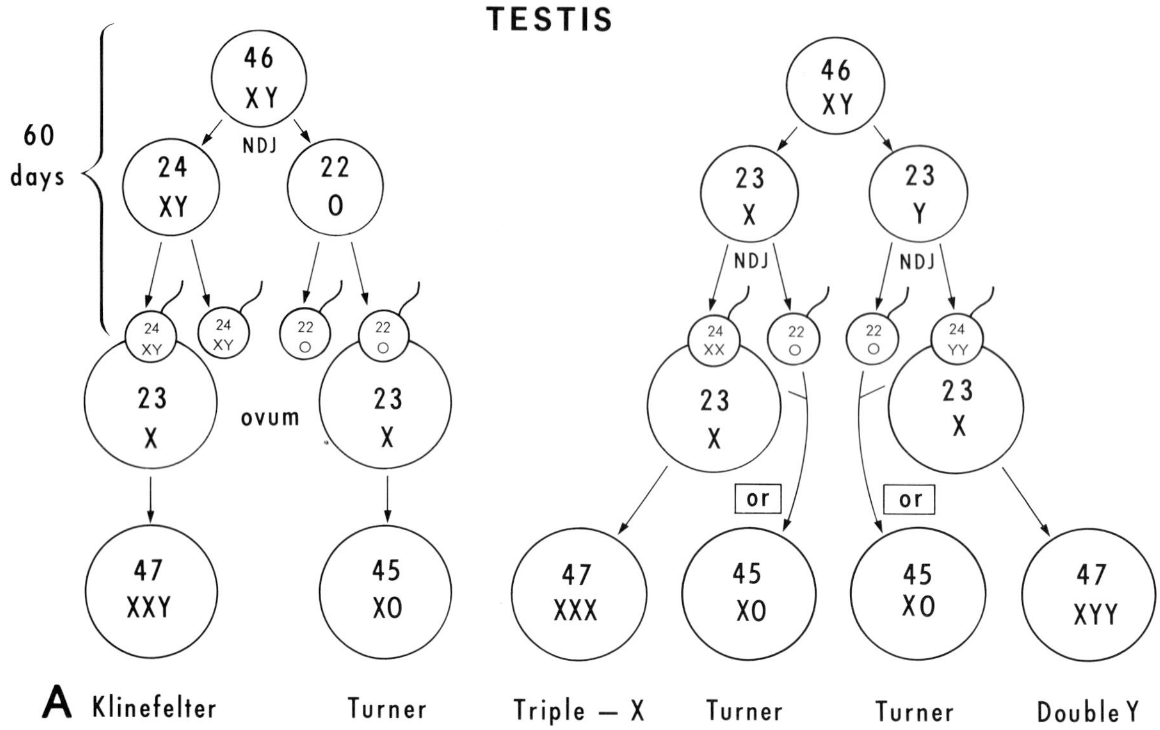

Fig. 11-11. Role of nondisjunction in common sex chromosome abnormalities (Klinefelter's, Turner's, triple X and double Y). Stages of meiosis with nondisjunction (*NDJ*) producing abnormal numbers of chromosomes during spermatogenesis **(A)** and oogenesis **(B)**. Each circle represents a cell with its chromosome number and sex chromosome pattern within. Each vertically arranged group (or column) of circles depicts development from germ cell (*upper*) to gamete (*middle*) and zygote (*bottom*). Circles representing oocytes and zygotes are shown larger than developing germ cells. The smallest circles represent polar bodies in oogenesis and spermatozoa (*with tails*).

A. In the testis, nondisjunction error at first division of meiosis (*at left*) results in production of two spermatocytes with 24,XY and 22,O pattern, which by further divisions result in two spermatozoa (24,XY) and two with 22,O pattern. When these fertilize normal 23,X oocytes, abnormal zygotes are formed, which may eventually become 47,XXY (Klinefelter's syndrome) or 45,XO (Turner's syndrome).

Normal first division of meiosis (*at right*) forms a 23,X and a 23,Y spermatocyte. A nondisjunctional error at second division of meiosis results eventually in three classes of spermatozoa: 24,XX, 22,O, and 24,YY. When these fertilize a normal 23,X oocyte, abnormal zygotes are formed: 47,XXX (triple-X); 45,XO (Turner's syndrome); and 47,XYY (double Y syndrome).

B. In the ovary, first and second divisions of each oogonia eventually result in one oocyte and polar bodies. Nondisjunction at either the first or second meiotic division results in 24,XX or 22,O. When these are fertilized, the chromosomal pattern in the zygote will depend upon whether the spermatozoa carries an X or a Y chromosome and will result in: 47,XXY (Klinefelter's syndrome); 47,XXX (triple X); or 45,XO (Turner's). A 45,YO embryo has never been detected and is presumed to be incompatible with survival (nonviable).

chapter in the section on the Y chromatin test (fluorescent Y).

An editorial[10] states: "The technique (fluorescence) not only permits visual typing of the 3,D group, and Y chromosomes, but the identification of all chromosomes by fluorometric tracings . . ."

Another editorial[11] states: "At the least, the

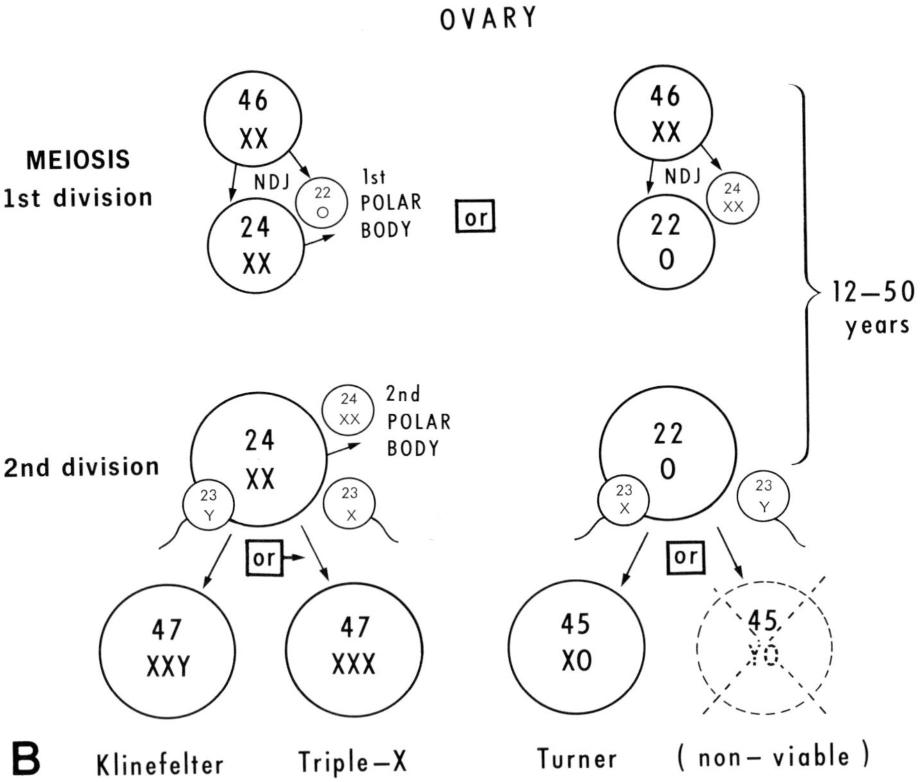

new technique will hasten the rate of progress in human cytogenetics and with any luck the next five years should see a number of fresh insights opened into the behaviour of chromosomes in cells . . . Important discoveries seem to be emerging rather faster than they can appear in print . . . The acridine dyes certainly hold a lot of interesting secrets in store and in the coming months laboratories throughout the world will doubtless be fluorescing with excitement to find out just what these may be."

Types of Chromosome Abnormality

These consist of abnormalities of chromosome number (aneuploidy), the presence of two or more cell patterns (mosaicism or chimerism), and structural chromosomal changes.

Most aneuploid patterns are usually due to nondisjunction in the parental gonad (Fig. 11-11) and have 47 chromosomes—XXY, XYY, XXX in sex-chromosome abnormalities, and an additional No. 21, 18, or 13 in autosome abnormalities (Table 11-4). In XO sex-chromosome abnormalities and in some translocations of chromosomal material between two chromosomes with loss of a centromere, the chromosome number is 45.

Abnormalities of chromosome number may be complicated by the presence of several patterns as in mosaicism, which is the presence in one individual of two or more chromosomally different cell types derived from one zygote (Fig. 11-12). A chimera is similar to mosaicism, but the cells are derived from two zygotes, as in transfusions or exchange of cells between certain twins. Mosaicism is important because, in a chromosomally abnormal individual, the presence of

Table 11-4. Incidence of Common Chromosome Abnormalities

Karyotype	*Conception**	*Ending in spontaneous abortion*	*Newborn*	*Adult*
Sex chromosomes				
Turner's & variants	1:80	98	1:5000	1:5000
Klinefelter's XXY	1:500	0	1:500	1:500
XYY	1:?500	0	1:?500	1:?500
Triple X	1:1000	0	1:1000	1:1000
Autosomes				
Mongoloid	1:200	70	1:700	?1:1200
D/D translocation	1:1000	0	1:1000	1:1000
D syndrome	1:3000	70	1:10,000	0
E syndrome	1:5000	0	1:5000	0
Cri-du-chat	1:50–100,000	?99.9	0	0
Triploids	?1:80	0	1:50–100,000	?1.:1200

* These figures are based on (1) estimates that at least 10% of all conceptions end in early spontaneous abortions; and (2) the observations that 30% of spontaneous human abortuses have chromosomal abnormalities.

some normal cells may modify the expected clinical findings and make diagnosis difficult; and, in an apparently normal individual, the presence of a few abnormal cells, particularly in the gonads, may produce defective gametes and result in some abnormal offspring.

Structural chromosomal abnormalities include translocations, inversions (rearrangement of

Fig. 11-12. Role of postzygotic nondisjunction errors and anaphase lag. Circles in upper row represent zygotes which are normal (*a-d*) and abnormal (*e*). Nondisjunction of anaphase lag at first mitosis will result in daughter cells with two different chromosome patterns derived from one zygote and mosaicism results (*upper row, b-d*). If one of the cell types is nonviable, as in the 45,YO cell formed (*a*), mosaicism will not occur. If nondisjunction occurs later than the first division, the original nondisjunction can produce mosaicism (*bottom row, a*) or formation of three cell types, XO, XY, XYY (*bottom row, b*) and XO, XX, XXX (*bottom row, c*).

In another mitotic error (*d* and *e*), anaphase lag (*AL*) produces mosaicism: when a chromosome (in this instance, X) does not move with the other chromosomes and is not included in the nucleus of a daughter cell. Anaphase lag can also result in cells with a normal chromosome pattern from an abnormal zygote (*f*).

The results of mosaicism depend upon the proportions of each cell present, the stage when the mosaicism developed, the organs or tissues involved, and whether the zygote was originally normal (*a-d*) or abnormal (*e*).

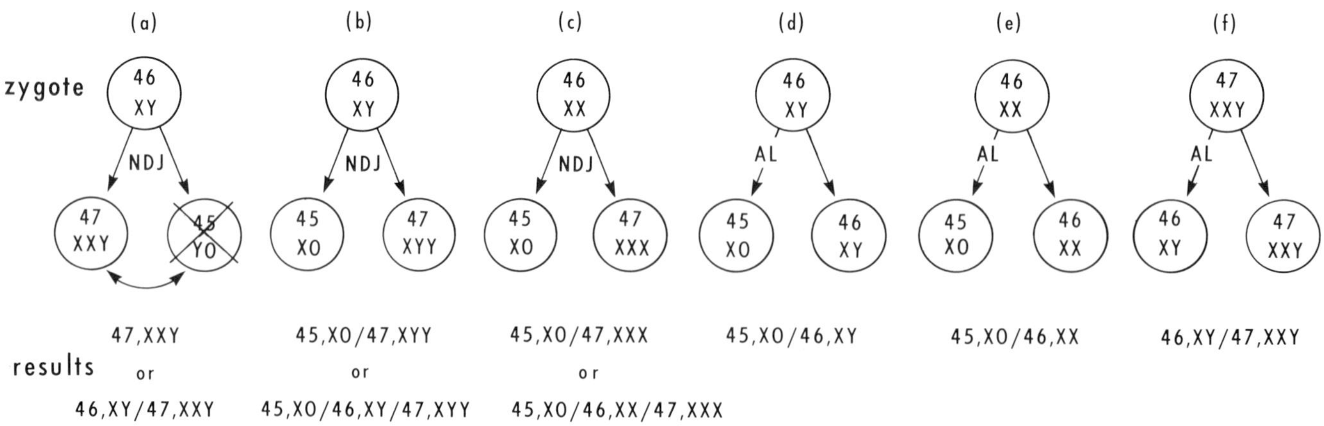

material within the chromosome), and deletions and rings—loss of part(s) of a chromosome (Figs. 11-13 and 11-14).

Consequence of Chromosome Abnormalities

One chromosome of each pair contains the maternal, and the other the paternal, contribution. To be normal, a person must have the normal amount of DNA in each cell.

The effect of excess DNA, usually manifested as 47 chromosomes, depends on the nature of the additional chromosome: an additional autosome is frequently associated with multiple malformations, mental retardation, and death in fetal life, infancy, or early childhood. Most people with an additional sex chromosome reach maturity (Table 11-4). The morphologic identification of the additional chromosome is often supported by the clinical features of the patient—e.g., in mongolism due to trisomy (presence in triplicate) of a No. 21 chromosome.

The effect of deficiency of DNA also depends upon the chromosome and amount of DNA involved. Persons with small deficiencies of part of an autosome are usually severely mentally retarded whereas one entire sex chromosome can be lacking and produce fewer developmental abnormalities. Total absence of an autosome has not been found in spontaneous abortuses, presumably because if the cells have such a loss of DNA, the embryo seldom survives even to fetal life. This observation suggests that in patients reported to have total absence of an autosome (usually of group G), an undetected translocation is a more likely explanation of the missing autosome.

A person with the normal amount of DNA *abnormally* distributed among his chromosomes (Fig. 11-15) is usually physically and mentally normal, because each cell has a complete set of genes (Fig. 11-13, except at *lower left,* and Fig. 11-14, except *C*). However, such a person would have a greatly increased risk of producing abnormal offspring (Fig. 11-15).

Biological Fitness and Male Vulnerability

Biological fitness implies that, as judged by clinical and laboratory tests, the individual is "normal" and that growth, lifespan, and reproductive fitness will be normal. This last assessment is based on his fertility—i.e., ability to

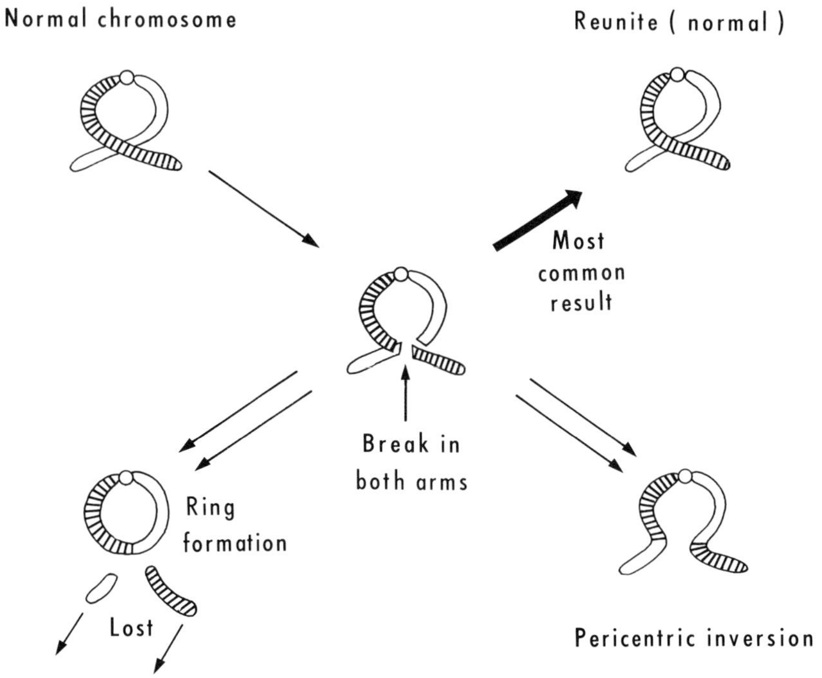

Fig. 11-13. Production of structural chromosome abnormalities (Part I). Normal No. 3 chromosome (*upper left*) has been drawn with overlapping arms, one crosshatched and one open so that breakage and recombination can be followed.

Chromosomal breakage by an ionizing particle, etc., at point of overlap (*center*) will produce a break in both arms.

After breakage these arms usually reunite with no morphologic evidence of damage (*upper right*).

In abnormal recombinations, either the proximal ends of both arms unite to form a ring and the terminal portions of the chromosomes are lost (*lower left*), or the proximal ends unite with the opposite terminal portion to form a pericentric inversion (*lower right*). The latter results in no loss of chromosome material but leads to abnormal chromosome pairing at meiosis.

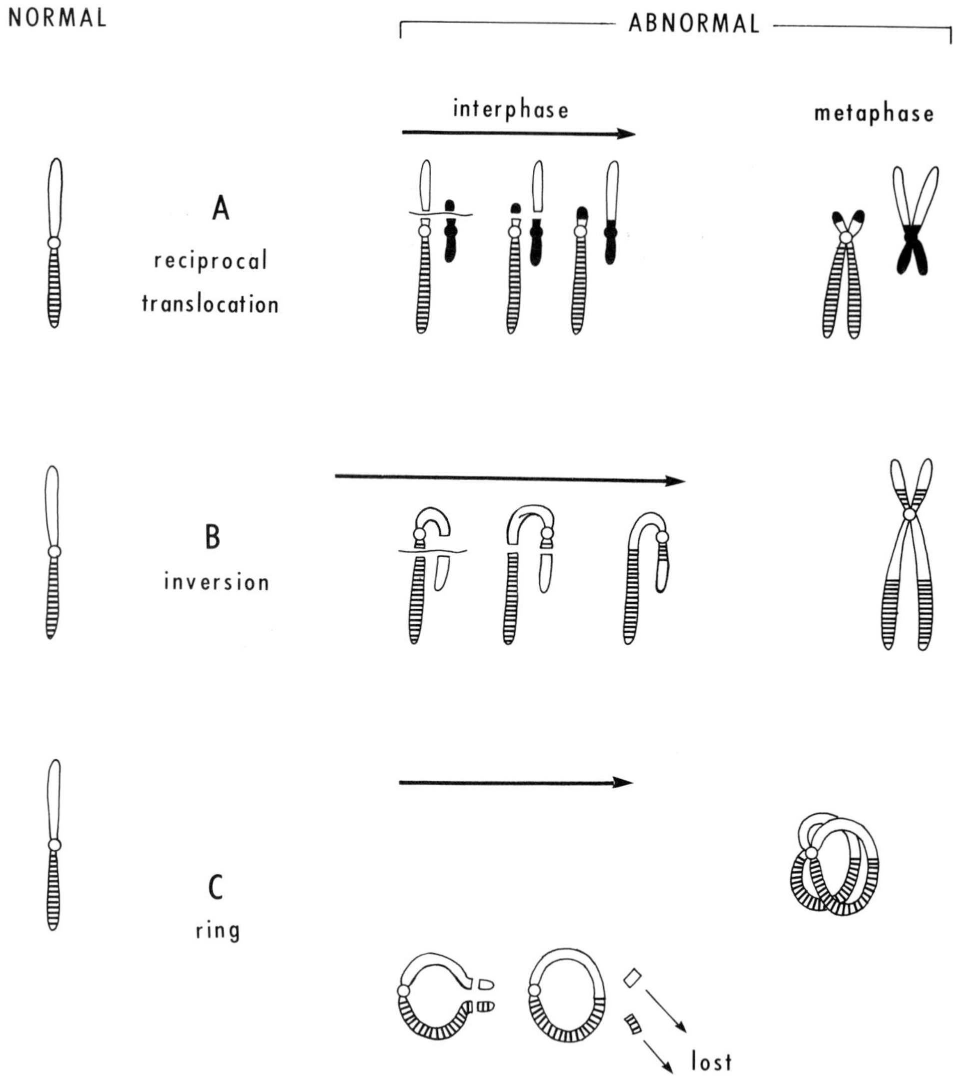

Fig. 11-14. Production of structural chromosome abnormalities (Part II). Normal No. 3 chromosomes at single chromatid (G_1) stage (*left*) have one arm cross-hatched to follow the breakage-recombination sequence (shown in the interphase part of the figure), No. 21 chromosome is drawn solid black.

A. A reciprocal translocation with exchange of terminal portions of chromosome between two chromosomes—the No. 3 and No. 21 (*solid black*). Note change in size and shape of these chromosomes. Each cell will contain the correct amount of genetic material, but abnormalities will occur at meiosis.

B. Pericentric inversion which is morphologically recognizable (in contrast to that in Fig. 11-13, *lower right* and to all paracentric inversions) because in this case the centromere position has altered, as shown in the metaphase stage (*right*).

C. A ring with loss of different amounts of the terminal portions of both chromosome arms compared with that in Fig. 11-13, *lower left,* although this cannot be determined morphologically.

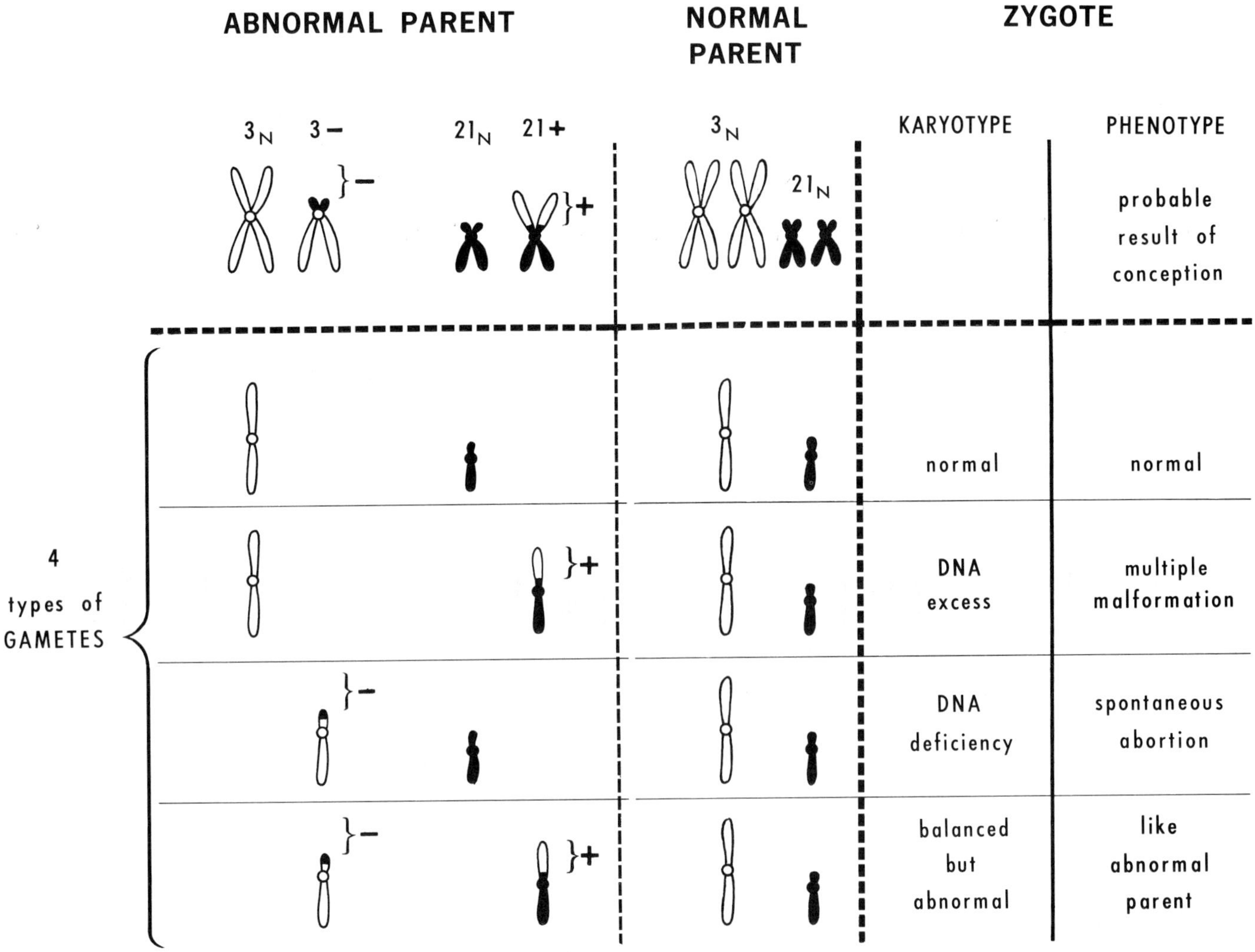

Fig. 11-15. Abnormal offspring of a parent with a balanced translocation. The upper row left shows two chromosome pairs from the parent with a translocation. One normal 3 (3_N) and one normal 21 (21_N) contrast with two other chromosomes which are abnormal because of translocation involving their short arms. This results in an abnormal 3 (3—), DNA deficiency, and an abnormal 21 (21+), DNA excess.

Because the gametes formed by this parent have equal chances of containing the 3_N or the 3—, or the 21_N or 21+, four types of gamete may arise from these two chromosome pairs (*left* below the *broken line*).

Assuming that these gametes are fertilized by normal gametes from another parent (*center column*), the karyotype of the zygote and the probable result of the conception (phenotype) are those shown (at *right*).

DNA deficiency is usually more deleterious than DNA excess so that early spontaneous abortion or earlier unnoticed loss of the embryo is frequent, particularly when an autosome is involved.

produce offspring that are "normal" and of an expected sex distribution. Because most human families are small, it is difficult to determine sex distribution. Each "normal" individual has 3–5% of deleterious (mutant) genes, but these are usually not expressed because of normal alleles (genes at the same locus) present on the homologue (matching chromosome of the pair).

Because the Y chromosome has very few genes, males have little chance to balance deleterious genes on the X chromosome and are therefore more likely to manifest disorders due to such genes. If the effect of the deleterious gene resulted in fetal death in these males, the presence of an abnormality could be detected in a large kindred because there would be only half the expected number of males.

Size of X and Y Chromosome

In most mammals, including man, the X and Y chromosomes differ greatly in size because, during mammalian evolution, genetically important material was transferred (translocated) from the Y chromosome to other chromosomes. Because the X and Y chromosomes share so few alleles, they pair end-to-end at the short arms during meiosis in the testes and thus greatly restrict the exchange of sex-determining factors (Fig. 11-16). Unless they disposed themselves in this way, intersex individuals would be produced more frequently, and because these individuals are sterile, the reproductive fitness of the species would be greatly reduced.

The Lyon Hypothesis: Gene Inactivation

Because of the great difference in the size of the X and Y chromosomes, female cells have more genetic material than male cells. To explain the limited effect of this excess material, workers have postulated that, in the female, most of one X chromosome is inactivated. The discovery of the sex-chromatin mass (Barr body) provided an explanation of this inactivation (Figs. 11-17 and 11-18). Because, in the female, one of the two X chromosomes is heterochromatic during most of the cell cycle, we believe that this tightly coiled chromosome cannot contribute much RNA and hence cannot influence the cell.

Lyon postulated that:

1. In most cells of the embryo, one of the X chromosomes is inactivated when the X chromatin mass forms.
2. The paternal or maternal X chromosome is inactivated at random.
3. In the progeny of each of these cells, the same paternal or maternal chromosome remains inactivated.

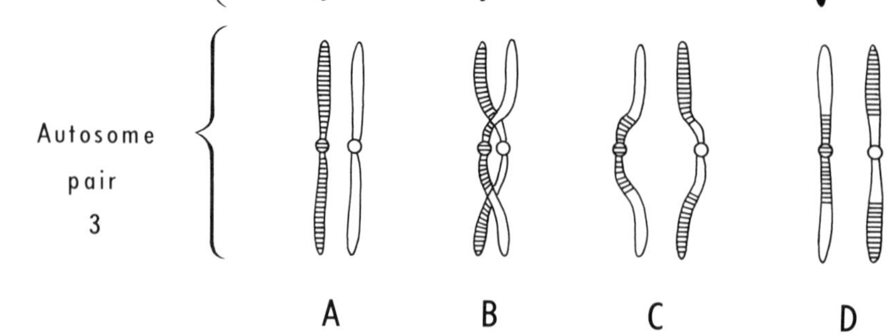

Fig. 11-16. Contrast between pairing of sex chromosomes and autosomes at meiosis in a male. An X chromosome (*upper line, solid black*) from the mother and a Y chromosome (*white*) from his father pair end-to-end (B) restricting exchange of genetic material.

On the lower line, an autosome pair, one (crosshatched) from the mother and one (*white*) from the father, pair side-to-side (A). They are in such close apposition as to exchange genetic material (B) and produce chromosomes with contribution from both parents (C *and* D).

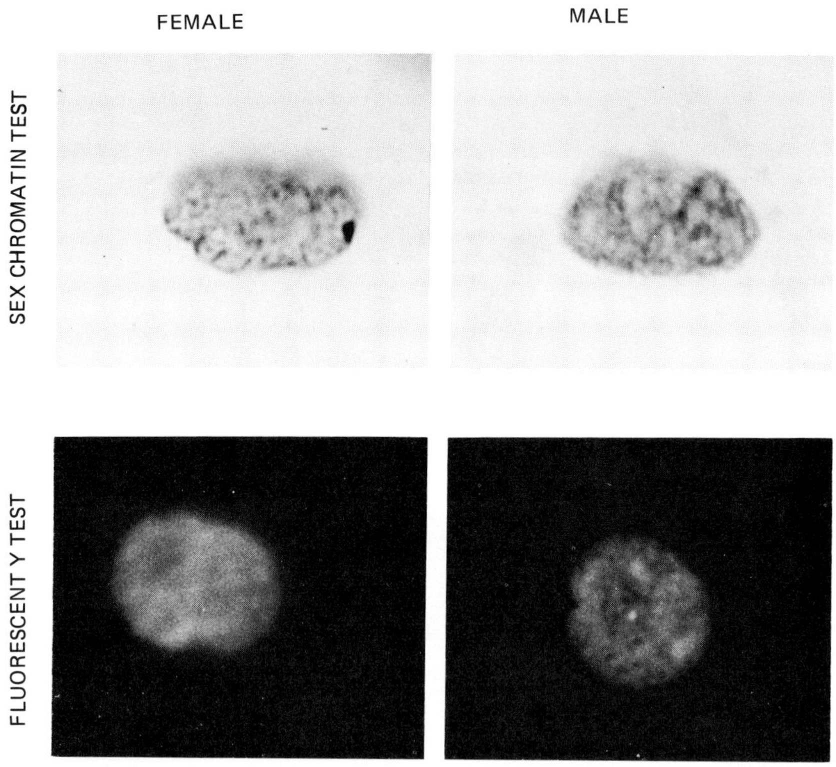

Fig. 11-17. Tests of nuclear sex. *Top.* X chromatin test is positive (cells contain a dark mass at the periphery of the nucleus) in most epithelial cells from females (*left*); and negative in most cells from males (*right*).

Bottom. Fluorescence reveals female lymphocyte nucleus negative (*left*) and male, positive (*right*), with a fluorescent bright spot within the nucleus. Results of both tests provide positive identification of the male (Y chromatin test) and female (X chromatin test). Positive X and Y chromatin tests would suggest Klinefelter's syndrome (XXY), and negative results for both tests would suggest Turner's syndrome (XO).

This hypothesis implies that with respect to the expression of genes on the X chromosome, females are mosaics: Their tissues are composed of some cells with a functional paternal X and other cells with a functional maternal X. In most females, approximately one-half of the cells have maternal and one-half have paternal functioning X chromosomes. However, in exceptional females, chiefly maternal X chromosomes will function and such females will be prone to some or all of the sex-linked genetic diseases usually found only in males.

Early studies of human material showed that X chromatin masses form about the tenth to twelfth day after conception, but more recent studies suggest that cells from females have twice as much enzyme activity as equivalent male cells as long as 10 weeks after conception, which implies that the second X chromosome is not completely inactivated until at least the third month of gestation. Serious differences apart from sex development would be expected between XO, XX, XY, and XXY individuals if all X chromosomes functioned during the embryonic period of human development because of activity of many genes on the X chromosomes and even more differences would be anticipated in individuals with many X chromosomes (Fig. 11-18). In fact, XXXX,

Fig. 11-18. Developmental anomalies associated with extra sex chromosomes. Some frequent sex chromosome anomalies (*Column 1, category*) and their sex chromosome complex (*Column 2*). At conception all chromosomes are presumed to be active and therefore extra or structurally abnormal X chromosomes produce developmental defects in those conditions (*enclosed in squares*).

During the first trimester, an X chromatin mass is formed in interphase cells by contraction of the second or additional X chromosomes (Lyon hypothesis, see text). The contracted X (*Column 3, stippled background*) is formed from a second or additional X's and any abnormal X's. At this stage the genetic influence of the extra X's is minimal or perhaps absent. *Column 4* shows the X chromatin patterns of a cell with a central uncontracted X and the maximum number of X chromatin masses.

This inactivation of X's is necessary to preserve some balance between the genetic action of X-linked genes in females (XX) and males (X). If the extra X's were inactivated completely at conception, there would be no abnormalities.

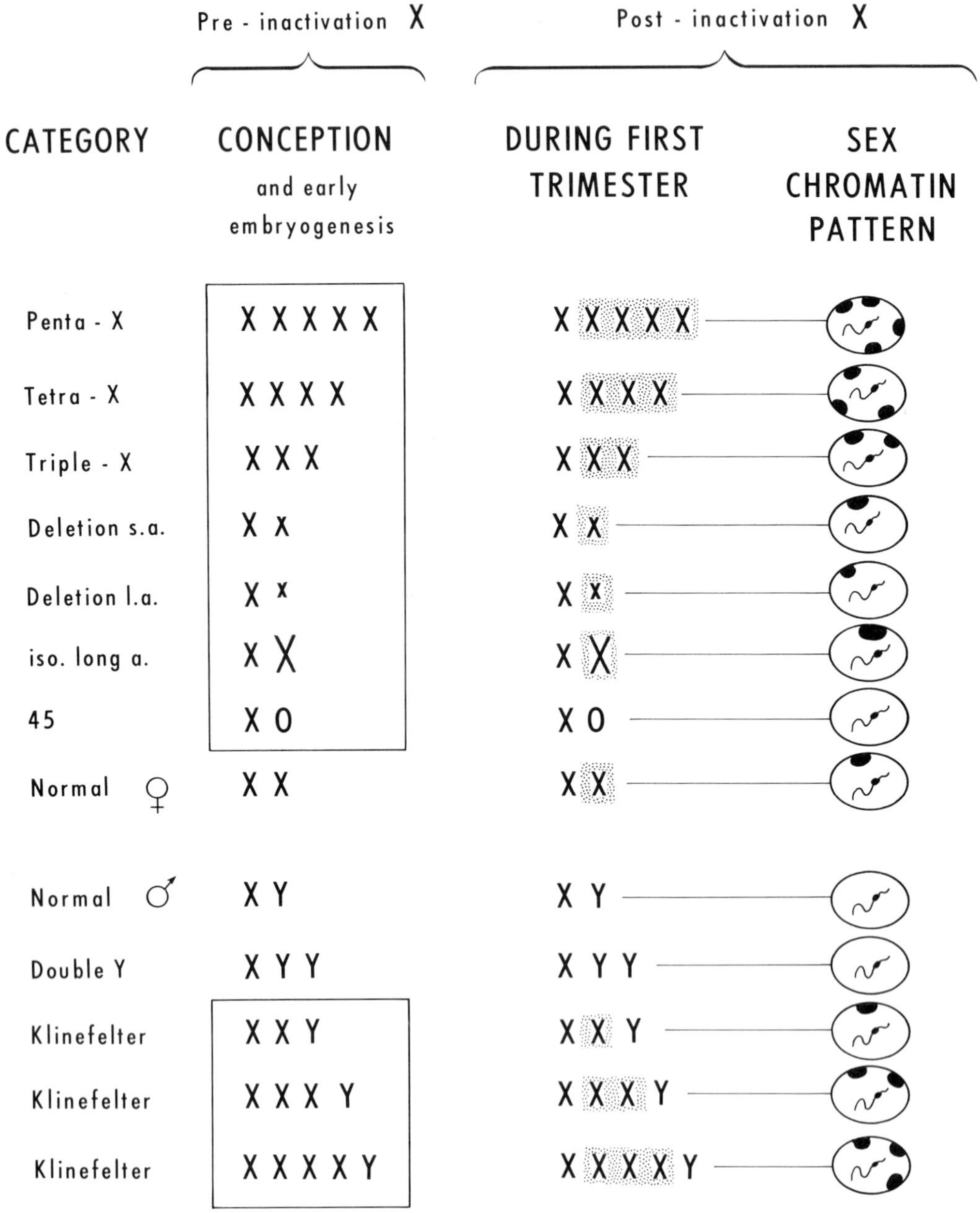

XXXXX, XXXY, XXXXY patients are mentally retarded and often have malformations. If all X chromosomes except one were inactive from conception onwards then XO, XX, XXX, XXXX, and XXXXX individuals would develop normally. Poly-Y individuals are seldom so affected because the Y chromosome contains few genes.

Additional Aids in Interpretation of Chromosomal Disorders

X Chromatin

The X-chromatin mass is a plano-convex, densely stained mass at the inner aspect of the nuclear membrane.[29] A single X-chromatin mass (Fig. 11-17) is found in normal females in about 25–50% of cells lining the inside of the mouth, in proportionately more cells from vaginal epithelium, and in almost 100% of amnion cells from placental membranes and in confluent fibroblast cultures (Fig. 11-19). The proportion of chromatin-positive cells is influenced by the mitotic activity of the tissue because, during mitosis and DNA replication, cells do not have a visible X-chromatin mass. Inflammatory lesions have many cells in mitosis and DNA replication, and therefore examination of cells from inflamed membranes lining the mouth or vagina may result in diagnostic problems because of a reduced incidence of chromatin-positive cells.

Nature of the X Chromatin. The X chromatin mass is formed by a tightly condensed X chromosome. One uncoiled X chromosome, indistinguishable in the interphase nucleus from the other chromosomes of the cell, must always be present so that one X chromatin mass implies two X chromosomes. The number of X chromosomes is, therefore, one more than the maximal number of X chromatin masses identified (Fig. 11-18). Real X chromatin masses are not found in normal males (Fig. 11-17), but a very low percentage of apparently positive cells (1–3%) may be scored as positive because of wrinkling of the nuclear membrane.

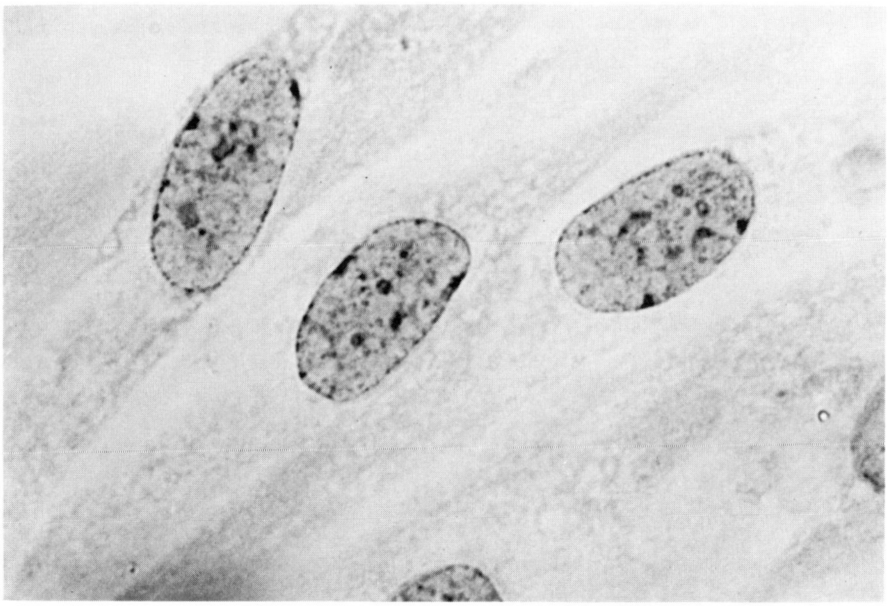

Fig. 11-19. Fibroblast culture. Two X chromatin masses in three cultured cells from an XXXY male. X chromatin masses are most frequent in nondividing cells. In tissue cultures, dividing cells are infrequent when the nutritive medium has not been changed for many days or when the cell growth is confluent [completely covers the available surface]. (Carbol fuchsin, × 1900.)

Preparation of Specimens. Smears are obtained by scraping the lining of the mouth or the vagina with a wooden or metal spatula, rubbing the cells onto a glass slide and immediately fixing them while wet. The preparations are then stained and mounted, and the cells examined for X chromatin. Rapid methods are available, using a wet mount, and cells can be examined a few minutes later. Cells must be scored by selecting only those with well-preserved nuclei and then focusing carefully with the microscope through the full depth of the cell to determine whether a mass is present or absent in the nucleus.

Similar tests can be made on solid tissues which have been fixed, embedded, and sectioned to provide slides for histology, but in these cells, X chromatin is not identified so reliably or so easily scored as in smears of epithelial cells. In addition, certain solid tissues are very difficult to "sex" accurately—e.g., cartilage cells—whereas others are more reliable—e.g., fibroblasts and smooth muscle cells.

Use of X Chromatin Tests. X chromatin tests have been useful in the rapid screening for sex chromosome disorders of patients in mental hospitals and in newborn and adult populations. The test is particularly helpful in testing whether an additional group C chromosome is an X chromosome. An abnormal X in those who have two or more X chromosomes always forms an X chromatin mass. This is known because the abnormal X is late replicating (shown by its radioactive labeling pattern with thymidine autoradiographs) in lymphocyte and fibroblast cultures, and the latter also show that all X chromatin masses in interphase nuclei are radioactively labeled.

Drumsticks in Neutrophils. Blood films have been used to determine the number of neutrophils with "drumsticks" (nuclear appendages with a narrow stalk and a rounded protruding mass approximately 1 μ in diameter). These drumsticks are found in a few cells from normal females but not from normal males.

Fluorescent Y Test (Y Chromatin)

Interphase nuclei from males when examined with a fluorescence microscope after staining with quinacrine contain a brightly fluorescent spot shown to represent the Y chromosome.[32] "The quinacrine test is the exact counterpart of the simple stain for the Barr body which shows up the presence of extra X chromosomes."[11]

The fluorescent Y test is already used as a diagnostic laboratory test to investigate intersex problems and screen males for the XYY condition. Cell preparations for tests of X and Y chromatin can be made and examined within a few minutes (Table 11-5). Results of both tests provide positive identification of the male (Y chromatin) and female (X chromatin). Positive X and Y chromatin tests would suggest Klinefelter's syndrome (XXY), and a negative result for both tests would suggest Turner's syndrome (XO). Excluding mosaicism and structural changes, all combinations of numerical sex chromosome abnormalities, including complex abnormalities such as XXXYY cells, etc., could be identified by these two simple tests alone, as shown in Fig. 11-20. However, apparently abnormal results should always be confirmed by chromosome analysis.

These tests of nuclear sex can be used on interphase cells in chromosomal preparations: the

Table 11-5. Comparison of Tests of Nuclear Sex

	Standard microscopy	*Fluorescence microscopy*
Advantages	Well-known ordinary microscope Ordinary stains *Positive identification of second X (Female)*	Test usable in tissues and conditions unsuitable for sex chromatin test Can be followed by Barr body test Positive identification of Y (male)
Disadvantages	Meticulous preparation essential Only vesicular nuclei testable Only 20–40% these nuclei positive	Fluorescent microscope method not well known Risk of retinal damage/strain

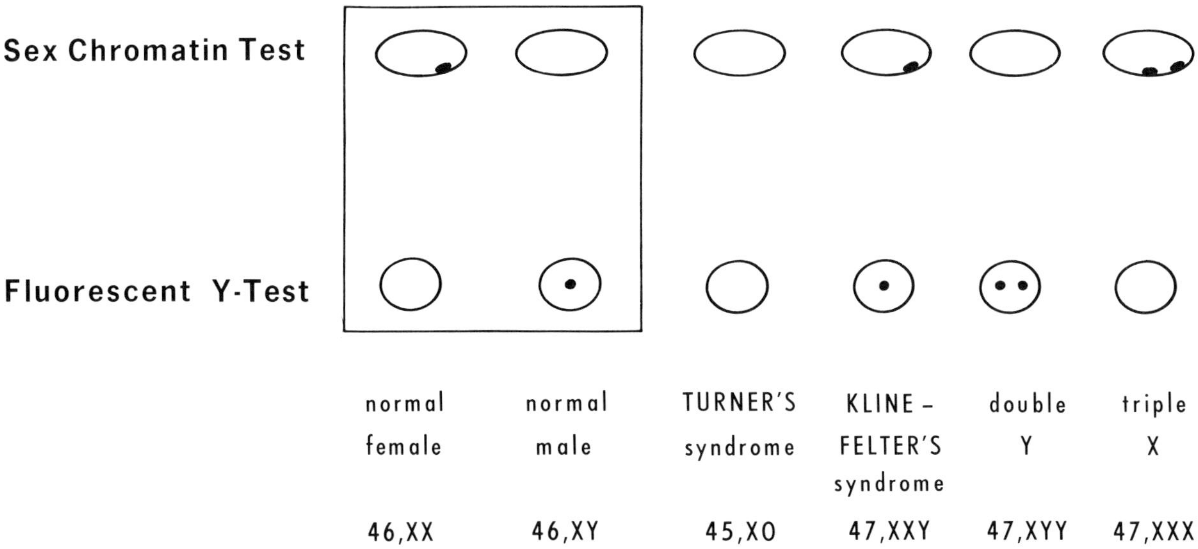

Fig. 11-20. Combined nuclear sex tests in normals and in various numerical X-chromosome disorders. The enclosed portion on the left of the figure shows the four cells seen previously in Figure 11-17. The remainder of the figure shows that the combined results of X-chromatin and fluorescent Y-chromatin tests can identify Turner's syndrome (XO), Klinefelter's syndrome (XXY), double-Y syndrome (XYY), triple X (XXX). In addition, other more complex sex chromosome disorders could thus be recognized, e.g., 49,XXXYY.

Y chromatin test on lymphocytes and fibroblast cultures and the X chromatin test on fibroblast cultures only. These can be made before chromosome stains are applied and also on old preparations stained with water-soluble Giemsa stain. Thus, retrospective studies could be made on cells with puzzling karyotypes by removing the coverslip, washing out the water-soluble Giemsa stain, and staining with quinacrine. Interphase cells can be examined by the fluorescent Y test, and identifications of individual chromosomes can be attempted on metaphase cells by their fluorescent banding patterns.

The sex of the fetus can be identified by examining amniotic fluid cells. Here the Y chromatin test is preferred because most amniotic fluid cells are unsuitable for X chromatin tests. The sex of the fetus may also be identified without amniocentesis by demonstrating Y chromatin in chorion cells in endocervical smears.

A wide variety of other interphase cells can be used for the Y chromatin test including those in frozen sections, provided the tissue is fresh or alcohol fixed. The Y chromosomes of man and gorilla fluoresce, but not those of other primates so far studied. Y-bearing spermatozoa can be identified in human sperm but not in cattle where breeders would like to use X-bearing sperm to increase the yield of female offspring.

Dermal Patterns

Dermal patterns (dermatoglyphics) are formed by small ridges (not to be confused with skin creases) on the palms, soles, and tips of the digits. Each ridge represents a mass of mesoderm with capillaries that presses against the epidermis. Sweat gland orifices form small dots along the ridges. The ridges develop at about 2–3 months gestation and, because they apparently remain unchanged during the life of the individual, are said to be the "frozen record" of that period of fetal development. For example, the 45,XO fetus is edematous, and swelling of hands and feet is often still present during the first few months of life. The amount of skin (hence, the number of ridges—"ridge count") necessary to cover a swollen fingertip will be greater than that on a

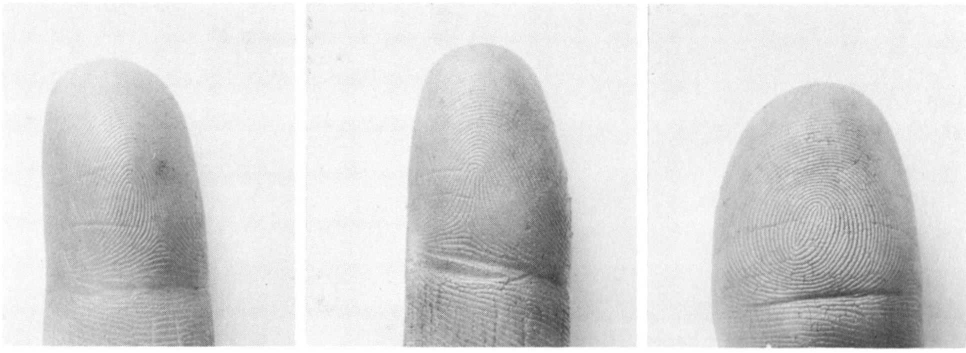

Fig. 11-21. Dermal patterns. Fingerprint patterns loop, arch and whorl (left to right).

normal digit. Fingertips of liveborn 45,XO infants are of normal size but contain many more ridges than normal.

Studies of other chromosome abnormalities show that the ridge count (number of ridges from the triradius to the center of the pattern on all 10 fingers) is inversely proportional to the number of X chromosomes. The fingertip ridges form patterns such as a loop, arch, or whorl (Fig. 11-21), easily seen on the fingers. These patterns and the skin ridge patterns on the palms and soles are useful in interpreting some chromosome abnormalities. The mean ridge count is: 170 in XO patients; 148 in normal males; 127 in normal females; and 115 in XXY patients. Preliminary examinations can be made by direct observation of the ridges with the aid of a magnifying glass, but counts, measurements, and detailed analyses are best done on pressure prints of the fingers, palms, and soles, like fingerprints made for police records.

Chromosomal Abnormalities and Variants Found in Normal and Random Samples

The Idea of "Normal"

In any study, the range of normal should be defined before abnormalities are examined. However, because chromosomal studies are laborious and most investigators are eager to find and study unusual cases, little attention has been devoted to surveys of unselected populations; hence we know little about the frequency of abnormalities and "variants" of normal in such populations.

In studies of several hundred "normal" adults, 0.5% had major structural chromosomal rearrangements, particularly those in which material was translocated from one chromosome to another, or chromosome material was "inverted" within one chromosome.[6, 21] Two to three percent had structural anomalies confined to one autosome, usually related to an area of secondary constriction; such areas are usually inherited and, hence, will be present in all cells. In 2–3% of males the length of the Y chromosome is unusual, most often longer than average.

Racial differences in chromosome morphology have been described: in Japanese males, the Y chromosome is unusually long; the incidence of elongated or absent short arms of acrocentric chromosomes is different in Negroes than in Caucasians.

Limitations and Advantages of Selected "Normal" Populations

In all populations studied thus far, certain chromosomal abnormalities appear to be particularly frequent, for example, 45,D/D translocation and 47, XXY and 47,XYY patterns in males (see Table 11-4). The chromosomal abnormalities found and their distributions will vary, depending on the population chosen for study. In adults, chromosomal abnormalities which shorten life will be diminished or absent; among university students, chromosomal abnormalities resulting in mental retardation will be absent. When the subject population is drawn from the armed forces or police, few individuals will be found with physical handicaps. The advantage of studies on adult populations is that one can collect data on fertility and type of offspring that is not yet available in younger populations.

Newborn Surveys

Surveys of randomly selected or consecutively delivered newborns give a true incidence of chromosomal abnormalities,[24, 39] but unfortunately, the full spectrum of physical and mental abnormalities may not be apparent until many months or years later or, if the infant dies, may never be determined. The approximate incidence of the more common chromosomal abnormalities in newborns is given in Table 11-4. In a city of 2 million with 40,000 livebirths per year, the following numbers of chromosomally abnormal babies would be born each year: 65 mongoloids; 40 with Klinefelter's syndrome; 40 with triple-X; 20–40, double Y; 15, Turner's syndrome; 8, E syndrome; 4, D syndrome; and 4, cat-cry syndrome. Two-thirds of the patients with mongolism and cat-cry syndrome, and probably all of those with the E and D syndromes, would die in infancy or childhood. Many of the remaining 140 patients would require regular or periodic medical attention.

Selected Abnormal Populations

The incidence of chromosomal abnormalities is, of course, higher in selected abnormal populations (Table 11-6). Mental retardates have many autosomal abnormalities, particularly those associated with mongolism, and many sex chromosomal abnormalities; tall and "aggressive" males show an increase in XYY syndrome; and infants with multiple malformations have general chromosomal abnormalities.

Studies of Spontaneous Abortions

Although it is possible to estimate the incidence of the chromosomal abnormalities by newborn surveys, the true incidence of abnormalities at conception can be estimated (Table 11-4) only by also considering the incidence of chromosomal abnormalities in spontaneous abortions:[3, 4]

Table 11-6. Selected Abnormal Populations with Chromosome Abnormalities

Group and disorder	*Percent afflicted**
Patients	
Multiple congenital malformations including F.L.K. ("funny-looking kid") syndrome	5
Retardation	
Mental (nonspecific)	5–10
Physical (very short girls)	10–20
Infertility problems	
Azoospermia	15–20
Primary amenorrhea	30–40
Early spontaneous abortuses	30–50
Tall aggressive males with behavior problems	5–25
Parents with a history of multiple spontaneous abortions	5

* Figures approximate and based on personal experience and/or published reports.

1. Of those tested, 25–30% have chromosome abnormalities, especially those who have early or malformed abortuses and those with empty amniotic sacs.
2. The most frequent chromosome abnormalities are:
   45,XO (the XO has an estimated incidence of 1:80 conceptions, 1:5,000 live births)
   Triploidy
3. Some have
   Tetraploidy
   D trisomy
   G trisomy
   No. 16 trisomy (not found among liveborns)
4. A few trisomics are found in spontaneous abortuses but not found in liveborns (e.g., trisomy No. 2).

Several abnormalities such as triploidy (69 chromosomes) and tetraploidy (92 chromosomes) are found only in aborted material, and frequently, in such circumstances, the amniotic sac is empty or contains only a minute nodule representing the deformed embryo.

The 45,XO chromosomal pattern found in patients with Turner's syndrome is frequent in spontaneous abortions. It appears that more than

95% of 45,XO conceptuses are spontaneously aborted, hence, the incidence of this condition in liveborn infants is low, although theoretically 45,XO should be more frequent than XXY and XXX. The possibility that all liveborn 45,XO individuals have mosaic cell lines should be considered because the presence of additional cell lines might confer a survival advantage. Chromosomal patterns identical with D syndrome (47, +13) and mongolism (47,+21) are also frequent in spontaneous abortions, a finding which suggests that 70% of these conceptions are aborted spontaneously.[3]

Sex chromosome abnormalities other than XO are seldom found in aborted material, and probably most infants with such abnormalities have a near-normal life span (Table 11-4). This observation demonstrates that sex chromosomes are relatively inert genetically compared with autosomes.

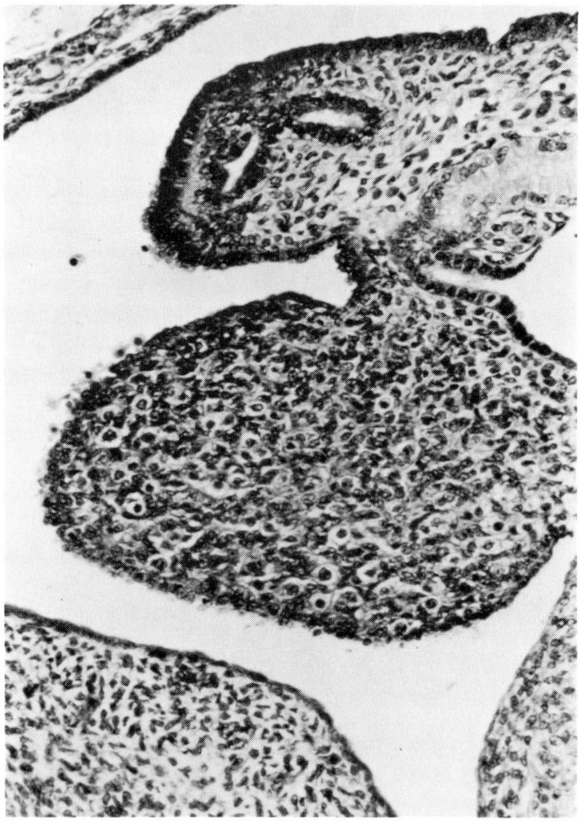

Fig. 11-22. Undifferentiated gonad. An undifferentiated gonad from a young human embryo/fetus of eight weeks gestational age (crown rump (CR) length 16 mm). The gonad consists of (a) germ cells, large cells with pale cytoplasm, (b) a stroma formed from the mesonephric mesenchyme and (c) a surface covering from the celomic epithelium (H & E × 225).

Gonadal Development

General

It should be remembered that in the first few weeks of life, the male and female embryos have identical primordia (undeveloped structures) which will later differentiate into gonads, ducts, and internal and external sex organs. In normal persons the structure and function of the gonads, ducts, and organs depends upon fetal development of some primordia and lack of development (regression) of others so that only the sex ducts and organs appropriate to the sex of the individual are formed. The external genitalia of young human fetuses are similar, but by 10–12 weeks the sexes can be distinguished easily.

The Undifferentiated Gonad

The human primordial (undifferentiated) gonad develops about the fifth week of embryonic life and consists of primordial germ cells in a mesonephric medulla covered by a peritoneal cortex (celomic epithelium). Primordial germ cells first appear beneath the endodermal yoke-sac epithelium at 24 days of fetal age and migrate to the gonadal ridges during the fifth week. The mesoderm of the gonadal ridge provides the stroma and the celomic epithelium the covering of the developing gonad. At 6 weeks, the histologic appearances of gonads in male and female embryos are similar (Fig. 11-22). The location of the gonads on the anterior surface of the mesonephros and the relationship of the genital ducts are shown in Figure 11-23.

Testes

The testes can be identified histologically from 7 weeks onward, by the following features (Fig. 11-24): (i) a single layer of celomic epithelium, (ii) a subepithelial connective-tissue layer that

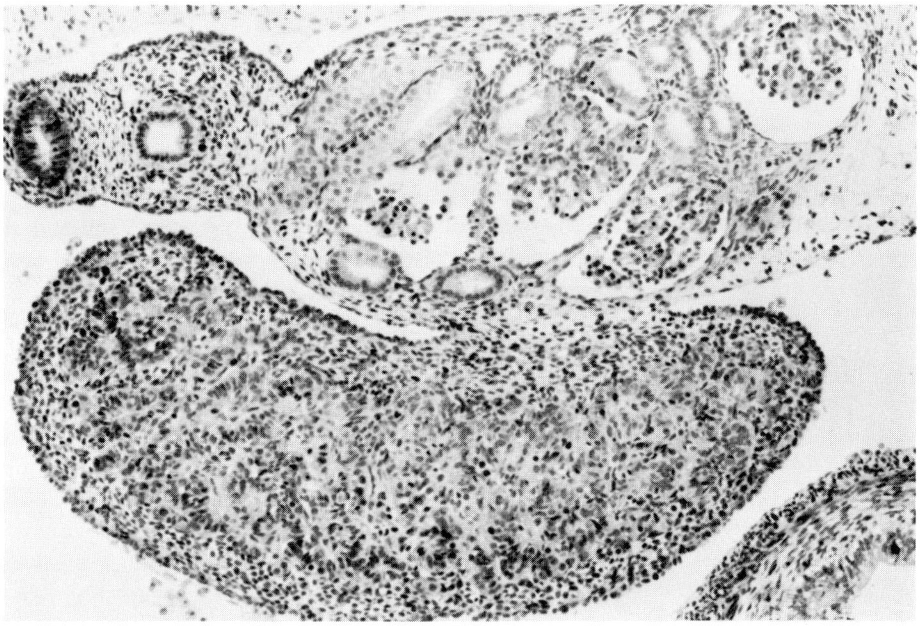

Fig. 11-23. Relationship of developing gonad and genital ducts to the mesonephros. This transverse section through the right testes of a young fetus shows the relationship of the gonad to the mesonephros (glomeruli identifiable) posteriorly, and the genital ducts posterolaterally (H & E × 225).

represents the tunica albuginea of the testis and (iii) many sex cords from which seminiferous tubules eventually develop (i and ii are most easily seen from 10 weeks on (Fig. 11-24 **B,** & **C**). The sex cords contain the germ cells which have abundant pale cytoplasm and resemble seminiferous tubules without lumens from 14 weeks on. At this stage the interstitial cells between the seminiferous tubules become larger and more numerous (Fig. 11-24**C**).

In the seminiferous tubules, germ cells form spermatogonia, which eventually produce spermatozoa; celomic epithelial cells form the Sertoli cells, which support and "nourish" the spermatocytes; and mesenchymal cells form the interstitial cells, which produce androgens. The seminiferous tubules are small in the newborn male testes (Fig. 11-25**A**), and become considerably larger at sexual maturity mostly because of active spermatogenesis (Fig. 11-25**B**) with increase in cell and fluid content.

The testes descend from the abdominal cavity to the scrotum about the seventh month of gestational age. The testes are still undescended at birth in about 20% of prematures and about 2% of term infants. In most cases the testes later descend spontaneously or following medical and/or surgical treatment at about 4–8 years of age, but about 0.2% of adults have one undescended testis.

Undescended testes in adults result in two important problems: (1) If both testes are undescended, spermatogenesis is absent (Fig. 11-25**C**) or grossly deficient, causing sterility, which is believed to result from the higher intraabdominal than scrotal temperature. (2) The risk of development of a gonadal tumor is considerably greater in an undescended testis, particularly in an individual with an abnormal karyotype.

Spermatogenesis begins about 12–13 years of age and continues, at a reduced rate, into old age. The progeny of spermatogonia divide and develop to form primary and secondary spermatocytes, spermatids, which mature into spermatozoa. Four spermatozoa, of equal size (in contrast to ova) are eventually formed 60-72 days after each divi-

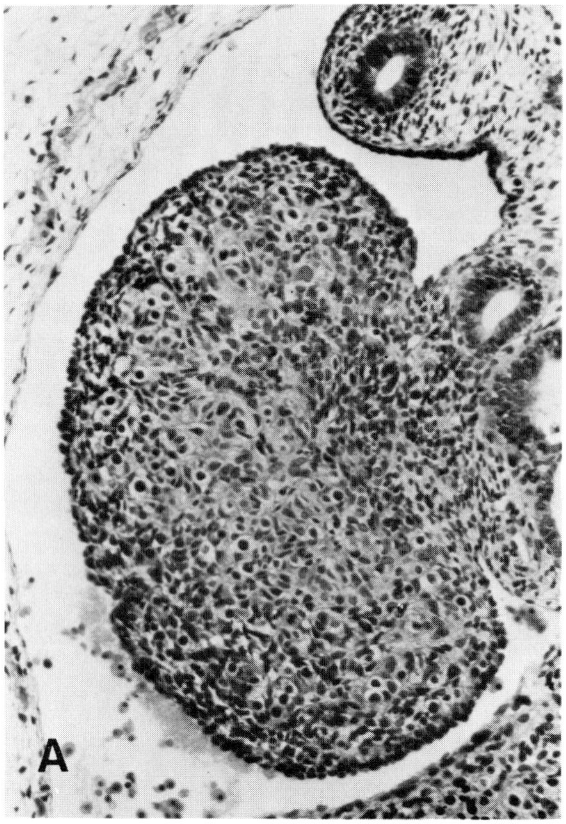

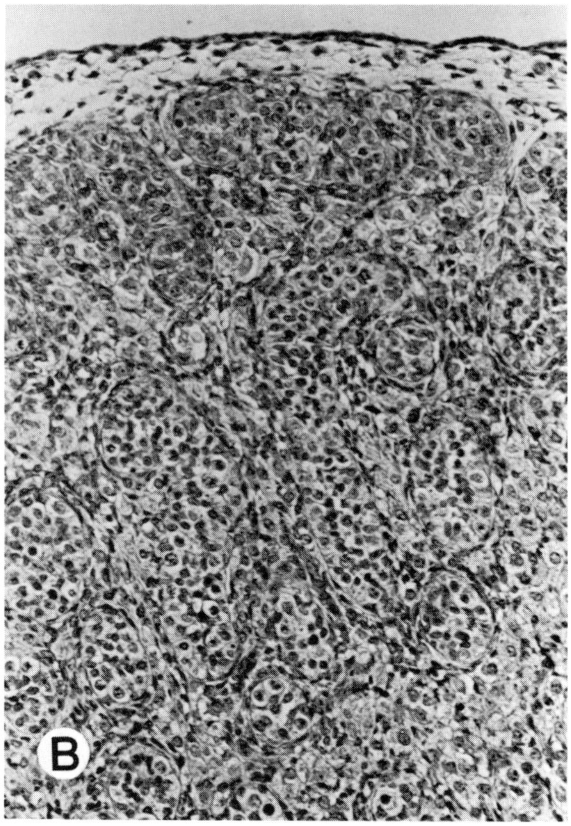

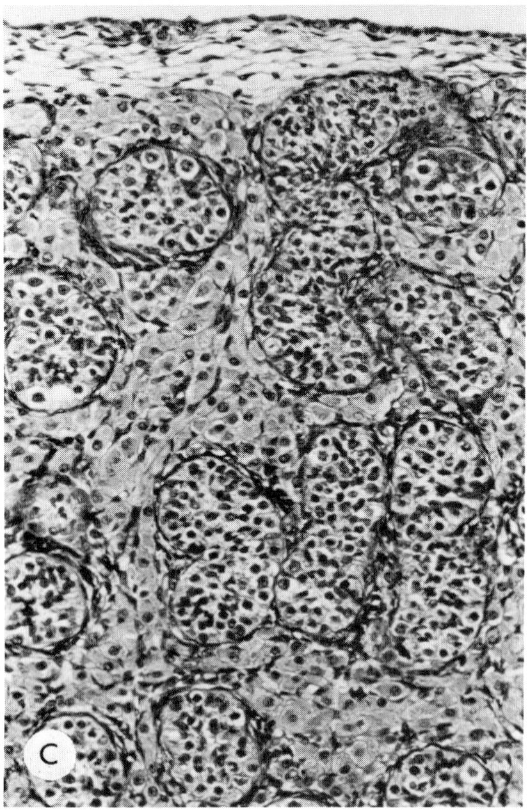

Fig. 11-24. Development of the Testis. These photomicrographs show three stages in the fetal development of the testes.

A. The large pale germ cells can be seen in the intertwining sex cords occupying the medulla of the gonad. These sex cords are separated from the celomic epithelium by a peripheral layer of small cells (future tunica albuginaea). 9 weeks (C.R. 24 mm)

B and **C.** The single layer of celomic epithelial cells and the loose connective tissue (tunica albuginaea) beneath are easily recognized (top of figures). The sex cords have formed tubules more easily distinguished from each other in C than in B because of the larger and more numerous interstitial cells between the tubules. B, 14 weeks (C.R. 75 mm), C, 16 weeks (C.R. 110 mm) (H & E $\times$ 225).

sion of a spermatogonia (Fig. 11-11). Genetic cells and sperm distend the seminiferous tubules and cause the rapid normal enlargement of the testes during puberty (Fig. 11-25). The slight diminution in testicular size in old men is due to reduction of spermatogenesis and some hyalinization of seminiferous tubules.

Ovaries

In developing ovaries[36] the germ cells, surrounded by epithelial cells to form follicles, are distributed uniformly without a particular pattern (Fig. 11-26). The stroma between follicles becomes progressively more dense by formation of twisted bundles of connective tissue. Probably the complete complement of follicles (approximately 200,000 per ovary) forms by the fourth to fifth month of gestation. Many of these follicles will degenerate during the late fetal and early infant life. Baker[1] has estimated there are 6–8 million oocytes in the midgestation fetus and only 2 million at birth. Of those that persist, only 350–400 will be released at ovulation, usually one per month, midway in the menstrual cycle, during the 30+ years (from age 13 to 45) of reproductive life in a woman. Ovulation usually begins within a few months to 2 years after menarche—onset of first menstrual cycles—and ceases before or around the menopause—when menstrual cycles end.

Mostly primary follicles (Fig. 11-27**A**) which consist of an immature ovum closely surrounded by a single layer of flat follicular cells, are seen until puberty. However, some maturation (Fig. 11-27**B**) of primary follicles to graafian follicles and cystic follicles can be found in the last three months of fetal development and in the newborn. This maturation is believed to result from chorionic gonadotropin, which comes mostly from the placenta although some gonadotropins come from the fetal and maternal pituitary.

Growing follicles mostly appear after puberty. In these, there is growth, differentiation, and maturation of the ovum, the follicular cells, and surrounding connective tissue. The follicles mature, usually singly, distend the surface of the ovary and rupture, liberating the ovum (ovulation). The wall and collapsed cavity of the follicle form the corpus luteum, a temporary glandular structure producing progesterone which prepares the uterine mucosa for attachment of a fertilized ovum. In the nonpregnant female, this structure degenerates (corpus luteum of menstruation) after about 10 days to form a white scar. If the ovum is fertilized (zygote) in the fallopian tubes, the corpus luteum enlarges and functions as a temporary endocrine organ during the first part of pregnancy. The mature ovary has a cortex with considerable amounts of intertwining connective tissue, small follicles (Fig. 11-26**C**), a few large mature follicles and many follicular scars.

The ovary has three unusual features: (1) The "excess of wasted oocytes" reminds us of the millions of eggs laid and fertilized by fish, except that, in women, few eggs can grow completely because of the long gestation period and the relatively short reproductive period. (2) Only one oocyte and three tiny polar bodies are produced from division of an oogonia (Fig. 11-11**B**). This allows development of extensive cytoplasm in the oocyte with organelles and stored nutritive material necessary for the developing zygote. (3) The oocytes proceed part way through the first (meiotic) division during midfetal life and complete this division only when they are released at each monthly ovulation. The second division begins in about 10 oocytes each month after puberty and is only completed in the one oocyte that is ovulated after it is penetrated by a sperm. The long mid-division interval (14–45 years) from fetal to late adult life is significant because of the sensitivity of oocytes in division and the risk that cell damage from many harmful agents such as X-rays, drugs, and viruses may result in defective ova and abnormal offspring. In contrast, sperm in adult males are formed relatively freshly.

Experiments Relevant to Gonadal Development

In general a sexual bipotentiality for developing genital structures has always been inferred, but this is not equal. In mammals the undifferentiated gonads would slowly become ovaries with subsequent female genital development *unless* maleness is imposed upon this system (by masculinizing genes on the Y chromosome). In birds the converse is true and masculine characteristics develop

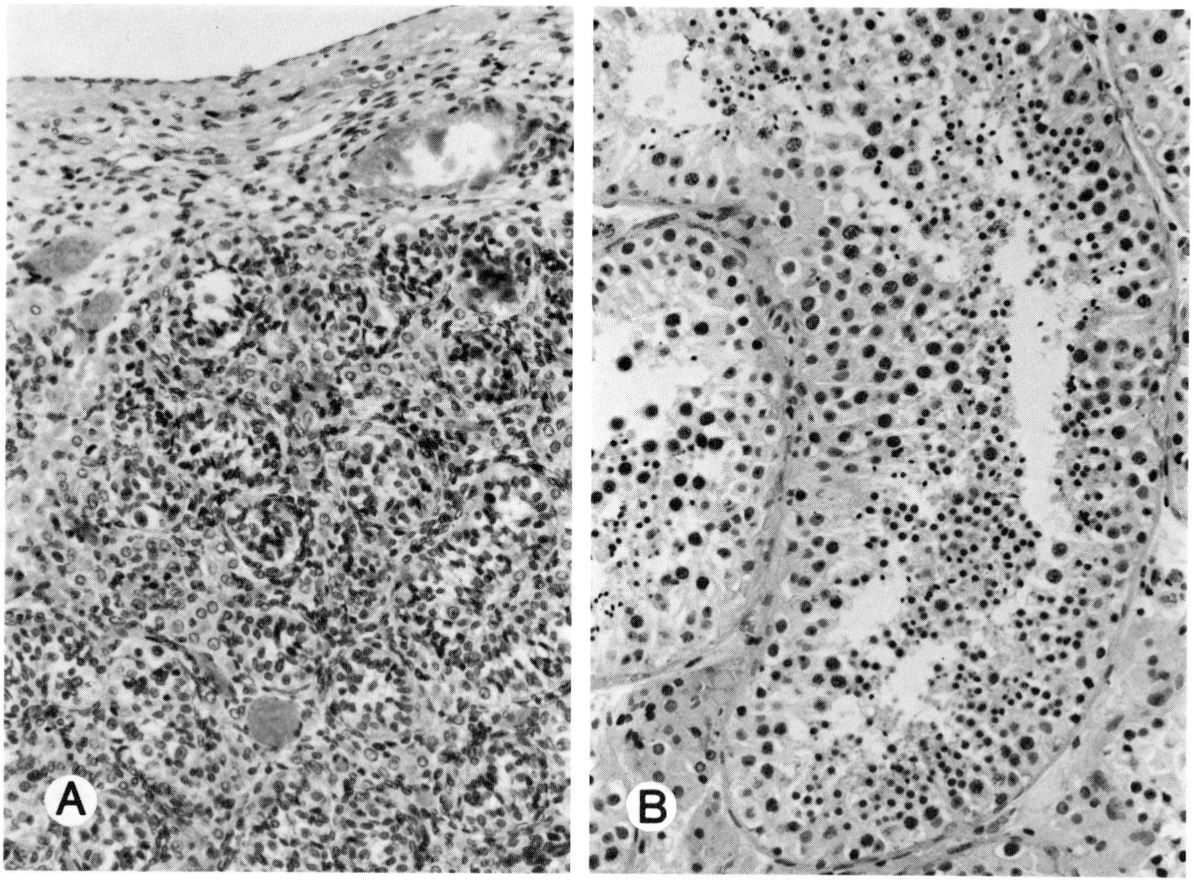
A
B

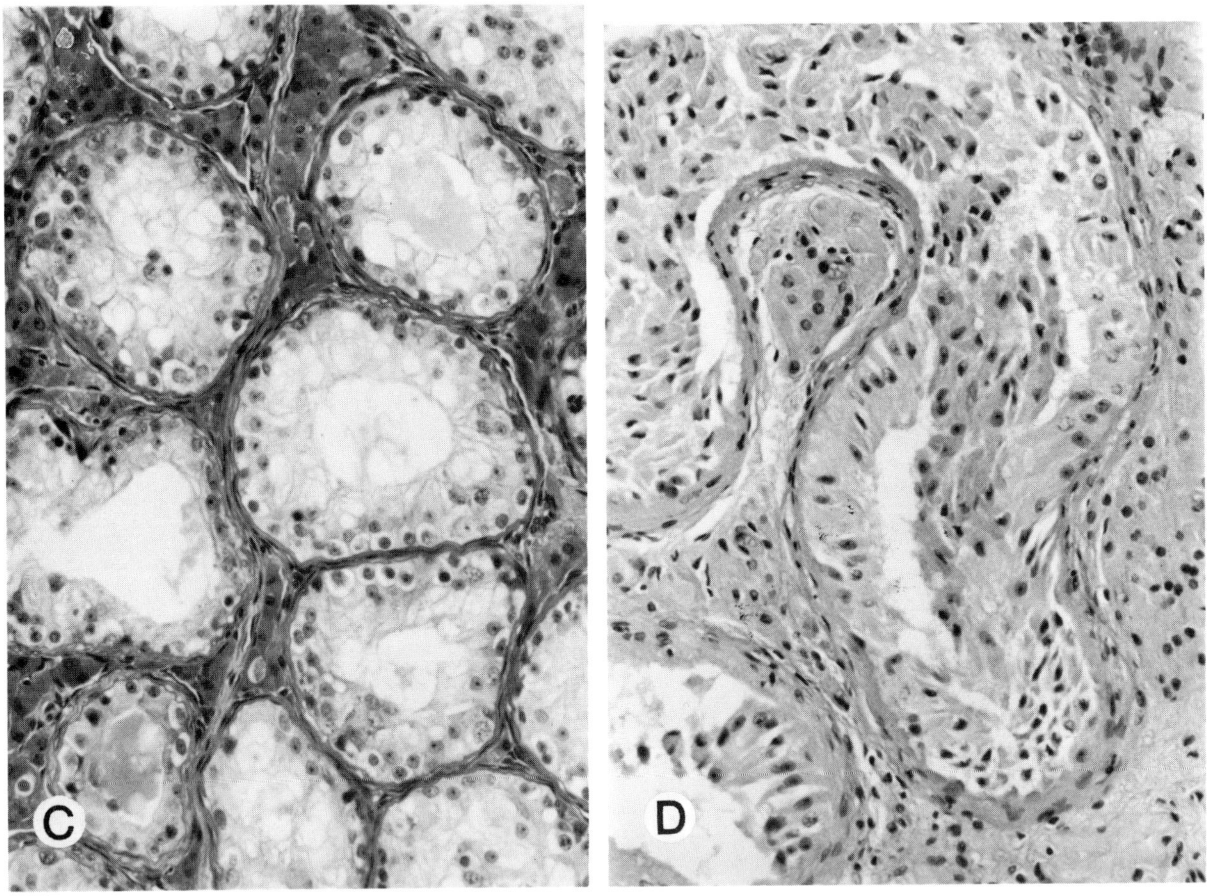

Fig. 11-25. Histology of the Testes. A. Normal newborn. This shows the closely packed, small diameter seminiferous tubules without spermatogenesis and the tunica albuginaea and thin epithelium.

B. Normal adult. The large diameter seminiferous tubules show active spermatogenesis with many dividing cells. Note the decrease in nuclear size from the periphery of the lumen, spermatogonia and Sertoli cells, through spermatocytes and spermatozoa. The walls of the tubules are thin and separate the tubule from the interstitial cells.

C. This is an undescended testes from a young adult with XO/XY condition who also has a streak gonad. The tubule is lined by inactive spermatogonia and Sertoli cells with no evidence of spermatogenesis. The interstitial cells are prominent.

D. Klinefelter's syndrome. This is a small, firm, descended testis from a youth with Klinefelter's syndrome. The tubules have thickened walls and are lined with Sertoli cells without spermatogonia or spermatogenesis (H & E $\times$ 225).

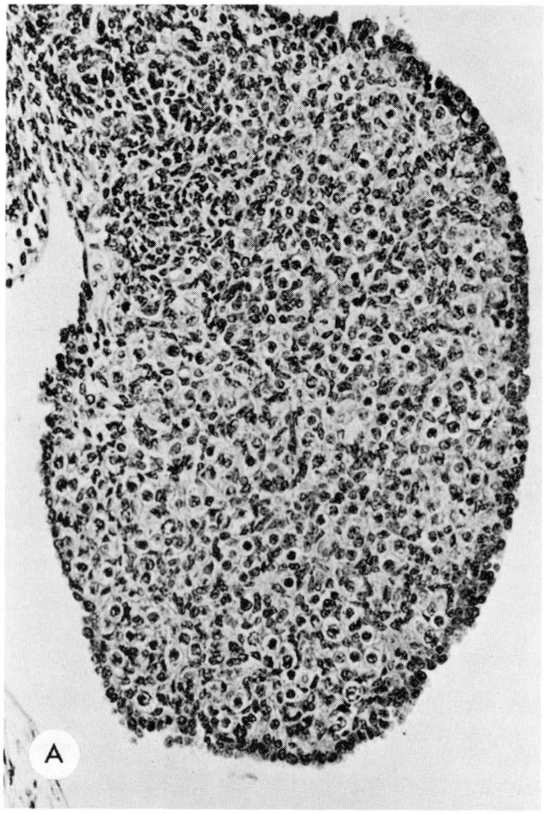

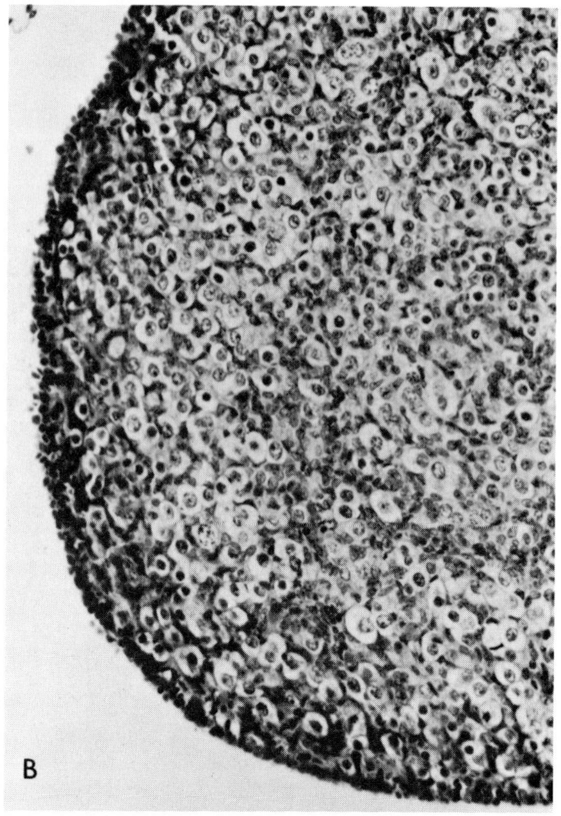

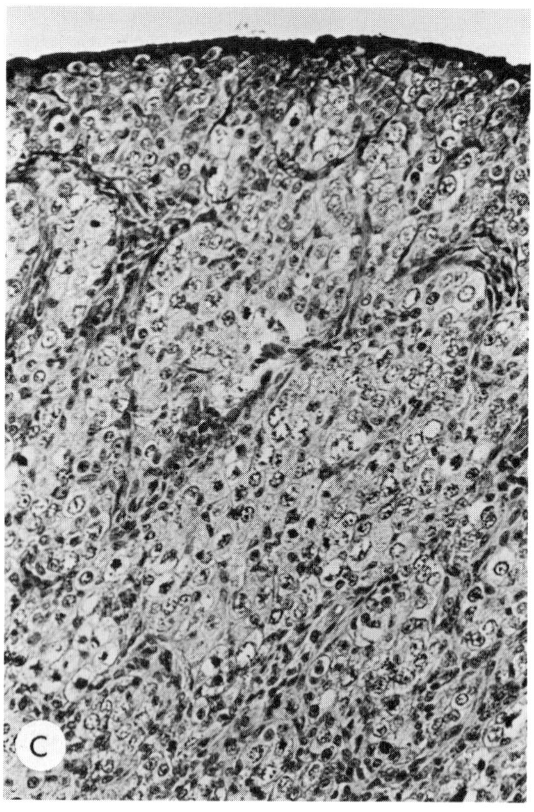

Fig. 11-26. Development of the Ovary. Three stages in the fetal development of the ovary.

A. The ovary has a thicker layer of celomic epithelium and the germ cells are evenly distributed in comparison with the developing testis. The gonad is recognized as ovary because it does not have the medullary localization of sex cords nor subepithelial fibrous tissue found in the testis. 10 weeks (C.R. 30 mm)

B and **C.** The thick germinal epithelium and uniform distribution of large pale germ cells without formation of sex cords is evident. B, 12 weeks (C.R. 52 mm), C, 16 weeks (C.R. 110 mm) (H & E × 225).

unless femaleness is imposed. These unequal bipotentialities remain even in adults: the feminine body characteristic frequent in eunuchoid men, and the masculine plumage developed by castrated adult hens. In mammal fetuses, these conclusions are strengthened by experiments that show (i) ovaries are unnecessary for feminine differentiation of the genital tract, that hypothalamic centers control pituitary function and affect sex behavior;[20] (ii) in cattle, influence of the male twin on the female but not *vice versa.*

The results of animal experiments provide considerable insight into the failure of normal gonadal development.

1. If a rabbit, 10 days pregnant, receives a single intravenous injection of nitrogen mustard, the offspring are sterile and have no germ cells in the gonads. The time of injection is important because most primordial germ cells are probably destroyed en route from the yolk sac to the gonadal ridge. Occasionally gonadal failure in humans may result when the mother is exposed to some injurious agent at a critical period of primordial germ-cell migration.

2. Jost[23] excised the gonads of rabbit fetuses at different stages of pregnancy and examined the internal and external genitalia of the newborn rabbits to determine the effect of castration in male and female fetuses.

Destruction of undifferentiated gonads leads to
- Development of müllerian ducts
- Suppression of wolffian ducts, producing
- *Neutral sterile female*

Unilateral destruction leads to
- Female differentiation of the genital ducts of that side

Variation in extent of destruction and in time of destruction leads to
- Intermediate forms of male-female differentiation

Males castrated early in fetal life had female differentiation of the internal and external genitalia. When male fetuses were castrated after wolffian duct development had occurred, the newborn had male internal genitalia but female external genitalia. Castration at any age had no effect on genital differentiation in female fetuses or in male fetuses after the external genitalia had begun to develop as male.

By these experiments, Jost established that in many forms of gonadal failure, the newborn will have female genitalia; such newborns represent a neutral state because male genitalia can only develop when the testis is normal.

These experiments have been confirmed (i) by female differentiation of genitalia after X-ray destruction of young fetal gonads, (ii) female differentiation of genital tract tissues from young fetuses cultured without exposure to hormones, (iii) masculinization of genital tracts in fetuses after testicular graft in vivo or addition to the in vitro culture.

Neumann and co-workers corroborated Jost's experiments when they injected pregnant rabbits and dogs with cyproterone acetate—a powerful anti-androgen; and produced profound effects upon the fetuses. The "feminized" (male) dogs produced by these injections showed histopathologic similarities to the human testicular feminization syndrome.

In cattle, an experiment of nature produces an opposite effect when twins of different sex have vascular placental communications. The female twin (freemartin) is sexually abnormal because the reproductive tract and genitalia are masculinized by testicular hormones from the male twin.[40]

Studies of early development of the gonads and reproductive tracts have been facilitated by use of organ cultures which have shown the secretory activity of the gonads (isolated in the culture system from the fetus) in relation to morphogenesis of the gonads and reproductive ducts.[35] Such experiments demonstrate that wolffian duct development depends on testicular hormones and that the müllerian duct development does not depend on ovarian hormones.

In adult rats, Pfeiffer showed the effects of neonatal gonadectomy or gonadal transplantation on gonadotropic hormone secretion. When an ovary was transplanted into an adult male rat, corpora lutea would form if the rat had been castrated as a newborn (this did not happen if the testes were transplanted into the neck of the newborn). Castrated newborn females had normal estrous cycles and formed corpora lutea in an ovary transplanted into them as adults. But when

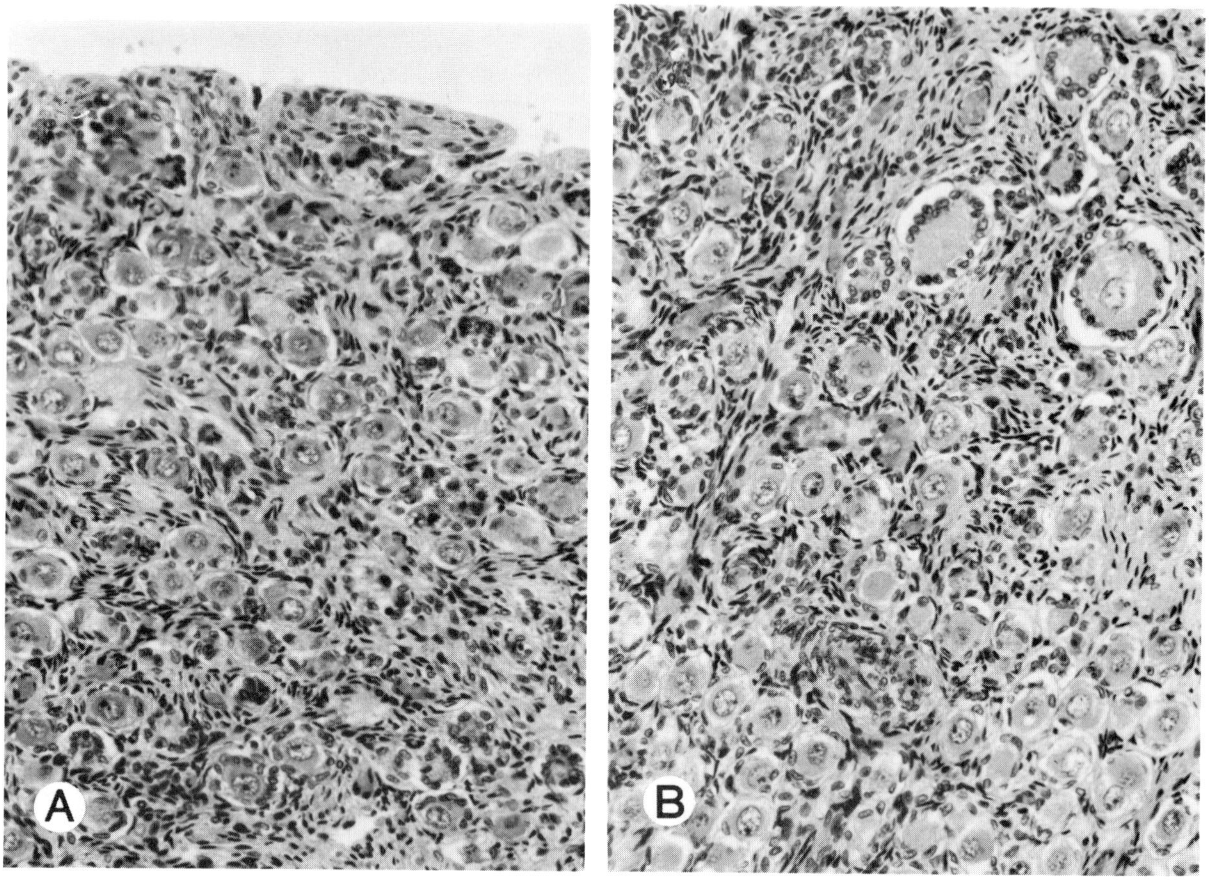
A
B

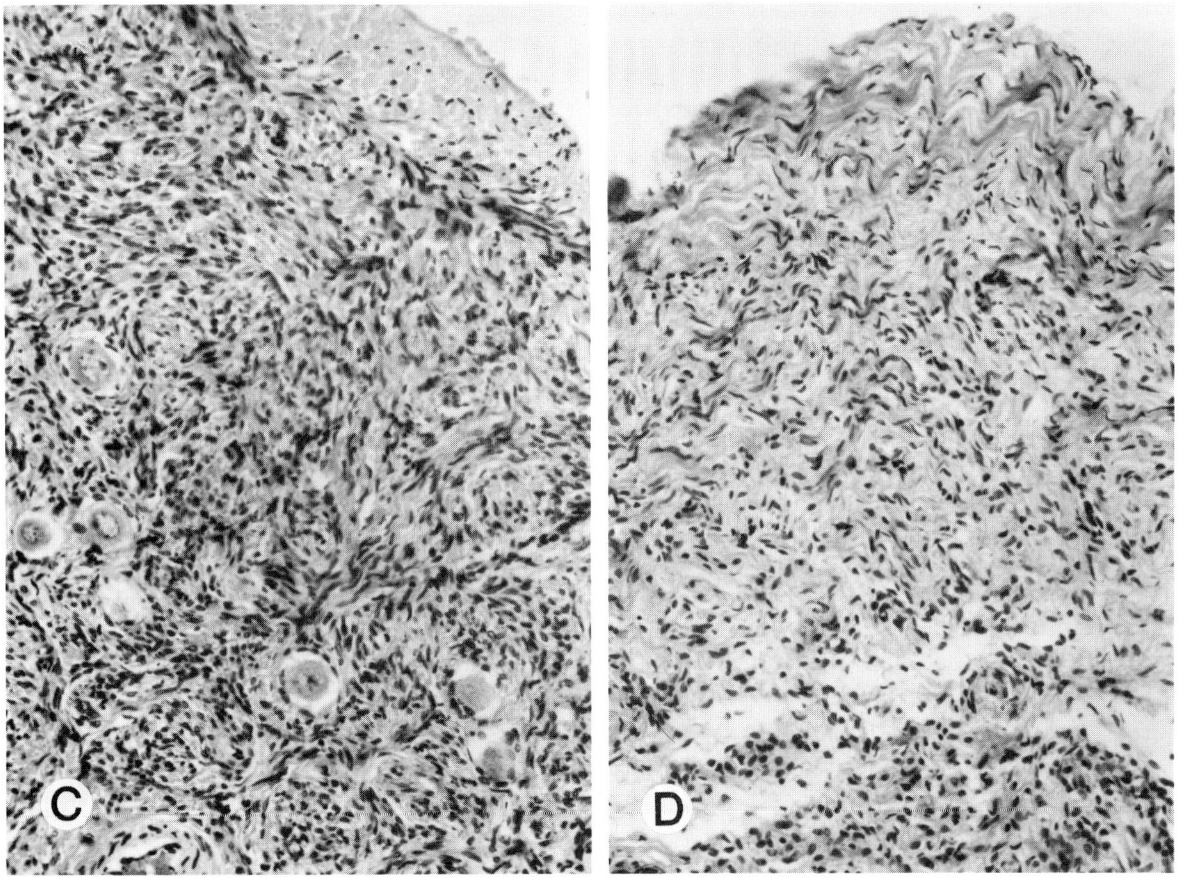

Fig. 11-27. Histology of Ovaries. A. and **B.** Normal newborn. Primary follicles consisting of an immature ovum surrounded by a single layer of follicular cells are distributed through the ovary including the subepithelial regions (top of A). A few follicles show maturation changes (right upper part of B) perhaps due to chorionic gonadotrophins from the placenta.

C. Normal adult. The cortex consists of a thick layer of intertwining connective tissue containing some follicles. Other areas would show all stages of follicular maturation and degeneration into graafian follicles which rupture (ovulation). The lining cells have a brief endocrine function (corpora lutea) and then involute, forming a white scar (corpus albicans). Most follicles do not develop completely and degenerate, forming small scars (atretic follicles).

D. Streak gonad (Turner's syndrome). This gonad is called a streak because it is as long as but thinner than normal. It is pale because it is composed of the dense intertwining connective tissue resembling that in the cortex of a normal ovary but the streak gonad contains no follicles or ova and no follicular scars which would be evidence of previous maturation of some follicles. (H & E $\times$ 225) newborn females were castrated and transplanted with a testis as newborns, they developed constant estrous and no corpora lutea after ovarian transplantation as adults.

Sex Chromosomes and Development of Gonads and Genitalia

If chromosomal abnormalities and gonadal histology are correlated in large numbers of human patients, some inferences can be drawn about the function of the genes carried on the X and Y chromosomes.

Because every individual with a normal Y chromosome has testes, a Y chromosome must carry gene(s) to form a normal testis. Other genes cause the müllerian duct system to regress so that the fallopian tubes and uterus do not form; the wolffian duct system continues to develop to form the vas deferens and seminal vesicles. When there is more than one X in addition to the Y, testes develop but are abnormal (Fig. 11-25**D**) and do not usually form sperm. Some other observations, correlations, and assumptions of function of the Y chromosome based on clinical experience are:

Observations and correlations:

- Great variation in length of Y chromosome
- Morphology inherited (? use in paternity test)
- Long Y usually not abnormal
- Very short Y found in some infertile men

Assumptions:

- Differentiation of testes
- Regression of müllerian ducts
- Aggressive behavior and tallness (poly Y syndromes)
- Few, if any, other genes

In the female, genes from two normal X chromosomes are necessary if a normal ovary is to develop (Fig. 11-27**C**). The müllerian duct system will develop from the mesonephric duct, and the wolffian duct system will regress. If one of the two X chromosomes is abnormal or absent, only a "streak" gonad with ovarian stroma, but without ova, will form (Fig. 11-27**D**) instead of a normal ovary. When one of two X chromosomes is abnormal, it forms the X chromatin mass (as shown by thymidine autoradiography); presumably this mass is inactive (?partially or totally), hence minimizing the effect of the chromosome defect on the individual.

Chromosomal Abnormalities and Related Disorders

Frequent or Important Chromosomal Intersex Conditions

Some of the more frequent sex chromosome abnormalities will be considered because they are clinically important and because they can illustrate the basic points just discussed.[33] These conditions are easier to consider if abnormalities and consequences are linked so that less needs to be memorized and more can be understood. To keep perspective, one should know for any condition:

1. Incidence in the general population
2. Effect on the development of gonads, ducts and genitalia
3. Whether the disorder is such that all or only some individuals will seek medical attention—e.g., a nun is unlikely to complain of infertility
4. The important diagnostic features
5. Age(s) of the patients and types of problems for which medical advice will be sought
6. Which of the problems can be treated
7. How much of the condition should be explained to the patient or parent
8. After treatment, what limitations the patient will have—risk of abnormal offspring, sterility, development of associated diseases and whether these can be prevented or minimized
9. Possibility of increasing scientific knowledge from more study of the patient without harm or distress and without loss of confidentiality to the patient.

Klinefelter's Syndrome

Klinefelter's syndrome (47,XXY), the most frequent chromosomal intersex condition in males, occurs in approximately 1:500 liveborn males (see also section on Clinical Syndromes of Hypogonadism in Chapter 9). Males with this anomaly are not detectable clinically until puberty although the condition is easily identified at any age by finding a sex chromatin mass in buccal smears and confirming the diagnosis by chromosome analyses. The condition does not cause spontaneous abortion, and hence the histology of the fetal XXY testis has not yet been described. However, even in infants, the testes are histologically abnormal; there are no spermatogonia, or they are extremely rare, and the seminiferous tubules are lined only by Sertoli cells. The internal and external genitalia are otherwise normal and the patients are reared as males.

During puberty, the testes do not enlarge and subsequently the seminiferous tubules progressively hyalinize (Fig. 11-25**D**; see also Fig. 9-2**A**, **B**). As a result, the testes are small, firm, and relatively insensitive. Urinary gonadotropin levels are abnormally high, indicating hyperactive pituitary function and gonadal failure. Testosterone levels are subnormal in many patients, and secondary sex characteristics may be poorly developed. After puberty, such patients have eunuchoid body proportions, high-pitched voices, scanty facial hair, and—commonly—gynecomastia. However, some of these patients have normal androgen production and therefore have normal secondary sex characteristics (Fig. 9-1). They are infertile because they produce no sperm but are often normally potent or have only slightly reduced libido.

The average intelligence of a group of these patients is lower than normal, and approximately 1:100 men in institutions for the mentally retarded has Klinefelter's syndrome. Although about 20% of XXY individuals may be so retarded as to require institutional care, many of those with normal or slightly low IQ have problems of personality and behavior which limit their achievement potential. Patients with Klinefelter's syndrome may have a slightly increased risk of death in early childhood and as adults are more prone to develop chronic pulmonary disease, varicose veins, and perhaps diabetes mellitus.

Comparison of chromosomal findings in surveys of male newborns or chromatin-positive newborns and adult patients with Klinefelter's syndrome show interesting differences (it should be noted that the latter have been selected because of their medical problems). In newborn surveys, approximately 25% of chromatin-positive males are mosaics with 46,XY and 47,XXY cell lines (Fig. 11-28). However, this mosaicism occurs in only 10% of chromatin-positive males found in surveys of the mentally retarded, and in less than 1% of those in maximal-security prison surveys. This suggests that the presence of the normal cell line modifies the effect of the 47,XXY cell line on the mental and behavioral development of these males.

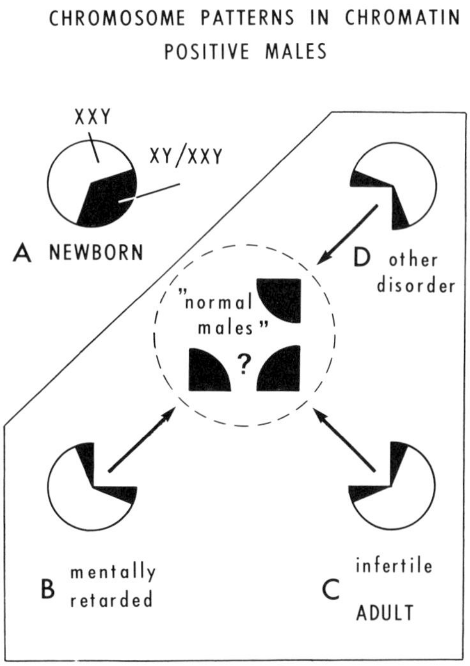

Fig. 11-28. Effect of mosaicism on chromatin-positive males. This figure contrasts the relative frequency among X chromatin-positive males of XY/XXY mosaics in (*A*) the newborn period, and (*B, C, D*) in adults with mental retardation, infertility, and/or other gonadal disorders. Because mosaic individuals probably survive to adult life, a random sample of "normal" males should contain several of these mosaics. Men with classic nonmosaic 47/XXY Klinefelter's syndrome are infertile and many are mentally retarded.

The presence of normal cells in mosaic (46,XY/47,XXY), chromatin-positive males may signify that some of these patients will be fertile since only 5–10% of adult chromatin-positive male patients studied because of infertility have this mosaicism. Such XY/XXY newborns may be "lost" to medical statistics as adults because they do not have the usual problems of the XXY individuals. It is therefore important to be cautious about the prognosis when discussing with the parents the consequences of an XXY pattern or particularly an XY/XXY finding in a newborn because the parents may believe they will not have grandchildren by that son. If the son were to have children, his parents will remember how wrong the physician was (while he may never know of his error), or they might believe that the grandchildren were illegitimate.

A difficult and important ethical problem arises when a baby boy is found to have 47,XXY Klinefelter's syndrome during a survey. The difficulty is whether to tell the parents that their apparently healthy newborn son will almost certainly be sterile, may be mentally dull or retarded, and will probably have learning and behavior problems. If the parents are not told, they will be spared some anguish until some of these events occur. The parents may be told if they are well adjusted and can understand the problem, particularly if the infant has any clinical abnormalities; or if they have provisionally decided to have no other children, they may then wish to re-consider that decision.

Variants of Klinefelter's Syndrome

Poly X with Y. Persons with three or four X chromosomes and a Y chromosome (48,XXXY or 49,XXXXY) have the clinical characteristics of Klinefelter's syndrome but are severely mentally retarded and usually have osseous abnormalities, particularly radioulnar synostosis and a prognathic mandible. Genital development is male because of the Y chromosome and despite the presence of three or four X chromosomes. The number of X chromosomes, and therefore the sex chromosome complex, can be accurately predicted by determination of the maximum number of X chromatin masses per cell (maximum number of masses per cell plus one equals the number of X chromosomes).

XX Male. This rare condition should be considered here because such patients have the clinical and sex chromatin features of Klinefelter's syndrome. The chromosomal findings may be regarded as one normal X (from the mother) and one morphologically normal X (from the father) which includes some Y chromosome material (X^Y). The latter is probably translocated from the Y to the X chromosome during end-to-end pairing of the X and Y chromosomes at meiosis in the father's testes.[14] (See also the section on True Hermaphrodites later in this chapter.)

Turner's Syndrome (45,XO) and Variants

These short, sterile females (see Fig. 11-2; see also Chapters 10 and 16 and Fig. 16-6) occur about 1 in 5,000 liveborn females and usually have a 45,XO chromosome pattern or variants that produce effective monosomy for the short arm of one X (Fig. 11-29)[7, 12, 13, 18, 19] or mosaicism that includes the XO type or an equivalent. Most patients are sex-chromatin-negative, but those with an isochromosome of the X chromosome are chromatin-positive.

These patients may come to the physician's attention:

1. *In the newborn period,* because of edema of feet and hands and certain characteristic anomalies, particularly skin webbing (Fig. 11-2) at the sides of the neck (from just below the ear to the shoulder), shield-like chest, coarctation of the aorta, multiple pigmented nevi, and other malformations
2. *In infancy or childhood,* because of retarded growth (Table 11-6) or sometimes because of disorders found in males—e.g., hemophilia, Duchenne muscular dystrophy
3. *At puberty,* because they do not develop secondary sex characteristics and do not menstruate
4. *In adult life,* because they are infertile. Their intelligence is usually normal and, at the time of their birth, their mothers were in the normal age range. Some prepubertal patients have

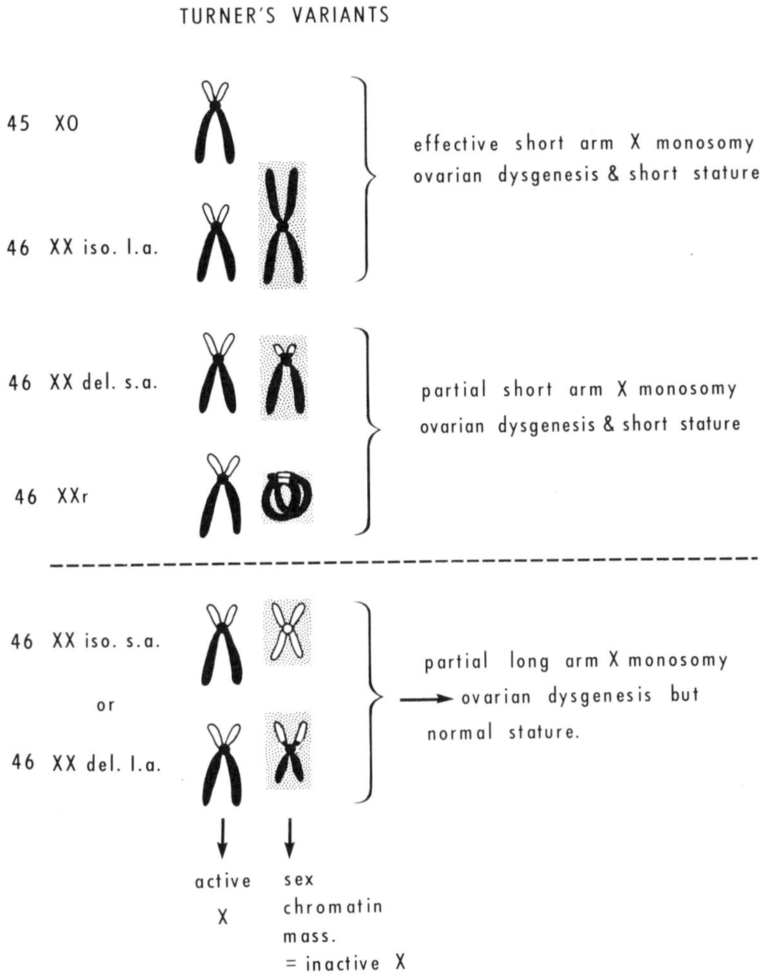

Fig. 11-29. Chromosome patterns in Turner's syndrome and variants. This diagram shows the X chromosomes (normal, *at left;* abnormal, *at right*). The long arm of the normal X is drawn black and the short arm white for clearer demonstration of the abnormality in the other X chromosome.

Patients with a defect in either the short or long arm of an X chromosome are sterile because of ovarian dysgenesis.

In the *top two rows,* one set of short arms of the X chromosome is totally absent, and in the *third* and *fourth rows,* part of the short arms is absent. These patients are always of short stature.

In contrast, the variants shown below the *dotted line* are of normal height; in them, the X abnormalities involve the long arm of an X. This and other evidence suggests that the short arm X chromosome bears a factor related to growth.

Isochromosome long arm (*iso. l.a.*); deletion short arm (*del. s.a.*); isochromosome short arm (*iso. s.a.*); deletion long arm (*del. s.a.*); ring chromosome (r).

no external abnormalities and are only identified by sex chromatin and chromosome studies.

Chromosome studies on spontaneous abortions show that 98% of XO conceptuses are lost in early pregnancy (Table 11-4). It has been postulated that those who survive must be mosaics with normal and XO cells who lost an X or Y chromosome by anaphase lag and therefore had XX or XY pattern in early embryogenesis.

Anatomic studies of chromatin-negative 45,XO spontaneous abortuses reveal considerable swell-

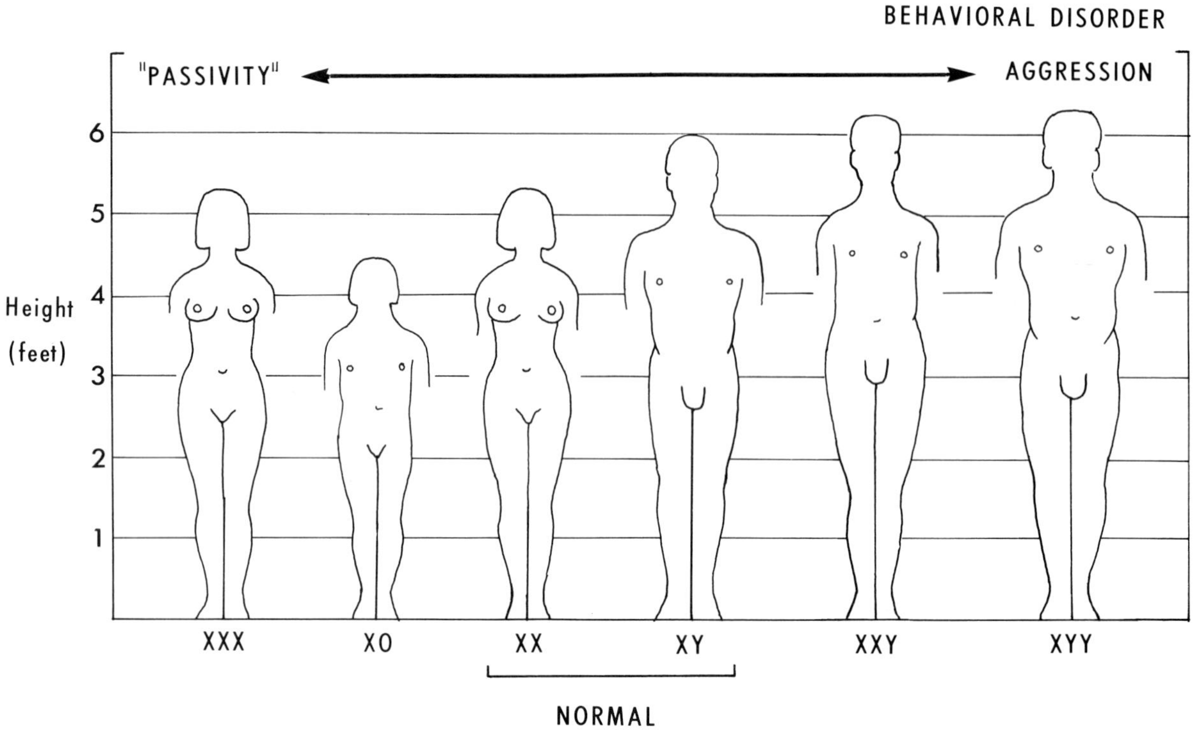

Fig. 11-30. Height, sexual development and personality. This figure shows the difference in height between the normal male and female, and the development of secondary sex characteristics. The XXY and XYY are both taller than average but the legs are disproportionately longer (eunuchoid feature) in the XXY than normal. This figure probably exaggerates the height of XYY individuals because tall men have usually been selected for this investigation and the true range of height is not yet established for the XYY individuals.

The XXX and normal female are indistinguishable physically, but the XO individual is very short with a thick neck and trunk and has no secondary sex characteristics.

The suggestion that XYY men are more aggressive than normal males and that XXX women are more passive than normal females is caricatured in this figure.

ing of the neck, mainly lymphatics, which probably causes the redundant skin folds present at birth (neck webbing).[42] The gonads in the first few months of gestation contain almost normal numbers of oocytes. These oocytes are assumed to degenerate during the last few months of fetal life because they are seldom found in such newborns at autopsy, and the ovaries are composed only of intertwining bands of connective tissue. These individuals develop primary sex characteristics of females, the müllerian duct system develops normally to form fallopian tubes and uterus, and the wolffian duct system regresses.

At birth, the internal and external genital organs of these patients are those of a normal female except for streak ovaries.[44] At puberty, secondary sex characteristics fail to develop. These girls do not menstruate spontaneously because they do not have the cyclic changes of hormone to build up a normal uterine endometrium; hence, the internal and external genital organs remain infantile.

With appropriate hormonal therapy, secondary sex characteristics can be partially developed and cyclical bleeding can be induced. Despite their handicaps, some of these patients wish to marry and, to avoid later disappointments, the fiancés should be told before marriage that these girls are almost always sterile because of lack of oocytes, follicles, and ova. However, they can enjoy normal sex relations and can be good mothers to adopted children.

Triple-X (47,XXX)

The first such patient reported did not menstruate and was infertile. In later reports, almost all triple-X females menstruated normally, had no physical defects, and were fertile with normal offspring. Most have no particular abnormalities that need medical attention, and therefore little is known about consequences of this defect, such as increased liability to certain diseases. Triple-X females can usually be identified only by sex-chromatin (Fig. 11-17 and 11-20) or chromosomal studies. Their incidence at birth is 1 in 1,200 liveborn females[2] (Table 11-4). These patients are alleged to be more passive (feminine) than normal females (compare with XYY and XY males in Fig. 11-30). The distribution curve of intelligence is shifted to the left compared with normal populations, and 1% of females in institutions for the mentally retarded have this disorder. The mean maternal age is above average.

Double-Y Syndrome (47,XYY)

The double-Y state is important because it is so frequent (about 1 in 500 newborn males).[39] However, we know relatively little about the condition, particularly about those 47,XYY males who are not unusually tall, criminals, or retardates. The incidence will be determined more accurately when results of many more newborn surveys are available. Newborns with XYY syndrome are now being followed through childhood and adolescence into adult life so that their growth patterns can be determined, because even in childhood many of them are unusually tall. They are also being followed in an attempt to find clinical "screening" tests and to study their behavior.

The syndrome is frequent in tall men in maximal security prisons and its identification in certain murderers has increased interest in this condition.[16, 22] In surveys, the incidence of XYY among tall males with normal behavior and short psychopathic males is little different from that in the newborn population. The aggressive behavior of the XYY male probably represents an exaggeration of that seen in the normal male; they are frequently described as "impulsive" rather than aggressive. Most XYY males studied to date have had personality problems from an early age and, because of their behavior, earned police records about 5 years earlier than the average criminal with a normal chromosome complement. Usually their crimes are against objects rather than individuals: Arson is particularly common. Sibling studies show that XYY individuals may be "genetic criminals" rather than environmental criminals because their brothers have a rate of criminal activity appropriate to their social class. The term "genetic criminal" has been applied to this condition on the assumption that such persons have more difficulties with society's rules, are less responsible for their actions than 46,XY criminals, should be punished less severely, and may be less likely to respond to therapy or be eligible for parole. If identified in early childhood, they might profit from special schooling or selection of occupations that may satisfy their aggressive tendencies without breaking the law, i.e., wrestling, boxing and certain occupations like lumbering.

Additional abnormalities have been reported in XYY males: fine tremors, clumsiness, and other minor neurological symptoms, an abnormal electroencephalogram pattern, severe acne, radioulnar synostosis and a long P-R interval on electrocardiograms. Minor defects of external genitalia, particularly hypospadias, have been found in some XYY patients, but development of gonads, ducts, genitalia, and sex characteristics are usually normal. The sex drive of these men appears to be normal, but because of their personalities, they frequently do not form firm attachments or marry, and proof of fertility is frequently not available. Meiotic studies on a few patients and mitotic studies on offspring of several patients showed normal patterns.

Until recently screening for the 47,XYY condition involved expensive, laborious, full chromosome analyses. Now, Caspersson and coworkers have found that certain fluorescent dyes "stain" the Y chromosome intensely in mitosis and in nondividing cells. The XYY condition can be suspected if two fluorescent spots (instead of the one in normal males) are found in many cells from buccal smears, amnion mounts, lymphocytes, and probably most cells (Fig. 11-17, 11-20).

ICSH (LH) levels in XYY males have been found to be elevated, but there are conflicting reports concerning increased testosterone secretion, which, if present, would require some alteration in the normal negative feedback regulation of androgen production. A more likely explanation of the increased gonadotropin levels is some relative insensitivity of the Leydig cells to pituitary stimulation.

It is of interest that killifish (small, live-bearing, aquarium fish) have been bred with two Y chromosomes by exposure to androgen in the water, which results in survival of a greater than normal number of XYY males, originating by paternal nondisjunction. These XYY fish are larger and sexually more active than killifish with a single Y.

True Hermaphrodites

In zoology, a true hermaphrodite is defined as an animal that functions as a male and a female at different stages of its life, as do some amphibians.

In medicine, this strict criterion does not apply, but a true hermaphrodite has both testicular and ovarian tissue and the condition is rare.[34] The testes may be abnormal (they are frequently intraabdominal; if so, they produce no sperm), and the ovaries must contain ova. Most of these individuals are chromatin-positive and have an apparently normal female chromosome pattern (Fig. 11-31). Because genes on the Y chromosome promote development of testes even in individuals with many X chromosomes (e.g., XXXY), true hermaphrodites have been carefully studied, usually without detection of a Y chromosome even in mosaic cell population. It is presently believed that exchange of material between the X and Y chromosome in the paternal testes may produce an X-bearing sperm which also contains Y chromosome material (X^Y—see also the section on XX male earlier in this chapter) that could therefore explain the paradox of Y effect with an XX pattern.[14] In such zygotes, inactivation (or "lyonization") of an unusual proportion of maternal or paternal X chromosomes might explain the considerable variation in gonadal and genital duct development. For example, if the zygotes are regarded as XX^Y then the X or the X^Y may have predominant effect, depending upon the proportions and distribution of such cells in relation to the developing gonads. The less frequent chromatin-negative hermaphrodites may have an XY pattern and/or other patterns.

Most patients will need medical advice during one or more of the following times:

1. Newborn period—ambiguous genitalia
2. Childhood–puberty—inguinal hernia containing an ovotestis, fallopian tube, or part of the uterus
3. Puberty—gynecomastia and/or menstruation
4. Adulthood—sterility

True hermaphrodites are usually reared as males, although the external genitalia are abnormal: The urethra may open onto the perineum, and the scrotum may contain only one gonad. At puberty their breasts may enlarge (80% of cases), and they may bleed periodically through the small perineal opening (50% of cases).

Rarely, true hermaphroditism may result from double fertilization (presumed to be an ovum and a polar body) by X- and Y-bearing sperms to form an XX/XY mosaic, in whom two populations of red cells may be found.

Pseudohermaphrodites

The pseudohermaphrodite has a phenotype and sex of rearing opposite to that indicated by gonadal type, sex chromatin, and sex chromosome pattern.[34] In addition to medical problems, in rare cases there may be other difficulties, such as inheritance of titles restricted to males and participation in athletic competitions (a female with male physique would have an unfair advantage in the Olympics).

Testicular feminization syndrome is one important type of *male pseudohermaphroditism* (see also Chapters 8 and 9). These patients have testes which are histologically normal but do not descend completely, usually only reaching the inguinal canal. Because of lack of end-organ

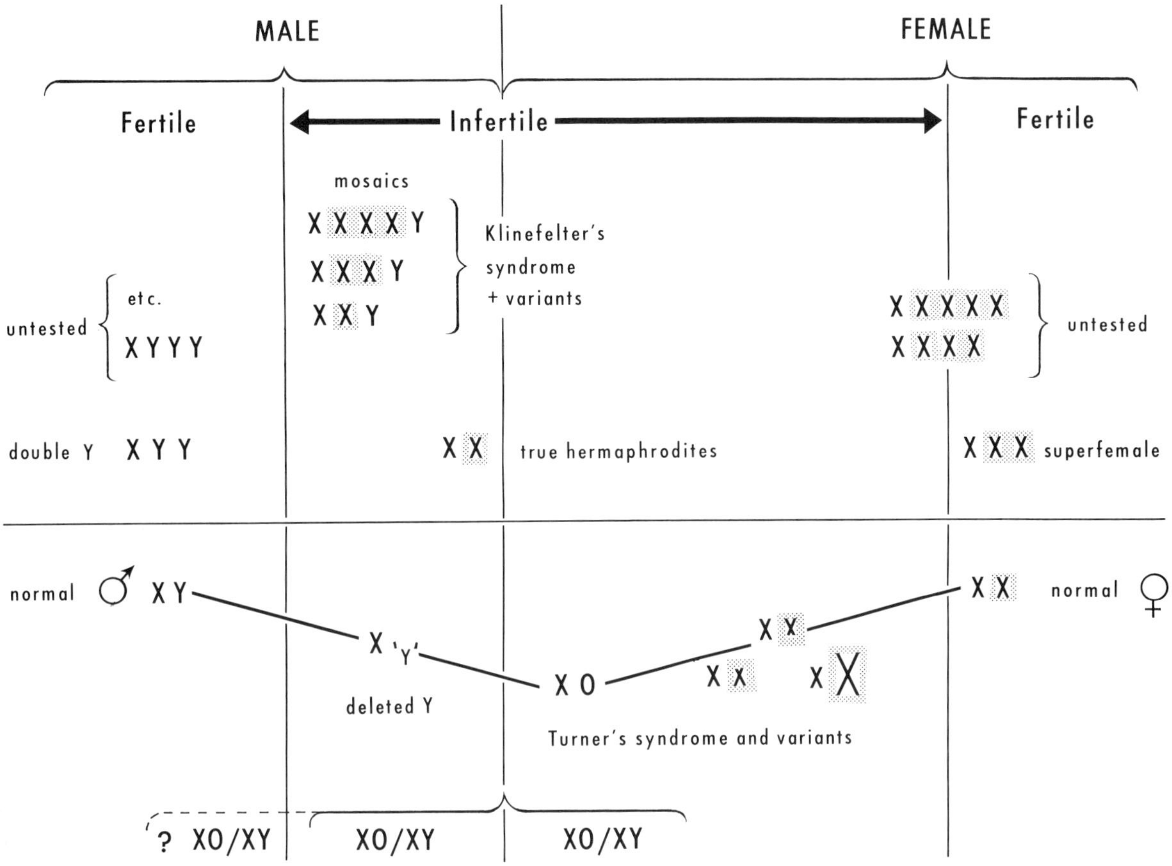

Fig. 11-31. Gender, fertility and karyotype. The basic theme of this diagram is the spectrum XY (fertile male)—XO (infertile intersex)—XX (fertile female). It also shows gender and fertility in individuals with normal and abnormal sex chromosome complements (patterns).

Extra sex chromosomes appropriate to the sex (i.e., extra Y's in males and X's in females) do not impair fertility as illustrated by XYY fertile males and XXX fertile females except perhaps when the number of extra sex chromosomes produces severe mental retardation or malformations.

Extra chromosomes inappropriate to the sex result in infertility as in Klinefelter's syndrome XXY and variants.

One of the variants of Klinefelter's syndrome is the "46,XX male with testes" in whom the paternal X chromosome is believed to contain some Y chromosome material as a result of a meiotic error. Some clinical features of true hermaphrodites may also be explained by similar exchange of material between the X and Y chromosomes in the paternal gonad which results in an abnormal sex chromosome (not presently recognizable morphologically) in the patient.

Structural abnormalities of an X chromosome often result in Turner's syndrome. The "XO/XY syndrome," often called 'mixed gonadal dysgenesis' may have the phenotype of Turner's syndrome, or male with abnormal genitalia, or possibly normal male (shown with dashed line in the fig.).

response to androgens, these individuals develop female external genitalia. However, the müllerian-duct derivatives regress so that the patients have no uterus or fallopian tubes. The presence of wolffian duct derivatives (vas deferens and seminal vesicles), which develop under the influence of testicular "organizers," proves that these organizers are not androgens.

These patients may be detected:

1. In infancy, when a partly descended testis may be found at operation for inguinal hernias
2. In childhood, if they develop X-linked diseases such as hemophilia and muscular dystrophies (limited to males)
3. In adulthood, because of failure to menstruate and infertility

They may also come to the physician's notice because there is a familial excess of females, many of whom are infertile.

Pseudohermaphrodites are of normal height and, at puberty, develop some secondary sex characteristics; they usually have breast tissue, but have scant pubic and axillary hair. When the testes are trapped in the inguinal canals, an operation may be necessary because the testes swell in this confined space. Because a tumor might develop in the gonads, these can be removed after feminization and the patient given supplemental female hormones.

Female Pseudohermaphroditism

Female pseudohermaphroditism has several causes, one of which is inherited as an autosomal recessive. The infant girls have a large clitoris (due to androgens from the hyperplastic adrenal) and may develop acute salt loss and die if the disorder is not quickly recognized and treated. When a mother has one affected child, doctors are forewarned and examine later-born babies very carefully to treat them early. Tests for pregnanediol in amniotic fluid from the late stages of a subsequent pregnancy in such a mother can facilitate diagnosis in the unborn baby and treatment with steroid injections into the affected fetus can be given.

Mixed Gonadal Dysgenesis (XO/XY Syndrome)

This uncommon mosaicism results from loss of a Y chromosome from some cells in an XY zygote soon after conception, resulting in XO and XY cells[41] (Fig. 11-12). The proportions of XO and XY cells in various tissues will affect the development of gonads, ducts, and genitalia and may result in a continuous spectrum of clinical findings from Turner's syndrome (XO cell predominant) to a "normal" male (XY cell predominant). The former but not the latter type of case has been reported (Fig. 11-31).

Patients with presumed predominant effect of XO cells have bilateral streak gonads, one of which may contain a small area of rudimentary testicular tissue, but this gonad remains undescended and does not produce male development of the genitalia. These patients are reared as females and are short and sterile.

Patients with presumed predominant effect of XY cells have one normal testis in the scrotum and an intraabdominal gonad, which may be a rudimentary testis or a streak. These patients may have otherwise normal external genitalia although hypospadias is frequent.

Chromosomal Abnormalities and Infertility

Fertility cannot be tested in many persons with autosomal abnormalities, particularly those associated with a shortened lifespan (trisomy 18, trisomy 13) and individuals with severe mental retardation. In patients with balanced translocations and other rearrangements, fertility (i.e., number of conceptions) is probably not reduced although the number of spontaneous abortions may be increased and result in fewer liveborns.

Fertility in persons with sex chromosome abnormalities (Fig. 11-31) can be studied more easily. In 45,XO pattern fetuses, primordial germ cells have been found until the fourth to fifth intrauterine month, when these cells degenerate. Consequently, from birth onward, these individuals have streak gonads without germ cells, and therefore cannot ovulate and are infertile. Fetuses with 47,XXY patterns have not yet been identified for histological studies of the gonads, but even infants with this syndrome have extremely few seminiferous tubules that contain spermatogonia. Therefore, these individuals produce no sperm and they are infertile although a few patients with the XY/XXY form of Klinefelter's syndrome might be fertile. Patients with Klinefelter's syndrome with more than two X chromosomes (XXXY and XXXXY) are infertile because of the same gonadal defects as the XXY type. They are also severely mentally retarded.

Males with two Y chromosomes (47,XYY) are presumably fertile. Females with an extra X chromosome (47,XXX) are fertile, but females with 48,XXXX and 49,XXXXX have such severe mental retardation that their fertility is not testable, although some of the 48,XXXX females menstruate.

Disproportionate Infertility in Males

Chromosomal abnormalities reduce fertility in males to a greater degree than in females. In Down's syndrome, pregnancies have been reported in more than 15 females, whereas fertility in a male has not been described. The latter might be difficult to prove, as in most cases of paternity, but it is probably a true finding because spermatogenesis is defective in most of these male patients.

The disproportionately severe effect on fertility in males can also be illustrated by hybrids resulting from mating between animals of different species—e.g., lions and tigers (chromosome number both 38). The female hybrids may be fertile, but males are sterile. In hybrids between species with different chromosome numbers—e.g., horse (64 chromosomes), donkey (62 chromosomes)—the offspring, a mule or a jenny, has 63 chromosomes and meiosis may be abnormal. Some female mules have shown evidence of ovulation on histologic examination of the ovaries, but male hybrids show no evidence of spermatogenesis.

Offspring of Fertile Patients with Chromosomal Abnormalities

Gametes formed by 47,XYY men and 47,XXX women should include equal numbers of 24,XY, 23,Y, 24,YY and 23,X; and of 24,XX and 23,X, respectively. Most offspring of XYY and XXX parents have normal chromosomes, a finding which suggests that selection operates against ova or sperm containing unbalanced haploid chromosome sets—i.e., 24,XX and 24,XY or 24,YY sperm. This is in contrast to pregnant females with Down's syndrome, who have had the expected equal incidence of normal or Down's syndrome babies following fertilization of 24,X+21 and 23,X gametes. This finding suggests that the normal 23,X and abnormal 24,X+21 ova are equally capable of fertilization.

"Artificial" Parenthood

Although infertile couples, including those with chromosomal abnormalities, cannot have children of their own, they often make excellent parents; therefore they may be encouraged to make use of artificial insemination, adoption, or less commonly, follicle-stimulating agents. Before this matter is discussed in detail, the relative roles of the normal male and female during pregnancy and labor should be considered: The male must be present at conception but plays only a supporting role during pregnancy and labor.

Artificial Insemination

When the husband is sterile, sperm can be "borrowed" from an anonymous normal male and used for artificial insemination of the female. This has enabled many couples to have a child. With some couples, the method has been technically successful in producing a child, but unhappiness has resulted from the disparity of the parental contribution and the confirmation of the fertility in the wife.

Adoption

At present, if the mother is infertile, or the father is infertile and artificial insemination is not acceptable, the couple must adopt a child. Although most adopting couples give their new child as much love as a natural parent, the child may notice a difference. In addition, the couple's desire to produce offspring is only partially satisfied, but some "subfertile" couples have subsequently had natural pregnancies after adopting a child.

Follicle-Stimulating Agents

Pregnancies have resulted after treatment with these compounds, particularly clomiphene, although there is a risk of multiple ovulations. Premature delivery of quintuplets has been reported following pituitary stimulation (see also Chapter 9).

Gonadal Tumors in "Intersex" Individuals

Tumors are more frequent in undescended than descended testes, and the risk is greatly increased for the patient who also has a sex-chromosome abnormality, particularly XO/XY syndrome and testicular feminization. The frequency of gonadal neoplasms reported in these syndromes may be overstated because many of these patients were investigated because of the tumor rather than the intersex problem. However, this is partly balanced by patients who develop gonadal tumors after investigation of their intersex problem (the gonadal tumor may therefore not have been described in the published report).

Gonadal tumors are usually formed of hyperplastic cells identifiable as testicular in origin, but frequently these tumors do not metastasize or spread beyond the gonad, they are seldom malignant in a strict sense. It is desirable to remove any tissue which may become malignant. However, the time when such tissue is removed is important, particularly in individuals with testicular feminization, because the testicular tissue can produce secondary sex characteristics "naturally" and malignant changes are rare until adult life. In some patients with testicular feminization, the testes increase in size at puberty, as in the normal male, but if the testes are in the inguinal canal, this increase causes extreme pain and tenderness, and the enlarging testicular masses are excised. These testicular masses, if they are intraabdominal, may become extremely large; the resulting "tumors" are given a variety of names. If, after puberty, such a patient has his abdomen opened for some other reason, the intraabdominal testes can also be excised.

In XO/XY syndrome, the patient with a descended gonad is usually reared as male although the intraabdominal gonad is probably a streak without testicular tissue. XO/XY persons without a descended gonad are reared as females, and one or both gonads may contain testicular material that may later become malignant. In such females, the gonad is unlikely to produce satisfactory feminization at puberty, and the gonads are therefore frequently excised during exploratory laparotomy in early childhood. In addition, the doctor can then say to the parents that the child is definitely a female and has no testicular tissue.

Nongonadal tumors and leukemia may also be increased in intersex individuals, but the number of proven malignancies and intersex patients at risk is too small for definite conclusions. Carcinoma of the breast has been frequently reported in males with Klinefelter's syndrome and can be linked with the hyperplasia causing gynecomastia in such patients.

Prenatal Diagnosis (Amniocentesis)

Many years ago some workers did X chromatin studies on cells from amniotic fluid of women from families with X-linked disorders, such as hemophilia and Duchenne muscular dystrophy, to detect samples with chromatin-negative cells which presumably signify a chromatin-negative (male) fetus. Such pregnancies are terminated because 50% of these male fetuses may develop the disorder although 50% of the males would be normal. Eventually tests will make possible the identification of affected male fetuses so that such pregnancies can be terminated (already possible with the rare Hunter and Lesch-Nyhan syndromes) and leave the normal male fetuses to be born. However, the routine abortion of males will only reduce the number of patients with the disorder in the next generation. The disorder could be eliminated from known carrier families if all female fetuses (or preferably only carrier female fetuses) were therapeutically aborted or if newborn females were tested and the carriers prevented from having male children.

Chromosome analyses and fluorescent Y tests done on cultured amniotic fluid cells have helped in "sexing" the fetus, because sex chromatin studies are difficult and frequently unreliable. By studying the enzyme activity and biochemistry of amniotic fluid cells, with and without culture, metabolic defects have also been recognized before birth.[26, 28] Little is known about normal enzyme levels at different stages of fetal development and less about these levels in the different types of cells found in early and late gestation.

However, studies of direct and cultured amniotic fluid cells and of concentrates from amniotic fluid can elicit much information. Already, a female pseudohermaphrodite can be recognized before birth, and death thus prevented in the first few days of life from salt-losing nephritis.

In families in which some members have testicular feminization, fetuses with XY karyotypes can also be identified; 50% of these will be liable to feminization and its attendant problems (see section on Pseudohermaphrodites earlier in this chapter; also see Chapters 9 and 10).

Change of Sex

It should be stressed that persons who request a change of sex rarely have an organic sexual disorder, in contrast to the vast majority who have psychological problems. These individuals are considerably outnumbered by homosexuals in both groups. In the future, only in rare circumstances will a person be reared in the inappropriate sex, but at present, a true change of sex might be contemplated in the occasional patient. Before any decision is made, such patients have to be investigated carefully using clinical and chromosomal studies. However, the most extensive studies should be psychological to determine how strongly motivated the individual is and how well he will adjust to the new sex. Most sex changes require extensive surgery and are usually performed by changing males to females rather than vice versa.

Although the number of patients in whom such a change is contemplated seriously is extremely small, the social, legal, and other problems involved can usefully be discussed because some of them might apply to other individuals with intersex problems. After a successful series of operations for change of sex, the patient must become accustomed to the new sex role. This is usually not difficult because he (or she) frequently has lived as a member of the opposite sex for some months or years. Legal requirements for registration of a new name, change of birth certificate, change of passport, etc., create many difficulties which can eventually be overcome.

However, it should also be remembered that the "changed" individual starts a new life, name and status, and would therefore usually lose the advantages of previously obtained favorable employment, business, or banking references. Finally, it should be stressed that the operation is bound to make the patient sterile because of the castration, but many of these individuals have been psychologically sterile and a few were sterile because of previous operations.

Chromosomal Abnormalities and Endocrine Disorders

Abnormalities of endocrine function or histology have not been thoroughly investigated in individuals with autosomal abnormalities associated with considerable reduction in lifespan. Many abnormalities have been described in Down's syndrome (trisomy-21 or equivalent), but as tests become increasingly sophisticated and diagnostic facilities improve, some of these abnormalities seem to be of less significance. Because these patients frequently have features shared by cretins—deep voices, large tongues, and dry skin—it may be difficult to distinguish between these two conditions. Thyroid and pituitary glands may have minor morphological abnormalities in Down's syndrome, although tests of pituitary function and many tests of thyroid function are abnormal in only a few. Although abnormal thyrcid function is not frequently found in tests, thyroid autoantibodies are common in these patients and their mothers.

About 50% of male mongoloids have undescended testes, and even in other male patients there is no evidence of fertility. In females, secondary sex characteristics appear later and are more poorly developed than in normals; these patients are probably subfertile. Serum calcium and protein levels are frequently low, and tryptophan metabolism is abnormal. Glucose tolerance test results are abnormal, particularly in older patients, who also have abnormal galactose tolerances, and some have abnormal insulin levels. Reports of adrenal function tests in patients with Down's syndrome are contradictory: On the basis of urinary steroid studies and eosinophil responses to corticotropin and epinephrine, some workers have reported that 50% of patients have adrenal insufficiency, while others have found no difference between these patients and controls.

The incidence of thyroid autoantibodies is increased in patients with Turner's syndrome. Hashimoto's thyroiditis and diabetes mellitus are unusually frequent in patients with Turner's syndrome, particularly those with an isochromosome long-arm X. Diabetes mellitus is more common in patients with Klinefelter's syndrome. Patients with this syndrome may also have somewhat depressed thyroid function (low protein-bound iodine, serum thyroxine, T_3 resin uptake, and radioactive iodine uptake, with poor response to thyroid-stimulating hormone) but usually without obvious hypometabolism.

Chromosomal Abnormalities and Growth

Growth is reduced in almost all conceptuses that have an autosomal abnormality (see also Chapter 15). In spontaneous abortion this suppression of growth is reflected in the empty amniotic sac, in which the embryo (fetus) is not recognizable or is represented only by a small nodule of tissue. In liveborn babies with autosomal abnormalities (trisomy 21, 18, or 13), the infant and the placenta are both small, despite the full gestational period. After birth, growth is subnormal: The infants do not gain weight or increase body length at a normal rate. In the few who do survive for several years, physical growth is greatly retarded. Patients with Down's syndrome (trisomy 21) are always short for their age; the growth rates of individuals with most other autosomal abnormalities cannot be determined because of their short lifespan.

The growth of patients with Turner's syndrome (45,XO and variants) is invariably slow after birth and is retarded in many other individuals with defects of an X or a Y chromosome. Sex chromosome abnormalities associated with defects of growth presumably are due to lack of genes concerned with regulation of growth. Such loci are believed to be on the short arms of the X and Y chromosomes because these chromosomes associate at meiosis by short-arm to short-arm pairing. Males with an abnormally small Y chromosome are sometimes very short although men with an abnormally long Y chromosome are of normal height. However, men with two Y chromosomes (47,XYY) are frequently tall. Those with Klinefelter's syndrome (47,XXY) and a few sterile persons with XY pattern reared as females are tall; but this height is attributed to the eunuchoidism, delayed epiphyseal closure, and consequently prolonged linear growth, particularly of the lower limbs.

In three relatively rare genetically determined disorders (Bloom's syndrome, ataxia-telangiectasia, Fanconi's anemia), the babies and placentas are low in weight despite term gestation. These short persons are especially liable to leukemia or malignant tumors. Lymphocyte or fibroblast cultures from these patients show a high incidence of chromosomal breakage and structural chromosomal rearrangements. The lack of growth of patients has been attributed to loss of cells in vivo following chromosomal breakage and misdivision, and the malignant changes, to chromosomal rearrangements following breakage ("new" cell types are formed, some of which may not be properly controlled by normal regulatory mechanisms).

New Approaches and Future Work

As chromosomal findings, X and Y chromatin, dermal patterns, and clinical findings in patients with intersex conditions are correlated, knowledge will continue to expand, though more slowly than in the past. Present hypotheses will continue to be tested against new genetic abnormalities. In the next decade greater insight will come chiefly through new approaches entailing refined studies on human specimens and elegant animal experiments that may lead eventually to "genetic engineering." However, even though exciting experiments are already possible in animals, many ethical, social, and legal problems must be solved before the techniques and results can be extended to man.

Studies on Man

Cultured Fibroblasts

Fibroblast culture has helped to elucidate many genetic disorders, particularly inborn errors of metabolism. The following procedures are used:

1. Histochemical techniques that demonstrate abnormal products in the cells
2. Studies of biosynthesis using radiolabeled precursors
3. Demonstration of specific enzyme defects through failure to incorporate the radiolabel (autoradiography)
4. Identification of two types of cells in mosaic individuals, particularly mothers of patients by enzyme histochemistry and autoradiography using radiolabeled precursors
5. Electron microscopic studies of fibroblasts cultured in normal media and in media containing material that the individual cannot metabolize (e.g., galactose in the culture medium produces changes in fibroblasts from patients with galactosemia whereas other sugars do not)
6. Biochemical estimations of specific substances in the fibroblasts (e.g., those in Hurler's and Marfan's syndromes contain abnormal amounts and distribution of mucopolysaccharides; in cystic fibrosis only the total amounts of mucopolysaccharides are abnormal)
7. Use of combinations of several of these studies, as when identifying different forms of gout

In endocrine disorders fibroblast cultures have not yet been used frequently except in studies of testicular feminization. Such patients produce excessive amounts of androgen(s) that are biologically active (in animals) but do not work in the patient. Androgens from other sources also produce no response in these patients, an indication that their end-organs are insensitive. This insensitivity has also been demonstrated by in-vitro studies of cultured fibroblasts.

"Transplantation" of Ova

A frequent cause of infertility in females is inflammation of the fallopian tube. The blockage thus caused prevents the normal passage of ova from the ovary to the uterine cavity or delays passage, with the result that the blastocyst is too far developed to implant when it reaches the optimal site in the uterus.

Females with gonadal dysgenesis, such as Turner's syndrome, produce no ova at all. As noted previously, with hormone supplements, women with Turner's syndrome will develop secondary sex characteristics, can engage in normal sexual relations, and can be satisfactory mothers. Such a woman could theoretically bear a child if her uterus had developed sufficiently through hormonal treatment to nurture a fertilized ovum placed in it. Transplantation of ova has been successful in animal experiments and might eventually be applied to selected human patients.

Animal Studies

A number of experiments have been conducted relating to early embryonic development, growth in utero, reimplantation, and gender role.

Artificial Fertilization

These experiments are done on animals of different coat color to permit instant identification of offspring. The normally fertilized blastocyst is washed from the tube of one animal and implanted into the tube of another animal. If the second animal is in the early stages of pregnancy or has a hormone-induced pseudopregnancy, the blastocyst will implant, develop, and an offspring of the "wrong" coat color will be born.

In-vitro Culture of "Artificial" Blastocysts

Ova can be obtained from the ovary and fertilized in a test tube by adding sperm. The zygotes will develop to the blastocyst stage if kept in special cultures at body temperature (37° C) for 2–3 days. The blastocysts can then be placed into the fallopian tube of an early pregnant or hormonally pseudopregnant animal of different coat color. The blastocyst then grows normally and differs from others at term only in coat color. These experiments were designed to test the effect on early zygotes and blastocysts of X-rays, toxic agents such as drugs, or other substances added to the culture media.

Previously it was impossible to evaluate this period of development because investigations were limited to histologic examination of the blastocysts. Now much more can be learned by determining whether the toxic agents seriously impair growth and further development of the blastocyst in a normal uterine environment. Use of pregnant animals provides "built-in" control blastocysts which, through the rest of pregnancy, would be exposed to the same milieu as test blastocysts. At birth and during rearing, the test animal is always recognizable by the different coat color.

These experiments might be applied to human problems. For example, if an ovum from a normal female, obtained during a pelvic operation or at laparoscopy, could be fertilized with the husband's sperm, the zygote would then be maintained for a few days in culture until it reached the blastocyst stage while the eventual, hitherto sterile, mother was made pseudopregnant. Finally the blastocyst would be transferred, perhaps via an amnioscope through the cervical canal, into the upper part of the uterine cavity.

Mice with Four Parents

During studies of cancer, mice were produced that were derived totally from two separate strains. A black mouse and a white mouse strain of low and high tendencies to spontaneous cancer were selected for study. The experiments are distinct from the ordinary mating between a black mouse and a white mouse in which each of the offspring has approximately one-half of the genetic complement from black or white mouse. In the cancer experiments, sperm and ova from the black mice and sperm and ova from the white mice were used to obtain black-mouse zygotes and white-mouse zygotes. When incubated together, after removal of the zona pellucida by gentle digestion with proteolytic enzymes, one black and one white "naked" zygote eventually "fused" to form a chimera. At the blastocyst stage, the mixed black-mouse and white-mouse cell chimeras were implanted in fallopian tubes of hormonally pseudopregnant animals that subsequently gave birth to the four-parent offspring. Although these experiments require meticulous work, several thousand of such four-parent offspring have been produced. In many animals resulting from fusion of XX and XY zygotes an interesting variety of intersex problems were found. Detailed study of genital development, fertility, and breeding experiments, if possible in such chimeras, will be of great interest.

Animal Models of Human Intersex Problems

In some species intersex conditions are relatively frequent—e.g., true hermaphroditism in goats. Other conditions are less frequent but easily recognized—e.g., tortoise-shell male cats which are sterile and have a chromosome pattern (39,XXY) comparable to Klinefelter's syndrome in man. XO mice have 39 chromosomes (normal 40) and are frequently fertile, in contrast to the XO condition in man.

Miscellaneous intersex conditions in animals resembling those in man are often reported in veterinary journals with detailed accounts of anatomical dissections and chromosome studies. Such animals are useless to breeders and are killed, but they would be valuable to scientists. Genital abnormalities without chromosomal disorders are frequent in certain pedigree animals—e.g., undescended testes in German shepherd dogs and dachshunds. Increase in knowledge will result when breeding experiments are made for assessment of normality of the offspring and to produce other examples of the animal intersex condition.

Studies of twin calves with a partially shared placenta have provided examples of masculinization of genitalia in the female when the other twin has been male. In rats a model of the testicular feminization syndrome of man has been reported after treatment of the pregnant rats with androgens. Double Y (XYY) killifish have also been produced by exposing mating fish to androgens (see section on the Double-Y Syndrome earlier in this chapter).

References

1. Baker, T. G. A quantitative and cytological study of germ cells in human ovaries. *Proc Roy Soc B 158:*417–433, 1963.
2. Barr, M. L., Sergovich, F. R., Carr, D. H., and Shaver, E. L. The triplo-X female: An appraisal based on a study of 12 cases. *Can Med Assoc J 101:*247–258, 1969.
3. Carr, D. H. Chromosome anomalies as a cause of spontaneous abortion. *Am J Obstet Gynec 97:*283–293, 1967.
4. Carr, D. H. Chromosomal errors and development. *Am J Obstet Gynec 104:*327–347, 1969.
5. Caspersson, T., Lomakka, G., and Zech, L. The 24 fluorescence patterns of the human metaphase chromosomes—distinguishing characters and variability. *Hereditas 67:*89–102, 1971.
6. Court Brown, W. M., and Smith, P. G. Human population cytogenetics. *Brit Med Bull 25:*74–80, 1969.
7. de la Chapelle, A. Cytogenetical and clinical observations in female gonadal dysgenesis. *Acta Endocrinol (Kbh) 40:*Suppl. 65, 1962.
8. Drets, M. E., and Shaw, M. W. Specific banding patterns of human chromosomes. *Proc Nat Acad Sci 68:*2073–2077, 1971.
9. Dutrillaux, B., and Lejeune, J. Sur une nouvelle technique d'analyse du caryotype humain. *C.R. Acad Sci (Paris) 272:*2638–2640, 1971.
10. Editorial Spotlighting chromosome types. *Med World News,* Sept. 11, 1970.
11. Editorial In pursuit of the Y chromosome. *Nature (Lond) 226:*897, 1970.
12. Engel, E., and Forbs, A. P. Cytogenetic and clinical findings in 48 patients with congenitally defective or absent ovaries. *Medicine (Baltimore) 44:*135–164, 1965.
13. Ferguson-Smith, M. A. Karyotype—phenotype correlation in gonadal dysgenesis and their bearing on the pathogenesis of malformations. *J Med Genet 2:*142–155, 1965.
14. Ferguson-Smith, M. A. X-Y chromosomal interchange in the etiology of true hermaphroditism and of XX Klinefelter's syndrome. *Lancet 2:*475–476, 1966.
15. Finaz, C., and De Grouchy, J. Le caryotype humain après traitement par l'x-chymotrypsine. *Ann Genet 14:*309–311, 1971.
16. Fox, R. G., XYY chromosomes and crime. *Australian and N. Z. J Criminology 2:*5–19, 1969.
17. George, K. P. Cytochemical differentiation along human chromosomes, *Nature (Lond) 226:*80, 1970.
18. Goldberg, M. B., Scully, A. L., Solomon, I. L., and Steinbach, H. L. Gonadal dysgenesis in phenotypic female subjects. A review of eighty-seven cases, with cytogenetic study in fifty-three. *Am J Med 45:*529–543, 1968.
19. Greenblatt, R. B., Rogers Byrd, J., McDonough, P. G., and Mahesh, V. B. The spectrum of gonadal dysgenesis. A clinical cytogenetic and pathological study. *Am J Obstet Gynecol 98:*151–172, 1967.
20. Harris, G. W. Hormonal differentiation of the developing nervous system with respect to patterns of endocrine function. *Phil Trans Roy Soc Lond B 259:*165–177, 1970.
21. Jacobs, P. A. "Chromosome Abnormalities and Population Studies," p. 284–290. In *Congenital Malformations, Proceedings of the Third International Conference, The Hague, The Netherlands, 7–13 September 1969.* Fraser, F. C., and McKusick, V. A., eds., New York, Excerpta Medica, 1970, pp. 284–290.
22. Jacobs, P. A., Brunton, M., Melville, M. M., Brittain, R. P., and McClemont, W. C. Aggressive behavior, mental subnormality and the XYY male. *Nature (Lond) 208:*1351–1352, 1965.
23. Jost, A. Hormonal factors in the sex differentiation of the mammalian fetus. *Phil Trans Roy Soc Lond B 259:*119–130, 1970.
24. Lubs, H. A., and Ruddle, F. H. "Applications of Quantitative Karyotyping to Chromosome Variation in 4,400 Consecutive Newborns." In *Pfizer Medical Monographs,* No. 5, Edinburgh, University of Edinburgh Press, 1970, pp. 119–142.
25. Manolov, G., Manolova, Y., and Levan, A. The fluorescence pattern of the human karyotype. *Hereditas 69:*273–286, 1971.
26. Miller, O. J. "Intrauterine Diagnosis." In *Congenital Malformations, Proceedings of the Third International Conference, The Hague, The Netherlands, 7–13 September, 1969.* Fraser, F. C., and McKusick, V. A., eds., New York, Excerpta Medica, 1970, pp. 349–358.
27. Miller, O. J. "Autoradiography in Human Cytogenetics." In *Advances in Human Genetics,* Harris, H., and Hirschhorn, K. eds. New York, Plenum Press, 1970, Chapt. 2, pp. 35–130.
28. Milunsky, A., Littlefield, J. W., Kanfer, J. N., Kolodny, E. H., Shih, V. E., and Atkins, L. Prenatal genetic diagnosis. I. *New Engl J Med 283:*1370–1381, II. 1441–1447, III. 1498–1504, 1970.
29. Moore, K. L. (ed.). *The Sex Chromatin,* Philadelphia, W. B. Saunders Company, 1966.
30. Neumann, F., Elger, W., and Steinbeck, H. Antiandrogens and reproductive development. *Phil Trans Roy Soc Lond B 259:*119–130, 1970.
31. Patil, S. R., Merrick, S., and Lubs, H. A. Identification of each human chromosome with a modified Giemsa stain. *Science 173:*821–822, 1971.
32. Pearson, P. L., Bobrow, M., and Vosa, C. G. Technique for identifying Y chromosomes in human interphase nuclei. *Nature (Lond) 226:*78–80, 1970.
33. Polani, P. E. "Chromosome Phenotypes—Sex Chro-

mosomes." In *Congenital Malformations, Proceedings of the Third International Conference, The Hague, The Netherlands, 7–13 September, 1969.* New York, Excerpta Medica, 1970, pp. 233–250.

34. Polani, P. E. Hormonal and clinical aspects of hermaphroditism and the testicular feminizing syndrome in man. *Phil Trans Roy Soc Lond B 259:* 187–204, 1970.
35. Price, D. In vitro studies on differentiation of the reproductive tract. *Phil Trans Roy Soc Lond B 259:*133–139, 1970.
36. Pryse-Davies, J., and Dewhurst, C. J. The development of the ovary and uterus in the fetus, newborn and infant: A morphological and enzyme histochemical study. *J Path 103:*5–25, 1971.
37. Schnedl, W. Banding pattern of human chromosomes. *Nature (New Biol) 233:*93–94, 1971.
38. Seabright, M. A rapid banding technique for human chromosomes. *Lancet 2:*971–972, 1971.
39. Sergovich, F., Valentine, G. H., Chen, A. T. L., Kinch, R. A. H., and Smout, M. S. Chromosome aberrations in 2159 consecutive newborn babies. *N Engl J Med 280:*851–855, 1969.
40. Short, R. V. The bovine freemartin: A new look at an old problem. *Phil Trans Roy Soc Lond B 259:* 141–147, 1970.
41. Sohval, A. R. "Mixed" gonadal dysgenesis: A variety of hermaphroditism. *Am J Hum Genet 15:*155–158, 1963.
42. Singh, R. P., and Carr, D. H. The anatomy and histology of XO human embryos and fetuses. *Anat Rec 155:*369–383, 1966.
43. Sumner, A. T., Evans, H. J., and Buckland, R. A. New technique for distinguishing between human chromosomes. *Nature (New Biol) 232:*31–32, 1971.
44. Teter, J. Morphology of the gonads in Turner's syndrome (a histological and clinical study of 11 cases). *Pol Med J 3:*118, 1964.
45. Van der Hagen, C. B., and Berg, K. Studies of human chromosomes by DNA-binding fluorochromes. I. The normal chromosome complement. *Clinical Genetics 1:*263–271, 1970.

Recommended Readings—Reference List

Human Chromosomal Disorders

1. Carr, D. H. Chromosomal abnormalities in clinical medicine. Chapter 1 in: *Progress in Medical Genetics,* Vol. 6, New York, Grune & Stratton, 1969.
2. Bartalos, M., and Baramki, T. A. *Medical Cytogenetics,* Baltimore, Williams & Wilkins, 1967.
3. Hamerton, J. L. *Human Cytogenetics,* Vol. II. *Clinical Cytogenetics,* New York, Academic Press, 1971.
4. Turpin, R., and Lejeune, J. *Human Afflictions and Chromosome Aberrations,* Oxford, Pergamon, 1969.

General Human Genetics

1. Thompson, J. S., and Thompson, M. W. *Genetics in Medicine,* Philadelphia, W. B. Saunders, 1966.
2. Carter, C. O. *An ABC of Medical Genetics,* Boston, Little Brown, 1969.
3. Sutton, H. E. *An Introduction to Human Genetics,* New York, Holt, Rinehart and Winston, 1965.

12

Diabetes Mellitus

C. Kenneth Gorman

A disease is fully understood only when the mechanisms responsible for it are completely known. Diabetes mellitus, a multisystem disease, has been investigated with greater thoroughness than any other inherited disorder of metabolism, but the mechanisms responsible for it are not yet fully understood. The main defect appears to be an *insufficiency* of metabolically active insulin. We do not know how this "insufficiency" arises, or completely understand the action of insulin, nor do we understand the relationship, if any, between the availability of insulin and the development of long-term microvascular and neurological complications of diabetes. Our concept of diabetes mellitus is therefore still incomplete. To use an analogy, we are still climbing the mountain, and cannot yet survey the whole terrain from the peak. Since this is so, our understanding of diabetes must come from ground already explored, which lies in two main areas: (1) the contribution of insulin to the body's normal biochemistry and physiology, and (2) the pathophysiological changes in the individual with diabetes.

On the basis of these two areas of interest, two groups of students of diabetes have evolved: One has as its main interest the investigation of insulin and its properties in normal and diabetic states; the other concentrates on the investigation and management of clinical diabetes mellitus. These two groups are mutually beneficial, and many physicians work in both areas. This division of interest, though inevitable because of the size and complexity of the subject, is unfortunate because it is artificial. The whole field of diabetes must be considered as one if all its aspects are to remain in the proper perspective. Because diabetes mellitus is a syndrome which affects many of the bodily systems, it provides the physician with a great opportunity to practice "true applied physiology." By using a physiological material (insulin), he can correct an abnormal state (uncontrolled diabetes mellitus) and restore the individual to a state approaching normal. Hence, every physician, when he is dealing with any diabetic patient, needs basic knowledge of insulin physiology.

In this section, I have attempted to integrate some parts of the two approaches to diabetes. The first part deals with the endocrine pancreas, and its products, and the second part deals with clinical diabetes mellitus. When reading the second part, the reader may occasionally have to refer back to the first, because relevant basic biochemical information cannot be repeated in each clinical situation in which it is pertinent. At the same time, I have attempted to bridge the gap between the research laboratory and the patient, by discussing selected basic information when it is particularly relevant.

The first part provides a brief refresher course

on the endocrine pancreas: normal enbryology and structure, then a comment on histological changes seen in the islets of Langerhans in diabetes. This is followed by an account of the hormones produced by the endocrine pancreas, discussed in the order of their known physiological importance. All known pancreatic hormones are included, since there may be some interrelation between the secretion of the different hormones.

The pattern followed in the discussion of each hormone is as follows:

Cell of origin
Hormones
Physical, chemical properties and structure
Relation of structure to function
Synthesis
Release into circulation
Blood transport; measurement; degradation
Effects on intermediary metabolism

The Pancreas

Histology and Embryology

The pancreas consists of two types of tissue: the exocrine (acinar), and the endocrine (islets of Langerhans). Both tissues have the same embryologic origin. Differentiation of the specific cells takes place between 60 and 90 days of fetal life, when islet tissue separates from the acinar canaliculi, and the component cells can be recognized. Seven cell types have been identified in all species, but only four are seen in man: Delta (D) cells appear at the beginning of the period, alpha (A) cells at about the middle, and beta (B) cells at the end of the third month. The time when the clear (C) cells appear has not been determined. On electron micrographs, the cells are distinguished by the granule size and density. These granules store the secretory products of the cell; they are largest and least dense in the alpha cells, smaller and irregular in the beta cells, and of intermediate size and most dense in the delta cells. During intrauterine life, the islet cell/acinar tissue ratio is much greater than after birth.

In the fetus, the exocrine pancreas apparently secretes little because spontaneous proteolytic activity cannot be demonstrated until the eighth month. In infants with cystic fibrosis, the development of meconium ileus indicates that the tryptic, amylolytic, and lipolytic enzymes, which the exocrine pancreas produces, are needed before birth. Endocrine secretion from the islets of Langerhans may begin at the same time as, or even before, the different cell types can be identified histologically because, with the use of immunofluorescent staining techniques, glucagon and insulin have been identified in the pancreas before the third month.

The Pancreatic Islets in Diabetes

In most "new" diabetic patients, routine studies of the islets show no changes pathognomonic of diabetes. However, on rare occasions young patients with "acute onset" diabetes have a variable degree of lymphocytic infiltration of the islets.

Because LeCompte *et al.* found similar changes in the islets of heifers that received injections of bovine insulin in adjuvant (a complex substance used to prime the reticuloendothelial system to increase antibody production), this infiltration probably represents an immune reaction. However, this does not necessarily mean that similar changes, occasionally seen in human islets, are due to this type of reaction.

Patients who have had diabetes for many years do not show structural changes pathognomonic of diabetes in islet tissue, such as a reduced or absent beta cell population. Hyalinization of the islets has been reported, but this change is not specific for diabetes. Hydropic degeneration, which is occasionally seen, is due to glycogen deposition. The basement membrane thickening seen in so many tissues of the diabetic may also be seen in electron micrographs of the beta cell. In patients with hemochromatosis, the islet cells are destroyed by progressive fibrosis. In diabetes due to primary or secondary malignant invasion of the pancreas, islet tissue is demonstrably deficient.

Secretory Products of the Different Cell Types in the Islets of Langerhans

The Beta Cell

The beta cell secrets insulin. This hormone, first extracted by Banting and Best in 1921, has been studied more intensively than any other protein.

Structure of the Insulin Molecule

Human insulin, which has a molecular weight of 5,807, consists of 51 amino-acid residues, arranged in an A chain (21 residues), and a B chain (30 residues). These chains are joined together by two disulfide linkages between cysteine molecules. A third such linkage joins two other cysteine molecules in the A chain.

In different animal species, and sometimes in the same animal, the amino acid sequences of the insulin molecule vary slightly, but this variation does not significantly affect biological activity.

The tertiary (three-dimensional) configuration of insulin has not yet been completely determined, but it is known that part of extracted insulin is arranged in a helix. However, the following information indicates that the extraction process alters the molecular configuration of insulin.

Antibodies to beef-pancreas insulin are formed when it is injected into normal cattle. The formation of these antibodies shows that the beef reticuloendothelial system does not recognize the injected insulin as the same molecule as the endogenous insulin. This failure means the two molecules are not structurally identical. This lack of identity is most probably the result of changes in the tertiary structure of the insulin molecule due to damage during its extraction. If this hypothesis is true, then the insulin molecule has not yet been obtained in its natural form.

The Relationship of Structure to Function

Insulin derives its biological activity from certain critical relationships in its primary and tertiary structure. For example, removal of the eight-terminal B-chain amino acids in beef insulin does not affect its cross reactivity with pork insulin antibodies but does reduce slightly its glucose-lowering potency. Removal of the C-terminal amino acid from the B chain does not affect its hypoglycemic property and its immunoreactivity, but removal of the terminal aspartate molecule (a molecule that is vital to the tertiary structure of insulin) from the A chain destroys its biological activity and immunoreactivity. Biological potency and immunoreactivity can also be destroyed by disrupting the disulfide linkages between the A and B chains. Re-creation of these links restores the activity of insulin.

These alterations in function following structural changes show clearly that the biological potency of insulin depends (1) on the integrity of its tertiary structure, and (2) to a smaller, but still significant extent, on the integrity of the component A and B chains. Immunoreactivity depends on an intact tertiary structure, but persists even when several component amino acid residues have been removed.

Synthesis of Insulin

Insulin is synthesized in the ribosomal particles of endoplasmic reticulum. Proinsulin, the product of the first stage of synthesis, is found in the beta cells, blood, and commercial insulin. Figure 12-1 shows the proinsulin molecule, the subsequent insulin molecule, and the sites of cleavage which result in the formation of the C chain or remnant, and the A and B chains of the insulin molecule. The molecule is arranged in the form of a coil, the overlapping ends of which represent the A and B chains of insulin. Proinsulin contains 84 amino acid residues, the sequence of which is known, and has a molecular weight of 9,082. It is a single-chain polypeptide. Its physiological importance has not yet been determined.

After the proinsulin coil has been formed, appropriate disulfide linkages are created between the prospective A- and B-chain parts. When the center part of the coil is "resected" by enzymatic cleavage, proinsulin is converted to insulin. The enzymes responsible for this separation have not yet been identified.

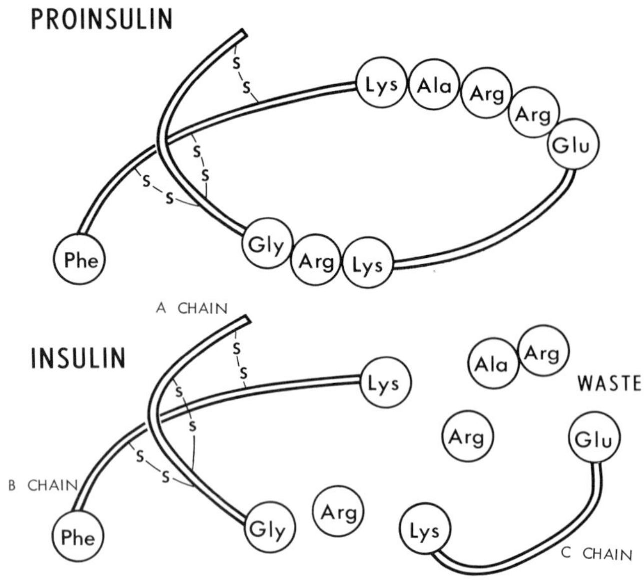

Fig. 12-1. Proinsulin molecule and subsequent insulin molecule. Cleavage results in formation of the C chain or remnant and the A and B chains of the insulin molecule. (From Steiner, D. F., *et al. Diabetes* 17:725–736, 1968. Reproduced with permission.)

The insulin thus formed in the ribosomal particles is stored in the beta granules of the islet cells, in the region of the Golgi apparatus. These granules, each of which is surrounded by a membrane, move toward the intercellular capillaries. Under appropriate stimuli they pass through the cell membrane into the circulation (Figs. 12-2 and 12-3); the cell membrane then reseals itself. The process is known as emiocytosis. Figure 12-3 shows this process in the rat pancreas during hyperglycemia. The beta granule (*arrow*) is being liberated into the extracellular space.

The physiological control of the formation of insulin and of its release into the blood is not fully understood. No pituitary regulating factor or direct feedback mechanisms have been identified. However, an increase of either growth hormone or glucose levels in the blood will stimulate insulin synthesis and will also increase the release of insulin into the blood. In view of the ability of growth hormone to stimulate the synthesis and release of insulin, its diabetogenic property seems somewhat paradoxical, as does the increased secretion of growth hormone which occurs during hypoglycemia. Further research is clearly necessary to resolve these questions. When injected into the pancreatic artery, many agents, such as sulfonylureas, glucagon, secretin, pancreozymin, isoproterenol, arginine, leucine, and free fatty acids, also increase insulin release but do not influence insulin synthesis.

Thus, many stimuli cause insulin release, but the problem is, which of these stimuli are physiologically important? Some recent observations may help to answer this question. The blood insulin concentration is higher after glucose is taken by mouth than when comparable hyperglycemia is caused by giving intravenous glucose. This indicates that an intestinal factor is acting to enhance the insulinogenic property of oral glucose. Three hormones may be responsible for this enhancement:

1. *Glucagon.* Extracts of mucosa from different parts of the intestine contain a "glucagon-like" material. This material is released into the circulation after a glucose meal, and purified samples of it do stimulate insulin release from the pancreas.
2. *Secretin.* When secretin and glucose are given together intravenously, the blood insulin rises to levels comparable with that produced by oral glucose. Under normal conditions, secretin induces pancreatic exocrine secretion. Therefore, it may also stimulate the release of insulin at the onset of postprandial hyperglycemia.

3. *Pancreozymin.* Like secretin, this hormone also stimulates insulin release and is also released into the blood from the intestine after a meal. In addition, this hormone may also stimulate glucagon production. If pancreozymin stimulates glucagon production to the extent that the increase can be detected in the peripheral blood, the local concentration in the region of the alpha cell (where it is produced) must be much higher. It is possible that this "local" high glucagon concentration may diffuse into the beta cells, and stimulate insulin release.

The importance of these hormones in the regulation of insulin release is not yet clear. For the present, it is important to remember that the most potent, most consistent stimulator of insulin synthesis and secretion is glucose. Many studies have confirmed the frequently direct relationship between the blood-insulin level and the blood-glucose concentration. Glucose thus appears to be the most direct physiological stimulus to insulin release.

In contrast to the large number of insulin-releasing factors, insulin release is inhibited only by epinephrine and other factors capable of stimulating the alpha receptors of the sympathetic nervous system, and by diazoxide. Small doses of epinephrine completely block insulin release. Diazoxide, which through some unknown mechanism inhibits insulin release from the beta cell, is used to treat patients with hyperinsulinism. Although this agent also stimulates catecholamine release, this does not completely explain its suppression of insulin release. When the alpha receptors have previously been blocked with compounds such as dibenzylene or phentolamine, sympathomimetic drugs, which stimulate both alpha and beta receptors, will cause insulin release. Pure beta sympathetic receptor stimulators (isoproterenol) stimulate insulin release.

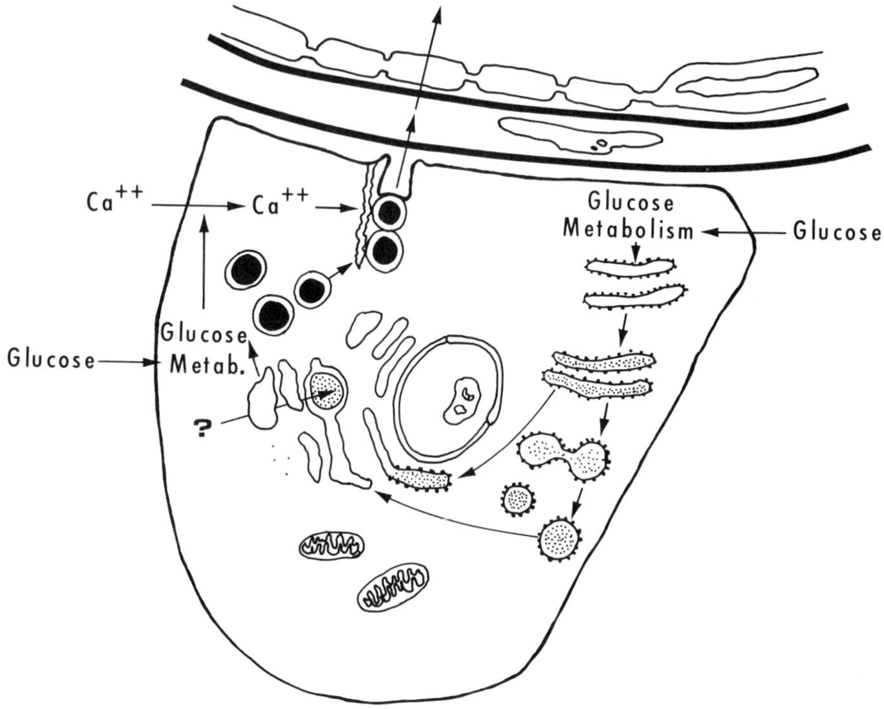

Fig. 12-2. Ultrastructural events in formation, storage, and release of beta granules in rat pancreas. In the process of emiocytosis, the membrane of the beta granule appears to fuse with the cell membrane. (From Lacy, P. E. *Diabetes* 19:895–905, 1970. Reproduced with permission.)

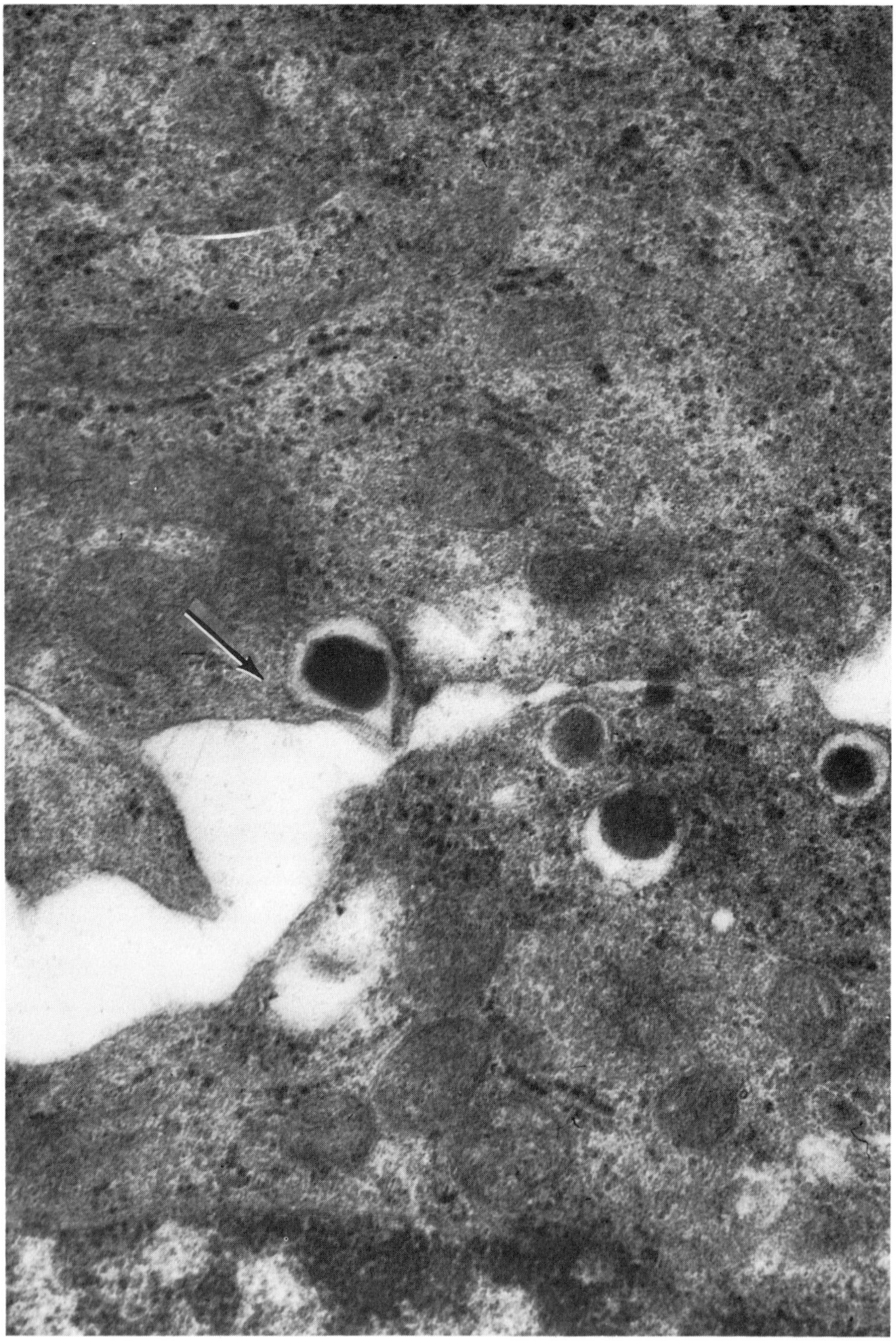

Fig. 12-3. Electron micrograph of part of a beta cell in the rat pancreas after production of hypoglycemia. A beta granule (*arrow*) is being extruded through the cell membrane. (From Lacy, P. E. *N Engl J Med 276*:187–195, 1967.)

The Physical State of Insulin in Solution

The physical state of insulin in solution depends on several factors: In low concentrations and a pH of less than 2, it is a monomer; in the presence of zinc at neutral pH, or at the pH of blood, it forms small polymers consisting of 6–12 insulin molecules. Insulin fibrils (very large polymers) are formed when a high concentration of insulin is present at a neutral or slightly alkaline pH.

Insulin has a short half-life in the blood—about 5–10 minutes. It is degraded rapidly in the liver through the action of the enzyme insulin transhydrogenase, which disrupts the disulfide bonds. Insulin does not appear to cross the placental barrier from the mother to the fetus. The hypertrophy of islets seen in infants of untreated diabetic mothers is almost certainly due to the hyperglycemic stimulus. It is not due to fetal insulin produced to regulate the maternal diabetes because fetal insulin probably does not pass into the maternal circulation in any significant quantity.

Factors Interfering with the Biological Action of Insulin

These factors include insulin antibodies, immunoglobulins produced by the reticuloendothelial system, and insulin antagonists. This latter term is used rather loosely, and includes factors (other than food) which will, by any means, cause the blood glucose level to change in a direction opposite to that which would be caused by insulin.

Insulin Antibodies. Anyone who repeatedly receives insulin by injection will develop insulin antibodies, but these are usually not present in sufficient concentration to interfere significantly with the action of insulin. When an antibody is present, it will, to some extent, bind the injected insulin, but the bound fraction is usually only a small proportion of the total dose. The fate of this bound insulin is unknown, but it probably loses its physiological activity. Occasionally, the antibody titer rises to a point where insulin resistance develops—a state arbitrarily defined as one in which the daily insulin requirement exceeds 200 units. When this happens, large doses of insulin are necessary to overcome the resistance. Alternatively, the physician may use porcine insulin or sulfated insulin, which has altered immunoreactivity but unaltered biological activity (see section on Insulin Resistance later in this chapter). In contrast to insulin, insulin antibodies do cross the placental barrier to the fetal circulation (see section on Physical Effects of Pregnancy on the Diabetic Mother later in this chapter).

Insulin Antagonists. In addition to insulin antibodies, other factors interfere with insulin action. These insulin antagonists include growth hormone, glucocorticoids, synalbumin, and other unidentified materials.

Growth hormone causes insulin resistance partly by mobilizing free fatty acids from adipose tissue. These fatty acids compete with glucose for entry into the cells. Cortisone increases protein catabolism and gluconeogenesis and, by raising the blood glucose concentration, increases the demand for insulin. Synalbumin is claimed to be an insulin antagonist and to be present in the serums of people with a strong family history of diabetes. It is isolated by dialyzing boiled serum albumin across boiled dialysis tubing. The necessity for an extraction technique of this nature casts doubt on the physiological nature of synalbumin, since the final product will have been altered grossly by the extraction process.

Growth hormone and glucocorticoids increase insulin requirements by altering glucose homeostasis. The mechanism of action of synalbumin and the unidentified factors is not known. The term "insulin antagonist" should probably be restricted to those materials which act directly against the insulin molecule. Thus the only true antagonists are insulin antibodies and perhaps the unidentified materials. Knowledge with regard to insulin antagonists and their pathophysiological role is still incomplete, and it is most important to keep an open mind on this, as well as the other questions related to insulin and diabetes.

Measurement of Insulin Levels in the Blood

The insulin concentration in the blood and elsewhere is expressed as units of biological activity, and not in metric units. This is necessary because the biological potency, in units per milligram, of different batches of insulin varies slightly. The international standard is 24 units per milligram of glucagon-free insulin.

The blood insulin concentration is now measured by bioassay or radioimmunoassay. Bioassay measures the effects of insulin on different metabolic functions in muscle (isolated rat or mouse diaphragm), or on adipose tissue (rat epididymal fat pads). Some of the parameters used as indexes of insulin activity are glucose uptake, glycogen synthesis, amino acid uptake, protein synthesis, carbon dioxide production, and free fatty acid uptake. However, different tissues give different values. For example, comparison of the glucose uptake by the isolated rat diaphragm caused by standard amounts of insulin and known amounts of human serum indicates that the average fasting human serum insulin concentration is about 50 μU/ml. However, with the adipose tissue assay, the value for human serum is about 200 μU of insulin per milliter.

Radioimmunoassay is at present the most useful technique. Here an insulin antiserum is first produced in a guinea pig, and after dilution, a quantity of this serum is incubated with mixtures of isotopically labeled insulin and known amounts of nonlabeled insulin. Because the labeled and nonlabeled insulins compete for the antibody-binding sites, only a small amount of labeled insulin will be bound to the antibody, if a large amount of unlabeled insulin is present in any one of the mixtures, and vice versa. Similarly, a large amount of the radioactive label will be present in the "bound" fraction if the concentration of unlabeled insulin is small. The amount of labeled insulin bound to the antibody must next be measured. To facilitate this, the bound insulin is removed by precipitating it with rabbit serum that contains guinea pig gamma globulin antiserum. The radioactivity of the precipitate is compared with that of supernatant to calculate the ratio of "bound-to-free" radioactivity. This ratio is inversely proportional to the concentration of unlabeled insulin. From such data, a standard curve is constructed, from which the concentrations of insulin in various biological fluids can be calculated. In fasting man, the amount detected—referred to as the immunoreactive insulin (IRI) concentration—is about 10–20 μU/ml.

As this brief summary indicates, the concentrations of insulin detected in the blood by the different techniques vary greatly. The fat-pad assay gives values 10 times greater than those measured by radioimmunoassay. For this reason, it has been suggested that adipose tissue responds to material with biological activity similar to, but different from, insulin. The source and physical nature of this material, called "insulin-like activity" (ILA) is unknown. It remains in the blood for long periods after total pancreatectomy and is therefore not insulin, nor is it related to it.

The human fasting blood insulin concentration detected by the rat or mouse diaphragm bioassay also differs from the radioimmunoassay—approximately 50 μU/ml as compared with 20 μU/ml. If sufficient insulin antibody is added to serum to neutralize all the IRI, the resultant serum can still promote glycogen synthesis in the diaphragm. This activity is called the nonsuppressible insulin-like activity (NSILA). Again the nature of this material is unknown. The biological importance of ILA and NSILA is open to question since they neither promote fat synthesis in vitro nor prevent ketosis after pancreatectomy.

Since the fat pad and muscle bioassays measure substances of questionable biological significance, these assays have lost favor, and currently the IRI assay is the best guide to insulin concentrations in the blood. However, even this method is open to question for the following reasons:

1. It measures the molecular concentration, and not biological activity of insulin. These terms, as indicated earlier, are not synonymous.
2. Radioiodinated insulin, which competes with the unlabeled insulin for antibody binding sites, is said to be without biological activity. If this is so, it may compete with unlabeled biologically inactive insulin for the binding sites. If so, the ratio of the bound to the free insulin will bear no relation to the biological activity of the insulin in the sample being assayed.

The ideal method for measuring insulin in the blood has not yet been developed. The present methods are good, but the frequently inexplicable results obtained with them show the need for improvement. Further progress will have to await technical advances.

Changes in Blood Insulin Levels

In fasting nonobese "normal" individuals, the concentration of immunoreactive insulin in the blood is between 10 and 20 μU/ml. The IRI virtually disappears from the blood during a prolonged fast. After a high-carbohydrate meal, it may rise to approximately 150 μU/ml. One gram of sodium tolbutamide or 1 mg of glucagon administered intravenously may raise the blood IRI to approximately 225 μU/ml. Much higher concentrations result from a prolonged intravenous infusion of glucose.

Obese patients have higher serum IRI levels than do normal individuals and have an exaggerated response to an oral glucose load, despite normal blood glucose concentrations. The amount of insulin produced in response to a glucose load by obese diabetics depends on the stage of their disease. Obese "chemical diabetics" (see section on Clinical Classification of Diabetes later in this chapter) release more insulin than obese nondiabetics. Obese overtly diabetic patients, although they have high fasting serum IRI levels, have a smaller insulin response to a glucose load than do obese nondiabetic patients, but a greater insulin response than normal weight nondiabetic patients (Fig. 12-4).

Prediabetics (those predisposed, on the basis of family history, to diabetes, but who have no demonstrable carbohydrate intolerance) have no consistent easily demonstrable abnormality in insulin secretion. Hyperinsulinemia is seen in laboratory animals with hereditary diabetes just before glucose intolerance develops, but this phase has not been detected in man.

Serum IRI usually disappears completely after "juvenile-onset" diabetes develops and also after pancreatectomy. It is also greatly reduced after suppressive doses of diazoxide—a drug capable of inhibiting insulin release.

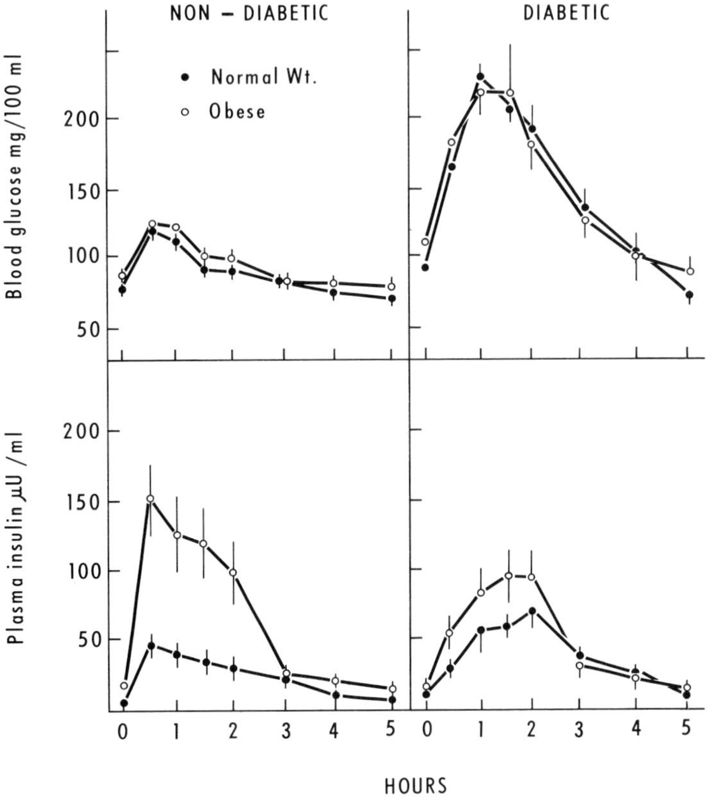

Fig. 12-4. Insulin secretion in response to oral glucose tolerance tests. Normal weight and obese nondiabetics, and normal weight and obese diabetic subjects. Note exaggerated plasma insulin responses in obese subjects, both normal and diabetic, even though the blood glucose concentrations are virtually the same. (From Perley, M., and Kipnis, D. M. *Diabetes* 15:867–874, 1966. Reproduced with permission.)

Effects of Insulin on Intermediary Metabolism

Insulin, a purely anabolic hormone, affects carbohydrate, fat, and protein metabolism (Fig. 12-5). It affects the transfer of substrates across cell membranes and also directly influences some of the anabolic processes inside the cell. The means through which insulin affects the enzymes responsible for these processes is not clear. Insulin may induce the formation of larger amounts of these enzymes by "de-repressing" their synthesis by RNA, according to the concept of Jacob and Monod, or it may "repress" the formation of enzymes which induce catabolism, such as adenyl cyclase. On the other hand, insulin may simply increase the activity of already formed enzymes. Current opinion is that all these processes play a part in the total effect of insulin. It has also been postulated that "translation factor" may be a necessary intermediate substance through which insulin affects the different metabolic processes. This factor is hypothetical and has not yet been identified.

Membrane Transfer. Levine initially postulated that insulin only affected glucose transport across the cell membrane—his "membrane permeability theory" of the action of insulin. When insulin was found to enhance the cellular uptake of free fatty acids and amino acids, he modified his theory to include these. He also proposed that all the intracellular effects of insulin were secondary to the increased concentration of the metabolites (glucose, free fatty acids, and amino acids) in the cell.

Intracellular Effects of Insulin. Although the influence of insulin on cell membrane transport remains undisputed, other properties of the hormone cannot be explained in terms of this transport; for example, insulin *directly* stimulates protein synthesis (as distinct from amino-acid uptake), ribonucleic acid synthesis, and the activity of glycogen synthetase, and inhibits the breakdown of triglyceride in the cell. These effects must be due to some intracellular activity of insulin.

Insulin may increase membrane transport through a direct effect, or secondarily through its intracellular actions. Recent work indicates that insulin can exert its biological effects only in the presence of active protein synthesis. The critical step appears to be the formation of a "translation factor"—the hypothetical "messenger stage" through which insulin affects intracellular metabolism. The formation of the "translation factor" does not depend on the formation of RNA from DNA because actinomycin, which blocks this stage, does not influence insulin action. However, cyclohexamide, which blocks protein synthesis from RNA does abolish insulin action, presumably by inhibiting "translation factor" synthesis.

The enzyme adenyl cyclase, another possible intermediary in the action of insulin, activates catabolic processes by converting adenosine triphosphate to cyclic 3′,5′-adenosine monophosphate (cyclic 3′,5′-AMP), which, in turn induces or activates enzymes such as lipase and phosphorylase. Because the intracellular content of adenyl cyclase is high, it is difficult to show significant changes in its concentration. Recent studies suggest that insulin reduces the activity of this enzyme in the liver and adipose tissue, thus reducing the catabolic effect and favoring anabolism. On the other hand, if insulin is withdrawn, cyclic 3′,5′-AMP activity sharply increases—a change that can be reversed by insulin administration. These findings suggest that adenyl cyclase may be an intermediary in the mechanism of action of insulin. It is possible that "translation factor" may inactivate adenyl cyclase, but this suggestion is hypothetical because "translation factor" has not yet been isolated. However, adenyl cyclase inactivation (?repression) cannot completely explain the action of insulin, because insulin has not been shown to affect the activity of this enzyme in muscle.

Other Actions of Insulin. The uptake of amino acids and free fatty acids by the cell under the influence of insulin is enhanced by, but not dependent on, the presence of glucose (Fig. 12-6). Insulin also stimulates lipid formation in the brain during growth, and increases the utilization of carbohydrate and lipid in the peripheral nerves. Insulin enhances glucose uptake by the brain by lowering the threshold at which glucose passes from the blood to the brain. However, insulin

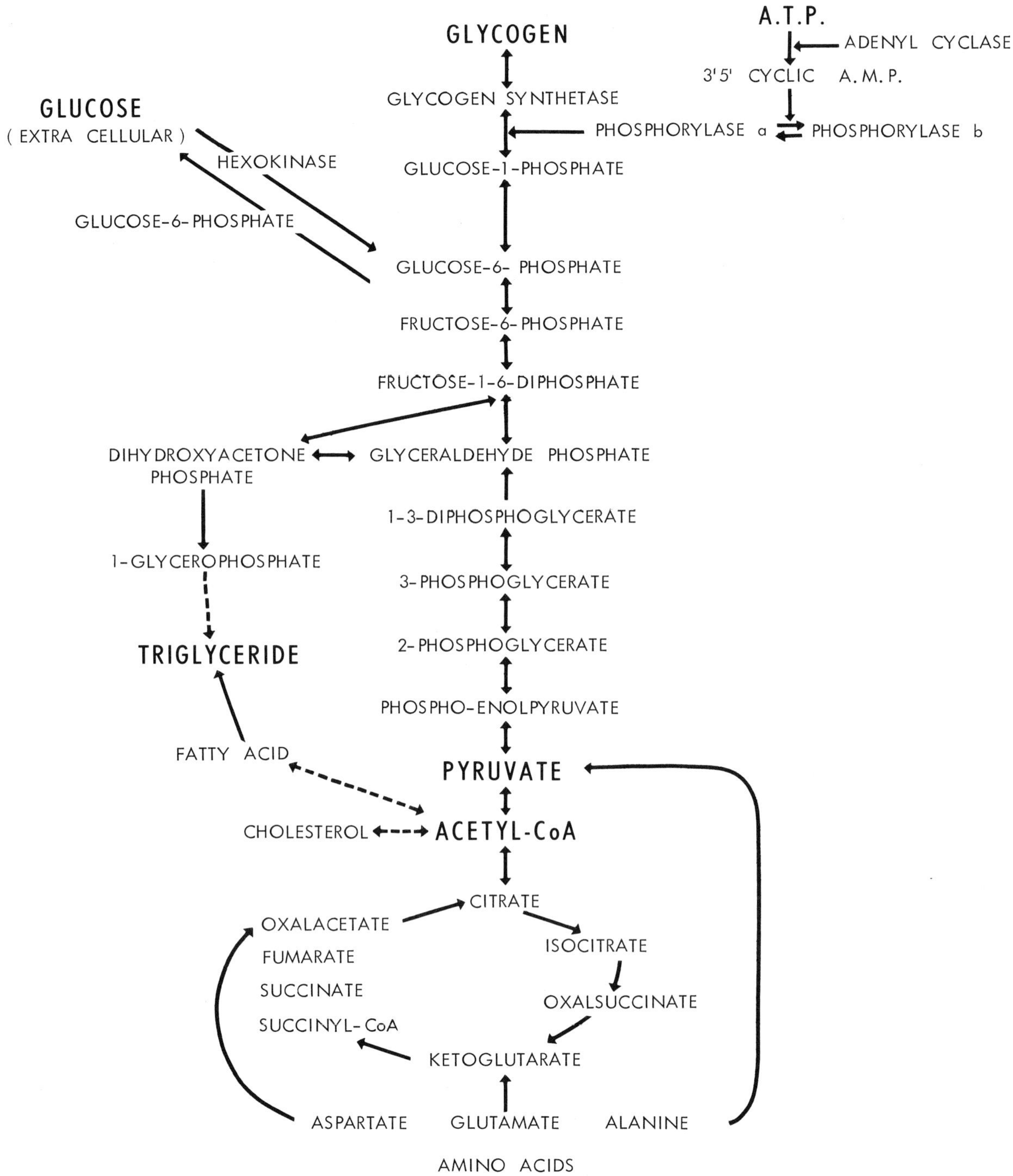

Fig. 12-5. Some metabolic pathways involved in carbohydrate metabolism. The pyruvate-acetyl-CoA stage is one of the major junctions linking carbohydrate, amino acid, steroid, and fatty acid metabolism. Below this stage lies the citric acid cycle, which is the major energy generating system in intermediary metabolism.

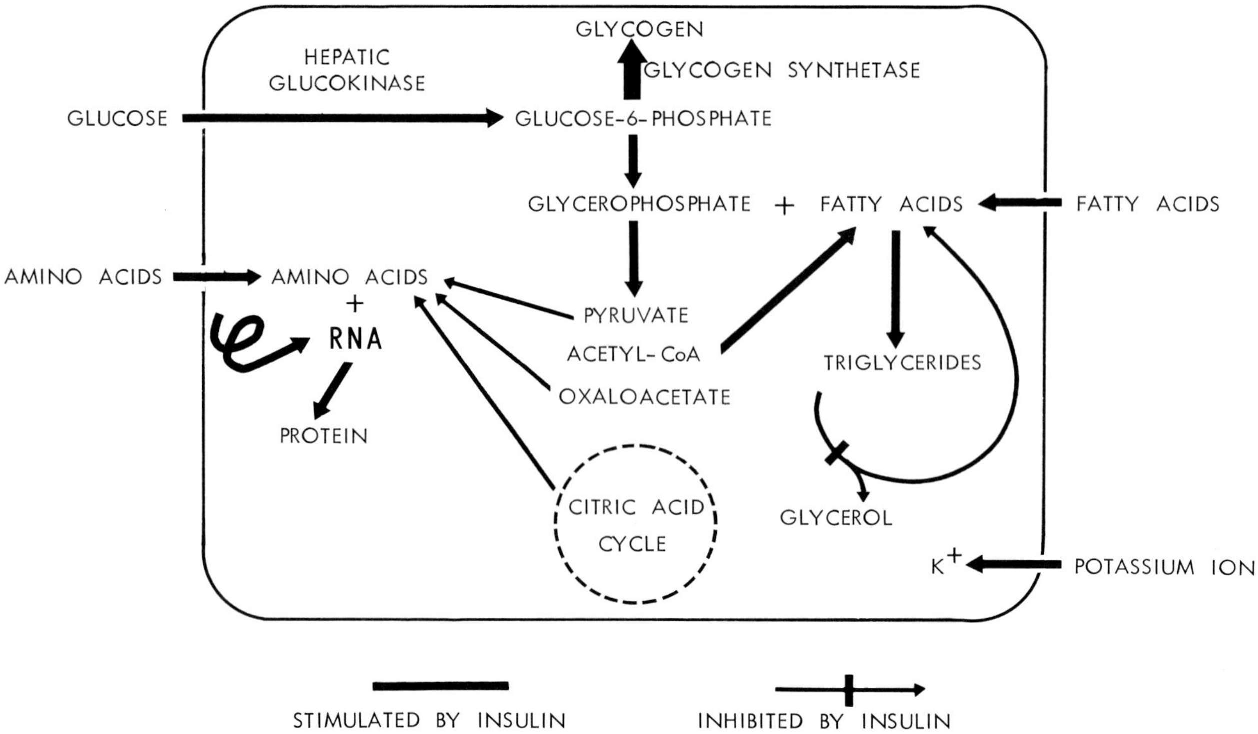

Fig. 12-6. Principal actions of insulin on intermediary metabolism. Insulin is primarily an anabolic hormone. It stimulates formation of glycogen, ribonucleic acid, protein, fatty acid, and triglyceride from their component units. Each tissue responds to the action of insulin in its own characteristic way.

does not affect active transport of glucose across the blood-brain barrier.

The various actions of insulin can be demonstrated in intact nondiabetic animals or in tissues obtained from them. Insulin action can be demonstrated more dramatically by acute insulin deprivation, by inducing alloxan diabetes, by total pancreatectomy, or by injecting a sufficient amount of potent anti-insulin serum to neutralize all the endogenous insulin. The last method is probably the best because it produces acute and complete, though transient, diabetes. Hyperglycemia, hyperketonemia, and increased blood free fatty acid concentrations rapidly develop, associated with a negative nitrogen balance, glycosuria, ketonuria, and acidosis. At the cellular level, glucose oxidation and acetyl CoA carboxylase activity (an enzyme involved in fatty acid synthesis from citrate) are decreased. Protein synthesis is decreased but gluconeogenesis is increased, as is the activity of phosphoenol pyruvate carboxykinase, an enzyme necessary for the first step in formation of glucose from oxaloacetate. Glycogen formation is decreased, and release of glucose and potassium ion from the liver is increased.

In summary, insulin acts directly on many aspects of intermediary metabolism. In nondiabetic animals, the activity of the enzymatic reactions directly affected by insulin varies within relatively narrow limits with the normal fluctuations in the blood insulin level. Because these reactions are essential to normal metabolism, an adequate supply of insulin, reflected by relatively normal blood glucose concentrations, is essential if metabolism is to be restored to a state approaching normal. This fact must always be borne in mind when the clinical management of diabetic patients is planned. A weak and half-hearted attempt to control the abnormal metabolic state of the diabetic produces a weak and half-living patient.

The Alpha Cell

Glucagon was isolated from the islets of Langerhans in 1923. The presence of a second hormone in pancreatic extracts was suspected because intravenous injection of crude insulin preparations caused an initial brief period of hyperglycemia, before the customary hypoglycemia. Staining with fluorescent glucagon antibodies confirms that this hormone is found only in the alpha cells of the pancreatic islets.

Structure of Glucagon

Glucagon, a single-chain polypeptide hormone, consists of 29 amino-acid residues and has a molecular weight of 2,852. It is not related to insulin, because it contains tryptophan and methionine (absent in insulin), and does not contain cystine, proline, or isoleucine (present in insulin). The primary structure of glucagon does not appear to differ significantly between the different animal species. As yet, nothing is known about factors regulating the biosynthesis of glucagon. No "proglucagon" molecule has been identified. Although the glucagon molecule has recently been synthesized, it is not yet known how changes in the structural formula affect the biological activity of glucagon. The formed hormone is stored in the alpha cell granules.

The only factors known to regulate the release of glucagon into the serum are hypoglycemia and high blood amino acid levels. Hyperglycemia, when induced by oral glucose administration, has a similar effect, but this is an artifact due to "glucagon-like activity" released from the intestine. This material is not glucagon, but has immunoreactive properties similar to glucagon, and cross-reacts with most glucagon antiserums. High serum glucagon concentrations inhibit glucagon synthesis. Glucagon does not appear to be bound to a carrier protein in the serum. It has a half-life of approximately 10–15 minutes, and is destroyed in the liver and kidneys and blood by nonspecific proteolytic enzymes.

Measurement of Glucagon

Blood glucagon concentration can be measured by biological or by radioimmunoassay methods. Bioassay is based on the ability of glucagon to increase the activity of liver phosphorylase, thus promoting glycogenolysis. This test depends on the ability of glucagon to increase the activity of adenyl cyclase, which promotes the conversion of adenosine triphosphate to cyclic 3′,5′-AMP, which in turn increases the activity of phosphorylase "a," either by inhibiting its conversion to phosphorylase "b," or by stimulating the conversion of phosphorylase "b" (inactive) to "a" (active). The blood concentration of glucagon by this technique is 8–12 mμg/ml.

Radioimmunoassay is the most practical method for measuring glucagon. The principle is the same as for the radioimmunoassay of insulin (see section on Measurement of Insulin Levels in the Blood earlier in this chapter). Two practical problems in setting up the assay have limited its use to a relatively few centers: (1) the difficulty in generating glucagon antiserum containing antibodies of high specificity and avidity; and (2) the tendency for proteolytic enzymes in the serum to destroy the glucagon during the incubation phase of the assay. A partial solution to the first problem is to increase the antigenicity of glucagon by binding it to a larger nonantigenic molecule, like albumin, or poly-l-lysine. The second problem is overcome by blocking the "kinin" activation of the proteolytic enzymes. "Trasylol," a specific kallikreinin inhibitor, is added to the blood or other fluid as soon as it is obtained for assay. Using this technique, the reported concentrations of glucagon equivalents in the serum are in the range of 0.5–3 mμg/ml.

The glucagon technique has the same weaknesses as insulin radioimmunoassay in that it measures the molecular concentration and not the biological activity. While immunoassay probably does measure true "active" glucagon in unknown samples, it usually also measures the concentration of intestinal glucagon-like material present in the blood at the same time, thus giving false results. Eisentraut *et al.* recently developed a glucagon antiserum that is specific for pancreatic glucagon and are therefore able to measure blood pancreatic glucagon levels. It is probable that most of the earlier reported blood glucagon levels represented the sum of both pancreatic glucagon and the intestinal glucagon-like material.

Actions of Glucagon

The physiological role of glucagon is not known. No glucagon-deficiency syndrome has been recognized, and only two patients with diabetes due to glucagon-secreting tumors have been reported. A review of its known properties suggests that glucagon (1) increase the peripheral availability of glucose, (2) stimulates insulin release from the pancreas, and (3) mobilizes free fatty acids from adipose tissue.

Increase of Peripherally Available Glucose. Glucagon has a significant action on carbohydrate metabolism only in the liver (Fig. 12-7).

The heavy lines represent metabolic pathways stimulated by glucagon. Four of its main effects

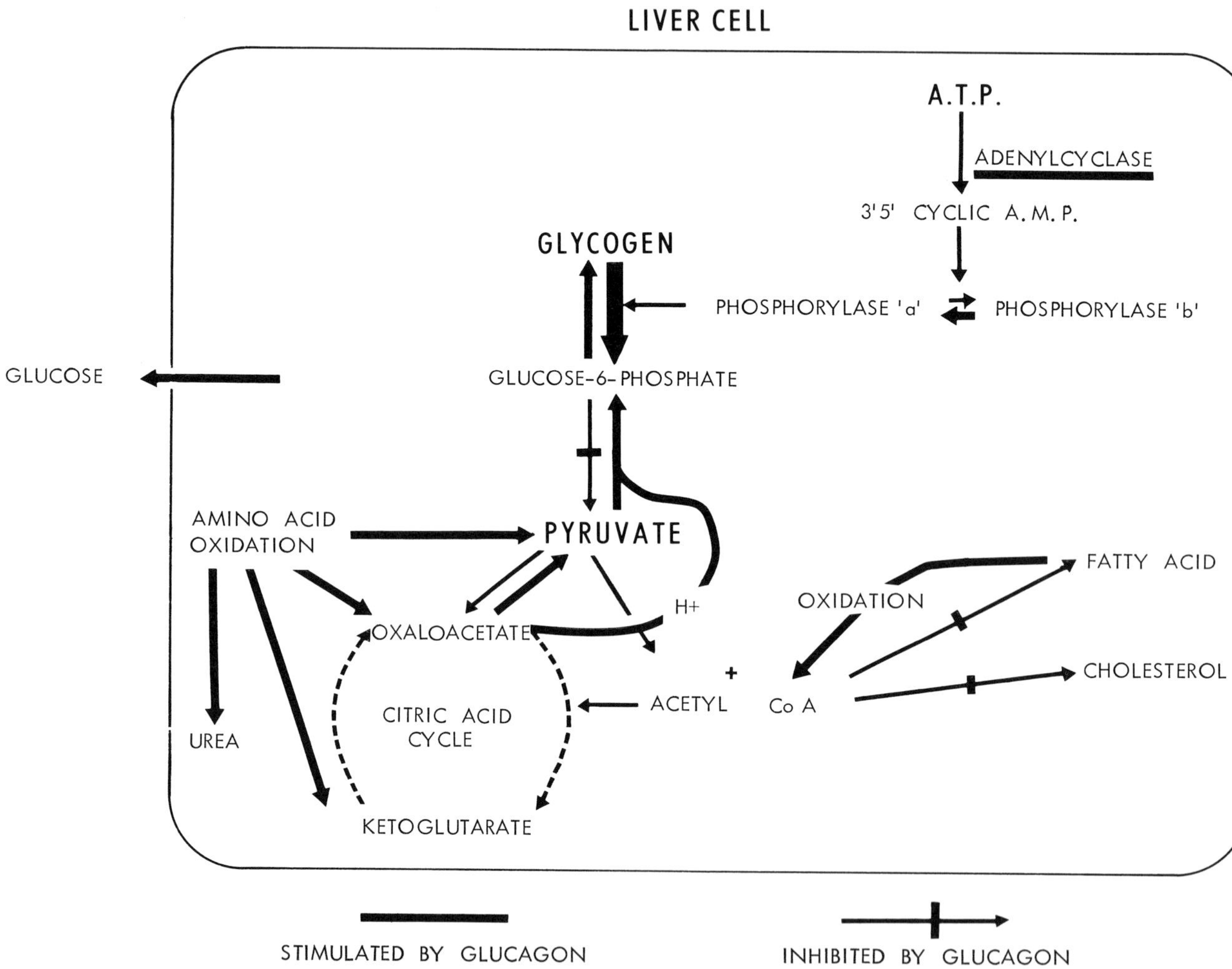

Fig. 12-7. Principal actions of glucagon on intermediary metabolism in the liver. Glucagon increases release of glucose from liver into the bloodstream (*upper left*). It acts on carbohydrate metabolism through a series of steps beginning with activation of adenyl cyclase (*upper right*) to increase glycogenolysis. Glucagon also affects protein metabolism by stimulating gluconeogenesis (*lower left*). Finally, it increases hepatic fatty acid oxidation (*lower right*), and thus facilitates gluconeogenesis by providing a ready supply of H+.

on intermediary metabolism affect glucose availability: (1) It increases glycogenolysis through activation of liver phosphorylase. (2) It increases the deamination of amino acids, and thus increases urea formation. (3) It increases fatty-acid oxidation, and hence increases hydrogen ion (H^+). The increased H^+ formation increases the efficiency of the conversion of the products of deamination (alpha-keto glutarate, oxaloacetate, and pyruvate) to glucose, since H^+ is necessary for the conversion of oxaloacetate to phosphoenol pyruvate. In the absence of another source, 1 mole of pyruvate has to be oxidized to provide sufficient H^+ for the conversion of 1 mole of oxaloacetate to phosphoenol pyruvate. Fatty acid oxidation supplies this need, and therefore spares pyruvate for conversion to glucose. (4) Glucagon inhibits glycolysis. This effect, though not completely understood, is probably achieved by inhibiting the conversion of glucose-6-phosphate to fructose-6-phosphate, or inhibiting the formation of fructose-1-6-diphosphate.

Through these four actions, which occur after a single injection of glucagon, the availability of glucose-6-phosphate is increased, which may then be converted to glucose and released into the blood. After repeated injections of glucagon, gluconeogenesis is so active that some of the newly formed glucose is converted to glycogen, and stored in the liver, possibly secondary to increased insulin availability.

Stimulation of Insulin Release from Pancreas. Glucagon may indirectly stimulate the peripheral utilization of glucose. Physiological amounts of glucagon have recently been shown to release insulin from the pancreas but the importance of this mechanism in the normal peripheral utilization of glucose is not known. Teleologically, this action would make sense, because it would allow the tissues to use the increased amounts of glucose made available by the hepatic actions of glucagon. However, it has not yet been demonstrated that glucagon, as an insulin-releasing hormone, has a role in normal human physiology.

Mobilization of FFA from Adipose Tissue. Glucagon influences fat metabolism by promoting lipolysis in adipose tissue and releasing free fatty acids into the blood. The fate of the released fatty acids appears to depend, to some extent, on the dose of glucagon used. Small doses increase blood free fatty acids, whereas large amounts reduce blood FFA, by stimulating their removal by the liver.

The inotropic action of glucagon on cardiac contraction, which has recently received much attention, is as yet unexplained. In any event, this effect is not produced by normal circulating levels—that is, pharmacological doses are needed to induce it.

The Clear Cell

The products of the C (clear) cells have not yet been determined. C cells have no granules and hence probably do not have secretory capacity.

The Delta Cell

The D cells probably secrete gastrin. In the Zollinger-Ellison syndrome (severe, multiple, recurrent peptic ulceration, an islet-cell tumor, and, in some patients, diarrhea), the pancreatic tumors contain large amounts of gastrin. The structure of the cell which characterizes this tumor is similar to that of the D cells.

Diabetes Mellitus

Diabetes mellitus, a common condition, occurs in about 3% of the population. It is rare in young children, but the incidence increases gradually until the age of puberty, after which it falls a little, and then remains at a plateau until about 30 years of age. From this age, the incidence increases steadily to a maximum between the age of 50 and 65 years (Fig. 12-8), followed by a decline in later years.

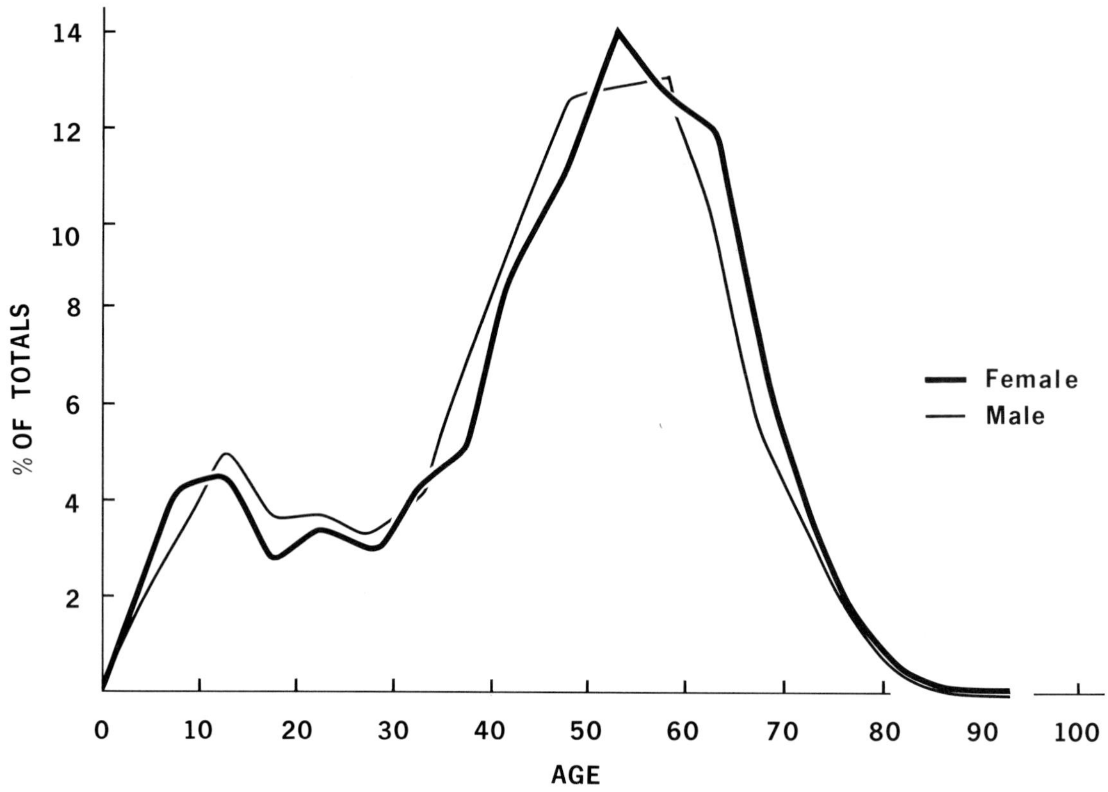

Fig. 12-8. Age at onset of diabetes mellitus. This figure illustrates the frequency with which diabetes develops in different age groups. The bimodal distribution, peaking at puberty (menarche) and at menopause may indicate that individuals are likely to develop diabetes at times of profound hormonal readjustment. (From Joslin, E. P., Root, H. F., Marble, A., and White, P. *Treatment of Diabetes Mellitus,* 10th ed. Philadelphia, Lea, 1959, p. 30. Reproduced with permission.)

Etiology

Diabetes is primarily due to one or more of the following:

1. Hereditary influence
2. Other endocrine diseases
3. Pancreatic destruction

Hereditary diabetes is the commonest variety. Endocrine diseases associated with an increased incidence of diabetes include acromegaly, adrenocortical hyperactivity, hyperthyroidism, and pheochromocytoma. Pancreatic destruction may be due to inflammation, neoplasia, or fibrosis, or to iron deposition, as in hemochromatosis.

Clinical Classification

Regardless of the predisposing factors, *clinical diabetes* may be classified in two main ways: (1) by the degree of detectable carbohydrate intolerance or (2) by the age of onset and the tendency to ketosis.

Classification Based on Carbohydrate Tolerance

Diabetic states based upon amount of carbohydrate tolerance are:

Prediabetes:
no demonstrable carbohydrate intolerance

Chemical (latent) diabetes:

Normal fasting blood glucose, but abnormal standard or cortisone-stimulated glucose tolerance

Overt diabetes:

Elevated fasting blood glucose

Prediabetes

Prediabetes, which is present in the affected individual from conception, is latent until detectable carbohydrate intolerance develops. The period of life before the development of abnormal glucose tolerance is referred to as prediabetes or potential diabetes. It can be predicted accurately only in the twin whose homozygous sibling has already developed diabetes mellitus. Prediabetes can be suspected when both parents have diabetes, or in women with certain characteristic obstetric and perinatal problems—e.g., mothers who have babies that weigh more than 10 lb at birth or babies that have a high mortality late in pregnancy or in the neonatal period.

Chemical Diabetes

The change from the prediabetic state to detectable abnormal glucose tolerance is subtle and is recognized only when specifically sought for. Initially, the abnormal glucose tolerance is reversible, and patients can swing from one group to the other for some time before becoming permanently diabetic. The fasting blood sugar level and the standard oral glucose tolerance test results may remain normal, and cortisone stimulation may be necessary to demonstrate carbohydrate intolerance. If the blood glucose level becomes abnormally high during the cortisone-stimulated glucose tolerance test (see below), this indicates latent chemical diabetes. Chemical diabetes is present if the fasting blood glucose is still normal while the blood glucose in the standard oral glucose tolerance test rises to higher than normal levels.

Overt Diabetes

Overt diabetes exists when the fasting blood glucose is elevated and, in addition, the glucose tolerance test results are abnormal. These patients usually have glycosuria and sometimes ketonuria.

A classification of diabetes based on glucose tolerance, though clinically useful, is not entirely satisfactory. Some patients develop histological changes, characteristic of long-term diabetes before carbohydrate intolerance can be detected. These changes (nephropathy and retinopathy) cannot be attributed to the effects of elevated blood glucose and must be due to some unidentified and probably inherited factor associated with the diabetic syndrome. In addition, in rare instances, abnormal glucose tolerance develops in conditions unrelated to diabetes.

Classification of Diabetes by Age of Onset

A useful classification of diabetes is based on age of onset: that is "growth-onset" and "maturity-onset." This clinical division serves to separate young, ketosis-prone, insulin-dependent diabetics, and elderly, often obese, diabetics who rarely develop ketosis. It must be emphasized that there is considerable overlap between these groups: There is no strict dividing line between them. Many elderly patients develop growth-onset diabetes, while some young patients have maturity-onset diabetes.

Inheritance of Diabetes

Diabetes mellitus may be inherited through a mendelian recessive system or through multifactorial inheritance. In the former, the progeny of two diabetic parents will all eventually develop diabetes. This predicted incidence does not always occur and is explained by the supposition that mendelian recessive genes responsible for the inheritance of diabetes mellitus have "variable penetrance." In other words, the diabetic gene will need to have a certain potency before it can transmit the defect.

In multifactorial inheritance, the gene or genes from each parent must "pair" in a specific and as yet undetermined formation to cause diabetes in the progeny. Since this is so, it is clear that transmission by this method will be theoretically weaker than with mendelian recessive transmission.

A weaker family history of diabetes will obviously give a proportionately smaller incidence of diabetes in the progeny with either form of inheritance.

Although the exact mode of transmission of diabetes mellitus is still uncertain, the multifactorial theory is currently favored for the following reasons:

1. If diabetes is transmitted by a mendelian recessive gene, the predicted incidence of the disease in the progeny of two diabetic parents would be 100%. However, studies in Canada and Great Britain have shown that the incidence in such circumstances is about 25%, a figure that would be expected with a mendelian recessive trait with very low penetrance or with the weaker multifactorial transmission.
2. The diabetic syndrome has several distinct pathological presentations. In some patients, pathological changes develop and progress faster than would be expected from the detectable severity of the metabolic defect. Admittedly, these patients are uncommon, but their existence does suggest that the unexpectedly rapid progress of the pathological changes is the result of genetic influences and is not just secondary to poor management. At present, the concept of multifactorial inheritance explains the clinical picture of diabetes better than a mendelian recessive inheritance.

Symptoms and Signs of Diabetes

In younger people, the onset of diabetes is often abrupt. In older patients it usually develops more gradually, but there are many exceptions to this generalization. The onset of diabetes may be defined as the time at which glucose tolerance changes from the normal to the diabetic type—a transition that cannot be detected in most patients.

When the onset of diabetes is rapid, the most common symptoms are polyuria and nocturia, thirst and dry mouth, weight loss, increased appetite, nocturnal cramps in the muscles of the legs and feet, and less commonly, decreased visual acuity. Women may have pruritus vulvae, and both sexes may occasionally develop severe skin infections, such as furunculosis and erysipelas. In the period shortly before the onset of symptomatic diabetes, especially after a prolonged fast, patients may have typical symptoms of hypoglycemia, such as hunger, faintness, and sweating. In patients with previously undiagnosed diabetes, symptoms may develop acutely after stress, such as an infection or sudden physical or emotional shock. In these patients, diabetes has been present in a latent form, and the stress has caused an exacerbation which gives rise to the symptoms. Often, however, no precipitating cause can be identified.

If the early symptoms of diabetes are disregarded, the patient may progress to diabetic acidosis and coma before medical advice is sought. Fortunately, such progression is now rare, because the public has been alerted through education and diabetes detection campaigns.

Diabetes, which develops gradually, presents greater diagnostic and therapeutic difficulties because there are often no symptoms to alert either physician or patient. The disease is often discovered when medical advice is sought for some other condition or during diabetes detection surveys. On close questioning, these patients may have had nocturia, or muscle cramps, or, in the male, impotence. Probably, clinical diabetes has been present at least as long as these symptoms, but its actual date of onset can usually only be estimated.

There are few abnormal physical signs in asymptomatic diabetes. Small, dark-brown, pigmented areas up to 1–2 cm in diameter are found on the shins (diabetic dermatopathy) more frequently in diabetics than in the normal population. The presence of one or more of the following conditions should always make one think of associated underlying diabetes:

1. Coronary artery disease in men under the age of 50 or in women before the menopause
2. Decreased visual acuity due to retinal changes characteristic of diabetes
3. Paresthesia due to peripheral neuropathy
4. Gangrene of the feet
5. Concurrent pernicious anemia and myxedema

Diagnosis of Diabetes Mellitus

The diagnosis of diabetes is based on the demonstration of an abnormal blood glucose concentration either in the fasting state or after stimulation with glucose or other carbohydrate. The most sensitive tests for abnormal glucose tolerance are (1) the blood glucose 2 hours after a meal and (2) the oral glucose tolerance test. A variety of other tolerance tests (intravenous glucose tolerance and tolbutamide tests and cortisone-stimulated glucose tolerance test) are occasionally used for detecting diabetes. Glycosuria, especially with ketonuria, helps to confirm the diagnosis, but is not essential to it.

Normal Blood Glucose Values

The normal fasting "true blood sugar" concentration is from 60 to 100 mg/100 ml. Formerly, the fasting range was said to be 80–120 mg/100 ml of blood. This higher range had been established because the Folin-Wu method for blood glucose measured the total reducing substance (which includes glutathione and vitamin C in addition to glucose). The result was referred to as the "whole blood sugar" content. Newer methods measure the blood glucose only, or "true blood glucose." In this section the blood glucose levels mentioned are true blood glucose values. Also, the term blood glucose, and not blood sugar is used, since the latter is not specific. The blood glucose is within normal limits if it is less than 100 mg/100 ml when fasting, or less than 120 mg/100 ml 2 hours after an average meal. Diabetes can be diagnosed if the blood glucose concentration is above 120 mg when fasting, or 140 mg/100 ml 2 hours after a meal.

The diagnosis of diabetes may be missed if only the fasting blood glucose is determined. It is easier to detect inadequate insulin production, and thus diabetes, after challenge with carbohydrates. The 2-hour postprandial blood glucose level is abnormal much more often than the fasting blood glucose and should be used routinely in screening tests. A useful diagnostic shortcut is to give the patient a normal meal plus 50 gm of glucose and measure the blood glucose level 2 hours later. If this value is greater than 150 mg/100 ml, the patient is diabetic.

A glucose tolerance test is the most satisfactory method for substantiating the diagnosis of diabetes. However, it is essential that the patients be adequately prepared for the test. They must have a diet containing 150–200 gm of carbohydrate per day for 3 days to ensure that their insulin production is at its optimum level at the time of the test. After an overnight fast, blood for fasting glucose determination is obtained. Then 100 gm of glucose is given by mouth in a lemon-flavored drink. Blood is taken for glucose determination and urine for sugar and ketone determination, ½, 1, 2, and 3 hours, and sometimes at 4, 5, and 6 hours after the glucose has been consumed. If each of the blood sugar values is below the following limits, the test results are said to be normal:

Time	*Mg/100 ml*
Fasting	110
30 min	150
1 hr	160
2 hr	120
3 hr	110

The glucose drink often causes nausea and vomiting. A new preparation, Glucola, which contains the necessary carbohydrates as dextrins, is more palatable. Although it contains only 75 gm of carbohydrate, it produces an increase in blood glucose similar to that produced by 100 gm of oral glucose.

In the nondiabetic patient, during the glucose tolerance test, the 3-hour blood sugar almost always falls below the fasting level. In early chemical diabetes it may fall even to hypoglycemic levels (associated with classic symptoms of hypoglycemia) 4 or 5 hours after the glucose was ingested, probably because of impaired control of insulin release at this stage of the disease.

Intravenous Glucose Tolerance Test

The intravenous glucose tolerance test is sometimes used to detect diabetes, but it does not add significantly to the information obtained from the oral glucose tolerance test (GTT). Preparation of the patient for the intravenous GTT is the same as for the oral test. After blood is taken for a fasting glucose determination, glucose (0.5 gm/kg) is given intravenously in a 50% solution over 3–4 minutes. Venous or capillary blood is then analyzed for glucose 10, 20, 30, and 60 minutes after the injection is completed.

The percentage utilization of glucose in milligrams per minute is calculated by determining the slope of the disappearance curve, by plotting the natural logarithm of the results, or by using the actual figures on semilogarithmic paper. A straight line is thus produced: the *K* value (slope constant), normally between 3.0 and 4.5, is calculated by dividing the time taken for the glucose concentration to fall by one-half, into 0.693 and multiplying the results by 100. That is:

$$K = \frac{0.693}{t\,½}\,(\text{glucose}) \times 100$$

A value below 2.5 is diagnostic of diabetes.

Other Diagnostic Tests for Diabetes

Sometimes, when the results of the oral and intravenous GTT are not decisive, the cortisone-stimulated oral GTT is used. The patient is given cortisone acetate, 50 mg by mouth 8 hours and 4 hours before the standard oral GTT. The criteria for normality are the same. Cortisone (or prednisone in equivalent doses) imposes a stress that unmasks the defect in glucose tolerance in the early chemical diabetic.

This test and the IVGTT are used mainly in research programs. In clinical medicine, when the diagnosis is in doubt, the standard oral GTT should be repeated at a later date.

An intravenous tolbutamide test is also used to detect diabetes. After the usual preparation, a fasting blood glucose is obtained and 1.0 gm of sodium tolbutamide is injected intravenously. Blood glucose concentrations are determined at 30, 60, and 180 minutes later. If the maximum fall in blood glucose is less than 20% of the fasting level, the patient is said to be diabetic, because the tolbutamide has been unable to release enough insulin to produce the expected degree of hypoglycemia.

In summary the patient is diabetic if he has: (1) fasting blood glucose greater than 110 mg/100 ml on three determinations; (2) 2-hour postprandial blood glucose concentration greater than 120 mg/100 ml on three determinations.

If the results of these tests are inconclusive, do an oral glucose tolerance test (OGTT). The intravenous glucose tolerance test (IVGTT) and the intravenous tolbutamide test (IVTT) are also described, but most information can be obtained from the OGTT.

Table 12-1. Tolerance Tests

Test	*Preparation*	*Dose*	*Time of sampling*	*Normal values*
OGTT	Diet to contain 150 gm carbohydrate, or more per day for 3 days before test	100 gm glucose or 75 gm Glucola	Fasting 30 min 1 hr 2 hr 3 hr	<110 gm/100 ml <150 gm/100 ml <160 gm/100 ml <120 gm/100 ml <110 gm/100 ml
IVGTT	Same	0.5 gm glucose per kg body wt	5, 10, 15, 30, and 60 min after completion of injection	K* value of less than 2.5
IVTT	Same	1.0 gm sodium tolbutamide	0, 15, 30, 60, and 180 min	Maximum fall in blood glucose concentration should be greater than 20% of preinjection value

* K is the disappearance coefficient for glucose.
Insulin immunoassays are of no value in routine investigation of diabetes mellitus at present.

Treatment of Diabetes Mellitus

With respect to treatment, diabetics may be divided into three groups: Group 1, those in whom dietary regulation alone keeps blood sugar levels within normal limits; Group 2, those who need oral hypoglycemic agents in addition to a diet; Group 3, those who need insulin and a diet. In all three groups, the object of treatment is, as far as possible, to keep the blood glucose within normal physiological limits.

Group 1—Diet

Dietary regulation is essential for all diabetics. Dietary restriction, by balancing the caloric intake against the available insulin, gets the maximum benefit from endogenous insulin in Groups 1 and 2 and from the exogenous insulin in Group 3. First, the patients' caloric requirements are determined from their daily energy needs and their weight. A physically fit construction worker of normal weight needs 3,500 calories or more per day to provide him with sufficient energy for his activity. At the other extreme, an obese inactive diabetic should receive a diet that will bring him or her back to an "ideal" weight. Such patients will initially need to be in a state of negative energy expenditure. This objective is often a source of frustration to their physician because only a few patients on a diet of 800–1,000 calories a day will cooperate for long. Those who do, need constant encouragement.

An easy guide to dietary requirements in children is 1,000 calories per day plus 100 calories for every year of age. Girls may want even less in their adolescent years. Adolescent boys, on the other hand, will demand and should get considerably more. Their caloric intake should be sufficient to support rapid growth and should be adjusted upward as along as they do not become obese.

The caloric requirement for adults of average weight and activity is between 1,500 and 2,500 calories per day, depending on sex and occupation. In the elderly, these requirements fall often to a level between 1,000 and 1,800 calories per day.

In most diabetic diets, 40% of the calories come from carbohydrates, 40% from fat, and 20% from protein. This provides a good balance and the calculation of carbohydrate, fat, and protein content is easy, once the caloric requirement has been established. From these figures the dietitian plans menus in which the patient takes approximately 80% of the calories in the three meals, and consumes the remainder in snacks, two between meals and one at bedtime.

Many patients use standard diet lists, based on the isocaloric food exchange lists published by the Canadian and American diabetes associations. With these, menu planning is easy.

There are six different exchange lists (Table 12-2).

Any two foods containing the same amount of carbohydrate, or fat, or protein may be substituted in an exchange. In this way, the type of food, but not the caloric content, can be varied as desired.

The diabetic diet can also be modified to meet the requirements of ulcer, low-sodium, and other types of dietary prescription.

The diabetic diet can be made up using foods normally available. The carbohydrate should come from starchy foods, and not pure mono- and disaccharides except for fruit and milk—for example, both bread and Coca-Cola syrup contain 50% carbohydrate by weight. However, because of the rate of absorption, the blood glucose increases much faster after 30 gm of Coca-Cola syrup than after 30 gm of bread. The caloric value of the fat should not exceed 40% of the total calories allowed in the diet. Although there

Table 12-2. Food Exchanges

Exchange	*Weight (gm)*	*Carbohydrate (gm)*	*Fat (gm)*	*Protein (gm)*
Bread	30	15	0	2
Meat	30	—	7	7
Milk	100	5	2.5	2.5
Fat	5	—	5	0
Fruit	100	10	0	0
Vegetable				
A	100	6	0	0
B	100	3	0	0

Taken from the Canadian Diabetic Association Meal Planning Guide for Diabetics.

is no conclusive evidence that polyunsaturated fatty acids are better than animal fat in the diabetic diet, excess of either will cause weight gain and upset the total calorie balance. Artificial sweeteners may be used and are useful in low-calorie beverages and canned fruit. In the latter, the carbohydrate content of the canned fruit is equivalent to that in the same weight of the fresh product.

Group 2—Oral Hypoglycemic Agents

In a limited number of diabetics, oral hypoglycemic agents can keep the blood glucose within normal limits. Several such preparations are available: tolbutamide, chlorpropamide, phenformin (DBI), acetohexamide, and tolinase. Carbutamide, the first widely used sulfonylurea (tolbutamide, chlorpropamide, and acetohexamide are also sulfonylureas) is no longer available in North America, but is still used in Europe. Except for DBI, these drugs lower blood sugar by releasing insulin from the pancreas. Hence, if these drugs are to be successful, the pancreas must have adequate reserves of insulin. The mechanism by which DBI lowers the blood glucose is as yet unknown.

Most diabetics who respond to the oral hypoglycemic drugs are in the older age groups. Patients over 40 years of age, who do not have ketones in the urine, who require less than 20 units of insulin per day, and have a postprandial blood sugar of less than 250 mg, stand the best chance of success with this form of treatment.

The choice of drug used is dictated largely by the preference of the physician. Tolbutamide, DBI, and tolazamide have a short half-life and must be taken up to 1–3 times per day. As a starting dose, 0.5 gm of tolbutamide may be given once or twice daily before meals; this can be increased to 1.0 gm 3 times per day if necessary. Usually, maximum benefit is obtained with a dose of 2.0 gm per day. DBI also has a short duration of action: 25 mg is given 1–4 times per day; 100 mg/day is considered to be the maximum dose, since above this level, gastrointestinal side effects (epigastric pain and nausea) become quite frequent. The 50-mg DBI (TD—time-delayed-release) capsules are probably more useful than the tablets and may be given twice a day. The maximum dose is again 100 mg/day.

Chlorpropamide, one of the most useful oral hypoglycemic agents, has a long duration of action—only one dose is given each morning. The maximum therapeutic benefit is obtained with 500 mg/day. With doses exceeding 500 mg/day, gastrointestinal side effects may develop.

The oral hypoglycemic agents are best taken before meals, but if epigastric pain and nausea occur with doses within the recommended range, the drug may be taken with meals.

The criteria for satisfactory control of diabetes with oral agents should be strict in middle-aged people. The fasting blood glucose should not exceed 100 mg/100 ml, and only rare glycosuria should be tolerated. In elderly patients, and especially those with limited life expectancy, a fasting blood glucose of up to 130 mg/100 ml can be accepted. In some cases, a combination of oral hypoglycemic agents may control the blood glucose when any one agent in maximum dose does not. Tolbutamide or chlorpropamide may be combined with DBI, and the dose may be increased to the maximum for each. This form of treatment is expensive and, although temporary control may be achieved, it may fail later and insulin must be started. I do not favor this combined treatment.

Patients who, on the basis of age and of pretreatment blood sugar levels, should theoretically respond to the oral agents may follow one of three courses: (1) success, (2) primary failure, (3) secondary failure. In primary failure, there is no satisfactory response to the oral agents. In secondary failure, there is initial success but the patient escapes from control later. This decompensation may be due to the following factors: The insulin-secreting capacity of the pancreas may decrease with the natural progress of the disease. (2) If patients do not keep to their diets and gain weight, the insulin released by the oral agents may not be sufficient to meet the increased demand. (3) Patients may also develop other illnesses such as infections or myocardial infarcts that increase insulin requirements, thus exceeding the limited capacity of the pancreas.

Table 12-3. Preparations Used in Treatment of Diabetes Mellitus

Drug	*Duration of action*	*Supply*	*Dosage*	*Max. effective dose**
		Oral agents		
Sulfonylureas				
Acetohexamide	12–18 hr	250 mg	1–2 every morning	1.5 gm/day
		500 mg	1–2 every morning and 1 every evening	
Chlorpropamide	24 hr	100 mg	1 every morning	0.5 gm/day
		250 mg	1–2 every morning	
Tolazamide	12–18 hr	100 mg	1–2 every morning	1.0 gm
		250 mg	1–2 tablets 1–2 times/day	
Tolbutamide	8–12 hr	500 mg	1–2 tablets 1–3 times/day	3 gm
		1 gm	1 tablet 1–3 times/day	
Biguanides				
Phenformin	8 hr	25 mg	1, 1–4 times/day	100 mg
Phenformin TD	12 hr	50 mg	1, 1–2 times/day	100 mg
Metformin	8 hr	500 mg	1–2, 1–3 times/day	3 gm

* Doses in excess of these limits will not increase the hypoglycemic effect of these drugs.

Complications with Oral Hypoglycemic Agents

Decompensation. When diabetic control is lost, acidosis and coma may develop, although this is rare. If the patients are selected carefully, and followed adequately, such decompensation should never happen.

Hypoglycemia. As many as 6% of patients on oral hypoglycemic agents may develop hypoglycemia. This complication, which is seen most frequently in the elderly, may be mistaken for a cerebrovascular accident. Fortunately, intravenous glucose is an effective cure. Sometimes the hypoglycemia may persist for several hours, so an infusion of 10% dextrose should be started if the patient shows any tendency to relapse.

Drug Allergy. This is uncommon, and usually presents as a generalized urticarial eruption. Very occasionally, thrombocytopenia may develop. In either situation, the drug must be stopped. If allergy to a sulfonylurea develops, DBI may be substituted, and vice versa.

Group 3—Insulin

Insulin is necessary if diet and the oral hypoglycemic drugs do not control the blood glucose level. It is essential in the management of growth-onset diabetics, and in older diabetics who readily develop ketosis. The object of treatment is to supplement or replace the patient's own insulin, so that the blood glucose is kept within physiological limits.

Hyperglycemia itself does not seem to produce organic change, but there is good evidence that chronic insulin insufficiency is harmful. Normal blood glucose concentrations are a good indication that insulin replacement is adequate. Every attempt, therefore, should be made to keep the blood glucose within the physiological range. Clearly, this program should be followed energetically in the otherwise healthy diabetic. It may be relaxed slightly in patients with preterminal illnesses that are not related to diabetes. When the patient has severe long-term complications of diabetes, adequate insulin replacement is most important, because the progress of the complications can sometimes be slowed (though not reversed) by good diabetic control.

It is obvious that efficient regulation of the blood glucose in the diabetic depends as much on the patient as on the doctor. The patient must be instructed in, and learn about, the conduct of the normal day-to-day diabetic routine. He must understand the various factors that affect his insulin requirements and how to cope with these factors. He must also be told how to care for his insulin syringe, needles, etc. The administration of insulin is easy, if the patient has received good instruction.

The various insulins can be classified into three groups according to their duration of action:

Short-acting. "Regular" or "soluble" crystalline zinc (CZ) and semilente insulins are one group. Crystalline zinc insulin, which is unmodified after extraction, has its maximum activity over 1–5 hours. Semilente insulin, an amorphous insulin-zinc suspension, has its maximum activity over 2–7 hours.

Intermediate. Lente and NPH (neutral protamine Hagedorn, or isophane) insulin are a second group. These insulins, which are comparable in their length of action, can be interchanged without altering the diabetic control. Lente insulin is a mixture of amorphous insulin zinc suspension (three parts) and crystalline insulin zinc suspension (seven parts). Each of the three insulin-binding sites on the protamine molecule in NPH insulin is filled, so that there is a 1:3 protamine/insulin molecular ratio. These insulins begin to have significant hypoglycemic effect within 2 hours of injection. They have their maximum effect in 4–14 hours and have some action for 16–24 hours. They are currently the most useful and most commonly used insulins.

Long Duration. The third group is the protamine zinc (PZ) and ultralente insulins. In PZ insulin, a 1:1 mixture of protamine and insulin, two potential insulin-binding sites per protamine molecule are unoccupied. The action of crystalline zinc insulin may be prolonged if it is mixed with PZ insulin because the former will combine to some extent with the free binding sites in the latter. Ultralente is the crystalline form of insulin-zinc suspension. These insulins have a significant hypoglycemic action 5–6 hours after injection, and some action for 20–36 hours.

"Actrapid" and "Rapitard" insulins (with short and intermediate durations of action respectively) are popular in the Scandinavian countries.

The duration of action of any insulin depends on four factors:

1. The form of the complex that is used to prolong its action (protamine and insulin zinc crystal preparations)
2. The injection site (Insulin given intravenously will have a much shorter duration of action than that injected subcutaneously. If the commonly used subcutaneous injection sites have become fibrosed, absorption of insulin will be delayed and its action prolonged.)
3. The extent to which injected insulin combines with fixed or circulating antibodies (This factor is important. Such a combination may both prolong the action and decrease effectiveness by destroying the insulin.)
4. The total dose of insulin (The larger the dose, the longer the action. This applies to all types of insulin.)

Insulin Mixtures

Since the unsaturated protamine molecule binds free CZ insulin (CZI), the latter should not be mixed with PZ insulin, but can be mixed with any of the others. NPH and PZ insulin should not be mixed with any of the lente preparations, because the phosphate buffers in the former disrupt the solubility of the insulin zinc suspension in acetate buffer. The risk of this happening should be remote since no advantage is gained by mixing two intermediate or long-acting insulins.

Selection of Insulin Type and Dose

Lente and NPH insulins are used most commonly. The proper dose can only be discovered by trial and error. A safe guide for the calculation of the initial dose of insulin for an adult is to divide the pretreatment fasting blood glucose by 10. The result is the estimated daily insulin requirement in units. This is injected subcutaneously about ½ hour before breakfast. In most cases, the dose will need to be increased in increments of 2–5 units per day, depending on the fasting and 2-hour postprandial blood glucose concentrations. The delayed action of the intermediate insulins may let the blood glucose rise above acceptable levels at midmorning. This escape can be controlled by adding CZI to the NPH or lente insulin; these insulins can be

Table 12-4. Preparations Used in Treatment of Diabetes Mellitus

Drug	*Duration of action*	*Supply*	*Dosage*	*Max. effective dose**
		Insulins		
Short-acting				
Crystalline zinc insulin (CZI)†	Short (6–8 hr)	40 or 80 U/ml	As necessary	None
Semilente insulin		40 or 80 U/ml	As necessary	None
Sulfated insulin		100 U/ml	As necessary	None
Intermediate-acting (globin insulins)				
Neutral protamine Hagedorn (isophane)	Intermed. (16–24 hr)	40 or 80 U/ml	As necessary	None
Lente insulin		40 or 80 U/ml	As necessary	None
Long-acting				
Protamine zinc insulin	Long (20–36 hr)	40 or 80 U/ml	As necessary	None
Ultralente insulin		40 or 80 U/ml	As necessary	None

* Doses in excess of these limits will not increase the hypoglycemic effect of these drugs.
† Insulin Toronto or regular.

mixed in the same syringe and given together. When CZI is added, it is often best to start with a dose of CZI that is about ¼ of the dose of NPH or lente insulin.

In many diabetics, the action of the intermediate insulins is not sustained long enough to cover the entire 24 hours. Such patients need supplementary NPH or lente insulin, before supper or at bedtime. In these circumstances, the initial evening dose should be about ⅙ to ¼ of the total daily requirements. A few patients who fall into this category will be controlled better with long-acting insulins (PZ and ultralente). However, if sufficient long-acting insulin is given in the morning to control the postsupper blood glucose, there is a high risk of hypoglycemia during the night. An alternative is to reduce the morning dose of long-acting insulin and give supplementary CZI before supper. The CZI prevents postsupper hyperglycemia, and the smaller dose of long-acting insulin prevents nocturnal hypoglycemia.

Some physicians believe that CZI given 2 or 3 times daily gives the most satisfactory control of diabetes. In my experience, however, this program is not satisfactory for most diabetics because it allows great fluctuation in the blood glucose, and associated disruption of intermediary metabolism (see section on Other Actions of Insulin earlier in this chapter). However, in the early stages of treatment, or when the patient has slipped out of control, supplementary doses of CZI should be given as often as necessary.

For young children, and particularly infants, the daily insulin requirement is much less than that for adults. The management of diabetes mellitus in children is discussed later, but the reader should note at this point that 2–5 units of CZI may be enough to control even severe hyperglycemia in the very young.

Adequacy of Insulin Replacement

The insulin dose is adequate if the patient's blood glucose concentrations are normal, or the amount of glucose in the urine represents less than 5% of the total 24-hour carbohydrate consumption in a patient receiving an adequate diet.

Blood Glucose Determination. The most useful values are the fasting, 11 A.M., and 3 P.M. blood glucose concentrations. The last two are measured approximately 2 hours after food. The normal ranges are 80–110 mg/ml fasting; and 100–130 mg/ml at 11 A.M. and 3 P.M. The fasting glucose level indicates the adequacy of either the intermediate or long-acting insulin given the previous day. The 11 A.M. blood glucose level is controlled by the CZI given the same morning, and/or by the intermediate-acting insulin given at the same time. The blood glucose level at 3.00 P.M. indicates whether the correct amount of the intermediate or long-acting insulin is being given. The interpretation of all blood glucose levels, of course, depends on a stable and constant dietary intake.

Urine Glucose Testing. The patient does not usually develop significant glycosuria until the blood glucose level is greater than 170 mg/ml, the concentration at which a significant number of renal tubules fail to reabsorb all the glucose in the glomerular filtrate—that is, the "renal threshold" for glucose is surpassed. However, this threshold varies from one patient to another, and also from time to time in the same patient.

The total amount of glucose passed in the urine each day is a very useful guide to treatment. If the 24-hour urine contains less than 5% of the previous day's carbohydrate intake as glucose, control is very good; between 5% and 10% of the total intake, control is fair; and if greater than 10%, control is unsatisfactory.

Commonly, only specimens of urine obtained before meals are tested for glucose. Shortly before the specimen is obtained, the bladder should be emptied completely. Urine secreted some hours previously will thus be removed and will not contaminate the specimen. The specimen can be tested for glucose with a variety of preparations, including Clinitest (which gives a positive reading with all reducing sugars), Clinistix, Testape, and Diastix (all of which depend on glucose oxidase and thus indicate only glucose). The results are recorded as either 0, ¼, ½, 1, or 2% or 0, 1+, 2+, 3+, and 4+. Color charts are provided with each testing material to help the patient interpret the results. A modification of the Clinitest method in which only 2 drops of urine, instead of 5 drops, is mixed with 10 drops of water before the addition of the Clinitest tablet is most useful. With this, urine glucose concentrations ranging from 0 to 5% can be detected. An appropriate color chart for interpreting these concentrations is available from the Ames Company, the manufacturer of Clinitest. Patients should periodically check their testing material against a glucose-containing solution, such as orange juice, to ensure that the test still responds to reducing sugars. When the diabetes is stable, urine need be tested for glucose only once a day but at different times each day. A complete record of the results is a great help to the physician when he is advising patients on their management.

If the patient has moderate to heavy glycosuria (1–2%), he should also test for ketones (β-hydroxybutyric acid, acetoacetic acid, and acetone), breakdown products of fatty acid oxidation that appear during severe insulin insufficiency. For this purpose, "Ketostix" strips or "Acetest" tablets may be used. Both depend on the Rothera nitroprusside reaction. The approximate concentration of ketones is indicated by the intensity of the purple color which develops.

Adverse Effects of Insulin Injection

Hypoglycemia. See section on Complications of Diabetes Mellitus later in this chapter.

Allergy. Allergy presents in two ways: One is local erythematous reaction at the injection site. This response, which may begin to appear as late as 2–3 weeks after treatment begins, consists of hard, red, painful, sometimes itchy lumps, 1–3 cm in diameter, at the injection site. Each lump disappears in 3–4 days. If the insulin treatment is continued, this local allergy disappears in 1–2 months. The second is generalized urticarial reaction due to circulating antibody, with possible anaphylaxis. This response is seen most often in patients who have received insulin on some previous occasion but who stopped treatment. Once the patient develops this type of allergy, further insulin can only be given after desensitization. This can be done quite rapidly by injecting an initially minute dose of insulin (0.001 unit) and increasing the dose by a factor of five at subsequent hourly injections. If this procedure is not successful, the physician can suppress the allergic response with prednisone, 10–20 mg every 8 hours. This can be withdrawn gradually over a week or 10 days unless the allergy recurs.

Insulin Resistance. The patient is insulin-resistant when the total daily requirement of insulin is greater than 200 units. Such resistance is most often due to circulating antibodies, but may develop in Cushing's syndrome, in hemochromatosis, or in the presence of chronic infection—e.g., pyelonephritis. Insulin resistance can be treated in three ways. (1) Prednisone (10 mg 3 times a day) may break the resistance by inhibiting antibody formation; if it succeeds, the results should be apparent within 4–6 days. (2) By using concentrated insulin (500 units per milliliter), an adequate dose can be given in a small volume and thus control may be reestablished. (3) Sulfated insulin may be used. When sulfate radicals replace some amino and carboxyl groups in the insulin preparation, the immunoreactivity of the insulin, but not its biological activity, is altered. Such insulin combines with antibodies to a much smaller degree, and a satisfactory hypoglycemic effect is thus obtained. Sulfated insulin, the newest material for treating insulin resistance, is the preparation of choice. In addition to specific treatment, predisposing conditions such as infection, should be treated vigorously.

Fat Atrophy. In many diabetics, particularly younger patients, subcutaneous fat may atrophy at the injection site (Fig. 12–9). The cause of this atrophy is unknown, but it is unlikely that it is due to insulin because this hormone promotes fat formation and deposition. It may be due to the small amounts of glucagon present in commercial insulins—up to 0.5% (glucagon has fat-mobilizing properties). The condition is self-limiting, although for several years it may cause severe disfigurement. There is no specific treatment. In addition, areas of fat atrophy should not be used as injection sites.

Fat Hypertrophy. If repeated injections of insulin produce a localized increase in fat deposition, this can be controlled by using different injection sites.

General Points in the Management of Diabetes

When the dietary and insulin requirements have been settled, the important smaller details that influence the life of the diabetic must be attended to. Ideally, the patient should be lean and healthy, with regular habits, and free from infection and foot problems. He may smoke if he must, and consume alcoholic beverages of the right kind (see below) in strict moderation. A short discussion with the patient about these points gives him more confidence.

Obesity

Obesity makes the management of diabetes more difficult, increases the insulin requirement, and may also predispose to vascular complications. Since the diabetic already has a tendency to vascular problems, any aggravating factor should be eliminated. The diabetic should be encouraged to maintain his body weight within the accepted range for his height and build, or preferably slightly under it.

Fig. 12-9. Severe insulin-induced fat atrophy. Atrophy has caused disfigurement at site of daily insulin injections in left thigh.

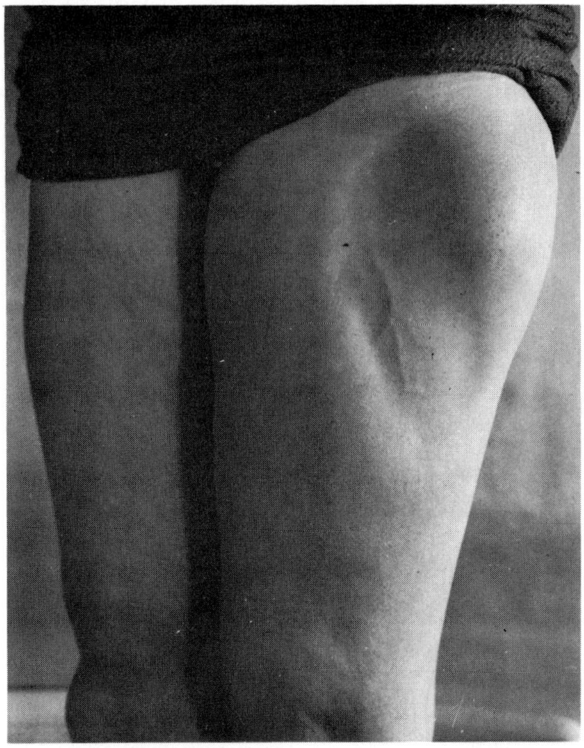

Exercise

Exercise can prevent obesity by increasing energy expenditure. It lowers the blood glucose by causing the active muscle to release "muscular activity factor" (MAF). This factor, a polypeptide with hypoglycemic properties, is still in the early stages of investigation. Exercise also increases the circulation and may help to prevent occlusive arterial and arteriolar disease. In addition to these benefits, the physical fitness from exercise may reduce intercurrent infections, such as colds, etc.

Regularity

The diabetic should take his insulin or oral hypoglycemic drugs and his meals at about the same time every day. A Sunday morning "brunch" is therefore out. However, if he is going out for dinner, he could take his bedtime snack about 6.00 P.M., and have dinner at 8.00–8.30 P.M.

Alcohol

Some physicians do not believe diabetics should drink alcohol. In my opinion, they can if: (1) they practice strict moderation, and (2) make suitable allowances for the carbohydrate content of the beverage. Dry wines and liquors contain little or no carbohydrates, but beers, sweet wines and many cocktails contain a significant amount. The latter should be avoided.

Infection

In poorly controlled diabetes, because the body's resistance to infection is decreased, furunculosis, wound infections, and erysipelas are more common. This tendency is attributed, in part at least, to the decreased motility of polymorphonuclear leukocytes in the presence of hyperglycemia. This complication can best be prevented by good diabetic control and good hygiene.

Foot Problems

Diabetics may have foot problems due to one or more of the following: infection, neuropathy, or ischemia. Most foot problems can be prevented by proper patient education. For example, an unnoticed minor injury to the foot, or an interdigital fungal infection can provide an entry for bacteria. This secondary infection may produce an indolent nonhealing ulcer, or, if the circulation is poor, gangrene. Both these lesions could have been avoided if the patient had been taught to inspect his feet regularly and promptly treat any minor lesions there or elsewhere. Pressure from poorly fitting footwear is hazardous and is a common cause of foot ulcers. Although a pair of specially made shoes costs about $50, this is less than a single day's cost for hospital care and much less than the cost of prolonged hospitalization sometimes necessary for treatment of diabetic foot lesions. It is also a small price to pay for the prevention of a foot problem which could lead to the loss of limb or a long stay in bed.

Complications of Diabetes

The complications of diabetes are the result of metabolic or vascular derangements, or both. The metabolic complications are mainly secondary to a rapid change in metabolic equilibrium, secondary to insulin excess (hypoglycemia) or insulin lack (ketoacidosis or diabetic coma). They can occur at any time during the life of the diabetic. The vascular complications are chronic and develop after diabetes has been present for a significant period. Diabetic retinopathy, for example, is rare in patients who have been diabetic for less than 10 years. The vascular changes involve the small and medium-sized arteries and cause retinopathy, nephropathy, coronary angiopathy, lower limb angiopathy, and certain types of neuropathy. However, enzyme defects are also present in diabetic neuropathy, so that both vascular and metabolic factors are involved.

Acute Complications (mainly metabolic in origin)

Hypoglycemia

Hypoglycemia may develop because the patient has taken too much insulin either by accident or design, or because of a late meal, or unaccustomed exercise. Symptoms appear when the blood glucose level falls to between 40 and 50 mg/100 ml and become more severe as the level falls further. Sweating, hunger, tremor, visual disturbance, and numbness of the fingers and lips progress to mental confusion, an unsteady gait and sometimes violent behavior. If untreated, the patient becomes unconscious. An occasional mild hypoglycemic episode (sweating, hunger, tremors, etc.) before a meal need cause no concern. If these episodes become more frequent and always occur before the same meal, the dose of insulin that has its effect at that time of the day should be reduced. Patients with coronary artery and cerebrovascular disease should avoid even mild hypoglycemia. In the former, a low blood glucose level induces increased myocardial irritability and ectopic beats, due in part to increased catecholamine secretion and hypokalemia. In patients with cerebrovascular disease, increased confusion and possibly temporary localized paralysis may occur. In any patient, hypoglycemia severe enough to produce unconsciousness, especially if it is prolonged, may cause permanent brain damage.

Prevention of hypoglycemia is the main object of treatment. Instruct your patients about the symptoms of hypoglycemia. Encourage them to carry identification cards or bracelets and some form of sugar or glucose for emergency use: 5–10 gm of carbohydrate by mouth (2–4 sugar cubes or a small glass of orange juice) will correct mild hypoglycemia. This can be repeated if necessary. Give the unconscious patient intravenous dextrose (50 ml of a 50% solution). He usually recovers rapidly. Glucagon (1 mg) can easily be injected subcutaneously and is very useful, especially in violent patients. After glucagon is given, oral or intravenous glucose must also be given as soon as the patient can cooperate because the hyperglycemic effect of glucagon is usually transient. The patient who does not recover consciousness even after the blood sugar has been raised to normal levels probably has increased intracranial pressure due to cerebral edema. This can be corrected by giving 100–200 ml of a 20% solution of mannitol intravenously over a 20- to 30-minute period. Mannitol is an osmotic diuretic which does not cross the blood-brain barrier. It increases the plasma osmolality, and thus draws water from the brain into the vascular compartment, and decreases cerebral swelling.

Diabetic Coma

Insulin coma and diabetic coma must be differentiated (Table 12-6). Diabetic coma is present when, because of insulin insufficiency, hyperglycemia and metabolic acidosis have developed, the plasma bicarbonate content is less than 10 mEq/liter, and the plasma ketones are markedly elevated. The term diabetic ketoacidosis is used to describe the state when diabetic control has been lost to the extent that blood ketones are increased and metabolic acidosis (plasma bicarbonate <10 mEq/liter) is present. Not all patients who fulfill the biochemical criteria of diabetic coma are comatose. The present definition, which is based on biochemical data, was evolved before the discovery of insulin, when patients with a plasma bicarbonate content of less than 10 mEq/liter usually died. Because biochemical data are still the best guide to the severity of diabetic coma, the original definition is still used, but all should recognize that the term coma does not always describe the level of consciousness of the patient.

Table 12-5. Treatment for Hypoglycemic Reactions in Diabetes Mellitus

Drug	*Route of admin.*	*Preparation*	*Dose*
Glucose	I-V	50% solution	50–100 ml
Glucagon	SC	1 ampule contains glucagon in dry cake form; 1 ampule contains diluent	1 mg
Epinephrine	SC	1:1,000 solution	1 mg

Table 12-6. Insulin Coma and Diabetic Coma: Differentiation

Insulin coma	*Diabetic coma*
History of long fast or of unusual exercise	History of insulin omission, complicating illness or of overindulgence in food
Rapid onset (1–3 hr)	Gradual onset (1–7 days)
Skin cool and moist	Skin warm and dry, dry tongue, and soft eyeballs
Fast bounding pulse	Fast, normal or thready pulse
Breathing may be stertorous, but is of normal depth and rate; no characteristic smell in breath	Breathing deep and fast, except terminally Strong smell of acetone in breath
Blood pressure normal or increased	Blood pressure normal but usually low
Hyperactive reflexes may have Babinski response	Reflexes normal or depressed

Diabetic coma, a critical medical emergency, still carries a mortality ranging from 4% to 15%. The mortality is higher in older patients, particularly if their diabetes is complicated by other illnesses.

In diabetic coma, the changes in acid-base balance and electrolytes are largely secondary to primary metabolic defects. The acidosis is mainly due to the high concentration of ketoacids, but is aggravated by the loss of base during osmotic diuresis, and by reduced tubular reabsorption of sodium due to the very high renal tubular flow and possibly impaired active reabsorption of sodium in the presence of insulin deficiency. Vomiting, which contributes to dehydration, also increases the ketoacidosis by two different mechanisms: (1) The stress caused by vomiting increases catecholamine release, which increases free fatty acid (FFA) mobilization. The FFA are then oxidized to produce ketones. (2) Persistent vomiting in effect results in a total fast, which is ketogenic. Hemoconcentration develops secondary to the fluid loss. The serum sodium and potassium concentrations may be normal or increased, but the body pool of both is greatly reduced. There may be a disproportionate increase in serum potassium in severe ketoacidosis, because the "sodium pump," which maintains the normal intra/extracellular sodium/potassium ratio, fails and intracellular potassium enters the extracellular fluid space. For these reasons, replacement of sodium and potassium is an essential part of the treatment of diabetic ketoacidosis.

Frequency of Diabetic Coma

Any diabetic patient can develop diabetic coma, but it is most common in insulin-dependent, ketosis-prone patients. Most such diabetics are young, and diabetic coma develops most commonly in young patients. Elderly ketosis-resistant diabetics may also develop diabetic coma but usually only under exceptional circumstances—for example, when the stress of a severe illness greatly increases insulin requirement.

Causes of Diabetic Coma

The ultimate cause of diabetic coma is always severe insulin deficiency, which may be precipitated by a variety of factors: (1) A new diabetic may fail to recognize the significance of early symptoms of diabetes. (2) Failure to take insulin for any reason—e.g., the diabetic who has nausea does not feel like eating and hence thinks he need not take his insulin. If a young diabetic omits his insulin (by accident) for one day, he may start a sequence of events that lead to ketoacidosis and coma. (3) Overeating: Although one would hope that patients would have more sense, overeating is still one of the more common causes of diabetic coma. (4) Insulin resistance: This usually develops slowly, but if it is not corrected vigorously, coma may result. (5) Severe acute illness or trauma of any kind such as gastroenteritis, sepsis, and myocardial infarcts. These events greatly increase the insulin requirement which must be met if coma is to be avoided.

Symptoms and Clinical Features of Diabetic Coma

Initially the symptoms are those of uncontrolled diabetes and the associated hyperglycemia—i.e. thirst, polyuria, and weight loss. The deterioration may progress rapidly or slowly, depending upon the cause; from 1 to 7 days or longer may elapse between the onset of symptoms and the development of the coma. Ketonemia and ketonuria develop early, and ketoacidosis follows. At this stage the patient feels tired and listless and begins to experience nausea, and you can smell acetone in his breath. Once vomiting starts, progress is more rapid because ketosis of starvation has been added to ketosis secondary to insulin insufficiency. By this time the metabolic acidosis is severe, and in an attempt to correct the acidosis by eliminating carbon dioxide, respiration becomes deep and faster—Kussmaul breathing. By now, the patient is acutely ill, with fast deep breathing, an intractable thirst, nausea and vomiting, and frequent retching and urination. Because of the strain of vomiting, and acute liver enlargement due to fat accumulation, he may have severe abdominal pains. Such patients are sometimes operated upon because of a supposed acute abdominal catastrophe; rarely, the two conditions may coexist.

The patient may lose consciousness when the plasma bicarbonate content falls below 10 mEq/liter, but the level of consciousness depends on the pH and on the state of dehydration. However, before the state of unconsciousness can be compared with these parameters (pH and dehydration in uncontrolled diabetes), many more data are needed. In the terminal stages of diabetic coma, the circulation collapses and the respiratory center is depressed: death soon follows.

Laboratory Data in Diabetic Coma

The urine contains more than 2% glucose and 4+ (strongly positive) ketones, and has an acid pH. There may be proteinuria (trace to 1+) and finely granular casts on microscopic examination. The urinary concentration of sodium and chloride is low, but the specific gravity is high because of the glucose.

The blood glucose is usually between 300 mg and 1,000 mg/100 ml, although it may go higher. The serum ketones increase to levels as high as 100 mg/100 ml of blood (normal 0.1–1 mg/100 ml). A semiquantitative nitroprusside test for serum ketones is a useful index of severity. If the test is strongly positive after the serum has been diluted 1:3 with water, the hyperketonemia is severe. The serum may be milky because of the increased concentration of lipoproteins. The plasma free fatty acid concentration is increased. The blood urea nitrogen may be normal but is increased if there is significant hemoconcentration.

The serum bicarbonate is decreased; in diabetic ketoacidosis, it is 10–20 mEq/liter and, in diabetic coma, below 10 mEq/liter. The blood pCO_2 will also be low and the blood pH will reflect the base deficit. In severe diabetic coma, the pH may fall below 7.0; if it falls below 6.8, the patient's chances of recovery are quite small.

In diabetic coma, hemoglobin and hematocrit values are either normal or increased, depending on the state of hydration. Leukocytosis is the rule, and is primarily polymorphonuclear, with a shift to the left. The total leukocyte count may be between 20,000 and 30,000 cells per cubic millimeter. Thus leukocytosis cannot be used to differentiate between diabetic coma and an acute abdominal catastrophe.

Management of Diabetic Coma

Replacement of insulin, fluid, and electrolytes must be started as soon as the diagnosis is made. In the case illustrated in Figure 12-10, treatment consisted of (1) large amounts of insulin, (2) large amounts of fluid, (3) adequate potassium replacement, (4) protection against hypernatremia, and (5) prevention of hypoglycemia in the later stages of treatment.

Insulin

The patient has a relative insulin resistance because of acidosis, increased free fatty acid concentration and hyperketonemia, and possibly, unidentified insulin antagonists. The adult should be given 50 units of CZI intravenously and 50 units CZI subcutaneously as soon as a blood sample is taken for the necessary laboratory studies. This dose should be repeated within 2 hours if the laboratory data indicate severe diabetic coma (pH 7.0 CO_2 content <5 mEq/liter and blood glucose >400 mg/100 ml). The blood glucose is then determined at three-hour intervals.

Fig. 12-10. Biochemical course and clinical management of diabetic coma in a 16-year-old diabetic. Treatment consists of large amounts of insulin, large amounts of fluid, adequate potassium replacement, protection against hypernatremia, and prevention of hypoglycemia in later stages of treatment.

Second graph from top. Note (1) very rapid fall in serum potassium after start of treatment (*solid line*); (2) development of hypernatremia (*broken line*). This was unexpected in view of severe dehydration. It was corrected by continuing fluid infusion, using half strength normal saline solution.

Third graph from top. Note (1) rapid correction of blood pH (*solid line*) after sodium bicarbonate administration; (2) the almost parallel rise in serum total Co_2 (*broken line*).

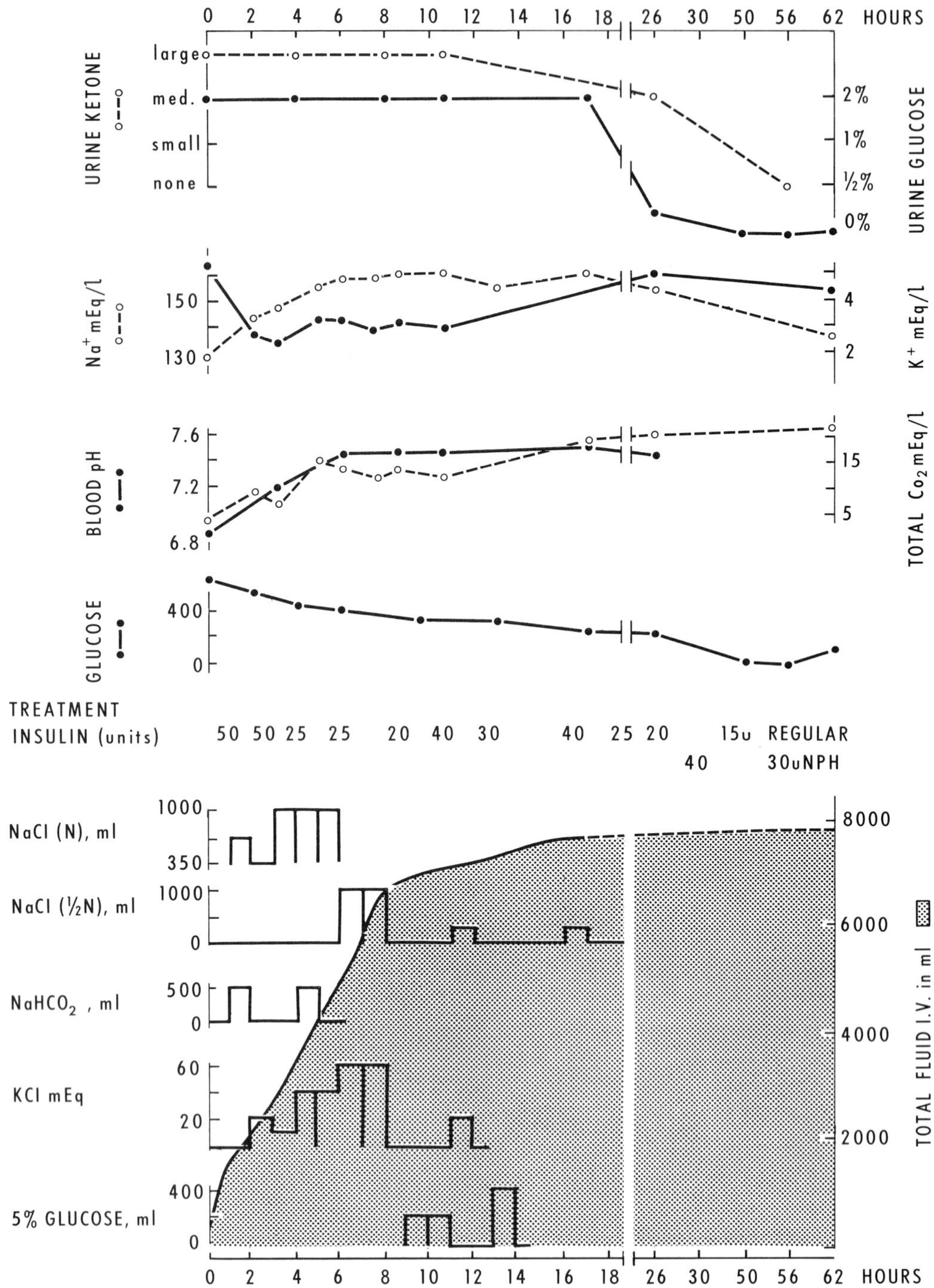

After each result is known, 50 more units of CZI is given intravenously until the blood glucose concentration decreases significantly—e.g., from 800 mg/100 ml to 500 mg/100 ml, or from 400 mg/100 ml to 250 mg/100 ml. This usually happens within 6 hours of starting treatment. When it does, 25 units of CZI should be given intravenously and the blood glucose checked 3 hours later. Final restoration of normal blood glucose is achieved by giving small doses (10–20 units) of CZI subcutaneously. The exact dose depends on the blood glucose level.

The blood glucose value is the best index of insulin requirement. If laboratory facilities are not available, there are two alternatives: (1) Determine the blood glucose with "Dextrostix" (a paper strip, glucose oxidase method for measuring glucose). This technique is highly useful even though the result is not as exact as a laboratory determination. If the initial glucose concentration is too high, the blood can be diluted. (2) Use the serum ketone concentration as a guide. If the Rothera test is still strongly positive after the serum sample has been diluted 1:3 or 1:4 with water, then 100 units of CZI should be given (50 units subcutaneously and 50 units intravenously). The serum should be tested again for ketones in 3 hours. Repeat the same dose of insulin if the Rothera test is still positive in serum diluted more than 1:2 with water, but give one-half the initial dose if the test is positive only at a dilution of less than 1:2. Neither of these techniques is as dependable as laboratory determination of the blood glucose, but they are useful substitutes. Determinations of urine glucose and ketone concentrations are of little value in the management of diabetic coma, except in making the initial diagnosis. Glycosuria and ketonuria persist for some time after the blood glucose has been corrected. They cannot be relied on as a guide for the treatment of diabetic coma.

On rare occasions, the first dose of 100–200 units of insulin does not lower the blood glucose. In this event, suspect insulin resistance and immediately give 100 more units of CZI intravenously. Then determine the blood glucose at two-hour intervals. The dose of intravenous insulin should be doubled after each determination until the blood glucose falls significantly. When diabetic coma is complicated by insulin resistance, massive doses of insulin (several thousand units) may be required.

Fluid and Electrolytes

Adequate rehydration is the only satisfactory method of correcting the hypovolemia and shock associated with diabetic coma. Physiologic saline contains the necessary sodium but potassium and, in severe cases, bicarbonate must be added.

Fluid and Sodium. Up to 5 or more liters of fluid may be needed in the first 2–4 hours. Initially, use normal physiologic saline. If hypernatremia develops (serum sodium greater than 145 mEq/liter), substitute half-strength physiologic saline. If there is uncertainty about the patient's ability to tolerate rapid fluid replacement, insert a central venous catheter, and adjust the rate of infusion to ensure that the central venous pressure does not rise. Solutions containing glucose should not be used in the early stages, because the increased blood glucose will further increase the extracellular osmolarity and thus increase the intracellular dehydration. When the blood glucose begins to approach normal levels, 5% dextrose in water should be substituted.

Potassium. Hypokalemia often develops during the early stages of correction of dehydration, but can be prevented by adding 20 mEq of potassium chloride to each liter of intravenous fluid after the first. More potassium should be added if there is laboratory evidence of hypokalemia, or if "U" waves appear in the electrocardiogram, since these may occur in the presence of hypokalemia. At the same time, hyperkalemia, which is equally dangerous, must be avoided. In the presence of renal damage, potassium should be replaced with particular care.

Base. In diabetic acidosis, the metabolic efficiency of insulin is reduced, the deep, fast Kussmaul breathing is an exhausting process in an already exhausted patient, and the normal mechanisms for maintaining acid-base balance may be impaired if there is renal disease due to diabetes or any other cause. For these reasons, when there is significant acidosis, give sodium bicarbonate early to reduce or correct this state.

The base deficit can be calculated using the Astrup technique and nomogram and making the appropriate correction. Another method is as follows: Determine the deficit in milliequivalents per liter of plasma bicarbonate and multiply this figure by the extracellular fluid volume (approximately 15–20 liters). The result will be the approximate total body deficit of bicarbonate. This deficit can be replaced with 5% sodium bicarbonate (580 mEq/liter). It is better to give slightly less than the total amount needed for total correction to avoid rebound alkalosis. The degree to which the patient's symptoms improve after the base deficit is corrected is most gratifying.

Other Emergency Measures

In the management of diabetic coma, other emergency measures may be necessary. In the early stages of treatment, nothing is given by mouth except small amounts of water. If the patient is vomiting, or if there is any evidence of acute dilation of the stomach, gastric lavage should be performed. If the patient is unconscious, an anesthetist should assist with the intubation. A urinary catheter should not be inserted unless renal shutdown is suspected (see below). Sympathomimetic drugs should not be used to correct hypotension. Instead, the volume of intravenous fluid should be increased. Any coincidental illness that may have precipitated the coma should, of course, be treated. Except in extreme emergencies, the patient should not be operated upon until he is rehydrated, the acid-base balance restored, and the diabetes brought under control.

It usually takes from 24 to 48 hours to correct the ketosis associated with diabetic coma. When nausea ceases, the patient can have fluid or soft diet with an appropriate caloric content. Intermediate or long-acting insulin should be started as soon as the initial hyperglycemia has been corrected. Until the proper dose has been determined, it can be supplemented with more frequent injections of crystalline zinc insulin. After 2 or 3 days, the patient can resume his normal diet. Bed rest is essential during the acute phase of the illness, but early mobilization is essential because phlebothrombosis is a constant threat during the hypovolemic phase.

Diabetic Coma: Complications

Dehydration and hypovolemia combine to produce most of the complications of diabetic coma. Many diabetic patients have arteriosclerosis and the blood supply to some vital organs may already be impaired. A fall in blood pressure in these patients may precipitate cerebral thrombosis, myocardial infarction, mesenteric thrombosis, or thrombosis in the arteries of the legs. Rapid and adequate rehydration is necessary to prevent these complications, especially in the elderly.

Occasionally, acute renal tubular necrosis develops. Such patients usually have severe infection as well, so that the tubular necrosis appears to be due to a toxin, combined with hypovolemia. If you carefully monitor the urinary output, you will recognize this complication early. If you suspect it, give mannitol (20–40 gm in a 20% solution) intravenously. This should produce a urine flow of at least 40 ml/hour. If it does not, start a renal failure program at once. (The 24-hour fluid allowance should be restricted to the fluid loss in the previous 24-hour period, plus 600–1000 ml of water to allow for insensible loss, and ensure an intake of 800–1000 calories per day. Urine volume, blood electrolytes, and glucose and urea nitrogen must also be checked daily.) Appropriate antibiotics should also be given to control concurrent infection. If the patient develops azotemia and acidosis, hemodialysis or peritoneal dialysis may be necessary. Hypokalemia may precipitate ventricular arrhythmias—a risk that is increased by coronary artery disease or a recent myocardial infarct. During the phase of massive fluid replacement, check the serum potassium each time a blood sample is drawn for glucose determination.

Hypoglycemia may be due either to overenthusiastic insulin administration or to an unexpected sensitivity to insulin. This can be prevented by starting an infusion of 5% dextrose in water (100 ml/hour) when the blood glucose has fallen to between 150 and 200 mg/100 ml.

Aspiration pneumonia is a great hazard in a vomiting, semiconscious patient. If the patient aspirates vomitus, 200–300 mg of cortisone hemisuccinate may be necessary to overcome the bronchospasm. A broad-spectrum antibiotic should also be started to combat secondary infection.

Acute diabetic neuropathy may develop during diabetic coma. The patient will recover completely, but this is a slow process.

Hyperosmolar Nonketotic Diabetic Coma

Hyperosmolar nonketotic diabetic coma (HNKDC), a relatively rare condition, has only recently been recognized. It is seen most commonly in middle-aged patients, some of whom may not previously have needed insulin. This type of coma may be precipitated by an acute illness or any condition that predisposes to dehydration. In one patient it was precipitated by an obviously unnecessary glucose tolerance test done when the fasting blood glucose was above 300 mg/100 ml.

The history of patients with HNKDC does not suggest the diagnosis although many have had symptoms of uncontrolled diabetes. On examination, the main findings are severe dehydration and glycosuria but no urinary ketones. In addition to signs of the precipitating illness (if any), some of these patients show a mild but unexplained bulbar palsy with dysphagia. The initial blood glucose is greater than 500 mg/100 ml, and values as high as 3,500 mg/100 ml have been recorded. The serum sodium and chloride are usually elevated (sodium > 150 mEq/liter and chloride > 110 mEq/liter). Undiluted serum gives a negative to 2+ positive reaction for ketones.

Patients with HNKDC are treated with fluid and insulin. Rapid rehydration with half-strength physiologic saline, and potassium chloride supplements if necessary, is vitally important. The central venous pressure should be monitored to prevent overloading of the circulation. The calculation of the insulin requirement is made in the same way as outlined for diabetic coma. Patients with HNKDC usually have a normal sensitivity to insulin. During the early recovery phase, some of these patients develop transient diabetes insipidus.

The pathophysiology of this disorder has not yet been worked out. Some suggest that these patients develop acute insulin insufficiency, but the reason for this is not known. After recovery, some of these patients may once more be managed by diet alone, indicating that the pancreatic insulin production is again adequate. Since comparable hyperglycemia in a nondiabetic animal does not produce the same dehydration and hyperosmolarity, some transient abnormality in renal function must have been present to create the gross osmolar imbalance seen in these patients. However, this abnormality has not been identified.

Complications Due to Diabetes of Long Duration

These consist of (1) microvascular, (2) large vessel, and (3) metabolic problems. There is probably a close connection between all three although the connecting links have not been identified. Microvascular disease plays a part in the production of all diabetic complications—in particular, diabetic retinopathy and nephropathy. In association with medium-to-large artery disease, it underlies coronary and peripheral vascular occlusive disease. Although the primary abnormality in diabetes is metabolic, an enzymatic defect can only be identified clearly in diabetic neuropathy. Almost certainly an unidentified metabolic defect produces the cataracts sometimes seen in young diabetics, and also the blood lipoprotein abnormalities.

Microvascular Disease

Diabetic Retinopathy

Diabetic retinopathy causes between 10% and 20% of blindness in Canada. It is primarily a disease of the capillaries in which the mural (support) cells disappear and the basement membrane thickens.

The patient has usually been diabetic for 8–10 years before retinopathy can be detected, and symptoms do not appear until the process is well advanced. Central vision is lost and visual acuity decreases when the macular area is affected. Vision may be lost suddenly from massive intraocular bleeding.

Early retinopathic changes can only be detected

when the pupil is properly dilated with homatropine or Neo-Synephrine. Mydriatics should not be used if there is any evidence of increased intraocular pressure. The first change is increased tortuosity and congestion of the retinal veins followed by the appearance of microaneurysms (Ballantyne aneurysms)—small dilations in the capillaries, which may be transient. Microaneurysms are often present before they can be seen with the ophthalmoscope; they can be seen when a bolus of intravenously injected fluorescein passes through the retinal circulation (Fig. 12-11). They appear first in the macular area and in the lateral part of the temporal region. Later, small, punctate, "pinhead" hemorrhages and small serous exudates in the nerve layer ("waxy exudates") develop. Hemorrhages and exudates may expand and cause scotomas. About this time or occasionally earlier, new blood vessels begin to appear. These fine, tortuous, and feathery vessels often appear first at the optic disc and may grow along the nerve layer or protrude into the vitreous humor. If these vessels rupture, they can cause large hemorrhages along the nerve layer or may burst into the vitreous. In either case, vision is impaired or lost, particularly if the macula is involved. Fibrous tissue, formed while the blood is being reabsorbed, is seen as white "sheathing" around the blood vessels or as bands of tissue in the vitreous. The combination of new vessel and fibrous tissue formation is called retinitis proliferans. When this fibrous tissue contracts, it often causes retinal detachment, with permanent loss of vision. The increase in intraocular pressure associated with this bleeding may induce glaucoma.

New vessels may also form around the ora serrata and involve the ciliary body. The canal of Schlemm is distorted and blocked, the intraocular pressure rises, and glaucoma develops. These new vessels may be seen growing through the iris, producing the condition known as rubeosis iridis.

In addition to the changes of diabetic retinopathy, flame-shaped nerve-layer hemorrhages and "cotton-wool exudates" usually appear when renal damage and hypertension are also present.

Treatment. There is no satisfactory treatment for diabetic retinopathy. It has been established that careful control of the blood sugar (and thus of the diabetes) does help to prevent this complication. However, the fact that it may develop even in patients with "well-controlled" diabetes indicates that other factors influence its development. On the other hand, in a few patients, the progress of the retinopathy can be halted or the process reversed when good diabetic control is restored. No drug therapy is of any help.

New vessel formation may be treated with photo- or laser-beam coagulation. This approach

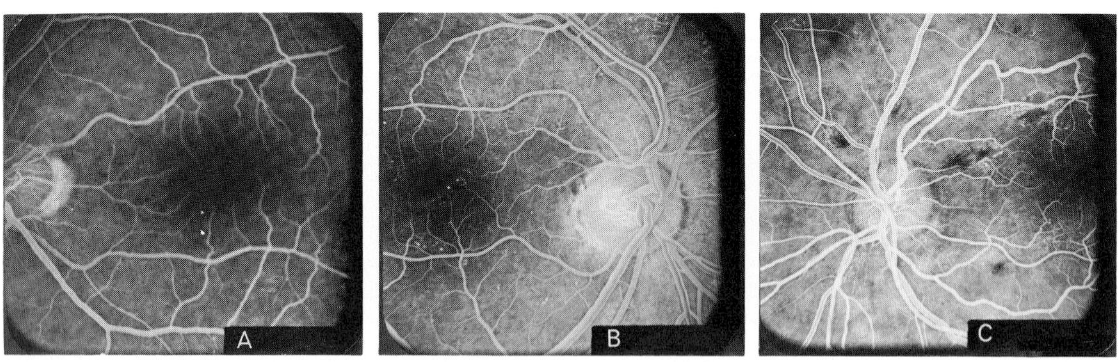

Fig. 12-11. Retinal photographs following intravenous fluorescein injection. A. In the normal eye, arteries and veins are filled with fluorescein. Note that there are no dilatations (microaneurysms). **B.** In the diabetic, fluorescein outlines microaneurysms arising from vessels of the retina. **C.** Also in the diabetic, the process in **B** has progressed, and fluorescein demonstrates a larger number of microaneurysms and some very faint feathery new vessels. (Photographs kindly provided by Dr. Clive Mortimer.)

is still experimental, but the results are encouraging, and it is at present the most frequently used type of treatment. When diabetic retinopathy is advanced and loss of vision threatens, hypophysectomy may be performed. In well-selected patients, this operation improves visual acuity in 50–70% of cases. Unfortunately, in some patients, the improvement is only transient, and this procedure is now rarely used.

Candidates for pituitary ablation must be very carefully chosen. The best results are obtained in patients under 40 years of age who have no cardiovascular, cerebrovascular, or overt renal disease. They should be well adjusted psychologically and must clearly understand the risks involved, including the possibility of failure. They must understand and accept that they will need permanent hormonal substitution therapy, including cortisone, thyroid hormone, and sex hormones. Posterior pituitary extract is needed initially to control diabetes insipidus, but only a few patients need it permanently. After pituitary ablation, the patient's sensitivity to insulin is increased and hence he must guard against hypoglycemic reactions. Each patient must understand that the cortisone dose must be increased during any illness or stress-producing situations.

The reason diabetic retinopathy improves after hypophysectomy is not known. The beneficial effect was discovered by chance, and for years the improvement has been attributed to the removal of growth hormone. However, this cannot be accepted as the final answer. Hypophysectomy does not benefit microvascular disease in other organs, and the life span of such patients is not increased by this operation. The transsphenoidal route is currently the best approach for hypophysectomy.

When the patient has intractable glaucoma due to hemorrhage or to rubeosis iridis, the eye must be enucleated.

Diabetic Nephropathy

Diabetic nephropathy is one of the common causes of death in patients who develop diabetes before the age of 15 years. In genetically transmitted diabetes, characteristic thickening of the basement membrane in the renal glomerulus may develop very early, even before glucose intolerance can be demonstrated. Rarely, symptoms of renal disease, which, on investigation, is histologically indistinguishable from diabetic nephropathy, appear before glucose intolerance develops. Symptoms do not develop until the renal damage is extensive. Polyuria and nocturia appear first and are soon followed by edema. The patient may have dysuria because of the almost invariably associated pyelonephritis. Later, weakness due to anemia (secondary to renal failure) and congestive heart failure develop.

The earliest clinical sign of diabetic nephropathy is proteinuria, which may be intermittent at first. It does not usually occur until 10–15 years after the onset of diabetes. Current evidence suggests that an individual with diabetic nephropathy will live 12–15 years after proteinuria first appears. The protein in the urine increases to values well within the limits of the nephrotic syndrome (>3.5 gm of protein in the urine in 24 hours) before tapering finally to much lower values, as renal failure develops. Microscopic examination of the urinary sediment will show hyaline and finely granular casts and doubly refractile fat bodies. If there is associated infection, pus cells and bacteria are also present. Hypoproteinemia and edema develop as a result of the massive protein loss. The anemia, which is normocytic and normochromic, may be due to decreased erythropoietin production. The urinary electrolyte content is normal in early diabetic nephropathy. Sodium excretion becomes excessive in the diuretic stage, but sodium retention begins with the onset of renal failure.

The cardiovascular system reflects the severity of the renal hypertension; the patient soon develops left ventricular hypertrophy. The cardiac failure seen in the late stages is due to hypervolemia secondary to sodium retention and due also to concomitant myocardial disease.

In the terminal stages, the patient has all the signs of uremia—i.e., weakness, edema, anemia, hypertension, azotemia, etc. Diarrhea, which can be troublesome, may be due to uremic colitis or diabetic enteropathy. In this state, patients are often aware of the hopelessness of the situation, and may develop severe anxiety and depressive psychoses.

In the later stages, in addition to the laboratory

findings already mentioned, the blood urea nitrogen may be deceptively low (50–80 mg/100 ml) when the serum creatinine is 10 mg/100 ml or higher. The creatinine clearance is greatly reduced.

The main pathological changes are in the small blood vessels; they consist of thickening of the basement membrane of the glomerular and mesangial cells and formation of eosinophilic nodules in the glomerular tufts. The nodular lesions are specific for diabetic nephropathy. These changes are progressive, and the degree of involvement is an index of the severity of the disease. Inflammatory cell infiltration and scarring due to pyelonephritis are almost always seen in advanced diabetic nephropathy.

Treatment. There is no specific treatment for diabetic nephropathy. Careful regulation of the blood glucose does help. (Renal biopsies from diabetic animals in ketoacidosis show acute basement-membrane thickening which resolves when diabetic control is restored.) The diet should contain adequate protein to replace urinary loss in the nephrotic phase. Infection should be treated vigorously with appropriate antibiotics, always remembering that in the presence of renal failure, the doses of some antibiotics must be reduced. Depending on the clinical state, fluid and electrolyte intake must be carefully controlled. Massive edema and hyponatremia, which occur in the later stages, must be treated by fluid restriction and not with hypertonic saline; the latter will only aggravate the situation. Hypertension and cardiac failure are treated with the standard methods.

Occlusive Disease of the Medium and Small Arteries

Although there is widespread involvement of the medium- to small-caliber vessels in the diabetic, narrowing of the coronary and leg arteries is most frequent.

Large Vessel Disease

Coronary Artery Disease

The only features which distinguish coronary artery disease in the diabetic and the nondiabetic are (1) earlier onset, (2) increased incidence, and (3) reversed sex ratio in the diabetics. In one group of patients who developed coronary thrombosis below the age of 50, 80% had a diabetic type of glucose tolerance, which was distinct from the decreased glucose tolerance present in the early stages of myocardial infarction (probably due to epinephrine release and other unidentified factors). Over 50% of all diabetics eventually die from coronary artery disease. Combined coronary artery and renal artery disease accounts for nearly 80% of all deaths in diabetics.

Symptoms of coronary artery disease are common in elderly diabetics and sometimes appear before the age of 40 in growth-onset diabetics. The symptoms progress more rapidly in the presence of renal disease. Sometimes these patients have no pain even after a myocardial infarct, probably because the pain-conducting autonomic fibers have been damaged by diabetic neuropathy. For this reason a silent infarct should be suspected when an elderly diabetic deteriorates rapidly without apparent cause.

Coronary artery disease cannot be prevented, but certain measures may decrease the morbidity associated with it. Hyerlipoproteinemia, which is often present in diabetics, is associated with an increased incidence of atherosclerosis. Good diabetic control (as judged by normal blood glucose levels, normal body weight, and a properly balanced diet) helps to reduce the serum lipoprotein concentrations toward normal. Over a period of years, this reduction may help the patient. There is as yet no absolute evidence that the ingestion of polyunsaturated fatty acids reduces the tendency to obliterative arterial disease. Regular exercise is said to prevent atherosclerosis and should be encouraged, but no properly controlled studies have been done to confirm this claim.

Treatment of Coronary Artery Disease in the Diabetic. This treatment is the same as for coronary artery disease in the nondiabetic. Hypoglycemia must be avoided because it increases the risk of ventricular arrhythmias, especially in the presence of hypokalemia. Potassium chloride should always be given with diuretics and may help to prevent arrhythmias after an acute myocardial infarct. There is often a temporary large increase in insulin requirement shortly after a "coronary." The blood glucose levels should be followed carefully and adequate supplementary CZI given to cover this increased need.

Lower Limb Arteries

In diabetics, particularly in the elderly, circulatory disease of the legs is 40 times more common than in nondiabetics. Young patients with diabetes of long duration may also be affected.

Patients with lower-limb ischemia complain of cold feet, nocturnal cramps in the calf muscles, and of pains in the calf muscles and occasionally in the gluteal region during exercise. When the ischemia is severe, the pain becomes constant. The patients will have noticed that healing is slow, an indication of decreased tissue vitality. Not uncommonly, these patients present with a painful gangrenous tip of a toe, the result of digital artery occlusion. The pain may be so severe that, even though the toe is not gangrenous, the patient requests amputation.

The signs of decreased blood supply to the legs appear early. The affected foot is cold, the skin dry and scaly, and the hairs will have disappeared from the dorsum of the toes and feet. The venous filling time is prolonged and a dusky redness will appear in the distal parts of the leg in the dependent position. Gangrene, when it develops, usually occurs in the toes, over the head of the fifth metatarsal, or in the heel. When such areas become infected, the lesion rapidly progresses. Initially, there is no clear demarcation line, and the inflammatory reaction may be poor because of the inadequate blood supply. At this stage, a radiograph may show bone destruction due to osteomyelitis, and tapering of the distal ends of the metatarsal bones secondary to neuropathy. It will also show calcification of the walls of the medium and small arteries.

Treatment. Every reasonable effort should be made to protect the foot from trauma. Shoes should fit well and socks should be free from hard rough areas. In addition, good foot hygiene, prompt treatment of any interdigital fungal infections, proper use of skin hardening or softening preparations, proper care of nails and calluses by a podiatrist, and prompt, skilled treatment of any abrasion of the feet are all important.

Should an ulcer develop in the foot, the patient should be put to bed. The affected leg should be kept in the horizontal position unless it is edematous, when slight elevation of the foot is helpful. Appropriate antibiotics should be used when necessary. Minor lesions will heal with these measures, though prolonged bed rest may be necessary. Unfortunately, such a course may be detrimental to the general health of elderly patients. If possible, the blood supply to the affected limb should be increased. Lumbar sympathectomy rarely helps the diabetic. In suitable patients, endarterectomy or a bypass procedure between the femoral and popliteal arteries may greatly enhance the blood supply to the foot, and allow healing.

Amputation becomes necessary when gangrene or intractable osteomyelitis develops. This ranges from removal of a toe to a midthigh amputation, depending on the extent of the lesion and on the age and general condition of the patient.

Long-Term Complications of Diabetes Due to Metabolic Disorders

Diabetic Cataracts

Cataracts sometimes develop in diabetic children if the blood glucose has been poorly regulated. The cataracts are characteristically flocculent, quite different from the "cartwheel" appearance of the early senile cataract. The latter type is seen in elderly diabetics, but is only slightly, if any, commoner than in nondiabetics. The metabolic defect responsible for the juvenile cataract has not been identified. Both types of cataract should be resected when they have reached a sufficient degree of maturity.

Diabetic Neuropathy

Diabetic neuropathy, a very common complication, presents with a wide variety of manifestations. It usually does not produce symptoms until 10–15 years after growth-onset diabetes appears, but may be the presenting feature in patients with maturity-onset diabetes; in these individuals, however, the duration of the illness is uncertain. Diabetes can cause sensory, motor, or autonomic neuropathy.

Sensory Symptoms. The sensory changes are those of a polyneural peripheral neuropathy, which involves the lower limbs primarily, but occasionally the upper limbs as well. The involvement increases with the duration of diabetes, especially if no treatment has been given. Paresthesias of the feet and legs, and a hot, burning sensation in the feet, are common. Patients may also experience hyperalgesia to light touch and "shooting bone pains" in the legs. These symptoms are usually worst at night, and may be associated with painful cramps in the feet, leg, or thigh muscles. Patients may complain of an inability to differentiate between hot and cold in their feet and later notice the loss of pain and touch. Trophic ulcers on the feet, which develop readily under these conditions, may bring the patient to the doctor (Fig. 12-12).

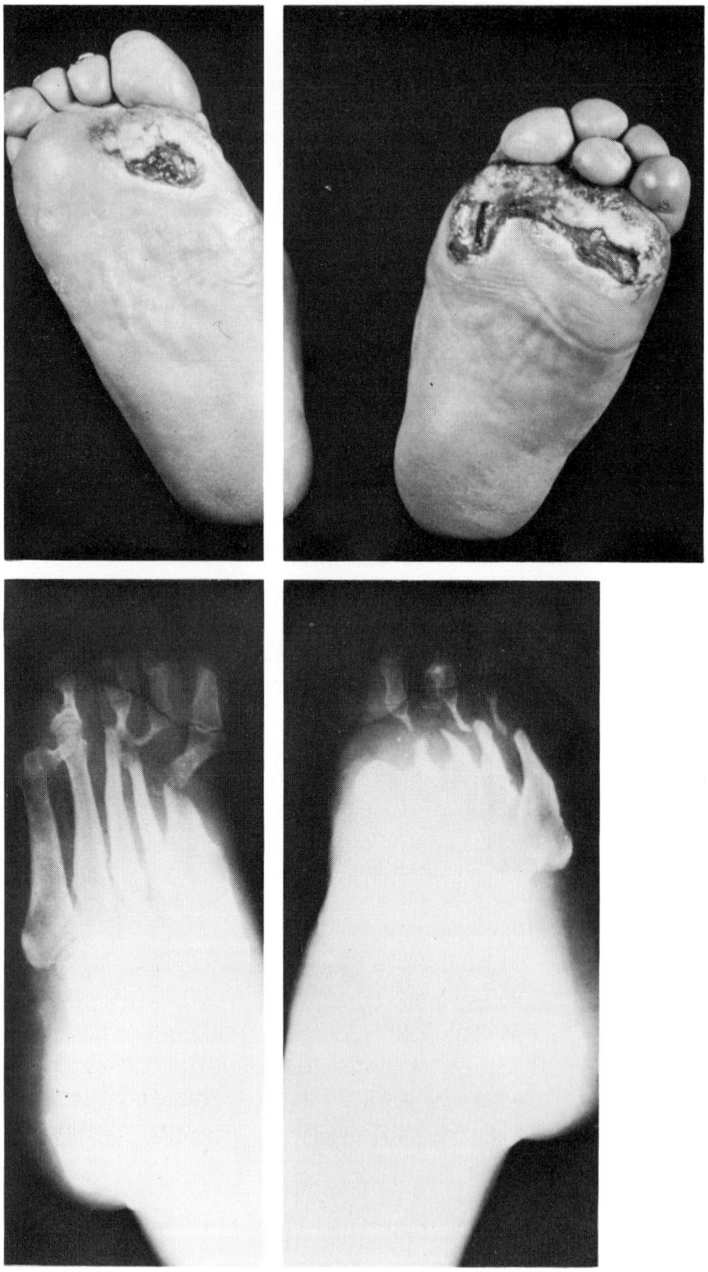

Fig. 12-12. Diabetic neuropathy, sensory type.

Top. Severe ulceration and deformation of feet secondary to diabetic neuropathy.

Bottom. Radiograph of the same feet, showing bone resorption and pathological fractures. Note marked tapering of metatarsal bones, a result of the neuropathy.

Motor Symptoms. Motor involvement is usually much more localized, involving one muscle or a muscle group supplied by one nerve. Paralysis may develop suddenly, or weakness of a varying degree can develop gradually. The nerves most commonly affected are the oculomotor, abducens, facial, femoral, and peroneal, and, less often, the radial nerve. Damage to these nerves causes (respectively): diplopia, ptosis, weakness of the facial muscle, and the iliopsoas and quadriceps femoris group, the peroneal muscle (foot drop), and the extensor muscles of the forearm (wrist drop). Individual trunk and upper limb muscles are rarely affected.

Autonomic Symptoms. Patients with lesions of the autonomic nervous system may complain of localized or generalized absence of sweating, faintness on standing up, a sensation of abdominal distention, indigestion, vomiting, constipation, and diarrhea, an ability to go for long periods without urinating, and impotence. One symptom usually predominates in each patient, but others are often present to a lesser degree.

Diagnosis of Diabetic Neuropathy. The diagnosis is based on physical examination. The earliest detectable change is loss of vibration (128 cps) sensation in the toes but becomes more extensive with increasing duration of the illness. Position sense may also be lost. Later, pain and temperature and touch sensations are lost in a "stocking and glove" fashion. The ankle and knee jerks are reduced or absent. Swelling, distortion, crepitus, and painless hypermotility in a joint indicates a Charcot type degeneration.

Weakness in dorsiflexion of the foot (foot drop) and in flexion of the hip indicate peroneal and femoral nerve involvement respectively. Involvement of the third, sixth, and seventh cranial nerves is indicated by weakness or paralysis of the muscle groups supplied by them.

Signs of autonomic involvement may be detected in the affected organs. In the eye, the pupil is constricted, and the light reflex reduced. Vasomotor tone is reduced, and the blood pressure may fall precipitously when the patient changes from the supine to erect position, producing dizziness or even collapse. Gross painless distention of the urinary bladder may occur.

Other signs of autonomic dysfunction require special investigations. Radiologic examination of affected bowel will show dilatation and ineffective peristalsis of the stomach, and dilatation of the small intestine, colon, and gallbladder. A cystometrogram will reveal increased volume, decreased contractility of the urinary bladder, and incomplete emptying. The resulting stasis predisposes to urinary-tract infections.

Electroneural studies show that, in diabetic sensory, motor, and autonomic nerves, the conduction rates are reduced, even before there are any clinical signs of diabetic neuropathy. The cerebrospinal fluid protein content is often above the normal upper limit of 40 mg/100 ml, even in the absence of intracranial disease.

Pathology of Diabetic Neuropathy. Our understanding of diabetic neuropathy has recently increased significantly. Histological examination of single diabetic nerve fibers shows two main changes: (1) demyelination, and subsequent remyelination, as indicated by the irregularly spaced nodes of Ranvier, and (2) axon degeneration, without recovery. Transient diabetic neuropathy is probably due to demyelination, while the more permanent type of neuropathy is attributed to axon degeneration.

These changes may be due to occlusion of small nutrient arteries causing ischemia or may be the result of specific enzyme deficiencies, which have recently been identified in peripheral nerves in diabetic patients. Specific changes in the vasa nervorum of diabetics have been recognized for many years, and electron microscopy has revealed that the basement membrane is thickened in the capillary endothelium, and also in the Schwann cells.

Enzyme defects and altered metabolic balances have been identified in nerve tissue taken from human diabetic subjects, and from alloxan-diabetic animals. Lipid synthesis in the myelin sheath is impaired, possibly as a result of a deficiency in acetic thiokinase—the enzyme responsible for conversion of acetate into acetyl coenzyme A, a basic unit in fatty acid and sterol synthesis. Carbohydrate metabolism within the myelin sheath is altered, secondary to the reduced activity of aldose reductase in the presence of normal sorbitol dehydrogenase activity. This causes increased carbohydrate metabolism, via the sorbitol pathway, and increased fructose formation. The exact mechanism through which these enzyme changes are brought about is not clear. Insulin treatment alone does not correct them in experimental diabetic animals, but cross-circulation between a diabetic and nondiabetic animal restores acetic thiokinase activity almost to normal in the latter. This recovery is therefore not due to insulin alone.

Treatment. In diabetic neuropathy, the first requirement is careful regulation of the blood glucose, thus ensuring adequate compensation for insulin insufficiency. Improvement almost always occurs, but may be very slow. Strong analgesic drugs may be necessary to relieve pain. Physiotherapy and adequate splinting are necessary when localized muscle weakness or paralysis has developed. If a Charcot degeneration has occurred, prolonged immobilization in a cast appears to give best results, but if the patient has septic arthritis, or osteomyelitis, amputation may be necessary.

Gastric atony does not respond well to any particular therapy. Creation of a gastrojejunostomy to relieve the obstruction is contraindicated. Occasionally, gastrostomy is necessary to allow feeding and, at the same time, prevent the accumulation of food and fluids in the stomach, with subsequent vomiting. Steatorrhea, the result of small bowel involvement, is treated in the standard way. Diabetic diarrhea may be improved with Lomotil (diphenoxylate hydrochloride plus atropine) or Periactin (cyproheptadine hydrochloride). The latter is an antihistamine with antiserotonin properties. Its action in diabetic diarrhea is attributed to its effect on serotonin.

The treatment of a diabetic neuropathic bladder consists of (1) precautions against, and treatment of, any urinary tract infections, and (2) regular voluntary voiding at 2-hour intervals during the day. There is no satisfactory treatment for impotence. Rarely, function may return after the diabetes is brought under strict control.

Postural hypotension may be treated by increasing the sodium intake. However, many patients with this symptom have associated diabetic nephropathy and sodium retention, thus contraindicating the administration of extra salt. These patients can control the hypotension by avoiding any sudden change from the recumbent to the erect position.

In summary, many aspects of diabetic neuropathy are managed by accommodating to the limitations imposed by it. However, the attempt must always be made to reduce the neuropathy by improving diabetic control.

Effects of Diabetes in Other States and Conditions

Pregnancy and Diabetes

Pregnancy is an intensely anabolic state. Insulin is necessary for anabolism, and in the normal pregnancy, enough is produced so that there is no demonstrable change in glucose tolerance and no decrease in blood insulin levels during glucose stimulation. In fact, in normal pregnancy there appears to be a greater increase in blood insulin levels after glucose administration than in the nonpregnant state.

When pregnancy and diabetes coexist, or when a pregnant woman has a tendency to become diabetic (history of large babies or previous gestational diabetes), the effects of pregnancy on diabetes, and vice versa, are manifested in physical and hormonal changes in both mother and fetus. The physical changes (see below) are probably not the direct result of hormonal changes, because the former can develop before there are any demonstrable hormone changes. (This statement obviously cannot be made without reservation, because methods for measuring hormonal production are, in some instances, still relatively crude.)

The net effect of these physical and hormonal alterations in the diabetic pregnancy is to increase maternal morbidity and to reduce the chance of fetal survival. The objective of the treatment of the pregnant diabetic is to reverse this tendency. Under ideal circumstances, fetal and neonatal loss in diabetic pregnancies is between 5% and 10%, which is only slightly greater than in normal pregnancies. Under moderately unfavorable circumstances, fetal loss can rise to 50–60%.

Hormonal Changes

Endogenous insulin production virtually ceases in growth-onset diabetes. Since there is good evidence that maternal insulin does not cross the placenta (this organ has a high concentration of insulin transhydrogenase), it is probable that fetal insulin does not cross to the maternal circulation. Growth-onset diabetic mothers are therefore dependent on exogenous insulin. The net insulin requirement in all diabetics usually increases during pregnancy.

In pregnant chemical diabetics, blood immunoreactive insulin levels are greater after glucose administration than in pregnant nondiabetics. This is somewhat paradoxical because glucose tolerance in these patients is decreased. These data are difficult to interpret because there are no accurate data on actual insulin production. Hoet has suggested that there is decreased pancreatic responsiveness. In semiquantitative studies, he found that during pregnancy, insulin secretion in prediabetics and normal patients is similar but is delayed in the former. The final answer to this problem is not yet apparent.

Some patients develop transient or gestational diabetes during pregnancy, and return to the prediabetic state after delivery. Such patients must be followed carefully for the rest of their lives because many of them will become overtly diabetic later. The full reasons for the deterioration in the diabetic state during pregnancy, though unknown, are probably related to increased protein synthesis and possibly also to increased placental lactogen production late in pregnancy. Other unidentified factors are almost certainly involved as well.

Pregnant diabetics become more prone to ketoacidosis, and hence their diabetic control is often more difficult. Diabetic coma may develop rapidly, especially in the presence of hyperemesis gravidarum, with disastrous results to the pregnancy. Hypoglycemic reactions and coma are most common in the first trimester but do not seem to have an adverse effect on the fetus.

Other hormonal changes peculiar to diabetic pregnancy are much less specific. There is said to be an increase in chorionic gonadotropin, and a reduction in estrogen and progesterone production. Present evidence suggests that these are the result of placental dysfunction and are not specific for diabetes. In the last trimester, most of the maternal estrogen comes from the placenta, and the ovary supplies only a small proportion of the total. The urinary estriol (derived from estrogen) may normally increase to 50 mg/24 hours in the last 6 weeks. Great use has been made of this increase in the past few years, because the urinary estriol content is a good indicator of the health of the placenta and thus also of the fetus.

Physical Effects of the Pregnancy on the Diabetic Mother

Except when it is grossly out of control, as in ketosis, or when the patient suffers from severe preterminal complications, diabetes does not affect fertility. The exact incidence of diabetes in pregnancies is uncertain. Estimates range from 1:1,000 pregnancies up to 1:200 admissions to a maternity hospital. These figures are probably quite comparable, because pregnant diabetics are admitted to hospital more frequently than nondiabetic mothers.

In the first trimester, the abortion rate is only slightly greater than average and is related to the same factors that affect the final outcome of the pregnancy. Clearly, a diabetic with multiple complications is less likely to complete her pregnancy than one who has no complications. In this respect, Dr. Priscilla White has developed a classification that is useful in making a prognosis. She divides her patients into the following:—

Class A: Mild chemical diabetics (high fetal survival, approaching normal)
Class B: Overt diabetes of less than 10 years' duration, which developed in adult life; no evidence of complications (67% fetal survival)
Class C: Diabetes beginning between 10 and 19 years of age, or diabetes of 10–19 years' duration, but without evidence of vascular disease (48% fetal survival)
Class D: Diabetes of more than 20 years' dura-

tion, with a high probability of vascular disease; or diabetes that began before the patient was 10 years old, or diabetes associated with mild retinopathy or leg-vessel calcification (32% fetal survival)

Class E: Pelvic vessel calcification on X-ray (13% fetal survival)

Class F: Diabetic nephropathy (3% fetal survival)

Class R: Severe diabetic retinopathy (high fetal loss)

In addition to the maternal diabetes, fetal survival is adversely affected by the maternal complications of pregnancy, which occur with greater frequency as one progresses from Class A to Class R.

Other changes in the pregnant diabetic include a lowering of the renal threshold for glucose, and an increased tendency to develop urinary infections. The blood glucose level at which significant glycosuria develops decreases in any pregnancy. Under no circumstances should glycosuria in a pregnant nondiabetic be regarded as normal until a fasting and a 2-hour postprandial blood glucose, and glucose tolerance test levels have been found to be normal and remain normal throughout the pregnancy. The lowered renal threshold for glucose in pregnant diabetics makes the interpretation of glycosuria more difficult and necessitates more frequent blood glucose determinations.

Urinary tract infections, which are common during pregnancy, are more common in pregnant diabetics. They exert a detrimental effect on the pregnancy by increasing uterine irritability and thus precipitating premature delivery. Such infections also have a detrimental effect on renal function, which may already be impaired by diabetic nephropathy.

Physical Effects of Maternal Diabetes on the Fetus

Maternal diabetes subjects the fetus to an increased risk of: (1) malformations, (2) marked hypertrophy of the islets of Langerhans, (3) large body size, (4) neonatal respiratory distress syndrome, and (5) hyperbilirubinemia.

The risk of fetal malformation is not affected by the stage of the maternal diabetes, and the actual incidence is only slightly, but significantly, higher than in nondiabetic pregnancies. Any system may be affected, but skeletal, cardiovascular, and genitourinary defects are the most common.

The term infant of a diabetic mother often weighs more than 10 lb (4.5 kg). This large size is due to a combination of excess fat, excess fluid, and large organs. Laboratory studies have shown that excess insulin, in the absence of growth hormone, can produce similar changes in the experimental animal. We can speculate that the maternal and thus fetal hyperglycemia stimulates islet growth and insulin release and that the combination of these two factors produces the large babies. Unfortunately, there is no documented evidence to support this speculation. Also, diabetic mothers with perfectly normal blood glucose levels during pregnancy may have big babies. Despite islet cell hypertrophy, these infants rarely have neonatal hypoglycemia.

Neonatal respiratory distress syndrome occurs more commonly in premature infants. This syndrome is relatively common in infants of diabetic mothers but is probably related to their prematurity. The prematurity arises because of the need for early delivery of the infant of a diabetic mother. After 36 weeks' gestation, the fetus runs an increasing risk of intrauterine death. Delivery at 36–38 weeks increases only slightly the risk of dying from prematurity; this date is therefore often chosen as the time for elective delivery of the diabetic mother. Hyperbilirubinemia is also more common in these infants but probably reflects only their prematurity.

Effect of Diabetes on the Placenta

Diabetes may affect the placenta in three ways: (1) It may cause relative placental immaturity, and a large size, when the pregnancy has been complication-free. (2) The placenta is susceptible to multiple local infarcts when preeclampsia or other complications develop. (3) Structural anomalies of the placenta are slightly more frequent than in normal pregnancies. There is no evidence that placental insufficiency contributes to stillbirths or abortions in diabetic mothers.

Diagnosis of Diabetes Mellitus in Pregnancy

The diagnosis of diabetes during pregnancy is based on the same criteria as in the nonpregnant women—i.e., the fasting and 2-hour postprandial blood glucose concentrations and the glucose tolerance test. The criteria for interpretation of the results are also the same. If the results of these tests are normal in patients in whom, because of their obstetric history, diabetes is strongly suspected, a cortisone-stimulated oral glucose tolerance test may be performed or, better still, the standard oral glucose tolerance test may be repeated at monthly intervals during the pregnancy.

Management of Diabetes and Pregnancy

Diabetics who are, or may become, parents often seek genetic counseling, and indeed, it should be offered even if they do not seek it. The physician's advice should be based on the probability of transmission of diabetes to their children (this, of course, depends on the strength of the diabetic trait in the parents; see section on Inheritance of Diabetes earlier in this chapter). There is no contraindication to parenthood in a couple in which either or both parents are diabetic, if they realize and accept the risks of diabetes developing in their progeny.

However, from a strictly medical point of view, a prospective mother should not become pregnant if she has severe diabetic complications—e.g., retinopathy, nephropathy, or coronary artery disease. If she does, therapeutic abortion may be necessary. On purely economic grounds, a prospective father who suffers from the more lethal complications of diabetes should be advised against procreation, since he may not live long enough to provide for his family.

A successful completion of pregnancy in a diabetic mother depends on: (1) her position in the White classification, (2) the proper care of her diabetes, (3) careful selection of date and mode of delivery, and (4) proper postnatal care of the infant.

As in all diabetics, the blood glucose concentration indicates the adequacy of treatment, and must be watched carefully throughout pregnancy.

In the first trimester, the mother's sensitivity to insulin increases. Hypoglycemic reactions may occur more often, and a decrease in insulin dose may be necessary. Prediabetes is unlikely to progress to chemical or overt diabetes in either the first or second trimester, during which insulin requirements usually change little. The mother's greatest need for insulin is usually in the third trimester. In this period, the physician should exercise care to preserve diabetic control and to detect chemical and overt diabetes in patients whose glucose tolerance has previously been normal.

He should see the pregnant diabetics every 2 weeks during the first 6 months and every week in the last 3 months. A blood glucose test and urinalysis should be done at each visit and the patient asked to bring a record of the urine tests she has done at home. Throughout the pregnancy, very close cooperation between the internist and the obstetrician is essential. The principles used for keeping the blood glucose in the normal range are the same as for other diabetics. Nocturnal hyperglycemia may be difficult to control, but can be achieved by twice-daily injections of lente or NPH insulin (see section on Selection of Insulin Type and Dose earlier). The diet need not be altered except perhaps to increase the protein allowance by up to 50%. The diabetes must be controlled, even if the mother must be put in hospital to achieve this control. At monthly intervals, or more often, a microscopic examination and culture of the urine should be done. If infection is present, it should be treated vigorously with antibiotics, but the tetracyclines and the neurotoxic antibiotics (and sulfonamides in the last 4–6 weeks of pregnancy) should be avoided.

The total daily excretion of estriol in the mother's urine should be measured for the last 6–8 weeks of the pregnancy. The urinary estriols are produced mainly by the placenta and the fetus and give a very good indication of the health of the pregnancy. The urinary estriol content rises gradually in the last 12 weeks from 4–8 mg/day to as high as 50–60 mg/day. Any sudden fall in the estriol excretion or a more gradual fall to less than 12 mg/day indicates that, unless the baby is delivered, it will almost certainly be dead within 48 hours.

The complications of pregnancy in the diabetic

mother are managed by standard methods. If she develops any of the symptoms or signs of preeclampsia, salt must be restricted and diuretics given.

Most patients are brought into hospital between 32 and 34 weeks of gestation and are delivered at 37–38 weeks of gestation, if no signs of fetal distress have been detected or the urinary estriol concentrations have not dropped to critical levels before then. In addition to normal obstetrical requirements (e.g., pelvic size and placental position), the mode chosen for delivery will depend on previous obstetrical history and on day-to-day signs of fetal health.

If an elective cesarean section is going to be performed, give only one-half of the *prepregnancy* dose of insulin on the morning of delivery, but start an intravenous infusion of 5% dextrose in water (1,000 ml/8 hours) at the same time. Give the remaining half of the prepregnancy insulin dose after the delivery when the mother has returned from the operating room, but watch her carefully for hypoglycemia due to the resumption of normal sensitivity to insulin.

If spontaneous or induced natural delivery takes place, the mother's blood glucose level must be watched carefully because she may not need any more insulin for 1 or 2 days. Usually, however, you can give the full prepregnancy dose as usual the morning after delivery. Thereafter, her insulin requirements are determined on the basis of her urine tests for glucose and her blood glucose concentrations.

The pediatrician should be present at the delivery and should supervise the care of the infant. The problems of the neonatal period are faced as they arise. The infant's respiration should be checked frequently because the respiratory distress syndrome is relatively common. Normally, these infants are not fed until 24 hours after delivery, but earlier feedings are now being recommended, since they reduce the incidence of hyperbilirubinemia and will of course be necessary if hypoglycemia develops. Hypoglycemia (blood glucose of 20 mg/100 ml, or less) is rare, but may develop more often in infants whose mothers are prediabetic. Hypocalcemia may also develop. The reason for this is not known.

Diabetes in Childhood

Diabetes mellitus is much less common in children than in adults. Although it is rare in infants, it can be dangerous because it is not expected. The incidence of diabetes increases gradually with age (Fig. 12-8). Diabetes in childhood is most common when one or both parents have growth-onset diabetes. Many children with diabetes, however, have no family history of this disorder.

Diabetes in children often comes on abruptly. They suddenly become thirsty, develop polyuria, weight loss, etc., and may progress rapidly to diabetic coma. When the onset is more gradual, these young children may fail to thrive. In older children gradual onset may be manifested as behavioral changes, poor performance at school, nocturia, and slow or interrupted growth. On rare occasions, children, particularly when they are overweight, may develop typical maturity onset diabetes.

After the acute onset, the disease may remit for a time, during which glucose tolerance and insulin secretion returns to normal. This stage (of variable duration up to 2 years or more) usually terminates in a rapid growth spurt, illness, or a period of overindulgence. From this point onwards, the child has permanent, insulin-dependent diabetes. Children have a greater tendency to ketoacidosis, and their general metabolic pattern is much less predictable. Infants are very sensitive to insulin, but this decreases toward adolescence. During puberty and in early adult life (the periods of major body growth), the individual requires large amounts of insulin, but this increased dose is matched by increased protein synthesis and increased food consumption.

Adolescence is a difficult period for diabetics, and they are called upon to make many adjustments. The complexity of their problems depends on the duration of diabetes, their success in managing their disease, the attitude of their family, the degree to which they have accepted responsibility for their own care, and their intelligence.

If their diabetes developed early, they will have accepted the constraints imposed by their disease as a matter of habit, and regard the diabetic program as a normal way of life by the time adolescence begins. Under these circumstances, the tendency to rebel against necessary limitations will develop only on rare occasions. However, diabetic adolescents will continue to experiment. If diabetes develops in adolescence, the youngster will feel a strong desire to conceal and deny diabetes and will reject the necessary restrictions. This pattern of rejection may persist until the patients marry and their new responsibilities force them to reconsider their way of life in the light of the security of their dependents.

The parents' attitude may aggravate the adolescents' tendency to deny their diabetes—e.g., they may be too repressive, or too lax in the management of diabetes, or fail to provide the necessary therapeutic regimen. Lack of understanding and tolerance by the physician will be harmful. Parents may occasionally partially reject the diabetic child as an "oddity" or may not give the child a sufficient opportunity to participate in his or her own care.

Youngsters may reject diabetes because of their immaturity, or because they are emotionally unstable. Any of these situations can create an environmental state in which stable control of diabetes is not possible. Severe emotional problems are not common, and many diabetic children have only a brief, inconsequential period of rebellion.

The prognosis in childhood diabetes varies. Most children can expect many years of good health. Some develop diabetic complications: retinopathy or nephropathy may appear in the late teens. Such complications seem most common in those who have rebelled most strongly against diabetes. However, multifactorial inheritance may play a significant part in the development of diabetic complications, but this is still speculative. It is almost certain that a variety of genetic factors influence the development of diabetic complications.

Management of Diabetes Mellitus in Childhood

The objective of the treatment of the diabetic child is to create a metabolic environment which will allow normal growth and activity and emotional development. The principles are the same as in the adult—specifically: appropriate diet, adequate insulin, regular exercise, and proper education. The parents must be actively involved in all phases of the management.

The basic caloric requirement is based on a general allowance of 1,000 calories to which 100 calories are added for each year of age. The diet, tailored to suit the preferences of the individual, should take into account the sex, physique, and general level of activity. Obesity must be avoided or, if present, controlled. Usually it is sufficient to adjust the diet upward every 6 months. The proportion of carbohydrate to fat and to protein is the same as in adults.

Almost every diabetic child needs insulin. The daily dose in infants is often small, but this "supersensitivity" soon passes, and the adolescents may need more than 100 units per day. When the child matures, the insulin requirement usually decreases. A problem arises during the "remission" (if it develops), when the insulin requirement may drop to zero. The physician should continue to give 1–2 units of insulin daily to these patients, for two reasons: (1) It will reduce or prevent the development of insulin allergy, so that when the remission ends, insulin can be restarted without hazard. (2) The daily injection is a very good reminder that diabetes is still present, and helps to prevent overindulgence, which may bring the remission to an end. During remission, the substitution of oral hypoglycemic agents for insulin does not affect its duration and is not recommended.

Specific Treatment

Insulins of intermediate duration give the best results; crystalline zinc insulin is added as necessary. About 70% of children need a small dose of NPH or lente insulin at supper or bedtime to prevent early morning hyperglycemia. This addition to the program reduces the chance of midafternoon reactions, which result when the doctor gives too much intermediate-action insulin in an attempt to prevent early morning hyperglycemia. The second injection also decreases the chance of night reactions, which may be severe when long-acting insulins (ultralente and protamine zinc) are used. At one time it was thought the biguanide drugs would increase the stability of growth-onset diabetes. Subsequent experience has shown that they do not.

Whenever possible, the parents should be taught how to adjust the insulin dose, on the basis of the urine glucose tests and insulin reactions. They must cooperate closely with the physician at all times, especially at the beginning of the institution of the diabetes treatment program.

Hypoglycemic reactions are more common in children than in adults because they are more sensitive to insulin, have a more varied and less predictable pattern of physical activity, and a more labile metabolism, with proportionately smaller energy reserves. In children, the symptoms of hypoglycemia include all of those experienced by adults, and, in addition, temper tantrums may occur. Reactions characterized by violent and convulsive activity are also commoner in children and adolescents. Hypoglycemia may come on rapidly, especially when precipitated by physical activity. Some workers report that many children who have convulsive hypoglycemic reactions also have borderline abnormalities in their electroencephalographic patterns. However, this has not been substantiated.

Treat hypoglycemia in children just as you do in adults—prevent it, but when it occurs, give carbohydrate by mouth or by vein, or inject epinephrine or glucagon subcutaneously to mobilize liver glycogen. Parents of diabetic children should be taught how to administer glucagon. As in the adult, the child must be given supplementary carbohydrate on recovery after glucagon or epinephrine has been injected.

When they are well, children should test their urine for sugar at least once a day, but at least four times a day when they are ill. Even minor illnesses, a cold or mild gastroenteritis, can induce ketoacidosis rapidly. This chain of events must be prevented, by adherence to the diabetic program, and by close cooperation between the family and physician. If an infant or young child develops diabetic coma, relatively small doses of insulin (1–5 units) and rehydration will control the condition. Adolescents in diabetic coma are treated by the same methods described for treating adults in diabetic coma (q.v.).

The blood glucose is determined during each visit to the physician, where possible using capillary samples. The times at which blood is obtained should vary to include both fasting and postprandial samples.

Judge the success of treatment by the results of blood and urine sugar determinations, and on evidence of the child's normal physical and mental development. The diabetic child's rate of growth and final physical development will lie within the normal average if the diet and insulin requirements are properly adjusted. The "diabetic dwarfs" once seen are now rare. They were small because they did not get sufficient calories and their diabetes was not regulated.

The psychological environment in which the diabetic child matures is most important. The child should, as far as possible, participate in daily events as a normal individual. The presence of diabetes must not be under- or overemphasized. Certain limitations have to be recognized; for example, the child cannot indulge in dietary fancies at will but can have occasional treats. Both the teachers and the parents of the child, and others with whom the child associates, should know about his or her diabetes, and what to do in an emergency. It is difficult to get children to keep candy in their pockets as a reserve, but the attempt should be made. They should carry personal identification, either a bracelet or a card.

The child must not be allowed to use diabetes as a means of getting attention. Any obvious willful lapses must be reprimanded. However, occasional temper tantrums may be due to high or low blood glucose levels; this should be borne in mind by all concerned.

As the child grows older, responsibility must be gradually transferred from the parents to the child. In this respect, camps for diabetic children help because they are designed to increase the camper's independence. By the age of 15, diabetic children should be able to manage their diabetes without parental help. Continued liaison between the child and physician is important. If severe rejection problems arise, psychiatric advice should be sought. There is no point in trying to frighten an adolescent into cooperating by threat or by demonstrating the complications of diabetes. Spend your time in trying to find out why the youth is rejecting diabetes. Is home life a problem? Is schoolwork or employment satisfactory? Is there trouble in "dating," etc? Open discussion of some of these points allows you to understand and help your patient.

Management of the Diabetic Surgical Patient

Diabetics who require surgery fall into two classes: (1) those who need elective surgery, and (2) those who require an emergency operation. In both groups, the patient's suitability for operation depends on the state of the patient's diabetes, and on his general health. Diabetics should not be subjected to elective surgery until they are under good metabolic control because an operation of any kind, including dental extractions, imposes stress that, in the poorly controlled diabetic, may precipitate ketoacidosis and coma. This reaction to operation is due to: (1) increased epinephrine release, (2) increased adrenocortical activity, and (3) fasting, if this is necessary. Healing is also impaired if the diabetes is poorly controlled. The risk of precipitating ketoacidosis during surgery in the well-regulated diabetic is very small.

The method chosen for regulating diabetes durthe major elective surgery depends on the treatment necessary under normal circumstances. When diet alone is normally sufficient, a slow infusion of 5% dextrose in water (1,000 ml/8 hours) should be given during the operation, and during the necessary postoperative period of fast. If the blood glucose tends to rise above 200 mg/100 ml, 10 units of crystalline zinc insulin should be added to each 1,000 ml of 5% dextrose and water. This combination will help to prevent ketosis.

If the patient takes oral hypoglycemic drugs in addition to diet, insulin should be used during the operation and convalescence. The routine for these patients is then the same as for those who require insulin—specifically:

1. Give nothing by mouth after the bedtime snack on the evening before surgery.
2. Give one-half of the normal total daily dose of insulin subcutaneously between 7 A.M. and 8 A.M. on the day of operation. At the same time start an intravenous infusion of 5% dextrose and water (1,000 ml/8 hr). Where possible, diabetics should be operated upon early in the day because this will minimize the period during which their normal diabetic control is disrupted.
3. When the patient is returned to the recovery room, the remaining one-half of the total daily insulin dose is given subcutaneously.

Fluid and electrolyte balance must be maintained in the diabetic, as in the nondiabetic, pre- and postoperatively. Because the diabetic must have carbohydrate available constantly, regardless of other factors, an intravenous infusion of 5% dextrose in water must be continued until the patient is once more able to take a normal diet. The insulin requirement in the days following operation must be based on blood and urine glucose concentrations. It will be the same as, or greater than, the preoperative insulin dose. Temporary loss of control, which may develop, especially if there is any sepsis or other complications such as thrombophlebitis, should be treated with extra CZI. The dose required is based on the blood and urine glucose tests. The patient usually returns to preoperative insulin requirements in 3–5 days.

A minor operation can be performed on a diabetic at any time, without causing much metabolic disturbance. However, if the diabetic is under good control beforehand, chances of success are much better.

Emergency Surgery

Diabetics who require emergency surgery usually have hyperglycemia and some degree of ketosis because of the stress of the situation that precipitated the emergency. Immediate surgery is necessary only in such catastrophes as hemorrhage from large blood vessels and some head injuries. In these patients, the acidosis is corrected with bicarbonate and the blood volume restored by tranfusion: These are the only measures absolutely necessary before operation. Steps must be taken to control the diabetic state, but the operation is begun before there is any laboratory evidence of success. Obviously the morbidity and mortality in such patients is increased.

In all other circumstances, any significant degree of acidosis must be corrected and definite evidence obtained that efforts to control ketosis and hyperglycemia are being effective. These patients may suffer from hypovolemia because of the osmotic diuresis associated with the hyperglycemia. Therefore, they must be rehydrated before the induction of anesthesia. The blood glucose concentration must be carefully monitored during the operation in these patients. It should be maintained between 100 and 200 mg/100 ml, approximately.

When the emergency is over and the cause corrected, and the patient has recovered from the operation, the amount of insulin needed will depend on the clinical state of the patient. If there is extensive infection or tissue injury, more insulin will be needed until this state has resolved. If healing is rapid, the insulin dose can be returned rapidly to normal.

Abnormalities of Subcutaneous Tissue Lipid Metabolism

Localized fat atrophy or hypertrophy at sites of insulin injection has already been discussed.

Occasionally, a generalized form of subcutaneous fat atrophy may be associated with diabetes. It may appear before or during insulin therapy but is not directly related to it. Subcutaneous fat may be lost from the whole body, or this loss may be localized to one area, such as the upper or lower one-half of the body. The syndrome lipoatrophic diabetes mellitus may be associated with insulin resistance. The cause of the abnormality is not known. No abnormality in fat synthesis has been detected, and these patients do not seem to be abnormally sensitive to any of the factors which normally induce lipolysis.

Necrobiosis lipoidicia diabeticorum is a localized patchy loss of subcutaneous tissue, usually confined to the lower limbs. Occasionally the purple bases of these areas may ulcerate. Histological and enzyme studies have shed no light on the cause of this condition. In patients with this disorder, glucose tolerance is always abnormal but may only be brought out by cortisone stimulation.

There is no effective treatment for subcutaneous fat atrophy. Cosmetic treatment is all that can be offered. The atrophic patches in necrobiosis often fill in with time.

Summary

This chapter is designed to show that diabetes mellitus is a syndrome which affects many systems. It is inherited. The probable major causative defect is an inadequate production of metabolically active insulin, resulting in altered carbohydrate, fat, and protein metabolism.

The best clinical classification of diabetes mellitus is based on whether the patient does or does not require exogenous insulin to maintain metabolic equilibrium. The patient with classic maturity-onset diabetes can be managed well with diet, with or without oral hypoglycemic drugs. The growth-onset diabetic must have insulin in addition to the diet. However, adults not uncommonly develop insulin-dependent growth-onset type diabetes, and children occasionally develop maturity-onset diabetes. The object of the treatment of diabetes is to provide the patient with a program that corrects (as far as it can be recognized) the biochemical abnormality and allows the patient to function normally in his social and occupational environment. The quality of the treatment is determined by the blood and urine glucose concentrations, the patient's weight, and his general health and energy.

Modern treatment has dramatically prolonged the lives of insulin-dependent diabetics. Nonetheless, serious complications do arise. These may develop acutely (hypoglycemia and diabetic coma), or over a long period (retinopathy, nephropathy, coronary artery disease, neuropathy, and enteropathy). The development of these latter complications is probably influenced in part by the degree of success of the treatment, and in part by inherited factors, which are at present beyond methods of recognition and control. Long-term complications are mostly due to alterations in the basement membrane, and the caliber of capillaries and arterioles, but enzyme defects may be the major cause of diabetic neuropathy.

Pregnant diabetic mothers, diabetic children, and diabetics who require surgery all present special problems requiring special management.

The successful management of all diabetics requires close cooperation between the patient and his physician. The patient must have sufficient lay knowledge, and the physician sufficient expert knowledge, about diabetes to allow them to deal with the day-to-day problems that can arise.

References

1. Eisentraut, A. M., Ohneda, A., Parada, E., and Unger, R. H. Immunologic discrimination between pancreatic glucagon and enteric glucagon immunoreactivity (G.L.1) in tissues and plasma. *Diabetes 17 (Suppl. 1)*:321, 1968.
2. Jacob, F., and Monod, J. Genetic regulatory mechanisms in the synthesis of proteins. *J Mol Biol 3*:318–356, 1961.
3. LeCompte, P. M., Steinke, J., Soeldner, J. S., and Renold, A. E. Changes in the islets of Langerhans in cows injected with heterologous and homologous insulin. *Diabetes 15*:586–596, 1966.
4. Levine, R. "Status of the Glucose Transport Theory of the Action of Insulin." In *On the Nature and Treatment of Diabetes Mellitus,* Leibel, B. S., and Wrenshall, G. A., eds. Amsterdam, Excerpta Medica, 1965, p. 250.

Additional Reading

5. *Diabetes: International Diabetes Federation, The Sixth Congress, 1967*. Oestman, J., ed. Amsterdam, Excerpta Medica, 1969.
6. Duncan, G. G. *Diseases of Metabolism,* 5th ed. Philadelphia, Saunders, 1964.
7. Marble, A., White, P., Bradley, R. F., and Krall, L. P. Joslin's *Diabetes Mellitus,* 11th ed., Philadelphia, Lea, 1971.
8. Leibel, B. S., and Wrenshall, G. A., eds. *On the Nature and Treatment of Diabetes Mellitus.* Amsterdam, Excerpta Medica, 1969.
9. Unger, R. H., Ohneda, A., Parada, E., and Eisentraut, A. M. The role of aminogenic glucagon secretion in blood glucose homoeostasis. *J Clin Invest 8*:810–822, 1969.
10. Williams, R. H., ed. *Diabetes.* New York, Hoeber, 1962.

13

Hypoglycemia

Robert Volpé

Hypoglycemia is arbitrarily defined as a true blood glucose level below 50 mg/100 ml. However, *symptoms* of hypoglycemia may occur at levels higher than this, when the blood glucose values drop precipitously; conversely, *symptoms* of hypoglycemia may be *absent* at blood glucose levels well below 50 mg/100 ml.

Hypoglycemia results from a failure of the homeostatic mechanisms that normally prevent an abnormal drop in blood glucose. The blood glucose level at any time is dependent upon an equilibrium between (1) the absorption of glucose from the gastrointestinal tract, (2) the hepatic uptake and release of glucose, and (3) the tissue utilization of glucose.[1]

Blood glucose is derived primarily from the intestinal tract and the liver. It may be derived not only from carbohydrate sources, but from fats and proteins; the absorption of foodstuffs from the gastrointestinal tract is the body's first defense against the development of hypoglycemia.

If man does not ingest or absorb food, after a few hours an increased amount of certain hormones is secreted that increase the blood glucose concentration: Glucagon from the pancreatic alpha cells stimulates glycogen breakdown by the liver by activating phosphorylase; epinephrine breaks down muscle and liver glycogen; and the lactate thus provided is converted into glucose. Lipolysis, which is activated by glucagon and epinephrine, and by *growth hormone and cortisol,* makes nonesterified fatty acids and glycerol available for gluconeogenesis, which is facilitated by the production of H^+ from the oxidation of released unesterified fatty acid. Cortisol and glucagon convert protein into glucose by catabolic actions. In addition, the peripheral utilization of glucose is retarded by cortisol and growth hormone, another mechanism for raising the blood glucose.

The hepatic stores of glycogen can meet the body's needs for no more than about 24 hours. Thus, during prolonged fasts, the glucose level is normally maintained by an increased rate of gluconeogenesis, the result of stimulation of the enzyme systems responsible for these processes.

The blood glucose concentration must be maintained within a narrow range because the brain cannot ordinarily extract significant amounts of energy from any other source than carbohydrate, chiefly glucose. The brain is almost unique among tissues in this regard; only kidney, red cells, and cells of the intestinal mucosa are similarly dependent on glucose. As is common knowledge, glucose is the best stimulant for increasing the release of insulin from the pancreatic beta cells. This effect is mediated partly through the right vagus nerve, but mainly through direct stimulation of the beta cells by the hyperglycemia itself. In addition to glucose, fatty acids and several amino acids can stimulate increased production and release of insulin. Gastrointestinal hormones (secretin, glucagon-like material, and pancreatin) also stimulate insulin release, which probably accounts for the greater rise in blood insulin levels produced by oral glucose compared with an equal amount of intravenous glucose.

Effects of Hypoglycemia

Metabolic

There is good evidence that in the normal individual, within 15–20 minutes of the development of hypoglycemia, the body increases its production of glucagon, corticosteroids, growth hormone, and its sympathetic nervous system activity (with epinephrine release). These mechanisms, as noted above, are regulatory, each an attempt to counteract the hypoglycemia.

The stimulation of sympathetic activity secondary to hypoglycemia results in a breakdown of fat stores and accumulation of acetyl coenzyme A (acetyl CoA), acyl coenzyme A (acyl CoA), and the ketone bodies. Acetyl CoA stimulates the conversion of pyruvate to oxaloacetate, while acyl CoA inhibits the conversion of acetyl CoA to malonyl CoA, the conversion of oxaloacetate and acetyl CoA to citrate, and the entry of glucose-6-phosphate into the hexose monophosphate shunt. These various changes may be interpreted as attempts to produce more glucose or at least to maintain the level of blood glucose so that the central nervous system can utilize it. In addition, the H^+ from fatty acid oxidation promotes gluconeogenesis.

Summary of Factors Necessary for Normal Glucose Homeostasis

1. Normal liver cell integrity
2. A supply of the appropriate nutrients, particularly glucose and amino acids
3. Glucocorticoid action, which promotes gluconeogenesis
4. Growth hormone
5. Stimulators of glycogenolysis: glucagon, thyroid hormone, and sympathetic nervous system action, with epinephrine
6. Autoregulatory reactions depending on the blood glucose concentration

Effects of Hypoglycemia on the Nervous System

The brain has a relatively high oxygen consumption. Since its major source of energy is glucose, hypoglycemia has a marked adverse effect on cerebral function. The response of various areas of the brain to hypoglycemia corresponds to their phylogenetic appearance: The later a given region of brain develops phylogenetically, the higher is its oxygen consumption, and thus the greater its need for glucose. The cerebral cortex is most sensitive, followed by the subcortical diencephalon. The mesencephalon, premyencephalon and myencephalon are progressively less affected, or conversely, show adverse effects only with more severe hypoglycemia. The adverse effects of hypoglycemia are related to anoxia, a state which stimulates the sympathetic nervous system but depresses the somatic nervous system.

Any preexisting brain lesion that contributes to anoxia will accentuate the symptoms of hypoglycemia. When the blood sugar falls quickly, more pronounced clinical manifestations result than when the blood sugar falls more slowly. The early manifestations (sweating, tachycardia, tremulousness, nervousness, and weakness) appear to be due to sympathetic nervous system discharge. Somatic nervous system manifestations include visual disturbances, confusion, and headaches. Later, as the hypoglycemia progresses, and other areas of the brain become involved, other manifestations may appear, such as sweating, twitching, restlessness, disturbed behavior, sensitivity to pain, erythemia, somnolence, hypotonia, stupor, coma, inconjugate ocular deviations, upgoing toes, and extensor spasms. Later, the coma may become profound, with bradycardia, miosis, atonia, hypothermia, shallow respirations, and hyporeflexia. Unless the hypoglycemia is reversed, permanent nervous system damage or death may result.

Repeated episodes of hypoglycemia, or even one severe prolonged bout may cause permanent changes such as mental deterioration, various psychoses, hemiplegia, aphasia, seizures, or choreiform movements.

Clinical Types of Hypoglycemia

Organic Primary

Excessive Secretion of Insulin

Neoplasms of the Beta Cells (Insulinomas)[1]

About 90% of insulin-secreting islet-cell tumors are benign, and 10% are malignant. These neoplasms may be located in various parts of the pancreas, particularly the body and tail; they occasionally may be outside the pancreas. Insulinomas occur most frequently between the ages of 35 and 55. About one-fourth of these patients have a family history of diabetes mellitus.

After onset, the condition may go undiagnosed for several months or even years. Patients may complain of various disorders of the nervous system, or may develop symptoms of epilepsy or even mental deterioration. Symptoms occur during fasting, often before breakfast or at night, and are characteristically improved by the ingestion of foods. About one-half the patients will lose consciousness at one time or another, and about one-third of patients will have convulsions. Even more severe symptoms may occur, similar to those already described above.

When patients discover that eating relieves their symptoms, they often gain weight; occasionally they become very obese.

In the recognition of hypoglycemia due to insulinoma, "Whipple's triad" may be characteristically recognized; the attacks must occur during fasting, the blood sugar levels should be below 50 mg/100 ml, and the episodes should be relieved promptly by the administration of glucose.

Laboratory Tests. Characteristically, the blood glucose is low during the attack. Sometimes, however, it is difficult to obtain a blood specimen during the attack and therefore the patient must be fasted; in some patients it is necessary to prolong the fast for as long as 24, 48, or even 72 hours before hypoglycemia is demonstrable. An intravenous sodium tolbutamide tolerance test may also help, because tolbutamide stimulates the release of insulin and, in patients with insulinoma, should cause a sharp sustained fall in the blood glucose levels. Occasionally, the hypoglycemia following tolbutamide may be prolonged, and it may be necessary to administer glucose. The intravenous sodium tolbutamide test should be carried out with caution in view of this hazard.

Plasma "immunoreactive" insulin (i.e., the insulin levels obtained by immunoassay) determinations are often helpful in diagnosis, but only if they are related to simultaneous blood glucose levels; thus, the plasma insulin levels will often be higher than expected for the given level of blood glucose.[4] Insulin levels are most helpful when determined in association with a glucose tolerance curve and an intravenous sodium tolbutamide test.

Treatment.[2,3] The only cure, surgical resection, may prove to be technically difficult; for this reason, the diagnosis must be established beyond doubt before exploration is recommended. Two hours before the operation, the patient is given an intravenous infusion of 10% glucose, which is continued over the next 8 hours. Intramuscular cortisone given before the operation may help to prevent hypoglycemia and hyperpyrexia. The insulinomas may be very small and thus difficult to find. About 10% of patients have multiple lesions; for this reason, the surgeon must mobilize the pancreas so as to examine it completely.

About 10% of these tumors are malignant, and, in such patients, a subtotal pancreatectomy is generally performed.

It is now possible to render patients with insulinomas normoglycemic by medical means, and this is helpful in patients with secondary carcinoma of the islet cells or in those who are otherwise not considered acceptable operative candidates. While such adjuncts as corticosteroids and a high-protein, high-calorie intake have previously been advocated in the management of insulinomas, the most useful modern therapy is diazoxide, a drug that is related to the sulfonamides, with marked hyperglycemic properties. Diazoxide simulates the known metabolic effects of adrenaline, although its precise mechanism of action has yet to be completely elucidated. At any rate, this agent has been used with considerable success to maintain patients with insulinoma at normal blood sugar levels.[3]

Diffuse Hyperplasia of the Beta Cells

This entity is rare, and possibly should not be separated from insulinoma. Because partial pancreatectomy does not greatly benefit such patients, continuous diazoxide therapy is the best treatment.

Extrapancreatic Tumors That Produce Hypoglycemia[4, 5, 6]

Recently a number of nonendocrine tumors have been described that appear to produce a variety of hormones. Doege in 1930 first proposed that nonpancreatic tumors might produce hypoglycemia (see Reference 4). Since then, workers have reported more than 100 extrapancreatic tumors that produce hypoglycemia. Most of these have been mesodermal tumors that are characteristically very large, weighing up to 9 kg. These mesodermal tumors arise in the retroperitoneal space, the mediastinum, the pelvis, attached to the diaphragm, or within the liver. Other tumors producing hypoglycemia include carcinoma of the adrenal cortex, primary hepatic carcinoma, and a few gastrointestinal carcinomas.

Although the mechanism through which the hypoglycemia is produced may differ in each of these tumors, much of the evidence suggests that these tumors produce a substance that has most of the actions of insulin but is immunologically distinct from it. In patients with hypoglycemia due to these tumors, both epinephrine and glucagon administration promptly increase blood glucose, indicating that they have adequate stores of hepatic glycogen and respond normally to these glycogenolytic stimuli.[5, 6]

Though these patients become hypoglycemic when fasted, their glucose tolerance curves are often (like a diabetic's) elevated in the first 2 or 3 hours after glucose is administered. Such curves suggest that the response of beta cells to the glucose load is deficient. Furthermore their immunoreactive insulin levels are generally very low throughout such glucose tolerance curves. Likewise, intravenous tolbutamide does not cause a sharp reduction in blood glucose or a concomitant rise in immunoreactive insulin; such results confirm that the response of the beta cells to their usual stimuli is hypoactive. Thus in these patients the prolonged hypoglycemia appears to have suppressed beta cell activity; there is no evidence that the beta cells are releasing normal, let alone excessive, amounts of insulin. Furthermore, on intravenous insulin tolerance tests, these patients have a normal sensitivity to insulin, ruling out the possibility that they are unusually sensitive to their own insulin.

Studies of glucose dynamics indicate that these patients produce glucose at a markedly diminished rate and that they use it at a relatively high rate. While some interpret this type of evidence to indicate that the tumor is using excessive amounts of glucose, the available evidence suggests that the tumor releases a humoral insulin-like factor, which acts like insulin on the liver and peripheral tissues. This action would explain the reduced rate of glucose production, the adequate liver glycogen stores, and the increased rate of glucose utilization by peripheral tissues.

Although this is not invariably true, insulin-like activity (by bioassay) can often be demonstrated in the plasma of these patients. On the other hand, assays of the tumors usually show no significant increase in insulin-like activity. However, these tumors are massive, and it may not be possible to demonstrate increased activity in the small unit of tissue. Another possibility is that the insulin-like substance is released as soon as it is produced; certainly there is no evidence that it is stored within such tumors.

The nature of the insulin-like substance is, as

yet, unknown. Some evidence suggests that tryptophan and/or its metabolites is responsible for the hypoglycemia associated with these neoplasms.

Clinical Features. The hypoglycemia seen in patients with extrapancreatic tumors does not differ from that seen with insulin-secreting tumors. Thus, Whipple's triad (i.e., attacks in the fasting state, blood glucose levels below 50 mg/100 ml, relief with glucose administration) applies equally well to patients with hypoglycemia due to known pancreatic tumors and to those with insulinomas. Furthermore, all these patients may present with confusing clinical features, the descriptions of their attacks are quite bizarre, and it may be necessary to fast such patients for 24 or more hours to establish whether they have true fasting hypoglycemia. In other patients, the extrapancreatic tumor may make itself known through mechanical effects—i.e., symptoms related to its size, site, displacement of other organs, or infiltration into adjacent organs.

Diagnosis. The tumor may be diagnosed by the mechanical presence of the direct or metastatic spread of the tumor. However, hypoglycemia may manifest itself before mechanical symptoms related to the size and site of the tumor appear. Fasting hypoglycemia per se does not distinguish nonpancreatic tumors from insulinomas. If the patient has persistently low immunoreactive insulin levels during a glucose tolerance test, he probably has a nonpancreatic tumor. Furthermore, in these patients, intravenous tolbutamide will usually not produce even a fall in blood glucose and will generally be associated with persistently low levels of immunoreactive insulin.

Treatment. This condition is cured by removing the offending tumor. However, this is often impossible, particularly when the tumor is massive, within the liver, or when it has metastasized widely. When resection of the tumor is not possible, the hypoglycemia can be controlled by high-protein diet, by corticosteroid administration to raise the blood glucose level, or by injections of growth hormone, which in some cases is quite effective. Glucagon has also been tried, but associated rebound hypoglycemia and nausea often present great difficulties. Occasionally, diazoxide has helped some patients with nonpancreatic tumors and hypoglycemia; however, more often the results with diazoxide have been disappointing in patients with extrapancreatic tumors, in contrast to its marked beneficial effect in patients with insulinomas.

Deficiency of Factors That Normally Counter Insulin Effects

Patients with severe hypopituitarism have a deficiency of several hormones that are necessary for normal glucose homeostasis. Thus, growth hormone, cortisol, and to a lesser degree, thyroxine all offset the effects of insulin. Cortisol has an additional effect of inducing gluconeogenesis and thus increases glycogen formation and storage. A deficiency of any or all of these hormones increases the patient's sensitivity to insulin and decreases his capacity to correct hypoglycemia. In these patients, the fasting blood sugar level is generally low; with an insulin tolerance test, the patients become hypoglycemic, and the state may persist 2 or more hours.

Glucagon has a powerful glycogenolytic effect. However, glucagon deficiency (alpha-cell deficiency) has not yet been demonstrated. This potential cause of hypoglycemia is mentioned only as a theoretical possibility. Epinephrine deficiency, however, has been described (Zetterstrom's syndrome).

Hypoglycemia Due to Inadequate Hepatic Storage or Release of Glucose

In patients with severe acquired liver disease, such as fulminating hepatic necrosis, the parenchyma cannot store glycogen. Thus, while glucose administration causes a sharp rise in blood glucose, the level during fasting will not be maintained near normal because this glucose cannot be stored. In this situation, the fasting blood sugar level is low, and the postcibal level is high and is associated with a proportionate rise in plasma insulin; this, in turn, is followed by rebound hypoglycemia that may persist during the fasting state.

Also, several congenital and familial disorders

are characterized by the deposition of a large excess of glycogen in various tissues, particularly the liver (von Gierke's disease). This glycogen accumulates because the patient lacks certain enzymes necessary for glycogenolysis. These defects generally become evident in infancy. Since glycogen cannot break down to glucose, the result is hypoglycemia, impaired growth, and other features associated with increased glycogen deposition. Different individual enzymes are deficient in the diverse varieties of this syndrome. One such entity is glucose-6-phosphatase deficiency; in another, there is a deficiency of certain "debranching" enzymes which are normally necessary for glycogenolysis. The accumulated glycogen may induce fibrosis and finally cirrhosis of the liver. Patients with glycogen storage disease cannot respond significantly to glycogenolytic drugs such as epinephrine and glucagon.

These patients require frequent feedings. There is some evidence that diazoxide is beneficial in this condition, although the rationale of this benefit is not clear.

Galactosemia, hereditary fructose intolerance, and maple syrup urine disease are also often associated with hypoglycemia. These are rare entities, and the associated enzymatic defects (of the liver) will not be discussed here. In these disorders, the hypoglycemia is due to an inability to convert precursor substance to glucose because the appropriate enzyme is inhibited, and therefore the precursors accumulate.

Secondary Hypoglycemia

In Adults

Hypoglycemia due to exogenous insulin administration is fairly common in diabetes mellitus. When hypoglycemia of unknown cause is being investigated, surreptitious insulin administration must always be borne in mind because it is exceedingly difficult to demonstrate that a person is taking insulin in this manner. Because of their emotional aberrations, such patients hide the insulin in unusual places (such as deep in a mattress).*

* See Appendix: Addendum to Chapter 13.

Oral hypoglycemic agents cause hypoglycemia by increasing the secretion of insulin or by other mechanisms. Many other compounds can cause hypoglycemia, including alcohol, nicotinic acid, iproniazid, propranolol, and others; these act through a variety of different mechanisms. Leucine produces hypoglycemia in children and adults, by stimulating insulin release. Central nervous system lesions, particularly in the region of the hypothalamus, may induce hypoglycemia, although the underlying mechanisms are not fully understood.

In Infants

In infants, leucine hypersensitivity is one of the more common causes of hypoglycemia; in these sensitive children, the leucine causes a marked release of insulin from the beta cells. Children with this disorder must avoid all foods containing leucine (particularly milk). Another secondary hypoglycemia occurs in infants born of diabetic mothers. In such children, the relatively high blood glucose levels in the late fetal life may stimulate insulin production and release by the fetal pancreas and thus induce transient postpartum hypoglycemia. As in adults, a variety of ingested compounds may cause secondary hypoglycemia in children.

Functional

Primary

Reactive Hypoglycemia

In this common disorder there is a sharp, somewhat excessive insulin response following elevation of the blood sugar (with meals or excitement). This physiological response should be sharply differentiated from the various organic hypoglycemias. Reactive hypoglycemia occurs in anxious persons, who usually show other somatic manifestations of anxiety. Following meals, the patients complain of weakness and faintness; and, in addition, tachycardia, tremulousness, and headache. However, they never become stuporous or comatose. If they eat carbohydrates, this generally relieves their symptoms, but this pattern leads to a vicious circle.

Aside from this history, the diagnosis is made in such patients by obtaining consistently normal fasting blood sugar levels. Following a glucose load, however, they have a rapid rise, followed by a precipitous fall in blood sugar. They show no exaggerated sensitivity to injected insulin.

Experience has shown that most patients referred for investigation of "organic hyperinsulinism" have functional hypoglycemia associated with emotional disturbances.

Although patients with reactive-functional hypoglycemia do well on a high-protein, high-fat, low-carbohydrate diet, psychotherapy and tranquilizers are even more beneficial.

Secondary Hypoglycemia

Alimentary. Following subtotal gastrectomy, patients commonly have mild postprandial hypoglycemia, which is due to the rapid deposition of ingested food, particularly sugars, into a large pool in the duodenum, from which it is rapidly absorbed. This rapid absorption causes a sudden rise in blood glucose, which induces a marked insulin response. This leads to a transient rebound hypoglycemia. In these patients, the fasting blood glucose level is consistently normal. Their symptoms are controlled by feeding frequent, dry meals.

Occasionally, hyperthyroidism may produce a similar clinical picture when, as a result of increased gastrointestinal motility, carbohydrates are rapidly absorbed, with a similar blood glucose response.

Early Diabetes Mellitus. A few patients have episodes of spontaneous hypoglycemia in the early phase of diabetes mellitus. These occur 3–5 hours after meals. Characteristically, in the glucose tolerance test, the 1- and 2-hour blood glucose levels are above normal, with a subsequent fall to below 50 mg/100 ml by 3–5 hours. Plasma insulin concentration rises more slowly than normal, but eventually reaches values well above normal; the subsequent decline of the plasma insulin is also much slower than normal. Insulin secretion appears to be delayed, but its response to the glucose load is also exaggerated.

When such patients are overweight, their caloric intake must be reduced, and an oral hypoglycemic agent is often beneficial.

Diagnostic Studies

A careful history is most important, especially to establish whether the symptoms are those of hypoglycemia and whether they occur when fasting or after meals. A history of drug ingestion and a psychological assessment are likewise very important. An accurate and detailed family history should be obtained because some of these disorders are familial.

Fasting hypoglycemic states must be differentiated from those that occur following the ingestion of food. Generally the fasting hypoglycemias are much more important, and these demand a complete investigation.

Thorough evaluation may include studies of the gastrointestinal tract, liver function tests, and tests of endocrine function and of the nervous system. It is usually necessary to determine the fasting blood glucose values, immunoreactive insulin, and free fatty acids. It will often be necessary to measure blood glucose and immunoreactive insulin changes following prolonged fasts and under a variety of other stimuli; these include the injection of such materials as tolbutamide, glucagon, and leucine. On rare occasions, it may be necessary to study specific enzyme defects, particularly in infants.

A word of warning is necessary here: *Even the best tests can be falsely negative.* Occasionally, for example, the tolbutamide test may be negative in a patient proved to have an insulinoma. Similarly, the immunoreactive insulin level may not be elevated in insulinoma, although such values should always be related to the actual level of blood glucose. If this is done, the immunoreactive insulin concentration will usually be found to be higher than expected for a given level of blood glucose. On the other hand, in functional hypoglycemia, in the presence of some drugs, and in the newborns of diabetic mothers, the plasma level of immunoreactive insulin may sometimes be higher than expected. Generally, in patients with hypoglycemia due to nonendocrine tumors, the immunoreactive insulin is low.

The aim of therapy is to relieve hypoglycemia and to cure or to control the underlying disorder. This may involve operative removal of an insulinoma or a mesenchymal tumor, but sometimes such operations are not successful. Furthermore, many types of hypoglycemia cannot be cured surgically.

In managing hypoglycemia itself, it may be possible to overcome an enzyme defect by withholding specific food (e.g., leucine or galactose). In the treatment of the hypoglycemia per se, a low-carbohydrate, high-protein diet, and frequent feedings may help. In acute emergencies, the administration of glucagon, epinephrine, or the glucocorticoids may be valuable. Diazoxide, alone or with trichlormethiazide, is useful and will often restore normal blood sugar levels in many, but not all, types of hypoglycemia. The use of diazoxide has been one of the more important recent advances in the therapy of hypoglycemia.

References

1. Arky, R. A. *Pathophysiology and Therapy of the Fasting Hypoglycemias: Disease-A-Month,* February 1968. Chicago, Yr. Book Pub., 1968.
2. Boshell, B. R., ed. Treatment of hypoglycemia. *Mod Treat 3:*329–426, 1966.
3. Black, J., Tabachnick, I. I. A., Loubatières, A. *et al.:* Diazoxide and the treatment of hypoglycemia. Conference papers 5, 6 Jan. 1967. *Ann NY Acad Sci 150:*194–203, 1968.
4. Marks, V., and Rose, F. C. *Hypoglycaemia.* Oxford, Blackwell, 1965.
5. Unger, R. H. The riddle of tumor hypoglycemia. *Am J Med 40:*325–330, 1966.
6. Volpé, R., Evans, J., Clarke, D. W., Forbath, N., and Ehrlich, R. Evidence favoring the sarcomatous origin of an insulin-like substance in a case of fibrosarcoma with hypoglycemia. *Am J Med 38:*540–553, 1965.

14

Obesity and Lipid Metabolism

George Steiner

Obesity is the major form of malnutrition seen today in North America. While two-thirds of the world is starving, Canadians and Americans spend vast fortunes on foods that are low in calories.

Although it has been difficult to reach a consensus on the definition of obesity, most physicians agree that obesity represents the presence of excess amounts of adipose tissue in the body. Thus, the first section of this chapter will deal with methods to measure the amounts of adipose tissue.

Basically, excess adipose tissue represents the end result of a disorder of homeostasis, in which energy intake (food) has exceeded energy utilization. When intake exceeds expenditure, a person is said to be in positive energy balance. When expenditure exceeds intake, he is said to be in negative energy balance. One pound of adipose tissue represents approximately 3,500 calories or kcal (see Fig. 14-1). Hence, a man will gain (or lose) 1 lb of adipose tissue when he achieves a positive (or negative) balance of this amount of energy. To date, all attempts to treat obesity have been aimed at producing negative calorie balance (i.e., to have a person take in less energy than he expends). The major question has been sidestepped: the cause of this energy imbalance. Because no one has yet discovered why an individual consumes more than his body needs, it is not possible to treat the true cause(s) of his obesity. In fact, treatment is only symptomatic, in the same sense that the treatment of hypertension with blood pressure-lowering agents is symptomatic. When treatment breaks down and the patient regains his weight, we blame him rather than our own ignorance. Astwood has pointed out that obesity, like venereal disease, is considered to be the patient's own fault.

Definition and Quantification of Obesity

Physicians find it hard to agree on a satisfactory definition of obesity. All might agree that most 225-lb men who are 5 feet 10 inches tall are obese. However, there might not be the same consensus if the man were a muscular football player. If the physician agrees that obesity means the presence of excess adipose tissue, he must assess the amount of adipose tissue in a patient in order to make the diagnosis.

A variety of research methods are available to measure adipose tissue mass, and lean body mass (that portion of the body which is not adipose tissue). These methods include:

Body density measurement. Density is the measure of mass, or weight, per unit volume. The density of adipose tissue is 0.90 gm/cc; that of lean body mass 1.10 gm/cc. An individual's body volume may be measured by immersing him in a tank of water and measuring the water displaced, or by weighing him both in air and in water. The more adipose tissue he has, the closer his density will be to 0.90 gm/cc. The inaccuracies of this technique derive from the corrections necessary for air in the lungs and intestine, and from the assumption that the density of lean body mass is constant.

Body water measurement. This technique attempts to estimate lean body mass by measuring body water. Because less than 10% of adipose tissue is water and approximately 73.2% of lean body mass is water, one can, by measuring total body water, estimate the per cent of the total body weight represented by lean body mass. The technique requires the use of water labeled either with deuterium or with tritium. It assumes that the tracer distributes as does the total body water, that it mixes completely with body water and that none of it is lost.

Exchangeable potassium. Another isotopic measurement, this technique estimates the potassium space of the body. By assuming that there is a fairly constant ratio of potassium to protoplasmic nitrogen, it is used to measure body protoplasmic protein.

Obviously none of these techniques can be applied in the office. However, there are three more practical but less accurate methods: visual inspection, reference to standard height-weight tables, and measurement of skin thickness. Visual inspection suffers because it is subjective, especially in the slightly obese. Height-weight tables also have serious limitations. They do not account for the "muscular individual," and they leave room for subjective interpretation, as the weights given for "light" and "heavy build" may vary over a range of as much as 30 lb. However, these tables do provide guidance to the doctor with a patient who has more than a 10–15% excess of adipose tissue. The best office method, the skin-thickness measurement, can be obtained by taking X-rays of soft tissues or by using skin calipers. Skin-fold thickness determined with calipers over the midtriceps area is perhaps the best, single, easy measure of obesity. However in using it, the physician assumes that adipose tissue mass increases uniformly in all areas of the body. The reader need only think of the male who tends to acquire most of his adipose tissue around the abdomen, and the female, around the hips, to realize the limitation of this assumption.

Etiology

Regulation of Energy Intake—The Appetite

Obesity develops when energy intake exceeds energy expenditure (positive balance). Its primary causes are those factors that allow this imbalance to develop. Unfortunately, it is here that our ignorance about obesity is greatest. Therefore, we blame the patient for his lack of self-control in allowing his food intake to increase. While, in many instances, this may be true, it is also possible that the obese individual has some alteration in his appetite control or that his body uses the energy from food more efficiently and stores the excess as fat.

The hunger drive, which originates in the "hunger center" in the ventrolateral nucleus of the hypothalamus, is modified by impulses from the cerebral cortex; these in turn may be set off by such stimuli as sight, smell, taste, and psychic influences. The "hunger center" may be inhibited by stimuli from the ventromedial area of the hypothalamus—the "satiety center." When the satiety center is destroyed in rats, the hunger center is released from inhibition. This uninhibited hunger drive results in hyperphagia and obesity. On rare occasions hypothalamic lesions in humans may also lead to massive hyperphagia. Sometimes a pituitary tumor, presumably by pressing on the hypothalamus, may lead to a voracious appetite.

Hypoglycemia is often associated with a sensation of hunger, which disappears when glucose is given. However, in the poorly controlled diabetic, or in the normoglycemic individual given glucose intravenously, the presence of hyperglycemia does not prevent the person from experiencing the sensation of hunger. Although hyperglycemia appears to inhibit hunger by increasing the impulses arising from the satiety center, the full role of blood glucose concentrations in regulating the appetite is not yet known.

The relationship between gastric activity and the sensation of hunger is also poorly defined. Gastric distention is often associated with satiety, and gastric contractions, with hunger. Some have suggested that the satiety center may inhibit gastric contractions, thereby abolishing the sensation of hunger, but no one has demonstrated whether gastric contractions cause, or result from, hunger. In some obese people the relationship between hunger and gastric contractions may become confused. They often lose the ability to appreciate the association of gastric contractions and distention as cues for hunger and satiety. Thus, when these involuntary controls are lost and food is freely available, many obese individuals must then regulate food intake voluntarily—a continuous effort that may produce great anxiety.

Low environmental temperature and exercise also stimulate the appetite. In rats, appetite increases with increasing exercise, but at both maximal and minimal levels of exertion, this relationship breaks down. Thus, with minimal exercise, appetite does not decrease in proportion to energy expenditure, and the animal may go into positive calorie balance.

Another factor that may regulate appetite is the individual's adipose tissue mass. When a portion of an animal's adipose tissue is excised, lipid is deposited in other areas. Furthermore, if animals are fasted and then allowed food ad libitum, they increase their intake until they return to their original adipose tissue mass. The converse also holds: If rats are force-fed to a point of obesity and then allowed food ad libitum, they decrease their intake until they return to their initial adipose tissue mass. Thus the basic amount of adipose tissue in the body may determine the overall food intake. This basic amount of adipose tissue (i.e., the size and number of adipocytes) may depend upon nutrition in infancy (see section on Fat Cells in Obesity later in this chapter). Although adipose tissue mass may not serve as an acute regulator of appetite, it may have a role in determining the long-term level of food intake.

Factors Determining the Availability of Calories from Food

The energy content of foods may be measured by determining the amount of heat produced when it is burned completely, in a bomb calorimeter. This is hardly a natural process. From a physiological and nutritional standpoint, it is more important to know the energy of food available to the body. Frequently, the energy available from a given nutrient is less than its energy content, as determined in a calorimeter. If completely burned, protein yields 5.5 kcal/gm. However, when the body oxidizes proteins, it cannot use the amino groups of the constituent amino acids, and thus does not burn the protein completely. The nonutilized groups, excreted as urea, represent a loss of 1.5 kcal/gm of protein. Hence, the energy available to the body from 1 gm of protein is 4.0 kcal. Because this is a constant phenomenon, protein is stated to have a nutritional value of 4 kcal/gm.

At times the energy available from a given nutrient may vary, depending upon the individual's metabolic state. An example of this situation occurs when fat is utilized. Normally, 9 kcal are available from each gram of fat. When fat is burned, ketone bodies—products of the incomplete oxidation of fatty acids—are produced. The body has a limited capacity to oxidize these ketone bodies, and this limits its capacity to utilize fat. In the ketosis of diabetes or starvation, the body's capacity to oxidize ketones, and hence to oxidize fat, is exceeded. The excess ketones are excreted and energy is lost—i.e., less than 9 kcal are derived from 1 gm of fat.

In other instances, as with cellulose, the energy available depends upon the animal species. Cellulose and starch, both polymers of glucose, differ only in the way in which the glucose units are linked. As the cell can only use carbohydrate as monosaccharide, these polysaccharides must first be hydrolyzed. Because the human intestinal tract contains enyzmes that break starch into its glucose units, man gets the full 4 kcal/gm from starch. However, his gut cannot hydrolyze cellulose into its glucose units—a task performed in the gut of ruminants by bacteria. Thus, although by bomb calorimetry, cellulose contains as many calories as starch, these are not available to man.

Calorie availability is also determined by the efficiency with which material is absorbed from the gastrointestinal tract. This, in turn, depends on the way in which the nutrient is presented, on the presence of intestinal disease, etc.

In addition to the factors just discussed, the availability of calories may be influenced by the efficiency with which the body uses them. This, in turn, may be related to the pattern in which they are consumed. If a rat is force-fed once a day he becomes fatter than if he is allowed to consume the same number of calories as several meals per day. This obviously must mean that more of the total energy content of the food consumed in the former manner is available to the body. The human counterpart of this may be seen in the variety of bizarre eating patterns which obese individuals may exhibit. Some nibble continuously; others consume small amounts at breakfast and lunch but eat huge evening meals; still others go on wild caloric binges or wake up at night to eat voraciously. Therefore, a physician must include an inquiry into eating patterns when assessing an obese patient.

Energy Utilization—Work

Positive calorie balance results not only from increased energy supply but also from decreased expenditure. Time–motion studies have shown that obese individuals undertake less physical activity than do the nonobese. Even when two individuals perform the same occupation, the obese expends less energy than does the nonobese—e.g., an obese secretary may not run to the filing cabinet as frequently as her slender colleague. Although an obese person may claim that he spends as much time in a given sport as another lean person, he often does so in a less active way. These observations, however, need not only mean that inactivity causes obesity. It may also be that the obese person exercises less *because* he is obese.

Balance of Energy Intake and Expenditure

A person becomes obese because he consumes more energy than he needs. However, all physicians are confronted, sooner or later, with the statement: "But, doctor, I eat less than my nonobese friend!" Although the patient frequently underestimates his food intake, his statement sometimes is true. A brief consideration of energy balance can indicate the reasons for this. While the patient was depositing fat, he was in positive energy balance (i.e., his food intake exceeded his energy needs). However, one does not continue to deposit fat forever, but eventually levels off. At this plateau of obesity, intake of energy must again equal energy expenditure. Frequently the obese person is less active than his slender counterpart (i.e., his energy expenditure is less). Thus he can maintain his plateau of obesity with less food intake than his nonobese friend.

The Energy Content of Tissues

Even though each gram of carbohydrate contains 4 kcal; protein, 4 kcal; and fat, 9 kcal; 1 gm of muscle does not represent 4 kcal and 1 gm of adipose tissue does not represent 9 kcal (Fig. 14-1). The energy content of a gram of tissue can only be determined when one allows for that portion of its mass that has no energy—tissue water. Tissues that contain mainly protein and carbohydrate, such as liver and muscle, have approximately 75% water. Thus 1 gm of these tissues has only 0.25 gm carbohydrate and protein. This represents only 1 kcal. By contrast, adipose tissue is 90% lipid and each gram, with its 0.9 gm of fat, represents 8.1 kcal. Thus, a given amount of fat-containing tissue has eight times more energy than an equal amount of a tissue which contains mainly carbohydrate and protein, even though pure lipid is only 2.25 times more efficient as an energy source than pure carbohydrate or protein. Hence, an 8-kcal deficit may result in the loss of 1 gm of adipose tissue or 8 gm of carbohydrate- or protein-containing tissue. Therefore, in response to a given negative calorie balance a patient will lose more weight if he loses lean-body-mass than if he loses adipose-tissue-mass. However, this greater weight loss is deceptive because much of it represents loss of water. This should remind the reader, once more, that changes in weight cannot be equated with changes in adipose tissue mass alone. The success of many crash reducing programs is misleading, as it results from rapid loss of lean-body-mass and water. Adipose tissue loss is slower and requires a deficit of 8 kcal for each gram (or 3,500 kcal for each 1 lb) lost.

Endocrine Causes (Fact or Fancy?)

Because "the cause" of obesity has not been found and because hormones affect metabolism profoundly, this disorder has frequently been

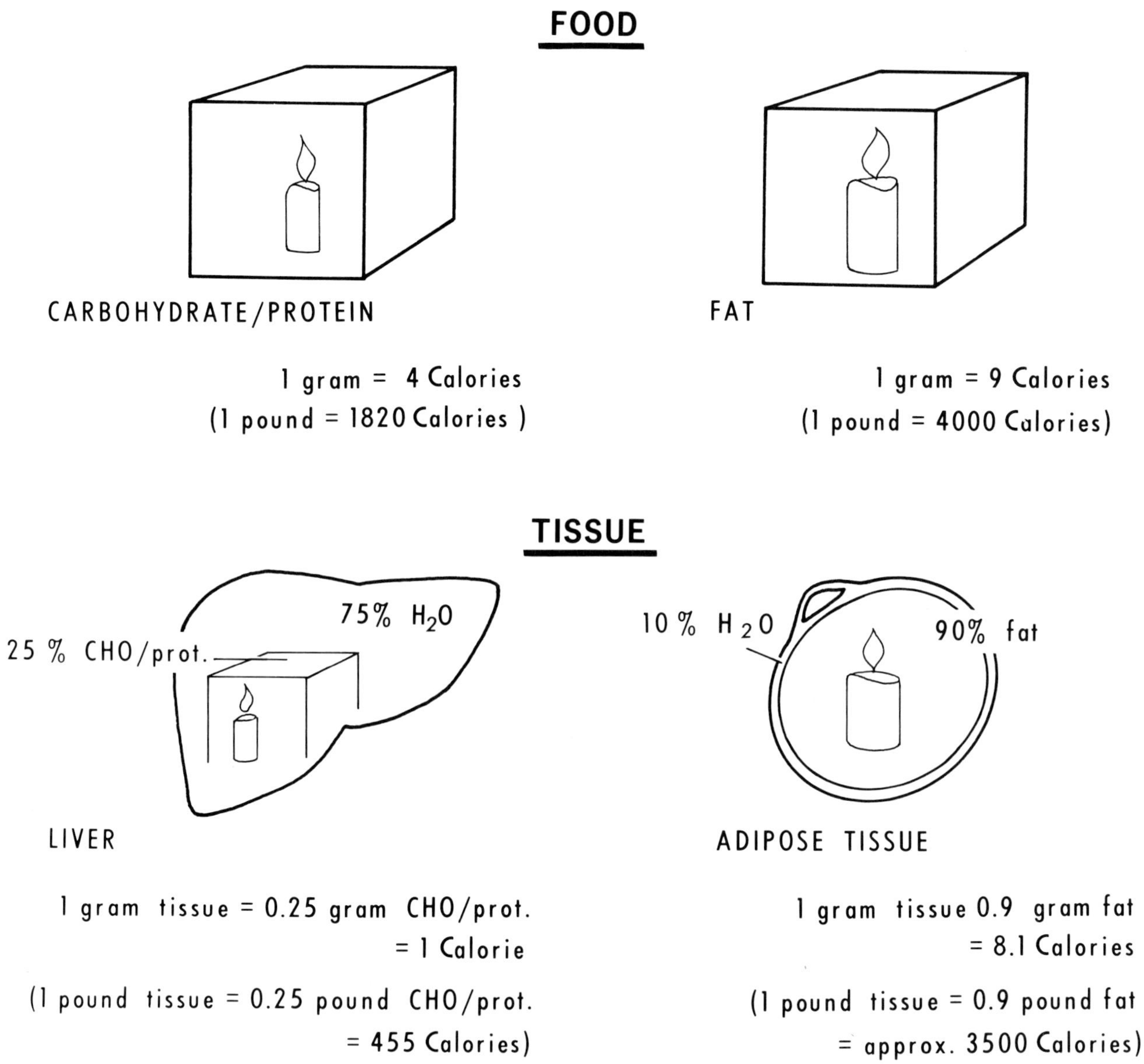

Fig. 14-1. Energy content of pure carbohydrate, protein, and fat compared with that of tissues containing these materials. The caloric ratio of pure carbohydrate or protein to pure fat is 4 to 9, whereas that of the respective tissues is 1 to 8, because tissues which contain mainly protein and carbohydrate—e.g., liver tissues have approximately 75% water. Adipose tissue on the other hand contains only 10% water.

blamed on the endocrine glands. The first gland so blamed was the thyroid, because hyperthyroidism is associated with hypermetabolism and, frequently, with weight loss. It was also because many obese people appear to have low basal metabolic rates, a finding commonly taken to indicate the presence of hypothyroidism. There are several flaws in this reasoning: (1) Hyperthyroid patients lose weight only if food intake does not meet energy expenditure. Furthermore, the weight lost is mainly from the lean-body-mass. (2) The low basal metabolic rate in obesity is misleading, as the metabolic rate is measured as a function of body surface area, a parameter that increases in obese individuals much more than does the actively metabolizing protoplasm. Hence, in obese patients, the basal metabolic rate is falsely "decreased."

The pituitary has also been said to be implicated in obesity. However, unless there is a disorder such as a tumor, which affects the hunger center or satiety center in the hypothalamus, there appears to be no such association.

Patients with hypogonadism may have excess adipose tissue, and hence be defined as obese. However, because they also lose lean-body-mass, they need not be overweight. This again points out that it is incorrect to define obesity in terms of body weight only. Women with Stein-Leventhal syndrome tend to be obese, for reasons not yet defined. In any event gonadal dysfunction can only account for obesity in an exceedingly small percentage of patients.

The role of the pancreas will be dealt with more fully when considering the relationship between obesity and diabetes. The patient with an insulin-producing tumor may also become obese, perhaps because the hypoglycemia stimulates the appetite (see section on Regulation of Energy Intake—the Appetite earlier in this chapter.)

Patients with Cushing's syndrome may also be obese. The development of obesity in Cushing's syndrome is again related to positive energy balance. It does not develop unless a patient increases his food intake. The obesity has a peculiar centripetal distribution. The reason for this distribution is not known. It appears that adipose tissue in different sites responds differently to a given hormonal stimulus. This is just one instance of the fact that adipose tissue from different areas of the body is not always the same metabolically.

Thus, if endocrine disorders account for obesity at all, they explain only an exceedingly small number of cases. The discovery of an endocrinopathy in an obese patient does not necessarily mean that it is the cause of the obesity. It may be another independent disorder, or it may even result from the obesity. Here, as elsewhere, obesity represents the imbalance between energy supply and utilization. Although endocrine activity may direct the path taken by the calories (i.e., to protein or to fat) it cannot increase the energy derived from a given amount of any food.

Genetic and Environmental Influences

Genetic studies in humans, difficult at the best of times, are especially difficult in multicausal disorders such as obesity. Obese parents more frequently have obese children than do nonobese parents. Obesity is more common among the children of two obese parents than among the children of one obese and one nonobese parent. Studies of identical twins reared in different environments and of children adopted by obese parents all indicate that obesity has some genetic basis. The patterns of such inheritance, however, have not been defined.

Environment also plays a vital role in determining food consumption. Certain individuals place a high value on eating; it may be an important part of their social or business life. For others, in a society in which undernutrition is the norm, overnutrition is a status symbol, a sign of wealth. Certain societies look upon obesity as a sign of health and beauty—e.g., the beautiful ladies painted by Rubens. Most of the world struggles against undernutrition and seeks the good fortune of overnutrition, but in North America, the general population is so overnourished that society places a high value on weight loss. Fortunes are spent on low-calorie foods and on supporting organizations whose avowed aim is to stop their patrons from eating.

Environment also contributes to obesity by influencing energy expenditure. Our society with its labor-saving devices (cars, floor polishers, power lawn mowers, etc.), its means of entertainment (television, spectator sports etc.), and its conquest of certain diseases, has allowed man to store more energy as adipose tissue. The environmental influences make it even more difficult to determine what contribution genetics makes to the difference, in amount of adipose tissue, between the wealthy North American and an Asian peasant.

Pathophysiology—Adipose Tissue Metabolism

Lipid is stored in adipose tissue as triglyceride —an ester of glycerol and three fatty acids. The amount of triglyceride in adipose tissue is a function of the amount deposited and of the amount mobilized (Fig. 14-2). Hence, one may divide the factors controlling adipose tissue mass into those controlling deposition of lipid (preformed lipid and de-novo synthesized lipid) and those controlling lipid mobilization.

Lipid Deposition

Lipid, deposited in adipose tissue, is derived either from preformed lipid brought to the adipose tissue or from lipid synthesized de novo from glucose within the fat cell (adipocyte). Preformed lipid arrives at the fat cell, either as free fatty acids, or as triglyceride in lipoproteins (Chapter 15). Before triglycerides can enter the cell, they must be broken down to their constituent fatty acids and glycerol, by the enzyme lipoprotein lipase. Little is known about the nature and localization of this enzyme. Its activity increases after heparin administration. In diabetes, its activity decreases but is restored by insulin. The normal physiologic control of this enzyme remains to be defined. After hydrolysis of the triglyceride, the adipocyte takes up the fatty acids. However, because the cell has no glycerolkinase, it cannot use the glycerol portion of the circulating triglyceride. Fatty acids that enter the cell can be esterified with α-glycerolphosphate. This must be made de novo from glucose and cannot be derived from glycerol per se. This is due, again, to the absence of glycerolkinase. Thus, anything which controls glucose entry into the fat cell, controls the availability of α-glycerolphosphate and, in turn, controls the amount of fatty acid that can be deposited as triglyceride. In addition to fatty acid derived from circulating triglyceride, the adipocyte can synthesize fatty acid directly from glucose at a rate which, again, reflects the rate at which glucose enters the adipocyte.

Thus one can see that insulin can regulate lipid deposition in three ways: (1) Insulin deficiency decreases lipoprotein lipase activity; (2) insulin increases α-glycerolphosphate synthesis; and (3) insulin increases de-novo fatty acid synthesis. The last two effects result from insulin's action to increase glucose entry into the cell. As will be indicated, insulin control of lipid in each fat cell not only increases lipid deposition, but also decreases lipid mobilization.

Lipid Mobilization

The second major determinant of the amount to triglyceride in the fat cell is the rate of mobilization. Just as intact triglyceride cannot enter the adipocyte, so it cannot leave; it must first be hydrolyzed. The lipase which controls the breakdown of intracellular triglyceride differs from lipoprotein lipase. It is activated by a variety of hormones (epinephrine, norepinephrine, glucagon, and several pituitary peptides) and is inhibited by insulin; hence its name—"hormone-sensitive lipase." Lipolysis goes on continuously within the adipocyte, producing fatty acids which may be reesterified, oxidized, or mobilized. The rate at which fatty acids leave the adipocyte depends on their intracellular concentration. This concentration, in turn, depends in part on the rate of lipolysis, and in part on the rate of reesterification. The latter is directly related to the amount of α-glycerolphosphate available.

Because both epinephrine and norepinephrine activate hormone-sensitive lipase, patients with pheochromocytomas mobilize lipid rapidly, have high plasma free fatty acid concentrations, and are rarely obese.

It may also be seen that, in addition to affecting lipid deposition, insulin decreases lipid mobilization: firstly, by inhibiting hormone-sensitive lipase and, secondly, by increasing the availability of α-glycerolphosphate. The latter increases reesterification and thereby decreases the intracellular concentration of free fatty acids and fatty acid mobilization.

Fat Cells in Obesity

Hirsch and his colleagues recently provided new insights into the metabolism of adipose tissue in

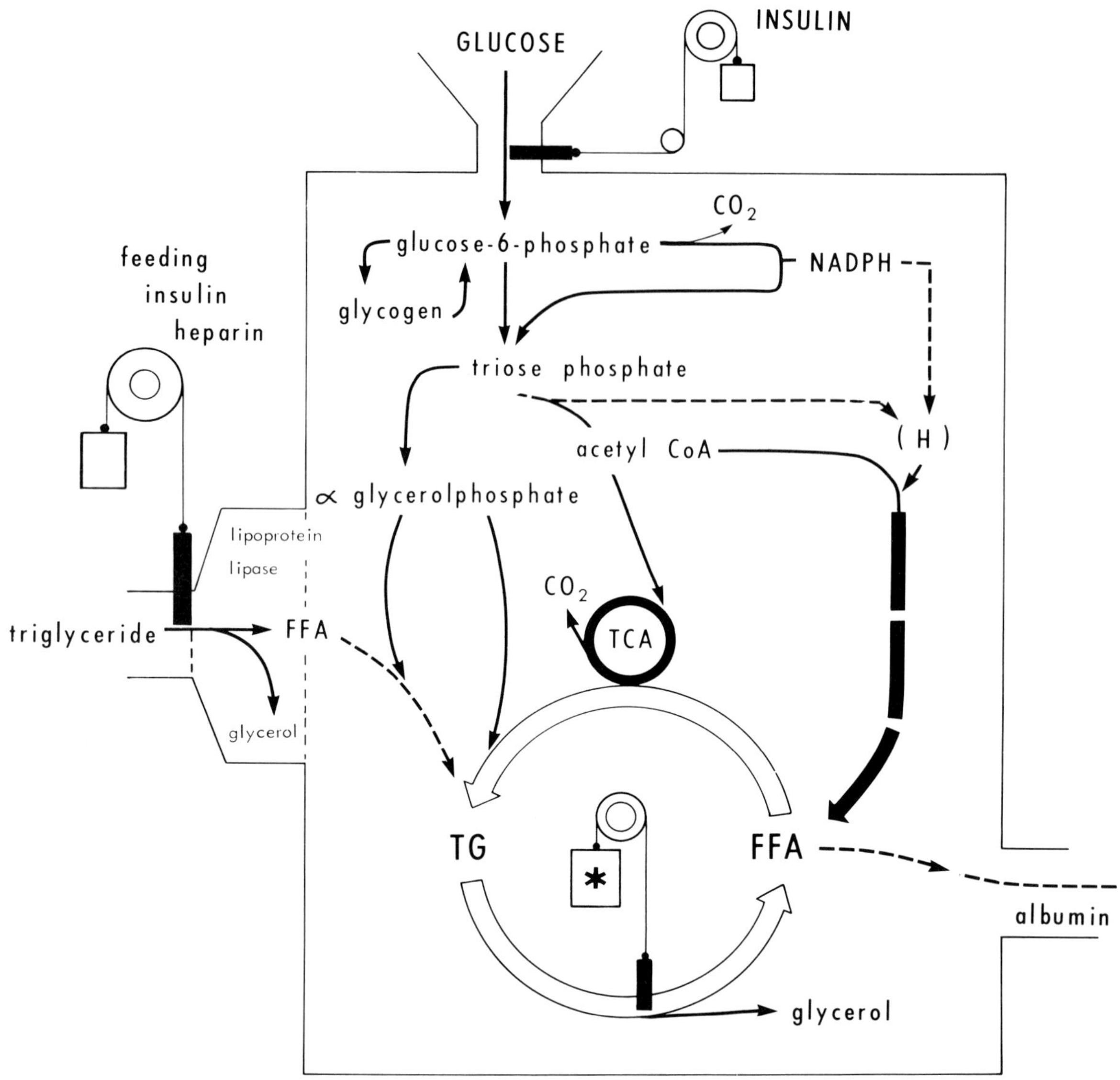

Fig. 14-2. Major pathways and key metabolic controls in fat cell. The three main control points, indicated as *black "gates,"* include (1) glucose entry—stimulated by insulin; (2) lipoprotein lipase—whose activity is increased following feeding and by heparin and is decreased in diabetes; and (3) hormone-sensitive lipase (*gate with asterisk*)—stimulated by norepinephrine, epinephrine, glucagon, and a variety of pituitary peptides, including ACTH and growth hormone, and inhibited by insulin.

Triglyceride (*TG*) within the fat cell arrives via two routes:

(1) Pre-formed lipid—the fatty acids are derived either from triglycerides, reaching the fat cell as lipoprotein, or as free fatty acid (*FFA*, bound to plasma albumin). If as lipoprotein, the triglyceride is hydrolyzed by lipoprotein lipase prior to entry into the cell.

(2) De-novo synthesis from glucose—the glucose may supply both fatty acids and α glycerol phosphate.

Intracellular triglyceride may be hydrolyzed by hormone-sensitive lipase (*) into fatty acid and glycerol. The former may be either relased from the cell, burned to CO_2 or reesterified. The latter cannot be reutilized and is released.

Tricarboxylic acid cycle (*TCA*).

obesity. Using elegant techniques to estimate the number and size of fat cells in the body, they showed that obese people have more and larger adipocytes in their body than do nonobese patients. When an obese individual loses weight, the number of his fat cells does not decrease, but the cells become smaller. It has been postulated that these "shriveled" cells refill very easily, just as a balloon, once inflated and then emptied, is easier to reinflate. They also showed that if rats were overfed during the neonatal period, the number of fat cells in their bodies increased and they became obese later in life. Early data in humans also suggest that overnutrition in infancy may produce increased numbers of fat cells in later life. In a person who became obese in childhood, the obesity is much more difficult to treat than that in someone who became obese in adult life; perhaps the former has more fat cells than the latter. The easy refilling of the shriveled cells postulated above may explain the frequent failure of the obese to maintain his weight loss after a reducing program.

Psychological Aspects

It is difficult to determine whether the psychological problems associated with obesity represent cause or effect. Frequently, the treatment and weight loss may create its own psychological problems in the obese patient. The physician who wishes to treat obesity successfully must study his patient's psychic make-up because this may influence the disorder at each of three levels: cause, effect, and treatment.

The obese individual has always been viewed as a jovial and jocular person. In *Julius Caesar,* Shakespeare pictured him in the following way:

> Caesar: Let me have men about me that are fat;
> Sleek headed men, and such as sleep o' nights.
> Yon Cassius has a lean and hungry look;
> He thinks too much: such men are dangerous.
> Antony: Fear him not Caesar; he's not dangerous;
> He is a noble Roman and well given.
> Caesar: Would he were fatter! But I fear him not.

Nothing could be further from the truth than these popular concepts of the obese personality. This is not to say that all obese people are neurotic; however, obesity frequently may be a physical manifestation of a psychological problem. Because most of the studies have been done in the grossly obese population, it is difficult to estimate the overall frequency of psychiatric disturbances in obesity. Virtually every form of psychic abnormality may be encountered in the obese patient. Obese children frequently relate poorly to other members of their family. The obese individual may have a disturbed body image and may assess himself unrealistically in relation to his environment.

To some, the size of the body itself has considerable significance. A large body may imply power and thus compensate for the patient's feelings of inferiority. On the other hand, other people find a large body loathsome, and thus the existence of obesity may just add to the patient's anxieties. Still other individuals find psychic significance in the act of eating. It may be a defense against a variety of anxiety-producing problems. If this anxiety includes guilt about overeating and about the state of obesity, a vicious cycle can develop, causing the person to eat even more. Another abnormality which may lead to overeating is depression.

As a class, the obese share many of the problems faced by minority groups. They are recognized on sight as different from the population at large. Special clubs are created for them. They attend special camps. They are excluded from certain activities. Magazine articles and books are written about their problems. They may have to buy their clothes in special stores. They are always the butt of jokes and caustic comments. Such factors separate the obese from their fellows and, of themselves, may induce anxiety or depression.

Treatment of obesity may produce its own problems. If eating is a defense mechanism, the physician may put his patient in a difficult position if he imposes a diet before he attends to the underlying emotional problems. If the patient's obesity and body size compensate for feelings of inferiority, a decrease in body size may produce a new set of difficulties.

The psychodynamics of obesity is too vast and specialized an area to be considered in other than a cursory manner. However, unless the physician is concerned with these aspects of his patient's problems he will be unsuccessful in treating the whole individual. Furthermore, in that success in weight reduction requires a high level of motivation, the physician's failure to appreciate any associated psychological problems will probably result in failure to treat the obesity itself.

Systemic Effects of Obesity

The busy physician will often wonder why he should spend time and energy in attempting to treat this frustrating problem. The effort is vital in order to combat the high morbidity and mortality associated with obesity. The harmful consequences of obesity are both physical and psychological. The latter have been discussed separately because it is often difficult to isolate the psychological abnormalities which contribute to obesity from those which result from it.

The death rate of obese individuals is higher than that of the normal-weight population, especially in the younger age groups. The major reason for this increase lies in the higher incidence, in obesity, of (1) atherosclerosis, (2) diabetes, (3) cirrhosis, (4) complications of surgery and anesthesia, (5) accidents, and (6) complications of pregnancy. There is also a higher incidence of perinatal death in the infants of obese mothers. The mortality risk often reverts to normal after weight reduction.

The Endocrine System

Adrenal Cortex. Obesity may produce changes in adrenal cortical function which resemble those seen in Cushing's syndrome. In both situations the urine may contain increased amounts of 17-hydroxycorticoids. The obese patient may even have some clinical similarities to the patient with Cushing's syndrome. In addition to the accumulation of fat, he may have striae and hirsutism. However, obesity may be differentiated from Cushing's syndrome by demonstrating that the elevated urinary corticoids may be suppressed with 2 mg of dexamethasone; that the plasma 17-hydroxycorticoids are generally low and display a circadian rhythm; and that the other features of Cushing's syndrome are absent.

Reproductive System. For as yet unknown reasons, obese women tend to have a high incidence of amenorrhea, hirsutism, decreased fertility, and complications of pregnancy.

Diabetes. Obese individuals have a much higher incidence of diabetes than those of normal weight, but it is not clear whether obesity causes, or results from, the diabetes. After weight reduction, the abnormalities of glucose metabolism may markedly improve. Adipose tissue is very sensitive to insulin's action in promoting the entry of glucose into the fat cell and hence its conversion to lipid. The basis for suggesting that diabetes causes obesity stems from the demonstration that plasma insulin levels are elevated in the early stages of diabetes, and from the increase in lipid deposition which occurs in the presence of insulin. These phenomena may combine in patients with early maturity-onset diabetes to divert most of the carbohydrate to adipose tissue, where it is stored as lipid. Neel has even suggested that the association of diabetes and obesity may have represented a developmental advantage to primitive man. He points out that primitive men ate after a successful hunt and starved for long periods between, a feeding pattern that required a very efficient method of energy storage. As energy is most efficiently stored as fat, the man who was able to store his energy in adipose tissue may have had a developmental advantage. Furthermore, the gene for diabetes, then, would not have become harmful until man adopted his current three-meals-a-day pattern. This interesting hypothesis might explain why a genetic trait, diabetes, which today appears to be harmful, did not eliminate itself over the ages.

The suggestion that obesity may cause, or aggravate, diabetes stems from the observation that abnormalities of glucose utilization frequently improve after weight loss and that obesity is associated with insulin resistance (Chapter 11). It has been indicated that the fat cells of the obese patient are larger and more numerous than those of lean individuals. Hirsch observed that large adipocytes are relatively resistant to insulin. Rabinowitz has also shown that the muscles of obese individuals are resistant to insulin. These observations allow one to understand how obesity can lead to insulin resistance and carbohydrate intolerance.

The Respiratory System

Obese individuals frequently complain of dyspnea on exertion. This may represent no more than the increased energy required to move a larger body about and the increased mechanical work expended in moving the diaphragm down against an obese abdomen. At times, the difficulty in breathing may be great enough to result in hypoventilation. We do not yet know whether the hypoventilation is just due to mechanical problems or is also due to fatty infiltration of the intercostal muscles or to changes in the respiratory center. In the severe form of obesity-related respiratory insufficiency, the "Pickwickian syndrome," the patient develops dyspnea, cyanosis, secondary polycythemia, right-sided heart failure, somnolence, CO_2 narcosis, and a decreased respiratory drive.

The Cardiovascular System

It has already been indicated that one of the reasons for the high mortality among obese people is the increased incidence of atherosclerosis. Stamler found that obesity is associated with an increased incidence of diabetes mellitus, hypertension, and hyperlipoproteinemia—all of which, on their own, increase the risk of atherosclerosis. However, he observed that the incidence of atherosclerosis in obese patients who do not have diabetes, hypertension, or hyperlipoproteinemia is no higher than that in the nonobese.

Other Systems

The obese patient may have a variety of gastrointestinal disorders—belching and flatulence, cholelithiasis, cholecystitis, and hiatus hernia. He may also show the mechanical effects of bearing excessive weight—namely, an increased incidence of osteoarthritis and of fractures. His skin may have numerous deep folds in which intertrigo may become established.

Treatment of Obesity

General Principles—Two Phases

There are two phases to the treatment of obesity: Phase 1—the loss of excess adipose tissue; and Phase 2—stabilization in the new nonobese steady state. Phase 1 is comparatively easily achieved by placing the patient in negative energy balance. This is accomplished by decreasing the supply of energy (calorie intake) or by increasing the energy utilization (work and exercise). Phase 2, unfortunately, all too frequently fails. In it, the patient must readjust his pattern of living, working, and eating in such a way that he will never go into positive energy balance. This requires a high degree of motivation and self-discipline.

Phase 1: Producing Negative Energy Balance

There is no mystery to Phase 1—the loss of excess adipose tissue. It merely requires the patient to be placed in a negative energy balance. Theoretically, approximately 1 lb adipose tissue should be lost for each 3,500 kcal that the individual burns up or does not eat. The basis for this approximation has already been given in Figure 14-1. Thus, if an individual consumes 500 kcal less than he needs each day, he should lose approximately 1 lb of adipose tissue per week. Unfortunately, this generalization has many pitfalls as one cannot direct one's body to lose adipose tissue only and not to lose lean body mass. A given calorie deficit would produce an eightfold greater weight loss, if lean body mass rather than adipose tissue mass were lost (1 lb of lean body mass has approximately ⅛ the energy content of 1 lb of adipose tissue, as shown in Figure 14-1). This difference is largely due to water loss.

Decreased Intake

Total Starvation. This form of therapy, which should be reserved for patients with extreme obesity, is hazardous and should be undertaken only in hospital. Furthermore, only the individual who is in good health should be subjected to total starvation. Some individuals have tolerated total calorie deprivation for several months in investigative situations. However, unless the circumstances are exceptional, the starvation period should not exceed 2–3 weeks. The patient is allowed fluid ad libitum and should receive appropriate supplements of vitamins, iron, calcium, sodium, and potassium. He may lose 5–10 kg during this time. Unfortunately, 65% of this may be accounted for by the loss of lean body mass and water. During the first few days, the patient generally loses his appetite, occasionally to such a degree that he will refuse to eat at the end of the fast. When the patient begins a low-calorie diet after the fast, he may quickly regain 25% of his lost weight. This largely represents retention of the water which was lost together with lean body mass. Frequently such a period of starvation will cause the patient to "reset his appetite" so that he will not eat excessively afterwards. As a continuation of this program after the total fast, some physicians advise their patients to fast for 1 day each week.

Frequently the patient undergoing total fast may complain of weakness and faintness, which results, in part, from the loss of sodium that occurs together with the loss of water. These symptoms frequently disappear when salt is administered. During total starvation the patient may also develop hyperuricemia due to decreased renal urate clearance. However, unless he already has gout, he rarely requires uricosuric agents. The greatest hazards of this program lie in cardiac problems that may develop; although rarely, some patients develop arrhythmias and congestive heart failure. In a few instances the cardiac complications have been fatal. For this reason, total starvation should not be undertaken in individuals with known myocardial disease. Another complication of treatment lies in the psychiatric problems which may develop. As has been discussed above, these may arise from such things as changes in the patient's body image, loss of his defense mechanisms, etc.

Gradual Dieting. A program of much wider application aims at producing a weight loss of 1–2 lb per week. Again, the general aim is to produce a negative energy balance but, in this case, more gradually. Unfortunately, the gradual method is less frequently successful than is the method of total starvation. The starving patient is closely monitored on a hospital ward, and thus, is less likely to consume excess calories than is the patient on the gradual regimen who is on his own. The latter individual requires a high degree of motivation as he must be the "policeman" of his regimen.

In designing a patient's diet the physician should follow certain general principles and take into account: (1) the patient's energy requirements; (2) the need for essential nutrients, such as vitamins and adequate amounts of protein; (3) a balanced distribution of calories; (4) the provision of three meals each day, none of which are omitted; and (5) the patient's life pattern.

In estimating the energy requirements the physician should consider the calorie intake that has kept the patient at a steady state, the patient's activity pattern, and the rapidity of weight loss desired. A diet which provides 500 kcal less than the daily requirement should produce a weight loss of approximately 1 lb (see section on Phase 1: Producing Negative Energy Balance earlier in this chapter). The patient should be started on such an estimated diet and his body weight should be followed. Should he lose more or less than anticipated, the calorie content of the diet should be appropriately altered. Both the patient and the physician should be aware that any person's weight may vary up and down a few pounds from one day to the next. Thus in assessing the success of a program, it is essential to follow the general weight trend over the course of several weeks.

Commercial calorie-restricted formula diets have the advantage that they provide essential nutrients and thus avoid one hazard of crash or fad diets. They also provide a fixed number of calories in a convenient form so that the patient does not have to learn diets and estimate food portions. However, in so doing, they merely delay the day when he will have to do this, as he will eventually return to eating normal foods. Of the current fad diets (high-fat diets, high-protein diets, citrus-fruit diet, drinker's diet, etc.), there is little evidence that one is any better than another. All of these diet programs are highly structured and thus provide support to aid the patient in attaining negative calorie balance. However, this support will be removed when the patient has lost his excess adipose tissue and returns to a more normal diet.

Thus the main features in designing a diet should be to provide a normal distribution of calories (40–50% from carbohydrate, 35–40% from fat, 15% from protein), in a diet whose total calorie content is restricted in such a way as to produce gradual weight loss. Obviously, the diet must provide all of the essential nutrients. Furthermore, with severe calorie restriction it may be necessary to increase the percentage of protein and to decrease the percentage of carbohydrate and fat.

Increased Utilization

Many an obese individual undertakes less physical activity than the nonobese, not only as exercise but also during his daily life, work, etc. A planned exercise program will help him to overcome this deficit. However, if the patient realizes that 1 hour of tennis consumes only 600 kcal (the energy of four slices of buttered bread), he will appreciate that he can produce his energy deficit more easily by lowering his intake.

Another way of increasing energy utilization is to induce hyperthyroidism by administering thyroxine. This produces weight loss, but the weight lost is mainly lean body mass and associated water, rather than adipose tissue. Furthermore, if the obese patient has latent coronary artery disease, the added stress of hyperthyroidism may be hazardous. The hypermetabolism may also be accompanied by increased nervousness, which may aggravate any existing psychological problems. However, as a crutch, thyroxine may ease the patient through Phase 1 of his treatment. Ultimately, however, the thyroxine must be discontinued and then, unless the patient is properly motivated and has gained some insight into any psychological problems, he will regain the lost weight and he will fail in Phase 2.

Phase 2: Maintenance in the Nonobese State

Phase 2 is a lifelong program. The patient must maintain himself in his new nonobese steady state. His energy intake should equal his energy expenditure. Because the patient's control mechanisms may not have set his appetite at the level required to maintain just this calorie intake, he may have to exercise conscious control over his food consumption for the rest of his life. He should also have a regular exercise program to maintain his energy expenditure. To achieve this new style of life the patient must be highly motivated. For his part, the physician must achieve a good rapport with each patient and pay appropriate attention to both the patient's psychic and somatic health.

Fads and Crutches

Because of the many difficulties and failures encountered in the treatment of obesity, both physician and patient have eagerly taken up a wide variety of "crutches" or supports. It should be realized that these are supports to the treatment of obesity and do not constitute treatment itself. Some crutches are dangerous and should never be used. Even those which are occasionally used must ultimately be discontinued. The crutches include fad and formula diets, which have been discussed above. Another crutch, the variety of clubs and societies devoted to conquering obesity, may help by providing much-needed motivation. On the other hand, the patient's early enthusiasm for such groups may frequently wane. Crutches like the amphetamines have distinctly harmful side effects. They have been used as anorexigenic agents and do succeed in curbing the appetite for a short time. This effect, however, soon disappears, leaving behind their other effects: nervousness, central nervous system stimulation, and addiction. The biguanide hypoglycemic agents also produce short-term anorexia but are less effective than was initially hoped. Finally, some surgeons have treated obesity by bypassing the ileum. This attempts to decrease fat absorption by breaking the enterohepatic bile salt cycle. Such an operation is a drastic crutch and is to be condemned except in exceedingly unusual situations.

Results of Treatment

Unfortunately, the results of treating obesity are not encouraging. Short-term weight loss, Phase 1, may be achieved in 25–50% of patients without great difficulty. However, over the long term, Phase 2, most clinics find that only 5% of patients maintain their weight at the ideal level for 5 years after the initial weight loss. The success rate is highest in patients with adult-onset obesity, in patients with no psychological problems related to their obesity or to weight loss, and in patients who have previously responded successfully to treatment for obesity.

Summary

The treatment of obesity is surrounded by ignorance because the factors that cause a patient's food intake to exceed his energy requirements are not understood. Therefore the symptom of this energy imbalance—obesity—is treated, rather than its cause. Therefore, the treatment is no more effective than that by the physician treating the hypertension of primary aldosteronism with antihypertensive drugs alone. The symptomatic treatment of obesity is approached by attempting, through diet, to produce a negative calorie balance. During the phase of weight loss (Phase 1) the prescribed diet contains approximately 3,500 kcal less than the body's need for each 1 lb of weight to be lost over an interval of time. It is not too difficult to achieve success in Phase 1 of treatment. However, failure is frequent in Phase 2, the long-term maintenance of ideal body weight. Throughout both phases the obese patient must do consciously that which his body is no longer capable of doing automatically: namely, regulate his food intake. This task requires the highest degree of motivation, understanding, and cooperation. As such, treatment can be supervised most effectively by a team consisting of a physician, dietitian, psychiatrist, and nurse. In designing the diet the physician and dietitian must consider the patient's life habits, ethnic background, and socioeconomic status. No patient will follow a program that he believes is unrealistic to his life situation.

In general, physicians and patients must avoid crutches. However, if such aids are not harmful and if they contribute to the patient's motivation, they may be used in certain instances. If they are used, the physician and the patient should be aware of what is being done and of the fact that at some point the crutch will have to be discontinued. Under no circumstances is the use of an anorexigenic agent justified. Until the cause of obesity is understood, the two most essential ingredients of therapy will remain the motivated patient and the dedicated treatment team.

References

1. Astwood, E. B. The heritage of corpulence. *Endocrinology 71*:337–341, 1962.
2. Bloom, W. L. Fasting as an introduction to the treatment of obesity. *Metabolism 8*:214–220, 1959.
3. Bloom, W. L., and Eidox, M. F. Inactivity as a major factor in adult obesity. *Metabolism 16*:679–684, 1967.
4. Brodoff, B. N., chairman. Adipose tissue metabolism and obesity. *Ann NY Acad Sci 131*:5–673, 1965.
5. Bullen, B. A., Read, R. B., and Mayer, J. Physical activity of obese and non-obese adolescent girls appraised by motion picture sampling. *Am J Clin Nutr 14*:211–223, 1964.
6. Chirico, A. M., and Stunkard, A. J. Physical activity and human obesity. *N Engl J Med 263*:935–940, 1960.
7. Duncan, G., Jenson, W. K., Fraser, R. I., and Christofou, F. C. Correction and control of in-

tractable obesity. Practical applications of intermittent periods of total fasting. *JAMA 181:*309–312, 1962.
8. Glucksman, M. L., and Hirsch, J. The response of obese patients to weight reduction; a clinical evaluation of behaviour. *Psychosom Med 30:*1–11, 1968.
9. Goldblatt, P. B., Moore, M. E., and Stunkard, A. J. Social factors in obesity. *JAMA 192:*1039–1044, 1965.
10. Hirsch, J., and Knittle, J. L. The cellularity of obese and nonobese human adipose tissue. *Fed Proc 29:*1516–1521, 1970.
11. Kannel, W. B., Le Bauer, E. J., Dawber, J. R., and McNamare, P. M. Relation of body weight to development of coronary heart disease. *Circulation 35:*734–744, 1967.
12. Karam, J. H., and Grodsky, G. M. Excessive insulin response in obese subjects as measured by immunochemical assay. *Diabetes 12:*197–204, 1963.
13. Marks, H. H. Influence of obesity on morbidity and mortality. *Bull NY Acad Med 36:*296–312, 1960.
14. Mayer, J. Some aspects of the problem of regulation of food intake and obesity. *N Engl J Med 274:*610–616, 662–673, 722–731, 1966.
15. Renold, A. R., and Cahill, G. F., Jr. *Handbook of Physiology,* Sect. V, *Adipose Tissue.* Washington, D.C., American Physiological Society, 1965.
16. Salans, L. B., Knittle, J. L., and Hirsch, J. The role of adipose cell size and adipose tissue insulin sensitivity in the carbohydrate intolerance of human obesity. *J Clin Invest 47:*153–165, 1968.
17. Seltzer, C. C., and Mayer, J. Body build and obesity —who are the obese? *JAMA 189:*677–684, 1964.
18. Stunkard, A. J., and Mendelson, N. Disturbances in body images of some obese persons. *J Am Diet Assoc 38:*328–331, 1961.
19. Withers, R. F. J. Problems in genetics of human obesity. *J Clin Invest 47:*153–165, 1968.

15

Lipoprotein Disorders

George Steiner

Misconceptions

Before proceeding, the reader should dispose of certain misconceptions that have clouded thinking in this area for many years.

Misconception 1:
"Hyperlipemias are disorders of lipid metabolism alone." It will be pointed out that lipids circulate in association with proteins, as lipoprotein, and hence these may, in fact, represent disorders of protein, as well as lipid metabolism.

Misconception 2:
"Hyperlipoproteinemia is a single disorder." Currently it appears that there are at least five different types of hyperlipoproteinemia. This chapter will review the basis for their differentiation. However, it must be realized that this classification is subject to revision, as knowledge changes.

Misconception 3:
"Normal plasma cholesterol rules out hyperlipoproteinemia." It will be indicated that many patients may have a marked elevation of plasma triglycerides with little or no elevation of plasma cholesterol, and vice versa.

Misconception 4:
"Hyperlipoproteinemia is always associated with early atherosclerosis." Although Types II, III and IV hyperlipoproteinemia are associated with early atherosclerosis, as yet, evidence of such an association in Types I and V is not strong.

Misconception 5:
"Treating hyperlipoproteinemia will prevent or slow atherogenesis." Although it is hoped that this is not a misconception, as yet there is no firm evidence for or against this proposition.

Misconception 6:
"A low-fat (and consequently high-carbohydrate) diet is beneficial in all forms of hyperlipoproteinemia." Not so. It will be indicated that in the carbohydrate-induced hyperlipoproteinemia, such a diet is precisely the wrong one to give.

Aims

This chapter reviews current knowledge concerning disorders of lipid transport in the circulation. To approach the diagnosis and management of abnormalities of circulating lipids rationally, the physician must understand certain theoretical aspects of lipid transport. These will be considered before approaching the clinical abnormalities. Certain controversial areas have been simplified for the sake of clarity. However, references are provided at the end of the chapter, for the reader who wishes to delve more deeply.

Many advances have been made in understanding hyperlipoproteinemias, as a result of the realization that they represent a group of several different disorders rather than a single disease. There are at least four types of lipoproteins in the plasma. Any one or more of these may either be elevated or absent. Fredrickson has classified the lipoprotein abnormalities into five different types of hyperlipoproteinemias and two lipoprotein deficiency states depending upon which lipoprotein is affected (Table 15-1). Each disorder has different manifestations and consequences, and each must be treated differently. Thus, to handle the patient with a lipoprotein disorder properly, the doctor must know the category into which his patient fits. We will deal with the different types according to their dietary behavior. It is hoped that this will provide a simple approach to understanding their pathophysiology and to planning therapy.

Lipoprotein Physiology

The Lipid Moiety

In examining lipoprotein physiology we will first consider the characteristics of the lipid moiety of the lipoprotein. Then we will briefly examine the way in which lipids, which are water insoluble, exist in an aqueous medium such as plasma. Next, the more specific properties of each lipoprotein species will be examined, and finally we will discuss the dynamic aspects of lipid turnover. In considering the lipid moiety of the lipoprotein, we will discuss the properties of four different fats: fatty acids, triglycerides, phospholipids, and cholesterol.

Fatty Acids

Fatty acids are aliphatic monocarboxylic acids. That is, they have a hydrocarbon chain with a terminal carboxyl radicle:

$$CH_3—(CH_2)_n—COOH$$

n represents the number of (CH_2) groups in a particular fatty acid, usually an even number.

With minor exceptions, the naturally occurring fatty acids have an even number of carbon atoms. Depending upon the number of carbon atoms, the fatty acids have been divided into two groups: the "medium-" and "short-" chain fatty acids and the "long-chain" fatty acids. The former group consists of fatty acids having less than 12 carbons. Their importance will be indicated later, when it is pointed out that they are absorbed from the intestinal tract directly into the portal circulation. This has allowed them to be used therapeutically in certain disorders of fat absorption. The long-chain fatty acids, those with more than 12 carbons, are more common in nature.

Table 15-1. Classification of Lipoprotein Disorders

	Fredrickson's classification	*Lipoprotein affected*	*Synonym*
Lipoprotein excess			
Fat-induced	I	Chylomicron	Exogenous hyperlipemia
Fat-induced (predominantly)	V	Chylomicron and pre-β	Mixed hyperlipemia
Carbohydrate-induced	IV	Pre-β	Endogenous hyperlipemia
Carbohydrate-induced	III	Very low density β	
Uncertain	II	β	Familial, or essential hypercholesterolemia
Lipoprotein deficiency			
Tangier disease		α	
β-lipoproteinemia		β	Kornzweig-Basen syndrome

Table 15-2. Nature and Distribution of More Common Fatty Acids

Name	*No. of carbons*	*No. of double bonds*	*% of the fatty acid of adipose tissue*
Palmitic	16	0	25–40
Stearic	18	0	7
Palmitoleic	16	1	2–3
Oleic	18	1	50
Linoleic	18	2	10
Linolenic	18	3	7
Arachidonic	20	4	Trace

Fatty acids may be further divided according to the presence or absence of double bonds—i.e., "saturated," no double bonds (see above) or "unsaturated," one or more double bonds as in:

$$—CH_2—CH{=}CH—CH_2—$$

The nature and distribution of certain, more common, fatty acids is shown in Table 15-2.

Triglycerides

Fatty acids may be esterified with glycerol to form glycerides. Most commonly, these glycerol esters have three fatty acids—triglycerides (Fig. 15-1). However, glycerol esters may have one fatty acid (monoglyceride) or two fatty acids (diglyceride). The largest amount of glyceride in animal tissue and in the circulation is in the form of triglyceride. Although mono- and diglyceride are only present in trace amounts, they play vital roles as metabolic intermediates, and help to stabilize nonpolar lipids in polar media.

Phospholipids

Phospholipids have the general structure indicated in Figure 15-2. Some special phospholipids such as sphingomyelin do not conform to this formula. It should be noted that the phosphoryl group and the "X" radicle are hydrophilic (water-liking) while the remainder of the phospholipid is hydrophobic (water-disliking). This gives them the ability to stabilize the water-insoluble lipids, such as triglycerides, in aqueous media such as plasma.

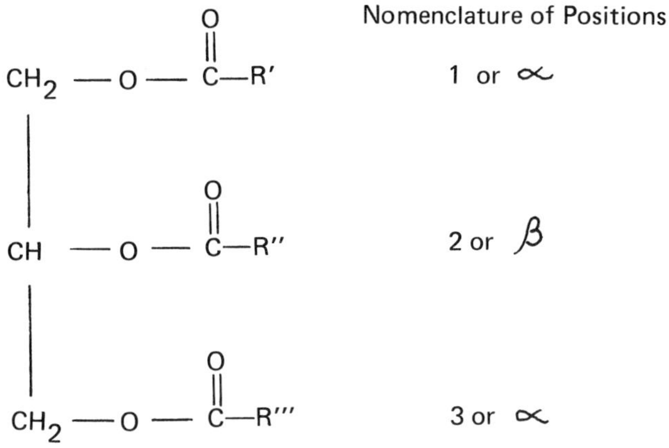

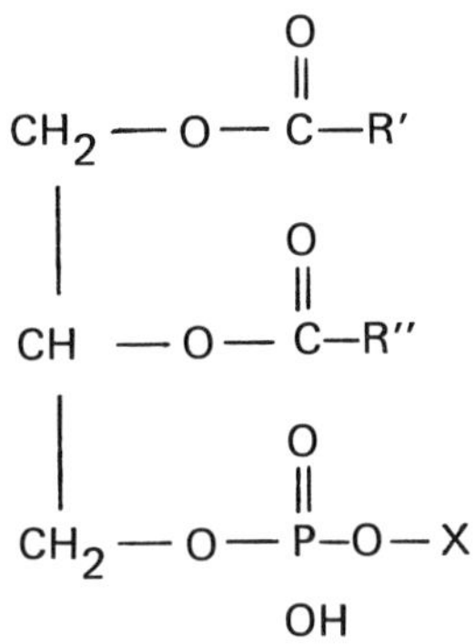

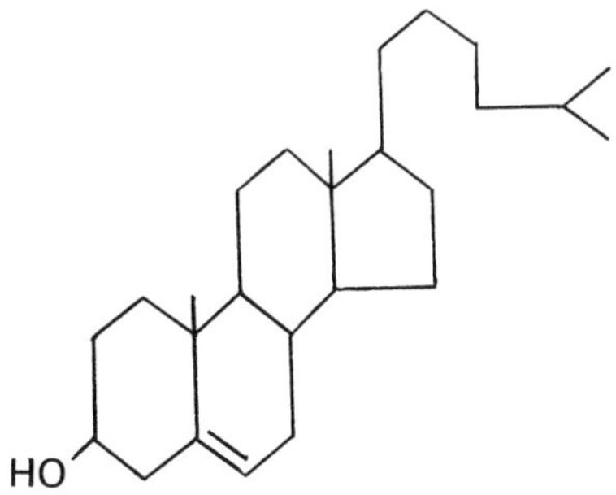

Fig. 15-1. General formula of a triglyceride. Two conventions of nomenclature to identify the glycerol carbons are indicated. *R*, fatty acid radicle.

Fig. 15-2. General structure of phospholipids. *R*, fatty acid radicle; *X*, nitrogen-containing base, such as (1) choline in phosphatidylcholine (lecithin), (2) ethanolamine in phosphatidylethanolamine, (3) serine in phosphatidylserine.

Fig. 15-3. Formula of cholesterol.

Cholesterol

For many years, because it was the only plasma lipid amenable to easy quantitation, cholesterol was considered to be the only lipid related to early atherogenesis. It is now recognized that other plasma lipids are of at least equal importance. Cholesterol's structure, like that of all steroids, is based on the cyclopentenoperhydrophenanthrene ring (Fig. 15-3). It may exist in the free form or with a fatty acid esterified to the HO radicle. The dynamics of cholesterol turnover in the body are beyond the scope of this chapter. Cholesterol in the circulation is derived mainly from that in the diet, and from that synthesized in the liver. It may be excreted as free cholesterol, or it may be converted to bile salt and excreted in this form.

Lipids in Polar Media

Triglycerides and cholesterol are insoluble in aqueous (polar, or electrically charged) media, such as plasma. They are therefore said to be hydrophobic. The reason for this hydrophobic nature is the presence, in the case of triglycerides, of three uncharged (nonpolar) fatty acids, and in the case of cholesterol, the nonpolar cyclopentenoperhydrophenanthrene ring. The monoglycerides, with only one fatty acid, are more polar than triglycerides. The phospholipids are also more polar than triglycerides, as a result of their phosphate groups and ethanolamine, serine, or choline radicles. In addition to their relative polarity, the monoglycerides and phospholipids are also amphiphilic (i.e., one end of the molecule is polar, the other is nonpolar). It has already been indicated (in Chapter 14 on Obesity) that the nonpolar nature of the triglyceride allows it to be stored in a stable form in adipose tissue. However, this creates problems for lipid transport in the circulation.

As plasma is polar, it cannot dissolve triglyceride. In order to keep the "solution" of lipid in plasma stable, the body has used a variety of amphiphilic materials (phospholipids and partial glycerides) and certain proteins to act as "bridges" between the plasma and the hydrophobic lipids. These all associate in specific proportions to form particles called "lipoproteins." There are at least four major classes of lipoproteins in the circulation. In each, the proportions of the specific components differ. When one measures plasma triglycerides, cholesterol, or phospholipid, one only measures the lipid moiety of the lipoprotein. Determination of the nature of the apoprotein (the protein moiety of the lipoprotein) is not yet a practically applicable procedure for the clinical laboratory. Certain properties of the whole lipoprotein particle, such as its electrophoretic mobility and density, can be examined more easily.

It has been indicated that a different lipoprotein is elevated in each type of hyperlipoproteinemia. Hence, the physician cannot diagnose and classify a hyperlipoproteinemic patient unless he characterizes the nature of the abnormal lipoprotein. To approach hyperlipoproteinemia knowing about the plasma lipid concentrations but not about specific lipoproteins would be similar to approaching leukocytosis knowing the total white cell count but not the differential count. Therefore, we shall now review the properties of the different lipoproteins, especially those properties that are most applicable to diagnostic procedures.

Specific Lipoproteins

There are four major classes of lipoproteins: the chylomicron, β-lipoprotein, pre-β-lipoprotein and α-lipoprotein. By strict definition there is a fifth circulating lipid-protein complex: the free fatty acid–albumin complex. However, by convention, the free fatty acid–albumin complex has been excluded from the term "lipoprotein." Each class of lipoprotein has fairly specific properties that are determined by the type and amount of lipid and protein in each, and by the size and density of the particles. By using a variety of chemical and physical techniques, one can separate lipoproteins from each other and characterize and quantitate them. The more commonly used of these techniques include: direct measurement of triglyceride, cholesterol, and phospholipid; electrophoresis; ultracentrifugation; and immunoelectrophoresis.

Chylomicrons

Chylomicrons, the largest lipoprotein particles, are produced by the intestinal mucosal cells during fat absorption. Of all the lipoproteins, they are the richest in triglyceride and the poorest in pro-

Table 15-3. Properties of Lipoproteins

	Chylomicron	*Pre-β-lipoprotein*	*β-Lipoprotein**	*α-Lipoprotein*
Synonym		Very low density lipoprotein	Low density lipoprotein	High density lipoprotein
Density	<0.95	0.93–1.006	1.006–1.063*	1.063–1.21
Sf	>400	>20	0–20	—
Composition (% dry wt)				
Triglyceride	80–95	50–80	10	Small amounts
Cholesterol	2–12	10–25	45	18
Phospholipid	3–15	10–25	22	30
Protein	0.5–2.5	2–13	20–25	45–55
Apoprotein	A, B, ?C	A, B, C	B	A
Size	0.1–5.0 μ		150 × 350 Å	300 × 50 Å

* This is the normal β-lipoprotein. In Type III hyperlipoproteinemia, the β-lipoprotein differs. Its characteristics are defined in the section on Type III hyperlipoproteinemia.

tein. Their exact composition is shown in Table 15-3. The chylomicrons are the largest of the lipoproteins, having a density of less than 0.95 (i.e., they will float through a medium with a density of 0.95 gm/ml). Another expression of the chylomicron's behavior in an ultracentrifugal field is the flotation rate. This is expressed as Svedberg units (Sf) and measures the rate at which particles float through a solution of NaCl of a density of 1.063 at 26° C. The Sf value is inversely related to the density. The flotation rate of the chylomicron is Sf > 400. Its size and charge is such that it has no mobility on electrophoresis (Fig. 15-4). Because of the difficulties created by the minute amounts of protein in the chylomicron, the apoprotein has been virtually unstudied.

Pre-β-Lipoprotein

The properties of the pre-β-lipoprotein (summarized in Table 15-3) differ only slightly from those of the chylomicron. The pre-β-lipoprotein is somewhat smaller, denser, poorer in triglyceride, and richer in protein. Because it migrates closer to the anode, or positive pole, on electrophoresis, than does the β-lipoprotein, it is called "prebeta." This lipoprotein is probably made in the liver. Its lipid is believed to be derived from lipid synthesized within the body. It is currently thought that the protein moiety of pre-β-lipoprotein is made up of several distinct apoproteins: that found in α-lipoprotein (the A-apoprotein), that found in the β-lipoprotein (the B-apoprotein), and at least two other peptides which are only partially defined.

β-Lipoprotein

This class of lipoprotein is the main carrier of cholesterol. As can be seen in Table 15-3, β-lipoprotein is smaller, poorer in lipid (especially triglyceride) and denser than the chylomicron or pre-β-lipoprotein. On electrophoresis the β-lipoprotein migrates just behind the pre-β-lipoprotein, in a position corresponding to that of the β-globulins. Once again, the liver appears to produce most of the β-lipoprotein. However, no one yet has demonstrated the direct release of β-lipoprotein, as such, from the liver. Rather, the β-lipoprotein seems to leave the liver as a part of pre-β-lipoprotein. It is then released into the circulation during the degradation of the pre-β-lipoprotein. It has also been shown recently that the intestine may make small amounts of β-lipoprotein. The protein moiety of β-lipoprotein is probably a single protein, called the B apoprotein.

α-Lipoprotein

The α-lipoprotein, the smallest, richest in protein, and most dense of the lipoproteins, is the

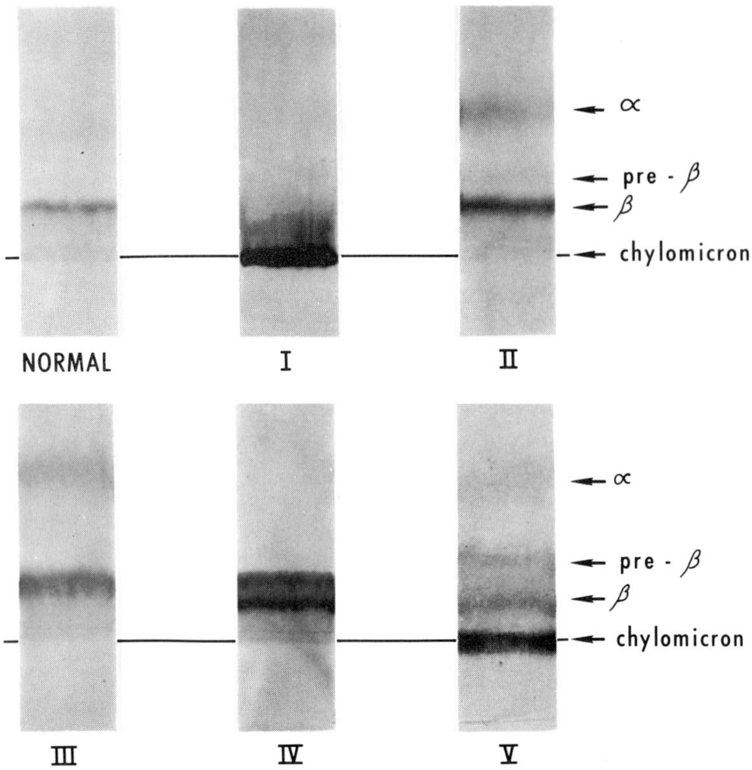

Fig. 15-4. Electrophoretic patterns in hyperlipoproteinemia. Six strips from the paper electrophoresis of fasting plasmas from patients with Types I–V hyperlipoproteinemia and plasma from a normal individual. The position of each lipoprotein is indicated on the *right*. Chylomicrons do not move from the origin (i.e., the point at which plasma sample was applied). In normal fasting plasma there are no chylomicrons, but the other lipoproteins may be seen.

most highly soluble in plasma. Its primary lipid constitutent is phospholipid. Because its density is greater than 1.063, it cannot be assigned a flotation rate (Sf) value. Its electrophoretic mobility is the same as that of α_1-globulin. It migrates ahead of pre-β-lipoprotein. It appears that the apoprotein of α-lipoprotein (A-apoprotein) is composed of several separate peptids.

Summary

Chylomicrons and pre-β-lipoproteins, the largest and lightest lipoproteins, are the primary carriers of triglyceride. The lipid in the chylomicron appears to originate mainly from the diet, and that in the pre-β-lipoprotein, from lipid synthesized within the body. β-Lipoprotein, the primary cholesterol carrier, is smaller, more polar, and denser than the chylomicron or pre-β-lipoprotein. α-Lipoprotein is the smallest, densest, poorest in lipid, and most polar.

Because all circulating lipid is carried as lipoprotein, we will henceforth speak of "hyperlipoproteinemia" rather than of "hyperlipemia." By now the reader should have realized that any given lipid may be carried by more than one type of lipoprotein. Thus hypertriglyceridemia may reflect hyperchylomicronemia, hyperpre-β-lipoproteinemia, or in certain rare circumstances, hyper-β-lipoproteinemia. Because the prognostic and therapeutic implications of each of these forms of hyperlipoproteinemia differ, the physician must measure not just plasma lipid levels but also must identify the specific lipoproteins in the circulation.

Lipoprotein Dynamics

If the amount of circulating lipoprotein is abnormal, one can conclude that homeostasis has broken down. The rate of supply to the bloodstream no longer equals the rate of removal. Hence, to understand the dyslipoproteinemias, one must understand the dynamics of lipoproteins (i.e., processes that govern supply and removal from the circulation).

Most is known about the lipoproteins that carry triglycerides, the chylomicron and pre-β-lipoprotein. Their lipid may be supplied from two sources: preformed lipid or lipid synthesized de novo. Preformed lipid is derived from fat in the diet (in Figure 15-5, a piece of butter); hence it is called "exogenous lipid." Lipid synthesized de novo from carbohydrate (in Figure 15-5, a lump of sugar) is made within the body, and hence called "endogenous lipid." The liver and adipose tissue are the tissues primarily responsible for de-novo synthesis. Lipid made and stored in adipose tissue as triglyceride may be released as free fatty acid after lipolysis. This free fatty acid may be carried to the liver and esterified there to form triglyceride.

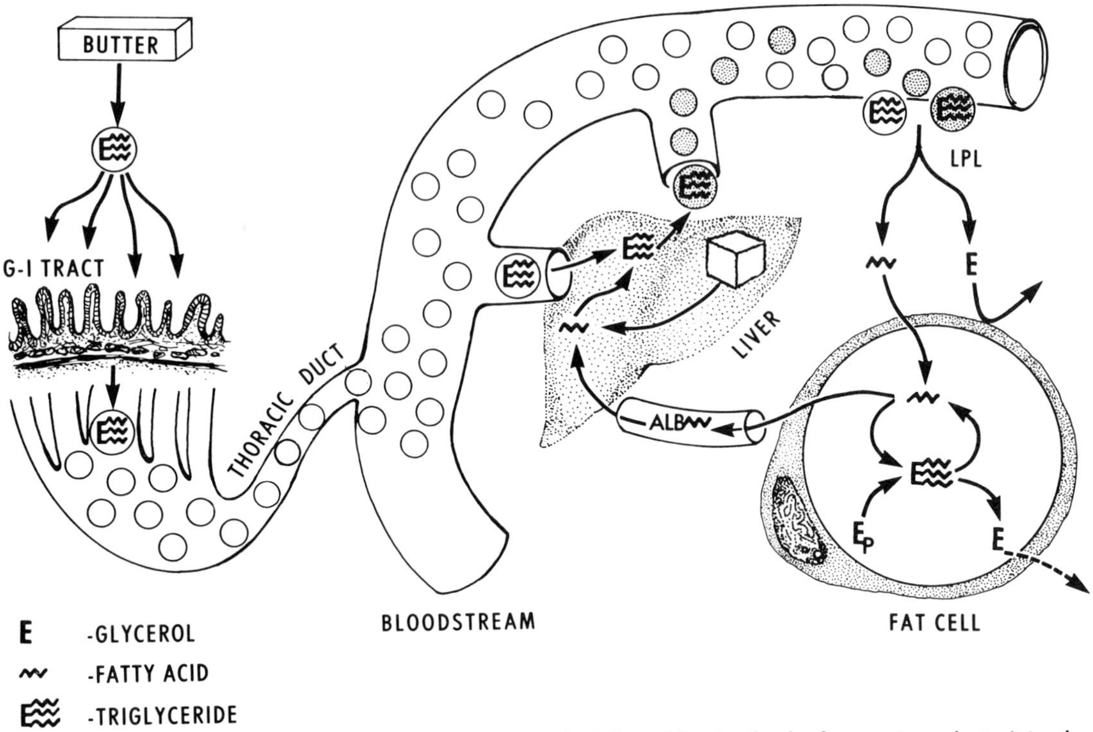

Fig. 15-5. Major pathways in turnover of triglycerides in the body. Fat (e.g., butter) is absorbed from the G.I. tract (*on left*) and passes as chylomicrons (*clear spheres*) via the thoracic duct into the circulation. The chylomicrons may then pass to the liver, or to peripheral tissues (e.g., the fat cell on the *right*). In the liver the chylomicron's triglyceride may be reprocessed into triglyceride in pre-β-lipoprotein (*shaded spheres*). The triglyceride of pre-β-lipoprotein may also be made from fatty acid. This fatty acid is derived either from plasma fatty acid (brought from the fat cell), or is made de novo from carbohydrate (the white sugar cube). The pre-β-lipoprotein is released from the liver and undergoes a fate similar to that of the chylomicron. Both are hydrolyzed by lipoprotein lipase (*LPL*). The resultant fatty acids enter the cell. There their fate is the same as that shown in Figure 13-2.

Fat Absorption (Exogenous Lipid)

Most natural dietary fat is long-chain triglyceride. Once ingested, it is mechanically emulsified in the stomach. This emulsified lipid then passes into the duodenum, where the triglycerides are partially hydrolyzed by pancreatic lipase to yield a mixture of fatty acids, glycerol, mono-, di-, and triglycerides. These, in the presence of bile salts, form micelles. The fat in these micelles is then absorbed by the intestinal mucosal cells. In the mucosal cell, the fatty acids and partial glycerides are reesterified to produce triglyceride. This triglyceride is then packaged with a small amount of phospholipid, cholesterol and protein, to form chylomicrons. The chylomicrons are extruded from the cell, picked up by the lacteals, delivered to the thoracic duct and carried to the bloodstream. If protein synthesis is blocked experimentally, or if the synthesis of apoprotein is defective as in a-β-lipoproteinemia, chylomicrons cannot be produced and fat absorption is impaired.

The absorption of synthetic medium-chain triglyceride differs from that of long-chain triglyceride. In the intestinal lumen, medium-chain triglyceride (MCT) is more readily hydrolyzed than long-chain triglyceride. It may be absorbed directly into the portal circulation without being incorporated into chylomicrons. Differences in digestion and absorption have therapeutic importance in certain disorders of fat absorption and of chylomicron synthesis and clearance.

De-Novo Lipoprotein Synthesis (Endogenous Lipid)

Another triglyceride-bearing lipoprotein (pre-β-lipoprotein) is primarily made in the liver. Its triglyceride may be directly synthesized there from carbohydrate precursors or may be made by esterifying fatty acid brought to it from adipose tissue. The latter fatty acids can also be synthesized de novo from carbohydrate precursors, but in this case in the adipose tissue. The triglyceride in pre-β-lipoprotein may also represent triglyceride which was originally in chylomicrons, but whose fatty acids have been reprocessed in the liver and incorporated into the pre-β-lipoprotein.

Triglyceride Uptake

Lipoprotein Lipase. Circulating triglyceride must be hydrolyzed to glycerol and fatty acid before it can be taken up by peripheral tissues. Although this hydrolytic (lipolytic) process appears to be important in most peripheral tissues, its role in regulating triglyceride uptake by the liver remains to be settled. For the sake of the present discussion, we shall take as an example of a peripheral tissue cell, the adipose tissue cell. The lipolytic process is catalyzed by an enzyme, lipoprotein lipase, whose nature and location is still uncertain. Some of this may be located on the fat cell membrane itself, some on the vascular endothelium.

An enzyme with properties similar to those of tissue lipoprotein lipase appears in plasma after administration of heparin (postheparin lipolytic activity—PHLA). It is not yet certain whether the enzyme in the plasma is the same as the tissue enzyme. However, because the PHLA is proportional to the activity of the tissue lipoprotein lipase, PHLA has been adopted as a measure of lipoprotein lipase activity. The physiologic role of heparin is also uncertain. Recently, patients have been described who have heparin-binding proteins in their plasma, a low PHLA and Type I or V hyperlipoproteinemia (forms of hyperlipoproteinemia associated with decreased lipoprotein lipase activity).

Intracellular Fate. Some of the adipose tissue cell metabolism has been reviewed in greater detail in Chapter 14 on Obesity. It may be recalled that this tissue has no glycerolkinase and hence cannot metabolize the glycerol released from circulating triglyceride by lipoprotein lipase. On the other hand, the fatty acids that are released from the triglyceride may enter the adipocyte and may be oxidized or may be esterified with α-glycerolphosphate. In the latter event, triglyceride is produced within the adipocyte. This triglyceride can be hydrolyzed by another lipase, hormone-sensitive lipase. The fatty acids produced from the adipose tissue triglyceride could then be oxidized, reesterified, or mobilized from the cell. If they leave the cell, these fatty acids, as indicated earlier, are bound to plasma albumin. One of the many possible fates of plasma fatty acids is to enter the liver, be reesterified and released as pre-β-lipoprotein.

Hyperlipoproteinemias

One cannot characterize a dyslipoproteinemia merely by examining the plasma lipid concentration. The lipoproteins must also be examined. Classification of the lipoproteins in plasma was a laborious task until Lees and Hatch described a paper electrophoretic method of separating them. This, and occasional ultracentrifugal characterization has allowed the hyperlipoproteinemias to be separated into five types. These five types are valuable, yet they are but guidelines. None is fixed, and with advancing knowledge they may be redefined or further subdivided. However, at present, this classification is the best approach to the hyperlipoproteinemias and has helped in gathering data on their natural history, predicting their course and complications, and planning rational therapy. Although the most straightforward way of discussing hyperlipoproteinemia is to list the types in numerical sequence, they may be more easily understood if they are divided on pathophysiological grounds—namely, fat-induced (Types I and V), carbohydrate-induced (Types IV and III), and unknown (Type II).

Clinical Features

Even when he does not have a sophisticated laboratory, the physician may predict, with reasonable accuracy, the type of hyperlipoproteinemia affecting his patient. Such "second guessing" depends on an accurate history and examination, particularly searching for features of hyperlipoproteinemia per se (xanthomas, lipemia retinalis, early corneal arcus, hepatosplenomegaly, and intermittent attacks of abdominal pain), for disorders that may underlie the hyperlipoproteinemia, listed here, and complications of the hyperlipoproteinemia.

1. Uncontrolled diabetes
2. Pancreatitis
3. Acute alcoholism
4. Hypothyroidism
5. Nephrotic syndrome
6. Biliary obstruction
7. Certain gestational hormones
8. Rarely multiple myeloma and other dysgammaglobulinemias
9. Idiopathic hypercalcemia of infancy
10. Lipoatrophy
11. Glycogen storage disease
12. Some lipidoses

Before deciding whether an individual patient has a primary or secondary hyperlipoproteinemia the physician must obtain a detailed family history and rule out any possible underlying disorders. Diabetes, latent or overt, is associated with certain hyperlipoproteinemias but not others. However, the presence, in one patient, of both diabetes and hyperlipoproteinemia does not necessarily mean that the former caused the latter. Although early atherosclerosis is a chief complication of hyperlipoproteinemias in general, the physician should be aware that this has not yet been observed in patients with Type I or Type V hyperlipoproteinemia. The doctor should now direct his attention to features influencing the hyperlipoproteinemia, such as obesity and weight changes, abnormal diets, and any medications.

Xanthomas. The xanthomas represent lipid deposition in the skin. They may be common to more than one type of hyperlipoproteinemia and therefore will be reviewed here as a group. With one exception (Type III hyperlipoproteinemia), they are not characteristic of any individual type of hyperlipoproteinemia.

1. The tuberous xanthoma is a soft, pedunculated, often cauliflower-like outgrowth which may be found over the knees, elbows, joints of the hand, or occasionally buttocks (Fig. 15–6).

2. The eruptive xanthoma is a yellow, papular lesion with a red, inflammatory, often painful, base which may be seen over the elbows, knees, thighs, or buttocks (Fig. 15–6).

3. The tuberoeruptive xanthoma has some characteristics of both tuberous and eruptive forms.

4. The tendon xanthoma is a hard, thickened lesion in the tendon. It is particularly common in the extensor tendons of the hand and in the Achilles tendons and is less frequent in other tendons (Fig. 15–7). It is detected by feeling or seeing it move under the skin when the tendon moves. If this movement is not observed, it may, at first glance, be confused with the swellings of arthritis.

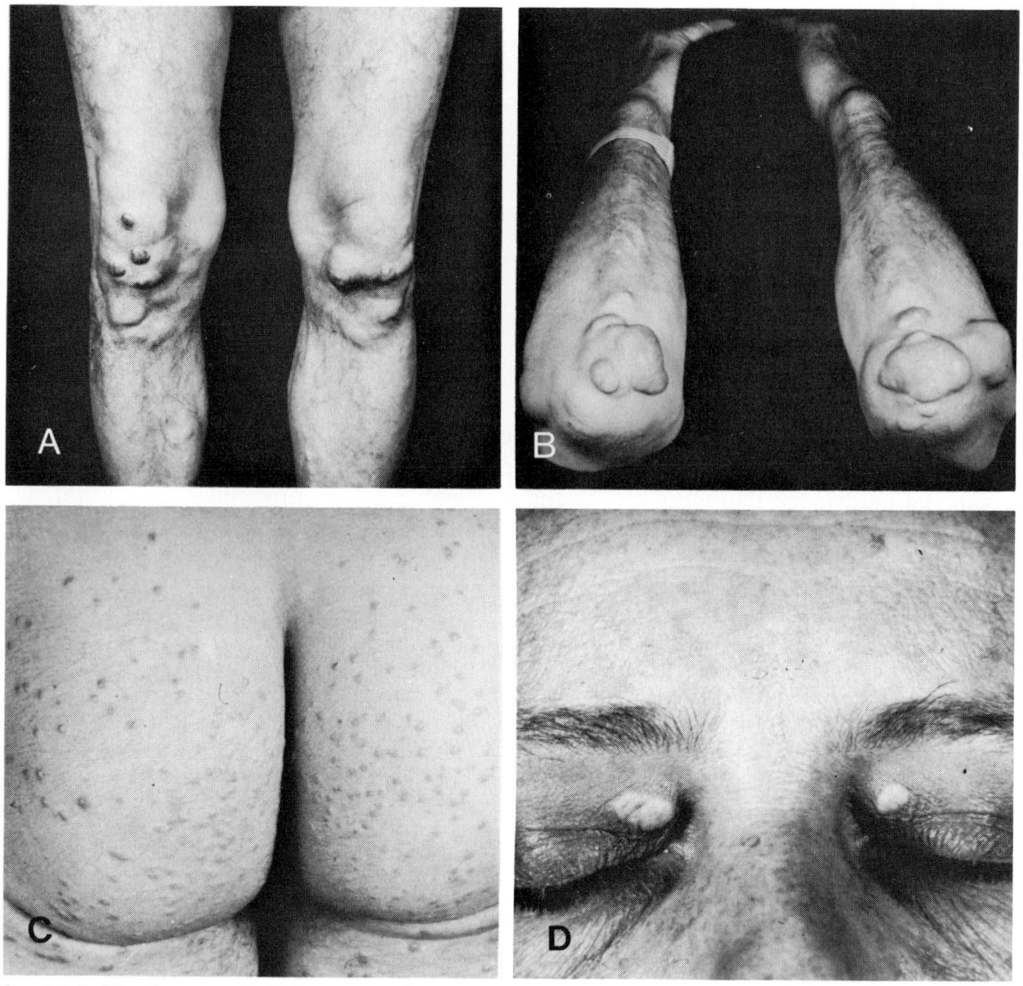

Fig. 15-6. Xanthomas. A. Tuberous xanthomas over the knees. **B.** Tuberous xanthomas over the elbows. **C.** Eruptive xanthomas over the buttocks. **D.** Periorbital xanthomas.

5. The palmar xanthoma occurs almost exclusively in Type III hyperlipoproteinemia. Although it is generally seen as flat, yellowish streaks in the palmar creases, it may also appear as flat, yellowish deposits elsewhere on the palm (Fig. 15-7).

6. The periorbital xanthoma is a soft, flat, yellow papule located around the eyes (Fig. 15–6). It has also been called the xanthelasma. About 50% of individuals with this have no measurable hyperlipoproteinemia.

Corneal arcus (*arcus senilis*). This has often mistakenly been assumed to indicate hyperlipoproteinemia. This is generally not the case unless the lesion occurs in young individuals.

Reticuloendothelial system. Lipid may deposit in the reticuloendothelial system, particularly in the liver, spleen, or bone marrow. This may lead to an enlargement of the liver or spleen. On histologic examination, these organs may contain many lipid-filled macrophages. The bone marrow may reveal foam cells. These findings are generally features in Types I, IV, and V hyperlipoproteinemias.

Lipemia retinalis. The retinal vessels have a pale, whitish appearance. This effect is produced because the vessels contain blood that looks like cream-of-tomato soup. The blood assumes this appearance because of very high levels of large, triglyceride-rich lipoproteins (i.e., chylomicrons and pre-β-lipo-

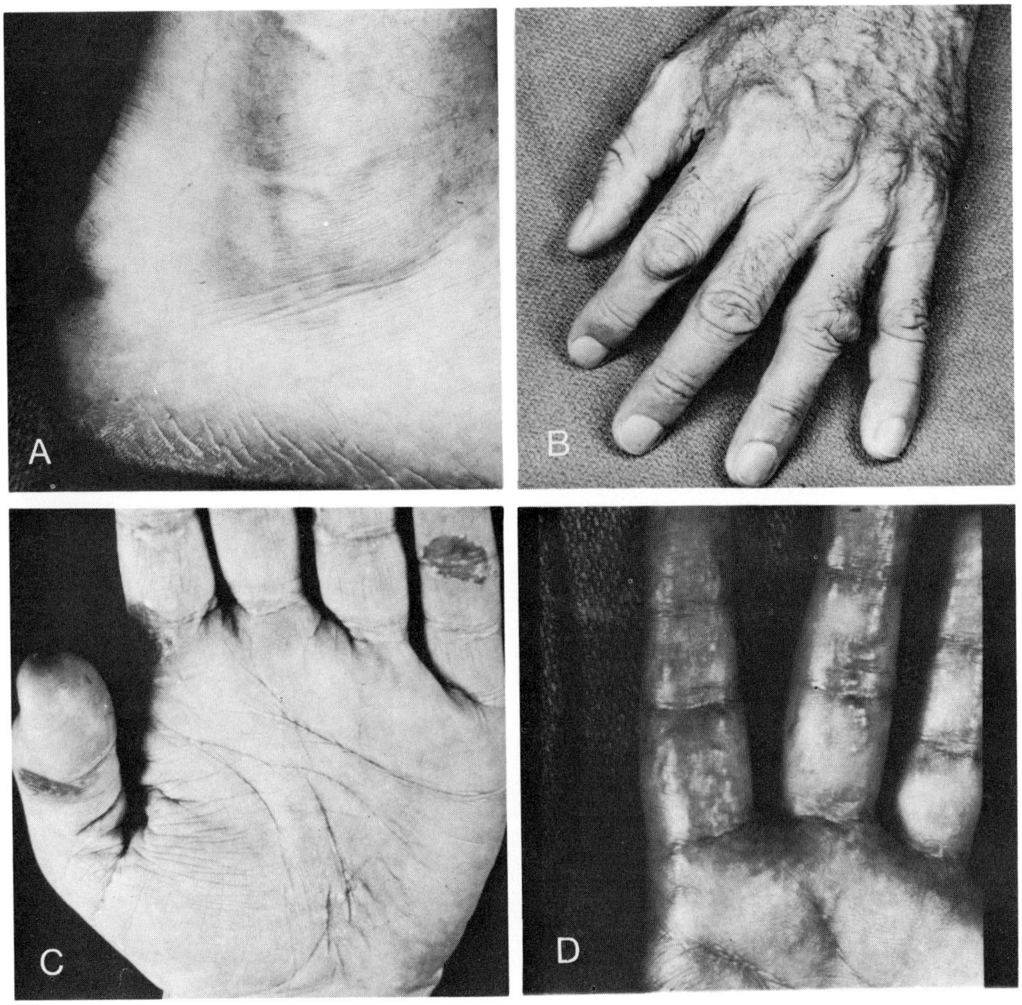

Fig. 15-7. Xanthomas. A. Tendon xanthomas in the Achilles tendon. **B.** Tendon xanthomas over metacarpophalangeal joints, and a tuberous xanthoma over the fourth proximal interphalangeal joint. **C.** Palmar xanthomas, white raised areas adjacent to skin creases. **D.** Palmar xanthomas predominantly on the fingers.

proteins). Therefore, lipemia retinalis is principally observed in Type I and Type V, and occasionally Type IV hyperlipoproteinemia.

By this time the physician should have a strong idea of the probable nature of the disorder. He can now begin to narrow it down by laboratory examination.

Laboratory Features

The laboratory examinations are of two kinds: those aimed at determining the type of hyperlipoproteinemia and those aimed at elucidating any underlying disorder or complication. This chapter will not review the latter group. However, this should not be taken to imply that the work-up is complete without it. Blood should not be drawn for lipoprotein examination unless the patient has been on a normal North American diet (carbohydrate, 40% of calories; fat, 40% of calories; protein, 20% of calories) for 1 week. If this precaution is neglected, significant abnormalities may be masked or mimicked. Because all postprandial plasma contains chylomicrons, blood should only be drawn after a 12- to 16-hour fast. To avoid alterations in the characteristics of the lipoproteins, it should be drawn into tubes containing 1 mg EDTA per milliliter of blood and the plasma should be kept at 4° C. Before sending the blood to the laboratory, the physician should inspect it visually. This office test is so important that no examination of hyperlipoproteinemia should be considered complete without it. On direct inspection, if the blood contains high amounts of large, triglyceride-rich lipoproteins, it may look like cream-of-tomato soup. By allowing it to stand for several hours in a refrigerator, one may determine whether the plasma is clear or lactescent and whether a layer of fat separates and floats to the surface of the plasma (Fig. 15-8). The significance of the appearance of the blood and plasma will be indicated when each of the different lipoproteinemias is discussed.

In the laboratory, the plasma should be assayed for cholesterol and triglyceride content and lipoprotein electrophoretic pattern. In addition, when a diagnosis of Type III hyperlipoproteinemia is suspected, the plasma must be characterized ultracentrifugally, to determine whether the density of the β-lipoprotein is less than 1.006. Occasionally, if one suspects Type I or V hyperlipoproteinemia, the plasma postheparin lipolytic activity should be determined. For this test, blood is drawn (into EDTA at 4° C) 10 minutes after an intravenous injection of heparin (0.1 mg/kg body weight). The postheparin plasma is then incubated with a standard emulsion of triglyceride and the rate of production of free fatty acid is measured.

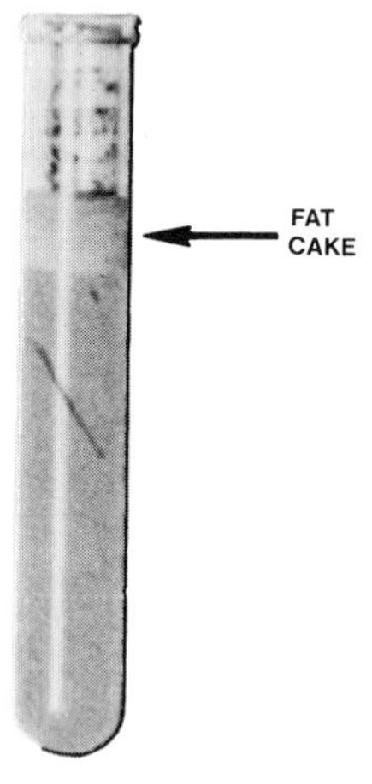

Fig. 15-8. Plasma from patient with hyperchylomicronemia. Note the fat cake, which floated to the surface after 2 hours.

Hyperlipoproteinemias Associated with Defects of Lipoprotein Lipase (Fat-Induced)

It has already been indicated that lipoprotein lipase appears to be involved with the clearance of triglyceride from the circulation. The activity of this enzyme in tissues appears to be mirrored by the PHLA of the plasma, although the exact relationship between these two is not clear. When lipoprotein lipase activity is low, triglyceride clearance from the circulation is impaired, and hence chylomicrons (which are so rich in triglyceride) accumulate in the circulation. This hyperchylomicronemia has been called Type I hyperlipoproteinemia by Fredrickson. Chylomicrons do not appear in the plasma if the individual is not absorbing fat. Hence this type of hyperlipoproteinemia disappears when fat is removed from the diet and reappears when it is consumed again. Thus Type I hyperlipoproteinemia has also been called fat-induced. Normal individuals may have chylomicrons in their blood after fat meals, but unless lipid clearance is impaired the chylomicrons disappear within 12 hours.

If triglyceride clearance is impaired, pre-β-lipoprotein, the second triglyceride-rich lipoprotein, may occasionally be elevated together with the chylomicron. This is not to say that elevated pre-β-lipoprotein levels always mean decreased lipoprotein lipase activity; indeed, they usually do not (see Type IV hyperlipoproteinemia). However, in one form of hyperlipoproteinemia, Type V, both chylomicrons and pre-β-lipoproteins are elevated in the plasma. No agreement has been reached about the PHLA in Type V hyperlipoproteinemia; however, fat tolerance is impaired. Because the pre-β-lipoproteins carry triglyceride generally thought to be endogenous in origin, and chylomicrons carry triglyceride generally thought to be derived from the diet, this has been called mixed hyperlipoproteinemia. However, the predominant dietary behavior is like that of a fat-induced hyperlipoproteinemia.

Type I (Hyperchylomicronemia)

Clinical Features. This disorder generally begins in infancy but may not be discovered until later in life. Although it may be found accidentally, when someone notes that the patient's plasma is grossly lipemic, the patient may come to the doctor's attention during an attack of acute abdominal pain. This pain frequently mimics acute pancreatitis, but unless there is concomitant pancreatitis, the serum amylase is not elevated and there are no other manifestations of pancreatic disease. The patient may give a history of recurrent attacks of abdominal pain with no apparent cause for its onset or remission. The pain occurs more frequently after a high-fat diet but can come on without an acute fat load.

Patients with Type I hyperlipoproteinemia may also display lipemia retinalis, xanthomas (usually eruptive), hepatomegaly, and splenomegaly. The liver, spleen, and bone marrow may contain lipid-filled macrophages. In Type I hyperlipoproteinemia, the incidence of carbohydrate intolerance is not greater than that in the general population. Although one generally associates hyperlipoproteinemia with early atherosclerosis, these disorders were not found together in the few well-documented patients with Type I disease.

Laboratory Manifestations. These, in the case of Type I hyperlipoproteinemia, can all be traced back to the presence of chylomicrons in fasting plasma. The large, very low density lipoproteins may impart a cream-of-tomato soup appearance to the blood and a milky appearance to the plasma. After standing a few hours at 4° C, they will float to the surface of the plasma, forming a fat cake (Fig. 15-8). On electrophoresis a lipid-staining band remains at the point of application —i.e., the origin (Fig. 15-4). Because chylomicrons are composed almost entirely of triglyceride, the plasma triglycerides will be very high, and the cholesterol will remain normal or only slightly elevated. The plasma PHLA will be low or absent. If fat is eliminated from the diet, the hyperchylomicronemia will disappear.

Causes. All hyperlipoproteinemias can be divided into two categories based upon their cause: primary or secondary.

1. Primary Type I hyperlipoproteinemia is not associated with any known underlying disorder. There may be a family history of this disturbance of lipid metabolism, and determinations of PHLA in relatives may detect individals with low activity of this enzyme. The exact pattern of inheritance has not been worked out.

2. Secondary Type I hyperlipoproteinemia may be associated with alcoholism, uncontrolled diabetes, acute pancreatitis, or rarely, certain gammaglobulinopathies. In the uncontrolled diabetic the hyperchylomicronemia disappears when the diabetes is brought under control. When it occurs with acute pancreatitis, it is difficult to decide which disorder is primary and which is secondary. Sometimes the matter cannot be settled until the patient recovers from the pancreatitis: If the hyperchylomicronemia then clears, it was probably secondary. Some of those rare patients with Type I hyperlipoproteinemia associated with gammaglobulinopathies have been observed to have a heparin-binding protein in their plasma. It has been postulated that the plasma of these patients binds endogenous heparin, thus producing a deficit in lipoprotein lipase. In these patients, the hyperlipoproteinemia clears when the gammaglobulinopathy abates.

In summary, the characteristics of Type I hyperlipoproteinemia are:

Elevation of chylomicrons
Triglycerides greatly increased
Cholesterol normal or slightly increased
PHLA decreased or absent
Onset in childhood
Xanthomas eruptive type
Hepatosplenomegaly
Abdominal pain
No early atherosclerosis
No carbohydrate intolerance
Fat-induced

Type V (Hyperchylomicronemia and Hyperpre-β-Liproproteinemia)

Clinical and Laboratory Manifestations. Clinically, Type V hyperlipoproteinemia resembles Type I except that it begins in the late teens and is frequently associated with carbohydrate intolerance. The laboratory manifestations also resemble Type I, except that pre-β-lipoproteins, as well as chylomicrons, are elevated (Fig. 15-4). This type of hyperlipoproteinemia best illustrates why it is necessary to obtain blood from patients only when they have been on a normal diet and have been fasting for 12–16 hours. If a patient with Type I hyperlipoproteinemia ingests a high-carbohydrate diet before the sample is taken, his plasma will have pre-β-lipoproteins in addition to chylomicrons. If a patient with Type IV hyperlipoproteinemia (hyperpre-β-lipoproteinemia) has been on a high-fat diet or has not been fasting, his plasma will contain chylomicrons in addition to pre-β-lipoproteins. The controversy over the nature of PHLA in Type V hyperlipoproteinemia has not yet been settled.

Causes. This disorder may be primary or secondary. Because Type V hyperlipoproteinemia is so rare, there are no good data on the patterns of inheritance. Secondary Type V hyperlipoproteinemia may appear in association with the same disorders which underlie secondary Type I—alcoholism, uncontrolled diabetes, acute pancreatitis, and in rare instances, certain gammaglobulinopathies.

In summary, the characteristics of Type V hyperlipoproteinemia are:

Elevation of chylomicrons and pre-β-lipoproteins
Triglycerides greatly increased
Cholesterol normal or slightly increased
PHLA ? (See text)
Onset in early teens
Xanthomas eruptive type
Hepatosplenomegaly
Abdominal pain
No early atherosclerosis
Frequent carbohydrate intolerance
Fat-induced

Carbohydrate-Induced Hyperlipoproteinemias

These hyperlipoproteinemias get worse when carbohydrate is ingested, and improve when carbohydrate is removed from the diet. Because the fatty acid portion of the circulating triglyceride is made up in the body de novo from carbohydrate, this group of hyperlipoproteinemias has been called endogenous, as opposed to the fat-induced or exogenous group. The carbohydrate-induced hyperlipoproteinemias include Types III and IV.

One can only understand the development of these hyperlipoproteinemias by piecing together data from studies both on humans and on animals. The fatty acids, which are later incorporated into circulating triglycerides, may be made either in the liver or in adipose tissue. If the fatty acids have been made in adipose tissue, they are released and carried, bound to albumin, to the liver. There these fatty acids, together with those made in the liver, are esterified to form triglyceride. This triglyceride is then "packaged" into pre-β-lipoprotein and released into the circulation. For a long time the carbohydrate-induced hyperlipoproteinemias have been regarded as being due to overproduction of lipoprotein. However, some recent evidence suggests that lipoprotein clearance may also be impaired.

Type IV (Hyperpre-β-Lipoproteinemia)

Clinical Features. Patients with the Type IV disorder, together with those with Type II, constitute the largest group of individuals with hyperlipoproteinemia in whom there is an association with early atherosclerosis. A recent study of lipoprotein patterns in patients with coronary vascular disease demonstrated that 50% of the hyperlipoproteinemics had Type IV disease and 50% had Type II. Frequently patients with Type IV hyperlipoproteinemia have no xanthomas. When xanthomas are present, one sees the eruptive form most frequently. On rare occasions patients with Type IV hyperlipoproteinemia may also have hepatosplenomegaly, lipemia retinalis, and even attacks of abdominal pain. In our experience, 80% of patients with Type IV hyperlipoproteinemia have abnormal carbohydrate tolerance. Frequently they also have hyperuricemia and occasionally, full-blown gout.

Laboratory Manifestations. The laboratory findings in Type IV hyperlipoproteinemia may be related to the elevated levels of circulating pre-β-lipoprotein. These large, very low density particles may make the plasma lactescent. However, in contrast to Types I and V, when the plasma is allowed to stand, the pre-β-lipoproteins rarely rise to form a fat cake at the top of the tube. Because the pre-β-lipoprotein is rich in triglyceride, the plasma triglycerides are elevated but the cholesterol is normal or only slightly increased. The PHLA is normal. Lipoprotein electrophoresis reveals pre-β-lipoprotein (Fig. 15-4). All of these changes decrease, or disappear when carbohydrate is removed from the diet.

Causes. Type IV hyperlipoproteinemia may be primary or secondary. The mode of inheritance of the primary (familial) form of Type IV hyperlipoproteinemia has not yet been fully worked out. Frequently other members of the family may be affected, but only one parent need have the disorder. The secondary form of Type IV hyperlipoproteinemia may be associated with the following disease:

1. Pancreatitis
2. Uncontrolled diabetes
3. Alcoholism
4. Idiopathic hypercalcemia
5. Certain dysglobulinemias
6. Lipoatrophic diabetes
7. Gaucher's disease
8. Niemann-Pick's disease
9. Hypothyroidism
10. Nephrotic syndrome
11. Renal failure
12. Glycogen storage disease
13. Progesterone, alone or in combination with estrogens
14. Pregnancy
15. Idiopathic hypercalcemia of infancy

In those patients who have Type IV hyperlipoproteinemia and diabetes, the diabetes, if uncontrolled, may underlie Type IV hyperlipoproteinemia. In other instances the Type IV hyperlipoproteinemia may persist even when the diabetes is brought into good control. In this latter circumstance the diabetes is probably not the cause of the hyperlipoproteinemia. In summary the characteristics of Type IV hyperlipoproteinemia are:

Elevation of pre-β-lipoprotein
Plasma turbid, no fat cake on standing
Triglycerides greatly increased
Cholesterol increased
PHLA normal
Early atherosclerosis
Frequent carbohydrate intolerance
Carbohydrate-induced

Type III Hyperlipoproteinemia

The plasma of patients with Type III hyperlipoproteinemia contains an unusual, very low density ($d < 1.006$) β-liproprotein (the normal β-lipoprotein has a density greater than 1.006). These two β-lipoproteins can be differentiated with the ultracentrifuge. After centrifuging the plasma at 100,000 $\times$ g for 16 hours, the normal ($d > 1.006$) β-lipoprotein will sediment (Fig. 15-9), whereas the very low density ($d < 1.006$) β-lipoprotein will float (Fig. 15-10). The β-lipoprotein in Type III hyperlipoproteinemia also differs from normal in its electrophoretic mobility; it migrates as a broad band that extends uniformly between the areas normally occupied by the pre-β and the β-lipoprotein (Fig. 15-5).

This very low density, broad-band β-lipoprotein is thought to be derived from pre-β-lipoprotein. The reader will recall that, among its other apoproteins, the pre-β-lipoprotein had A-apoprotein. Recent evidence suggests that the $d < 1.006$ β-lipoprotein is pre-β-lipoprotein which lacks A-apoprotein. The plasma from patients who have no A-apoprotein (Tangiers disease) has no pre-β-lipoprotein but does have a broad, $d < 1.006$ β-lipoprotein. Thus, one may speculate that patients with Type III hyperlipoproteinemia can break down pre-β-lipoprotein part way—i. e., they are able to remove the A-apoprotein but not more. This, together with the carbohydrate-inducible behavior of Type III hyperlipoproteinemia, would

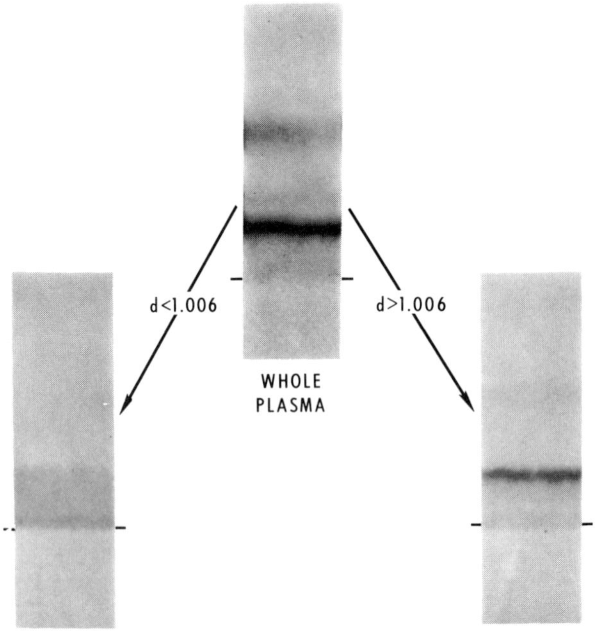

Fig. 15-9. Electrophoretic strip of normal whole plasma (Fig. 15-4) separated by ultracentrifugation into fractions. Density of one fraction is <1.006 (*lower left*) and the other, >1.006 (*lower right*). Note that the β-lipoprotein appears in the heavier fraction (d $>$ 1.006).

suggest some relation between it and Type IV hyperlipoproteinemia.

Clinical Features. Type III hyperlipoproteinemia manifests itself by xanthomas, early atherosclerosis and, in about 60% of patients, carbohydrate intolerance. Xanthomas may provide an important diagnostic clue. In addition to the xanthomas seen in other types of hyperlipoproteinemia, Type III patients may have palmar xanthomas (Fig. 15-7), lesions which are not typical of any other primary type of hyperlipoproteinemia.

Laboratory Manifestations. The laboratory findings in Type III hyperlipoproteinemia are related to the very low density β-lipoprotein. It carries cholesterol, as does the normal β-lipoprotein. However, it is also rich in triglyceride. Thus, the plasma levels of both triglyceride and cholesterol are elevated. Because the β-lipoprotein in Type III hyperlipoproteinemia is very low in density and large in size, the plasma may appear turbid. However, it does not develop a fat cake on standing. Electrophoresis of the plasma reveals a broad β-band (Fig. 15-5). Investigation of Type III hyperlipoproteinemia is not complete until one determines the density of the β-lipoprotein on the ultracentifuge. Although the xanthomas may disappear and the plasma triglyceride and cholesterol levels return to normal following carbohydrate restriction, the β-lipoprotein still has its unique very low density.

Causes. At the University of Toronto we have encountered only one patient with secondary Type III hyperlipoproteinemia; in her, the disorder was associated with myxedema and cleared on treatment. The mode of inheritance of primary Type III hyperlipoproteinemia is gradually being elucidated. We have examined the members of four generations of one family in our laboratory: Type III hyperlipoproteinemia was present in the index patient; some of her siblings, and members

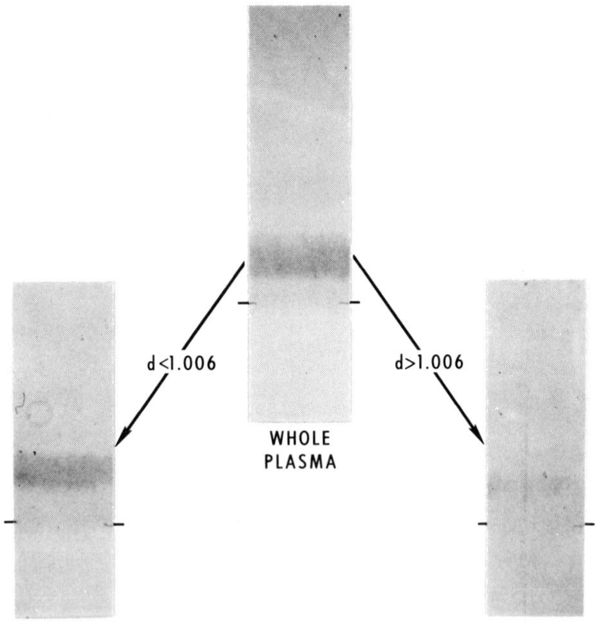

Fig. 15-10. Electrophoretic strip of plasma from patient with Type III hyperlipoproteinemia. Plasma has been separated by ultracentrifugation into fractions with density <1.006 (*left*) and with density >1.006 (*right*). Note that whole plasma has a "broad" β band. This *abnormal* β-lipoprotein appears in the lighter fraction (d $<$ 1.006).

of both the maternal and paternal sides of her family had Type IV hyperlipoproteinemia. This pattern suggests that the same genes may be responsible for both Types IV and III hyperlipoproteinemia; Type IV possibly representing the heterozygous state, and Type III, a homozygous state. In summary, the characteristics of Type III are:

Elevation of abnormal β-lipoprotein ($d < 1.006$)
Triglycerides increased
Cholesterol increased
PHLA normal
Xanthomas: palmar almost diagnostic
Early atherosclerosis
Frequent carbohydrate intolerance
Carbohydrate-induced

Hyperlipoproteinemia of Undetermined Nature

Type II Hyperlipoproteinemia

Because it displays no clear-cut response to dietary manipulation, in contrast to the other types of hyperlipoproteinemia, Type II hyperlipoproteinemia is classified as being of undetermined nature. This type of hyperlipoproteinemia has also been known as essential familial hypercholesterolemia, and is characterized by an elevation of β-lipoprotein of normal density—i.e., between 1.006 and 1.021 (Fig. 15-9). Because it is a main lipid constituent, considerable attention has been focused on cholesterol dynamics. Unfortunately, this has failed to yield much information about the cause of Type II hyperlipoproteinemia. The primary defect may lie, not in the lipid moiety, but in the apoprotein of the β-lipoprotein. However, until recently it has been impossible to obtain pure, undenatured B-apoprotein. At present, it appears that B-apoprotein is the same in normal individuals and in those with Type II hyperlipoproteinemia.

Clinical Features. Type II hyperlipoproteinemia may appear in childhood, and occasionally even at birth. The patients may have evidence of premature atherosclerosis. Of all patients with hyperlipoproteinemia, those with Type II have the most florid and varied xanthomas, especially the tendinous, tuberous and periorbital forms. Carbohydrate intolerance is not prominent, occurring in only 10% of Type II patients. In summary, the presence of tendon xanthomas and a strong family history of atherosclerosis should suggest the possibility of Type II hyperlipoproteinemia.

Laboratory Manifestations. The characteristic findings of Type II hyperlipoproteinemia are related to the presence of β-lipoprotein. Because this lipoprotein is smaller, denser, and more polar than those previously described, the plasma is clear. As β-lipoprotein carries cholesterol primarily, this disorder is characterized by very high plasma cholesterol levels, but normal or minimally elevated triglycerides. Electrophoresis of the plasma shows a sharp β-lipoprotein band (Fig. 15-4). Ultracentrifugation, though not generally necessary to reach the diagnosis, shows that the β-lipoprotein has a density greater than 1.006 (Fig. 15-9).

Causes. Primary (familial) Type II hyperlipoproteinemia is not associated with any underlying disorders. Generally Type II hyperlipoproteinemia is also found in at least one of the patient's parents. If both parents have the disorder, the offspring may manifest Type II hyperlipoproteinemia even more strongly and may have severe vascular complications in early childhood. Secondary Type II hyperlipoproteinemia is most frequently seen in association with hypothyroidism, nephrotic syndrome, and obstructive biliary disease. On rare occasions it has been associated with some dysgammaglobulinemias. In summary, the characteristics of Type II hyperlipoproteinemia are:

Elevation of β-lipoprotein ($d > 1.006$)
Plasma clear
Triglycerides normal or slightly increased
Cholesterol greatly increased
PHLA normal
Xanthomas: especially tendinous, tuberous, and periorbital
Early atherosclerosis
No predisposition to carbohydrate intolerance
No dietary pattern

Hypolipoproteinemias

Tangier Disease (Deficiency of α-Lipoprotein)

This exceedingly rare disorder, first observed in families from Tangier Island in Chesapeake Bay, shows, as its hallmark, the massive deposition of lipid in the reticuloendothelial system. These patients may have huge, orange tonsils, splenomegaly, and lymphadenopathy. Lipid may also be deposited in the skin, cornea, and blood vessels. Fat absorption from the gastrointestinal tract is normal, although transport of the fat through the circulation may be defective. The plasma level of cholesterol is low, and that of triglyceride slightly elevated. On electrophoresis, in addition to the absence of α-lipoprotein, one sees a broad β-lipoprotein band and no pre-β-lipoprotein. The broad β-lipoprotein has a density less than 1.006, and thus resembles the very low density β-lipoprotein observed in Type III hyperlipoproteinemia. Recently, it has been suggested that patients with Tangier disease may not have a total absence of α-lipoprotein but may have very low levels of immunologically different α-lipoprotein.

A β-Lipoproteinemia (Kornzweig-Basen Syndrome)

Patients with this rare disorder appear to be incapable of making B-apoprotein. Hence they have no β-lipoprotein in their circulation. Because β-lipoprotein contributes to chylomicron formation, these patients may have impaired lipid absorption. They also have acanthocytosis (crenated red blood cells) and neurologic deficits, specifically signs of cerebellar and posterolateral column degeneration, muscular weakness, and retinal pigment degeneration.

Treatment of Patients with Hyperlipoproteinemias

Diet

Diet is the mainstay of therapy. Other treatment is merely adjunctive. The general dietary principles are outlined here, but each patient's diet should be tailored individually. The distribution of calories, to be described, may have to be adjusted for the actual calorie content of the diet—e.g., it may be impossible to restrict fat to 10% of the total calorie content when the diet contains only 1,000 kcal. Although the practical design of the diet should be drawn up in cooperation with a dietitian, two guiding principles should be employed: weight reduction, and restriction of those constituents that aggravate the particular type of hyperlipoproteinemia. Weight reduction by itself will ameliorate most hyperlipoproteinemias. In the fat-induced hyperlipoproteinemias (Types I and V), fat intake must be severely curtailed. One should aim at a diet with 10–15% of the calories derived from fat. Obviously, under these circumstances, carbohydrate intake may have to be increased to supply the patient's total calorie needs. Such an increase in carbohydrate intake in individuals with Type V hyperlipoproteinemia may result in an increase in pre-β-lipoproteins, thereby preventing the complete return of triglyceride to normal levels.

Patients with either of the fat-induced hyperlipoproteinemias should avoid alcohol. In the carbohydrate-induced hyperlipoproteinemias (Types III and IV), in addition to aiming at weight loss, the diet should minimize carbohydrate intake. There is some evidence that patients ingesting simple sugars, especially those containing fructose (e.g., sucrose) have higher plasma triglyceride levels than those ingesting equicaloric amounts of polysaccharides (e.g., starch). Therefore, the carbohydrates should be supplied largely as polysaccharides. In general, not more than 30% of the total calories should come from carbohydrates. When this restriction is applied, the balance of the calories may have to come from fat, 60% of which should be polyunsaturated fat. Again, alcohol should be avoided. The carbohydrate-induced hyperlipoproteinemias thus represent forms of hyperlipoproteinemia for which the diet need not contain restricted amounts of fat. Indeed, in this large group of hyperlipoproteinemias, restricting fat and supplying the balance of calories with carbohydrate may be harmful. This reemphasizes one of the misconceptions outlined earlier in the chapter.

The dietary management of Type II hyperlipoproteinemia is the most difficult and least satisfactory of all. If fat intake is reduced to 30 gm (of which 20 gm are polyunsaturated) and cholesterol intake is reduced below 300 mg, one may hope for a lowering of plasma cholesterol by 20–25%.

Ancillary Therapeutic Measures

Because dietary management alone frequently corrects the hyperlipoproteinemia, it should be tried before any form of drug therapy is attempted. Even when drugs are added, the patient should continue his diet.

Cholestyramine (*Questran*)

This agent binds bile salts and prevents their reabsorption, thereby interrupting the enterohepatic cycle and producing bile-salt deficiency. This deficiency in turn leads to: (1) impaired fat absorption and (2) increased conversion of cholesterol to bile salts and hence increased cholesterol excretion. The same rationale underlies ileal bypass operations, which had been suggested because bile salts are reabsorbed in the ileum. The operation has lost favor, but cholestyramine is still used. Although this drug lowers plasma lipids, the patient generally does not accept it. The dose (12–24 gm/day) is bulky and bad-tasting and produces some intestinal discomfort. Patients with asymptomatic hyperlipoproteinemia often find this treatment worse than their disease.

Nicotinic Acid

This drug, given in a dose of 1.5–6 gm/day, appears to decrease cholesterol synthesis and increase cholesterol excretion. It also decreases hepatic triglyceride synthesis and decreases the mobilization of free fatty acids from adipose tissue. Though often effective, it produces distressing side effects: flushing and burning skin, itching, and gastrointestinal upset.

Dextrothyroxine

This drug is given in a dose of 4–8 mg/day. Contrary to early hopes, its action in increasing cholesterol catabolism does not seem to be divorced from its effect on metabolic rate. Increased metabolism is, of course, undesirable in patients with coronary vascular disease.

Chlorphenoxyisobutyric Acid (*CPIB, Atromid-S, Clofibrate*)

This agent is given in a dose of 500 mg 4 times a day. At the moment it appears to be the most promising drug and has no major side effects. Two of the many suggested modes of action are: (1) a block in cholesterol synthesis at a point beyond β-hydroxymethylglutaryl CoA, and (2) partial displacement of thyroxine from its plasma-binding protein. Because CPIB appears to make the individual more sensitive to the coumarin anticoagulants, in patients on such treatment, prothrombin times should be measured repeatedly and anticoagulant doses appropriately adjusted. Occasionally, patients taking CPIB may develop muscle pain, elevation of serum glutamic-oxaloacetic transaminase, glutamic-pyruvic transaminase, and creatine phosphokinase. The syndrome clears if the drug is stopped. CPIB is effective in Types III and IV hyperlipoproteinemia. Unfortunately, it is only slightly effective in Type II hyperlipoproteinemia, the type most resistant to dietary measures. Types I and V hyperlipoproteinemia do not respond to CPIB.

Summary

Hyperlipoproteinemia is not one disorder but a family of disorders. At present five types of hyperlipoproteinemia are recognized. However, this classification may change at any time. Recognition of these types has allowed the adoption of a more intelligent approach to diagnosis, prognosis, and management, and the discard of some previous misconceptions. These misconceptions include: (1) "A normal plasma cholesterol rules out hyperlipoproteinemia." (2) "All hyperlipoproteinemia is associated with early atherosclerosis." (3) "All hyperlipoproteinemia should be treated by a low-fat, high-carbohydrate diet." When a physician understands the lipoprotein abnormalities, he can make an intelligent guess, even without sophisticated laboratory tools, about the type of disorder affecting a specific patient. On the basis of family history, evidence of early atherosclerosis, diabetes, xanthomas, lipemia retinalis, abdominal pain, and *the appearance of the fasting plasma,* he can frequently reach a reasonably accurate diagnosis.

If he is to provide effective therapy, the physician must know which type of hyperlipoproteinemia the patient has. This will determine the diet he prescribes and will allow him to predict the efficacy of pharmacologic agents. If an accurate diagnosis cannot be reached, he should prescribe a 2-week trial of diet, bearing in mind that the two most common hyperlipoproteinemias are Types II and IV. Type IV should respond to carbohydrate restriction within this period. It must be reemphasized that diet is the keystone of therapy and all else is ancillary. Despite growing knowledge concerning lipid transport in the circulation and the association of certain hyperlipoproteinemias with atherosclerosis, the reader should recognize that there is, as yet, no proof that the treatment of hyperlipoproteinemia will prevent or slow the progress of atherogenesis.

Diagnosis of Hyperlipoproteinemias

The diagnosis is made on the results of:

1. Inspection of blood and serum obtained after a 12-hour fast
2. Serum cholesterol and triglyceride determinations
3. Serum lipoprotein electrophoresis

The results are interpreted according to the criteria outlined in Table 15-4.

Table 15-4. Diagnostic Criteria in Hyperlipoproteinemia

Class	*Lipoprotein elevation*	*Plasma appearance*	*Triglyceride**	*Cholesterol†*
Fat-induced				
Type I	Chylomicron	Milky with fat cake	Very high	Normal or slight increase
Type V	Chylomicron and pre-β	Milky with fat cake	Very high	Normal or slight increase
Carbohydrate-induced				
Type IV	Pre-β	Turbid	High	Slight increase
Type III	Very low density, "broad" β	Turbid	High	High
Unknown				
Type II	Normal β	Clear	Normal	High

* Laboratory values for triglycerides: Normal adult, <150 mg/100 ml.
† Laboratory values for cholesterol: Normal adult, 150–250 mg/100 ml.

References

1. Beaumont, J. L., Carlson, L. A., Cooper, J. R., Fejfar, Z., Fredrickson, D. S., and Strasser, T. Classification of hyperlipidaemias and hyperlipoproteinemias. *Bull WHO 43:*891–908, 1970.
2. Dietschy, J. M., and Wilson, J. D. Regulation of cholesterol metabolism. *N Engl J Med 282:*1128–1138, 1179–1183, 1241–1249, 1970.
3. Fredrickson, D. S., Levy, R. I., and Lees, R. S. Fat

transport in lipoproteins—an integrated approach to mechanisms and disorders. *N Engl J Med 276:*32–44, 94–103, 148–156, 215–226, 273–281, 1967.
4. Greenberger, N. J., and Skillman, T. G. Medium-chain triglycerides. Physiologic considerations and clinical implications. *N Engl J Med 280:*1045–1056, 1969.
5. Heinle, R. A., Levy, R. I., Fredrickson, D. S., and Gorlin, R. Lipid and carbohydrate abnormalities in patients with angiographically documented coronary artery disease. *Am J Cardiol 24:*178–186, 1969.
6. Senior, J. R. Intestinal absorption of fats. *J Lipid Res 5:*495–521, 1964.
7. Shumaker, V. N., and Adams, G. H. Circulating lipoproteins. *Ann Rev Biochem 38:*114–136, 1970.
8. Steiner, G. Biosynthesis, physiologic role and normal patterns of lipoproteins in normal human plasma. *Acta Diabetol Latina* 9: 1972 (in press).

16

Hormones and Growth

John D. Bailey

The physical, intellectual, and sexual function and the emotional stability of the normal adult depend on adequate endocrine development and activity in childhood and adolescence. The child with an endocrine disorder will usually show a temporary or permanent disruption of physical growth, sexual differentiation and maturation, intellectual progress and/or emotional stability. It is because of these aberrations of growth and development that patients with excess or deficient growth and precocious, delayed, or abnormal sexual development are referred to pediatric endocrinologists.

This chapter outlines the contribution of both endocrine and nonendocrine factors to physical growth. The differential diagnosis and treatment of growth retardation is described in some detail. Excessive growth, a rarer medical problem, is reviewed at the end of the chapter.

Growth is a dominant characteristic of the living organism from conception to maturity. It should be emphasized that functional capacity and physical size often increase at different rates; for example, the brain is almost fully grown by 2 years of age but does not attain optimal function until several years later. During fetal life, infancy, and childhood, the rate of growth of individual body components varies a great deal. Some body tissues such as the skeletal muscles of a male continue to increase in bulk after linear growth has ceased; others such as the fetal adrenal cortex and the thymus reach their maximum at birth or in early infancy and then atrophy.

The factors that limit growth are not clearly understood. The electrolyte changes noted with cellular aging suggest that the control is biochemical. Many body cells, however, retain their growth potential and can begin to grow again when conditions require compensatory hypertrophy—e.g., the remaining kidney after one has been removed. If they are not inhibited by bony fusion, many tissues of the adult acromegalic enlarge to an abnormal degree.

Ultimate size is proportional to both the rate and duration of growth. During early life, the height of a child with sexual precocity will increase rapidly, but because accelerated skeletal maturation causes early epiphyseal fusion, he will be short at maturity. On the other hand, the individual who is short because of hypopituitarism may continue to grow for more than 30 years and may eventually, without treatment, reach a height beyond 5 feet.

Growth is dynamic. The term "growth retardation" is used to encompass a variety of conditions in which the child does not reach the height appropriate to his chronological age. This term covers (1) children whose short stature is temporary and who, without treatment, will achieve a normal height—e.g., delayed adolescence; (2)

those who will achieve a normal height only if they receive specific therapy—e.g., the cretin; and (3) those children who will be permanently short—e.g., the achondroplastic dwarf.

There is no completely satisfactory term for a person of abnormally small size. "Dwarf" is used widely to describe a person, animal, or plant much below a normal size, but unfortunately, the term often carries the implication of disproportion or deformity with its strong affiliation with pathological conditions such as achondroplasia. The term "midget" is used to describe individuals with small size who are well-proportioned and otherwise normal. The term "ateliotic dwarf" is a synonym and these terms are used interchangeably. In the following discussion, "growth retardation" refers to the individual who is below the third percentile for height.

General Factors Affecting Growth

Before maturity, growth is a cellular function and many factors affect this function, directly or indirectly.

Genetic Factors

Each species appears to have an inherent mechanism for controlling its eventual body size. In the human, these ill-defined processes are responsible for the differences in the adult height of various races, and differences within families with a common racial background.

Nutrition

Tissue growth requires large supplies of nitrogen derived from protein. Adequate calories supplied from carbohydrates and fats are also necessary, otherwise dietary protein will be used for energy instead of growth. Vitamins and minerals supply specific needs such as calcium and vitamin D for normal bone growth. For physiological function the cell also needs a sufficient supply of oxygen. A deficiency of any of these elements in pre- or postnatal life will impair growth. Growth failure in conditions such as fetal malnutrition, malabsorption states, or cyanotic congenital heart disease can all be related to nutritional deficiencies.

Infection

Prolonged infection may cause growth failure in several ways. With appetite decreased and caloric requirements increased because of fever, a nutritional deficit develops. Certain intrauterine infections such as rubella inhibit cellular growth and may severely affect the development of specific organs such as the brain. The stress of infection may also increase adrenal glucocorticoid secretion, accelerating the catabolic rate. Because some children with chronic or recurrent infections grow at a normal rate, the direct causal relationship between infection and growth failure has been seriously questioned. However, radiological evidence of decreased bone growth and the negative nitrogen balance during infection support the hypothesis.

Metabolic and Renal Defects

Metabolic disorders may interfere with growth in a variety of ways: through a deficiency of specific enzymes, through inadequate cell nutrition, or by creating an unfavorable environment such as acidosis, which inhibits cellular activity. Abnormal renal function depresses general body metabolism either through accumulation of waste products and/or a loss of essential substances because of inadequate tubular reabsorption. Metabolic defects are usually genetically determined, as in cystinosis, but may be acquired as in postnecrotic cirrhosis of the liver.

Hormones

Both growth and maturation depend on hormones. Growth retardation is prominent in either thyroid or growth-hormone deficiency. Insulin and androgens stimulate growth. Adrenal glucocorticoids inhibit growth and skeletal maturation. Cortisol interferes with the peripheral action of growth hormone but does not appear to inhibit its secretion. Estrogens increase the rate of skeletal maturation and possibly inhibit linear growth.

General Concepts of the Hormonal Control of Growth

Hormonal Control of Cellular Growth

The investigations of Cheek and others have emphasized that growth should be studied at the cellular level. Gross increase in body or organ size depends on an increase in number of, or size of, the individual components—the cells. Cheek's investigation showed that caloric insufficiency slows the multiplication of cells while protein deficiency reduces cell size. Growth hormone appears to increase the rate of DNA replication; hence cell number increases. Thyroid hormone seems to act differently in the newborn (and probably the fetus) than in older children. In hypothyroidism that has developed after infancy, body cells are large but do not multiply at a normal rate. In thyroid deficiency of infancy, on the other hand, both cell size and multiplication are decreased. Insulin produces its effect on growth by increasing individual cell size, a process that is associated with increased transfer into the cell of amino acids and glucose. Androgens seem to stimulate cell multiplication and also increase cell size, while estrogens probably inhibit cellular multiplication.

Influence of Hormones on Growth at Various Periods of Life

Intrauterine Growth

In the fetus, endocrine abnormalities appear to have little effect on physical growth. At birth, congenital apituitarism is associated with hypoplasia of the adrenal cortex, poorly developed genitalia in the male, but normal body size. Rimoin, Merimee, and McKusick have described a father, mother, and offspring who had isolated growth-hormone deficiency, but the child was of normal size at birth. In this infant, fetal or maternal sources produced no growth hormone. The mother was able to produce prolactin normally as demonstrated by milk production.

Human placental lactogen or human chorionic "growth hormone-prolactin" has biochemical, immunochemical, and biological properties resembling growth hormone. The levels in maternal serum of placental lactogen are decreased in intrauterine growth retardation with a small placenta, and increased in pregnant diabetic women and twin pregnancies. Serum levels in the fetus, however, are low, and there has been no demonstration of placental lactogen having a direct role in the control of fetal growth.

In apituitarism, the size and cellular structure of the thyroid is usually normal, indicating that, in utero, the thyroid develops with considerable autonomy. On the other hand, the thyroid and pituitary must have some organic connection because thyrotrophs appear in the pituitary at the 13th week of gestation and TSH has been demonstrated in the anterior pituitary cells as early as the 12th week. The tenth week, or even earlier, has been noted as the time when the fetal thyroid gland first becomes capable of taking up radioactive iodine, which also suggests that these glands are interdependent in early fetal life.

Clinically, congenital thyroid deficiency is difficult to recognize at birth. Although the placenta does not transfer thyroxine and triiodothyronine efficiently from mother to fetus, the infant does not usually show the clinical stigmas of cretinism until he is 3–4 weeks old. Athyrotic newborns weigh slightly more and are slightly longer than the average for their gestational age. Retarded bony maturation in utero is shown by the lack of a distal femoral epiphysis on radiographs. Even when thyroid replacement therapy is started early, these infants probably do not develop to their full intellectual potential.

Infancy and Childhood

Growth may be retarded by either growth hormone or thyroxine deficiency. Excess adrenal glucocorticoids, either endogenous or exogenous, markedly delay growth. The child with poorly controlled diabetes mellitus usually has a decreased rate of linear growth. Pseudohypoparathyroidism is associated with dwarfism and skeletal abnormalities; however, these changes do not appear to be related to the decreased parathyroid function.

Excess growth in infancy and childhood may be due to abnormal androgen production either from complete isosexual precocity or to disease of the adrenal cortex. Gigantism can be caused by a pituitary adenoma but occurs very rarely. Hyperthyroidism produces an increased growth velocity.

Adolescence

Acquired lesions of the hypothalamic-pituitary area such as a craniopharyngioma may cause growth-hormone deficiency in the teenager. Impairment of thyrotropin and gonadotropin secretion will increase the growth deficit.

Delay in the onset of puberty is a common cause of temporary growth retardation at this age; permanent gondadotropin deficiency of genetic origin or that due to hypothalamic lesions is rare. In gonadotropin deficiency, skeletal maturation is delayed, but if there is no associated deficiency of growth hormone or TSH, the individual may eventually reach a height greater than average as a result of the prolonged growth period.

Acquired hypothyroidism due to thyroiditis or other causes is an occasional cause of adolescent growth failure. In this age group, certain patients with mild defects of thyroid hormonogenesis may come to the physician because they are short; they will have a goiter that may have been unnoticed by the patient or his family.

Short stature is a constant feature in Turner'

Fig. 16-1. Growth charts showing percentile height standards **(A)** for girls, and **(B)** for boys from birth to 19 years. Numbers at *upper right inside* represent the percentile—the percentage of the appropriate population whose height falls below this value at each age. Plotted on this chart, the height of a 9-year-old boy with a height of 120 cm (47.25 inches) will fall on the third percentile (*lowest broken line*); compared with 100 boys of the same age, this lad is third shortest. On these special charts, serial measurements of the child's height at regular intervals show that with respect to height, the range of normal increases as the child grows older. Eighty per cent of children will have a height that falls between the tenth percentile (*lowest solid line*) and the eightieth (*upper solid line*). (From Tanner, J. M., Whitehouse, R. H., and Takaishi, M. *Arch Dis Child* 41:454–471, 1966. Reproduced with permission.)

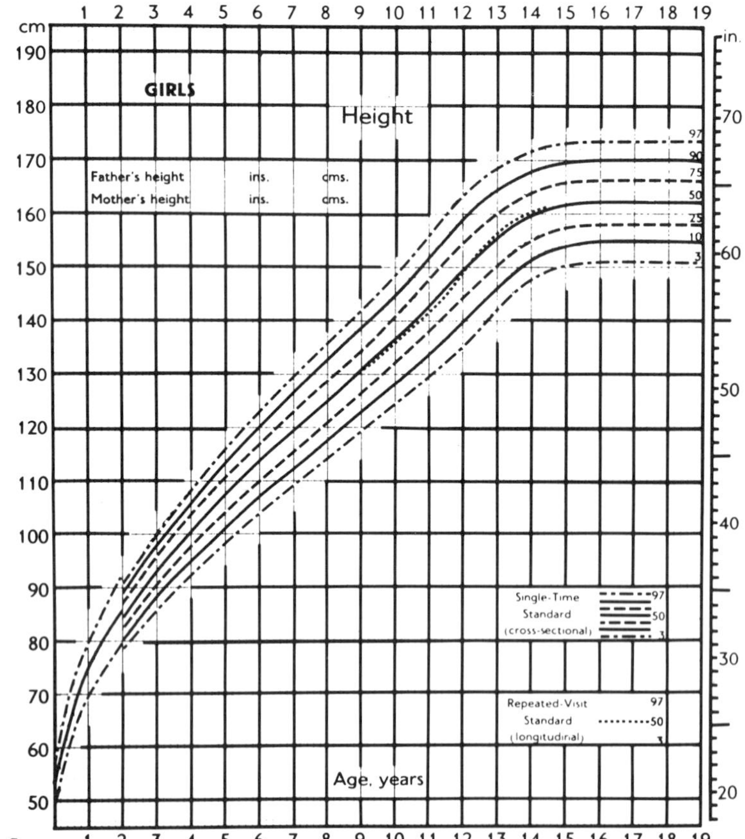

A

syndrome. The growth deficit is not due to gonadal dysgenesis or other known hormonal factors. Dwarfism is not a feature of other types of primary gondal insufficiency; boys with Klinefelter's syndrome, for example, may grow to be taller than expected from their genetic background.

Methods of Assessing Physical Growth and Development

Height and Weight Measurements

The physician can only assess the effects of endocrine abnormalities on growth and evaluate the effects of his treatment if he has accurate measurements and records of height and weight. With such measurements, the individual's progress can be compared with the standard for the specific population. Repeated examinations give the most useful data, and over a period of time, growth velocity can be calculated. From height and weight data, one can determine whether the child with short stature is falling further behind, catching up, or remaining parallel to his own age group.

Heights of infants and toddlers should be measured with the subject lying with feet fixed on the base of a special measuring board that has a movable head board. Older subjects are measured standing against a fixed device with movable horizontal bar that rests on the top of the head. Without such aids, two height measurements made by the same individual may vary as much as 2 cm. Other useful measurements include crown-to-pubis and pubis-to-heel distances. Sitting height gives similar information with greater accuracy but requires special equipment. The arm span and head circumference are also valuable in determining growth proportions. To make comparisons more valid, if possible, repeated measurements should be made by the same examiner.

Several types of growth charts are available. At the Hospital for Sick Children we use those developed by Tanner, Whitehouse, and Takaishi at the Institute of Child Health, London (Fig. 16-1), which show percentile channels of height and weight for boys and girls from birth to 19 years. Velocity charts are also available, which allow growth rates to be compared at various ages for both sexes (Fig. 16-2). The physician using these charts should remember that these standards were developed in London, England, and that adjust-

B

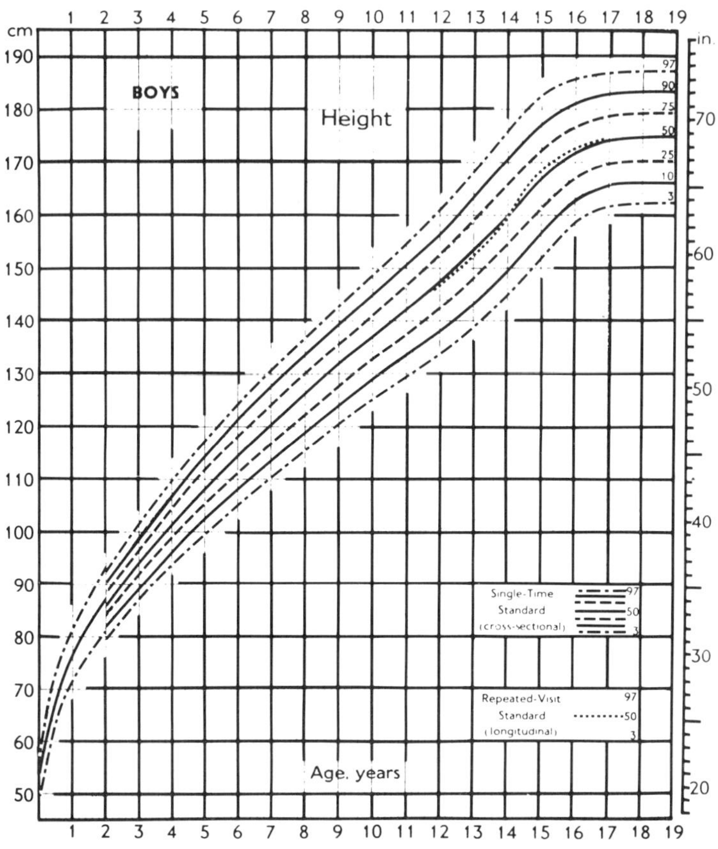

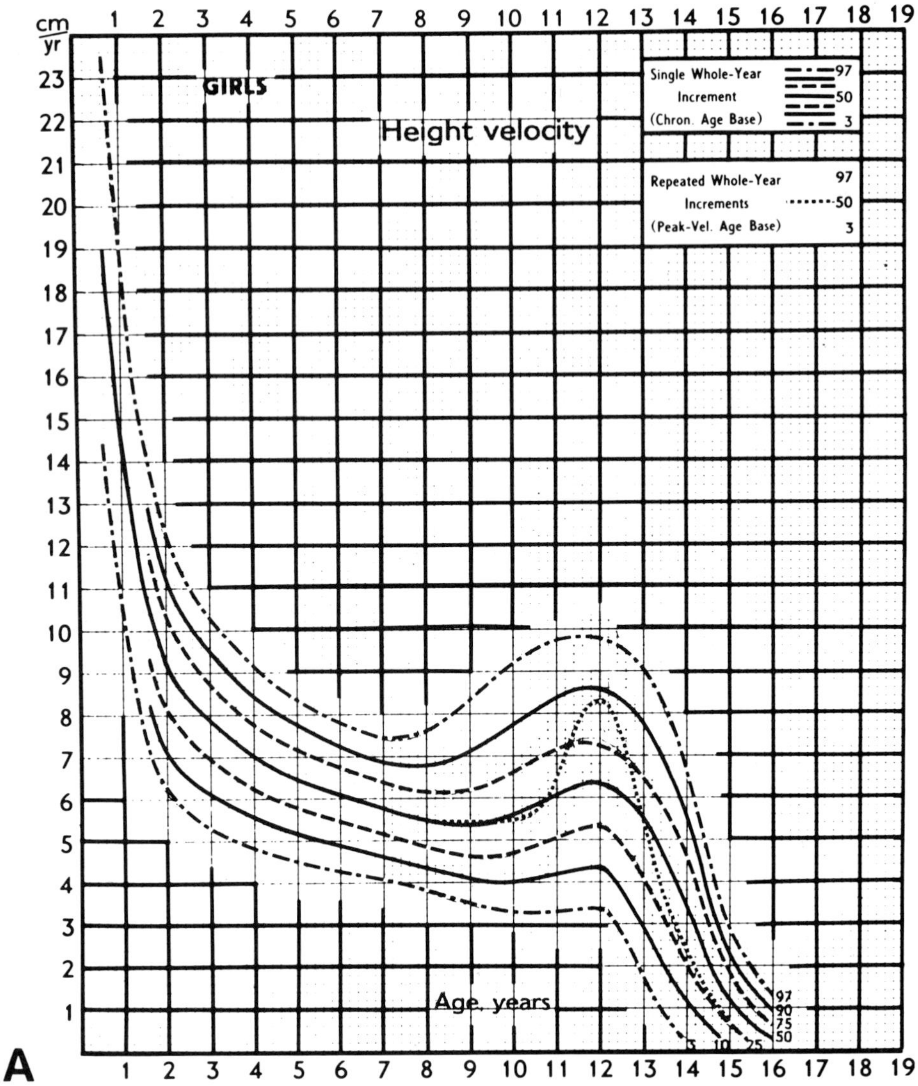

A

Fig. 16-2. Height velocity charts **(A)** for girls, and **(B)** for boys. Note that these charts show more distinctly the variations in growth rate throughout childhood. Height velocity provides a measure of growth rate. Scale *at left* indicates growth rate calculated in centimeters per year. Until puberty, the range of normal is fairly narrow; variations in age of onset of the pubertal growth spurt produce wide fluctuations in the range of normal. These *variations* can be seen after age 8 in girls and age 10 in boys. Growth takes place rapidly in the early years: on the average (*solid fiftieth percentile line*) a 7-month-old infant grows at the rate of 19 cm/year. Her velocity at age 16 had dropped to almost zero because her epiphyses had closed. (From Tanner, J. M., Whitehouse, R. H., and Takaishi, M. *Arch Dis Child 41*:613–635, 1966. Reproduced with permission.)

ments may be necessary if there are significant racial or other differences in the local population. Children whose height is below the third percentile for age must be carefully assessed to determine if their constitutional growth pattern is normal or abnormal.

Roentgenographic Studies

In children with abnormal growth, skeletal maturation should be compared with chronological age. With standards derived by Greulich and Pyle, radiographs of the hands and wrists can be

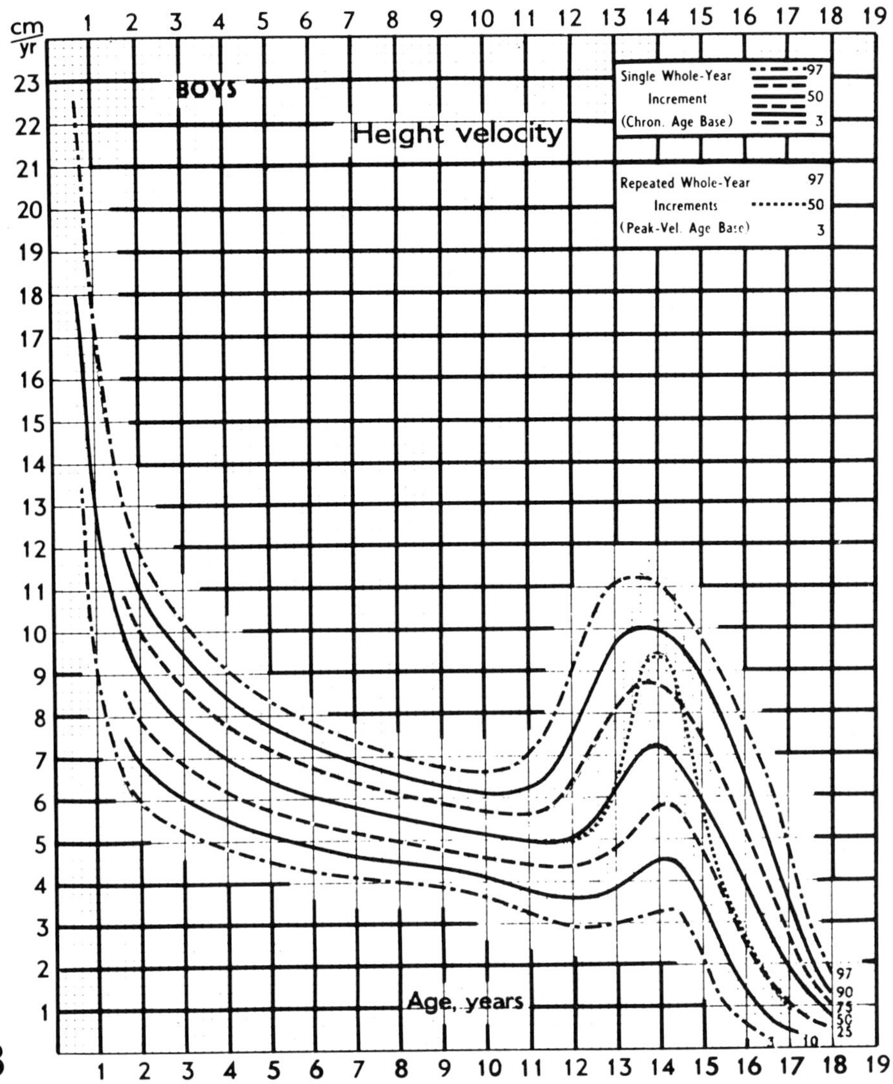

B

used to estimate skeletal maturation (bone age). Roentgenograms of the skull are often valuable in patients with linear growth abnormalities; delayed skeletal maturation can be demonstrated by delay in fusion of the synostoses at the base of the skull. The pituitary fossa should be examined for enlargement, calcification, and changes in the clinoids suggestive of tumor. A small pituitary fossa is not usually significant. Signs of increased intracranial pressure may indicate a tumor or other space-occupying lesion but could represent a rapidly growing brain in a small skull. In some growth studies, stereotaxic roentgenograms of the lower limbs have been used to record growth more accurately. These special views, however, do not generally have any place in clinical practice. Roentgenograms should be made of the spine in patients with disproportionate short stature, which occurs in conditions such as osteochondrodystrophy.

Assessment of Sexual Development

In children with growth problems, sexual development should be observed closely and recorded accurately. In young children, inspection

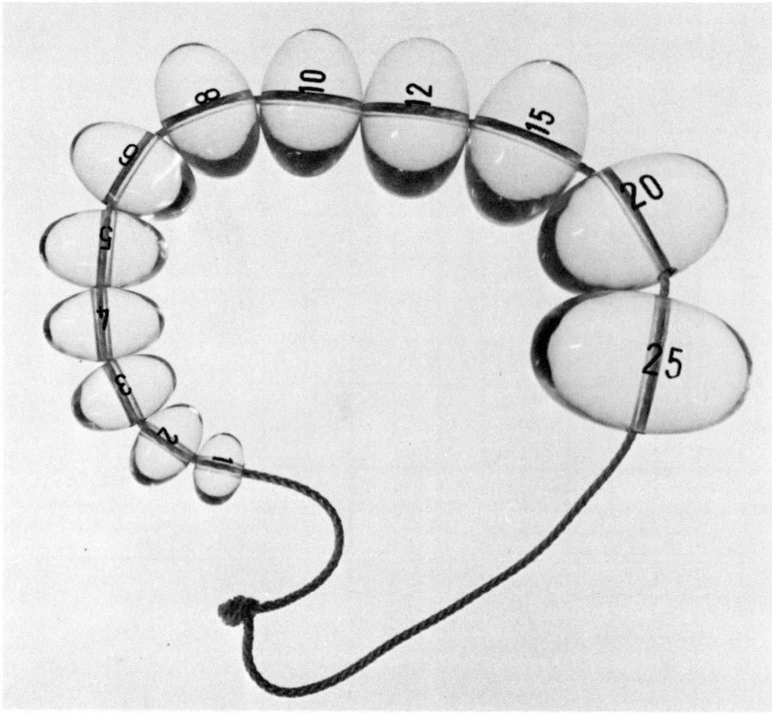

Fig. 16-3. Orchidometer devised by Prader for comparative measurement of testicular size. This device was designed using data such as that shown in Table 16-1. Figures on plastic ellipsoids represent volume in cubic centimeters (From Prader, A. *Triangle* 7:241, 1968. Reproduced with permission.)

provides most of the information. In boys, the physician should determine whether the testes are descended and are of normal size. Prader devised a method for measuring testes by comparing their size with plastic ellipsoids of various sizes. Thus, the child's testicular development can be compared with the standard for his age (Fig. 16-3, Tables 16-1 and 16-2). With sexual maturation, the plasma levels of testosterone and serum levels of FSH and LH increase in normal males as shown in Table 16-3 (normal values of Winter and Faiman).

Table 16-1. Volumes and Diameters of Testes in 300 Healthy Boys and 300 Men*

Volume (ml)	*Longitudinal Diameter (cm)*	*Transverse Diameter (cm)*
1	1.68	1.07
2	2.11	1.34
5	2.87	1.85
10	3.61	2.30
20	4.55	2.90

* Derived from Prof. A. Prader[10] and used with his permission.

Breast development in either sex is determined by noting the size of the nipple and areolar tissue. The examiner should also determine the amount of true breast tissue and distinguish this from fat. The amount and distribution of sexual hair should be recorded. Tanner has described the various degrees (Stages 1–5) in the development of pubic hair (Fig. 16-4). In females with suspected abnormalities of sexual development, the physician should also do a rectal examination to determine the size of the uterus and to exclude the presence of enlarged ovaries or other abnormal masses. For further details of female sexual development, see Chapter 10 on The Ovary.

Nitrogen and Other Balance Studies

The child can grow only if the amount of body protein increases. Linear growth is slow, and it is

Table 16-2. Developmental Stages in Bodily Growth, the Growth of Pubic Hair and the Size of the Testes in Healthy Individuals.*

Age (Years)	*Growth*	*Pubic Hair*	*Testicular volume*† *(ml.)*
0–11	rapid at first then slowing	none	0.5 to 2
12			2 to 5
13	pubertal growth spurt	beginning to grow	5 to 10
15		grows rapidly	15 to 25
18	growth ceases	male distribution pattern	15 to 25

* The developmental stages for the 12- to 18-year group may be completed up to 3 years earlier or later than the ages indicated.
† Comparative palpation using models in the form of ellipsoids of revolution.

Table 16-3. Normal Values of Plasma Testosterone, Serum FSH and Serum LH in Male Children and Adolescents*

		Plasma Testosterone (ng/100 ml)		*Serum FSH (μg LER-907/100 ml)*		*Serum LH (ICSH) (μg LER-907/100 ml)*	
Age	*n*	*Mean*	*Range*	*Mean*	*Range*	*Mean*	*Range*
0–2	11	13	(4–37)	7.0	(4.3–12.1)	1.2	(0.6–1.8)
2–4	7	11	(5–16)	7.5	(4.8–9.0)	1.3	(0.6–2.1)
4–6	13	20	(8–40)	7.8	(5–12.9)	1.5	(0.7–2.2)
6–8	22	14	(6–28)	10.0	(6.1–13.5)	1.7	(1.1–2.9)
8–10	25	21	(9–50)	10.3	(6.9–21.3)	1.9	(1.1–3.0)
10–12	53	41	(8–290)	12.6	(8.5–28.3)	2.0	(1.0–3.0)
12–14	51	130	(5–757)	13.6	(8.9–23.5)	2.5	(1.4–4.9)
14–16	26	328	(90–560)	15.8	(9.7–25.5)	3.1	(2.2–4.9)
16–18	10	532	(264–732)	15.7	(11.6–25.5)	4.1	(3.0–6.5)
18–20	6	564	(400–724)	20.2	(11.7–25.3)	3.6	(3.0–6.5)
20–25	29	605	(336–1120)	17.0	(11.0–25.5)	4.2	(3.0–6.5)

* Adapted from Winter, J. S. D., and Fairman, C. Pituitary-gonadal relations in male children and adolescents, *Pediatr Res 6*:126–135, 1972.

difficult to detect changes over short periods. Now, because increased nitrogen retention reflects an increase in growth, in special centers nitrogen balance studies are used to determine growth response over short periods. This procedure requires prolonged hospitalization, during which the child is kept on a constant, regulated diet, and urine is collected continually. Nitrogen in the urine is measured during the control period and after giving an anabolic agent such as growth hormone. If the short patient responds to treatment, increased nitrogen retention will be reflected in a decreased nitrogen excretion in the urine. In addition to nitrogen, the body retains potassium, phosphorus, and magnesium during growth. Initially, growth hormone increases the excretion of calcium in the urine, but it also stimulates intestinal absorption; hence the trend to a negative calcium balance is reversed. The reader should note that, in many cases, there has been no good correlation between nitrogen retention and linear growth response to the administration of growth hormone.

Some investigators have used increased urinary excretion of hydroxyproline as an index of the effectiveness of growth hormone. This test, however, is difficult to standardize because hydroxyproline excretion in normal children varies widely from day to day. In addition, the child's diet must be restricted while he is on hydroxyproline collection because foods such as gelatin contain large amounts of this amino acid.

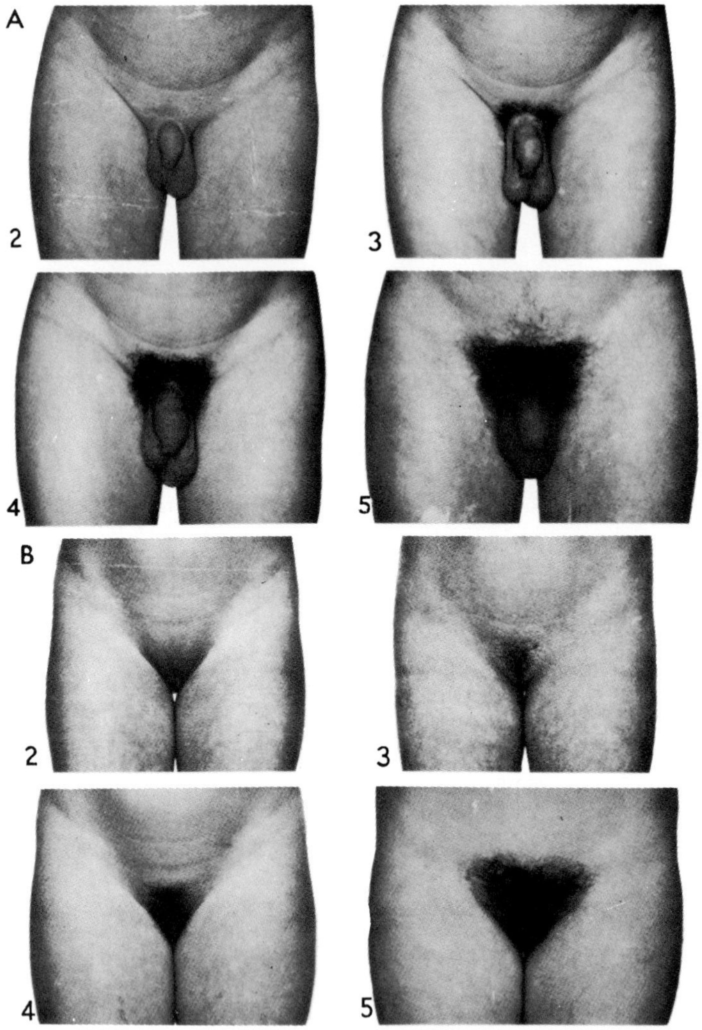

Fig. 16-4. Stages and development of pubic hair **(A)** for males, and **(B)** for females. In Stage 1, pre-adolescent (not shown) the hair over the pubis is not developed more than that over the abdominal wall—i.e., the subject has no pubic hair.

In Stage 2, there is sparse growth of long, slightly pigmented downy hair, straight or slightly curled, chiefly at the base of the penis or along labia.

In Stage 3, considerable dark or coarser and more curled hair is spread sparsely over the junction of the pubes.

In Stage 4, hair is now adult in type but covers an area still considerably smaller than in the adult. It will spread to the medial surface of the thighs.

In Stage 5, hair is adult in quantity and type and distributed in the horizontal (or classically feminine) pattern. It has spread to medial surface of thighs but not up linea alba or elsewhere above the base of the inverse triangle. (From Tanner, J. M. *Growth at Adolescence.* Oxford, Blackwell Sci., 1962.)

Growth Retardation

Growth failure may be evident at birth or develop in infancy, childhood, or adolescence. In each patient one must distinguish the underlying cause or causes, such as hormonal dysfunction, so that remedial conditions can be treated and distinguished from those in which no treatment is necessary or possible.

Growth Retardation at Birth and in the Neonatal Period

Small size recognizable at birth is almost never due to an endocrine abnormality. Because length is difficult to measure at birth, most diagnoses of growth failure are made on the basis of birth weight (Fig. 16-5).

Fig. 16-5. Mean weight (A) and mean length (B) compared to gestational age in weeks. In these charts, based on measurements made on 300 newborns at birth, the *heavy line* represents the mean, the *superior* and *inferior light lines* show +2 and −2 S.D. (approximately the 3rd and 97th percentiles). Those infants below are classed as having intrauterine growth retardation. (From Usher, R., and McLean, F. *J Pediatr 74*:901–910, 1969. Reproduced with permission.)

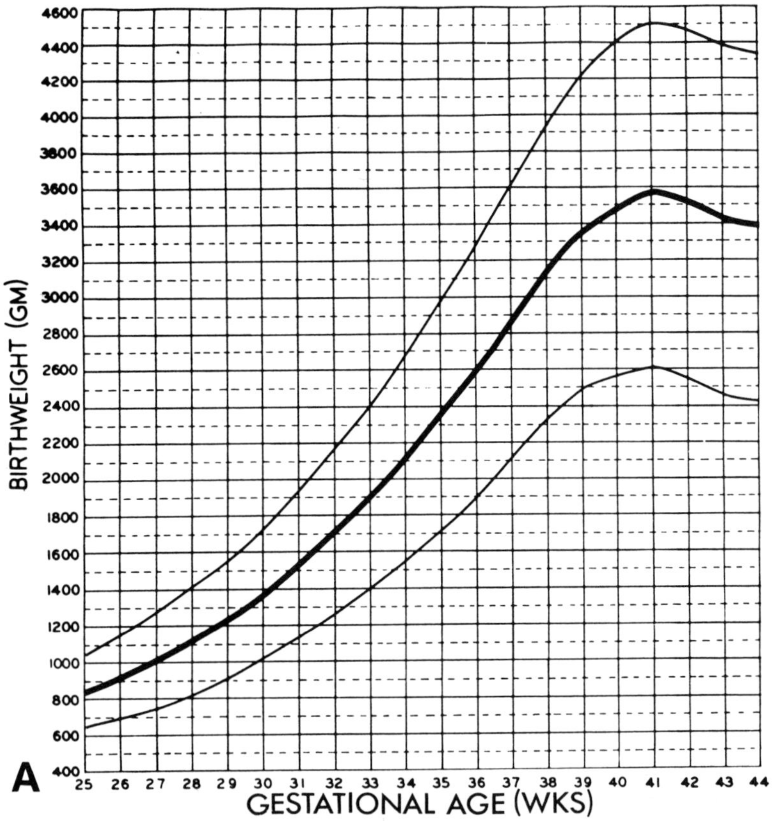
4600
4400
4200
4000
3800
3600
3400
3200
3000
2800
2600
2400
2200
2000
1800
1600
1400
1200
1000
800
600
400
BIRTHWEIGHT (GM)
25 26 27 28 29 30 31 32 33 34 35 36 37 38 39 40 41 42 43 44
GESTATIONAL AGE (WKS)

A

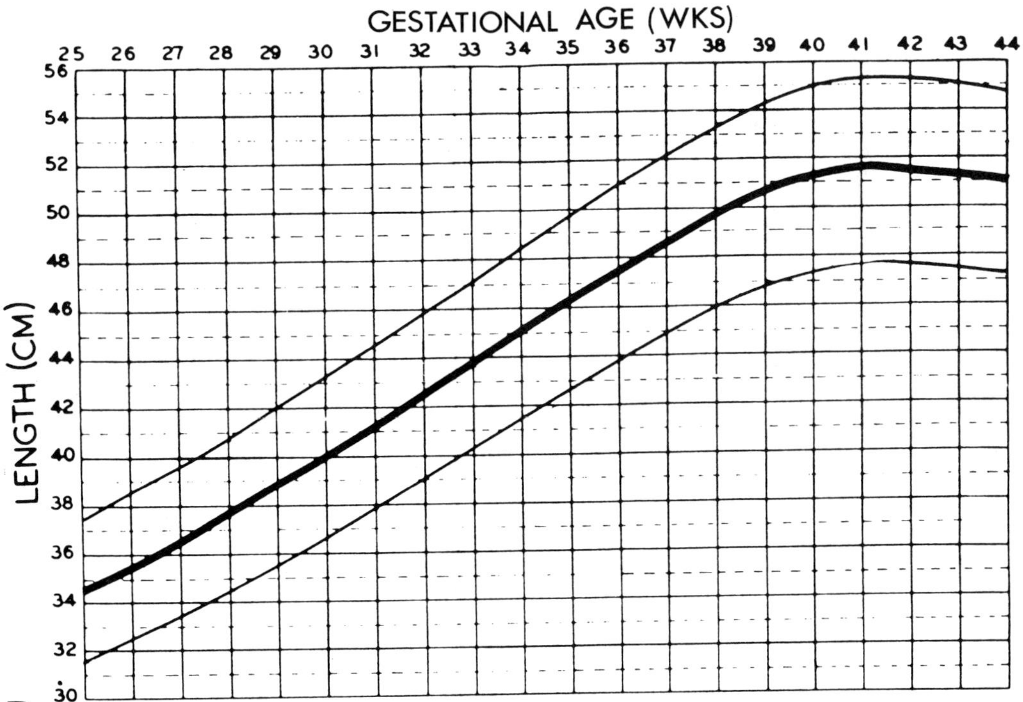
GESTATIONAL AGE (WKS)
25 26 27 28 29 30 31 32 33 34 35 36 37 38 39 40 41 42 43 44
56
54
52
50
48
46
44
42
40
38
36
34
32
30
LENGTH (CM)

B

Usually growth fails during intrauterine life because insufficient nutrients pass into the fetus from the mother. The placenta is usually small. Whether the baby has been premature, term, or postmature, he is smaller than expected for the period of gestation. Some investigators have used the term "fetal malnutrition" to describe the condition of these newborns. In many cases, the cause of the condition is obscure. In some, the reason may be obvious, such as in twin pregnancies when one twin has received less than his share of placental attachment. In addition, children with reduced growth may have a single umbilical artery and other associated anomalies. In mothers who smoke cigarettes during pregnancy, the incidence of low-birth-weight infants is increased. The mothers of some of these infants have been toxemic, but this seems more important if she is over 30 years of age and has chronic renal vascular disease. Thin mothers are more likely to have an infant with fetal malnutrition than one of average or increased weight. In future pregnancies, mothers who have borne a "small for dates" infant are more likely to produce a similar baby than the mother who has not.

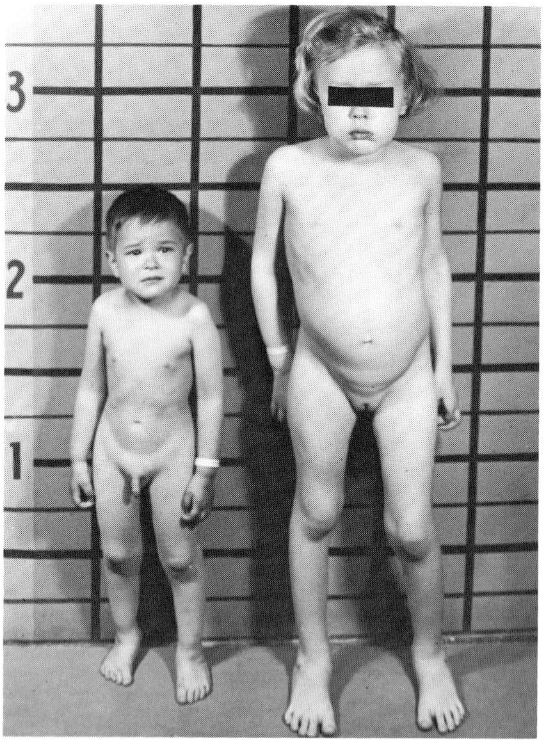

Fig. 16-6. A 4-year-old boy with Fanconi's anemia. He is shown beside a normal girl of the same age. This boy's weight was 2.4 kg after 40 weeks' gestation.

Certain noxious influences may attack the fetus or embryo and produce growth retardation. Infections such as rubella, cytomegalic inclusion disease, or toxoplasmosis produce a variety of stigmas in addition to growth failure. Teratogenic drugs or radiation of the mother in early pregnancy may also be responsible for fetal malnutrition.

Other types of intrauterine growth failure are due to "the seed" rather than "the soil." Several demonstrable chromosomal defects cause abnormal intrauterine growth. Infants with the D and E syndromes or mongolism, of which all are due to the presence of an extra chromosome or extra translocated chromosomal material, have low birth weights for gestational age. In Turner's syndrome, due to an absence of one of the X chromosomes, retarded intrauterine growth is a common feature. Other conditions that have a genetic basis, such as Fanconi's anemia (Fig. 16-6) and the syndromes of Cornelia de Lange or Bloom, show intrauterine growth failure. Certain infants with bony dysplasia such as achondroplasia may be recognized at birth, but the growth defect becomes more obvious with increasing age.

An uncommon but important condition associated with low birth weight for gestational age is Russel-Silver dwarfism.[13,14] Although these cases have been reported separately from two continents, their common features suggest that the patients each author described have the same syndrome. The description of these infants drew attention to the fact that all babies with a birth weight less than 2.5 kg were not premature in terms of gestational age.

Besides a low birth weight and decreased length, Russel-Silver dwarfs have a number of stigmas. The infant's appearance often suggests hydrocephalus; the skull tends to be large and the baby has a prominent forehead; the face is small and triangular (Fig. 16-7**A**). Body asymmetry, which is common but not present in all, may be slight, and the physician will have to search carefully and in some cases use roentgenograms to demonstrate this asymmetry. Syndactyly and clinodactyly may be present. In the neonatal period, the infants are prone to hypoglycemia, but infants with fetal malnutrition due to other causes may also have this tendency.

Unlike the true premature, the baby who is smaller than expected for gestational age has growth retardation that frequently persists through life (Fig. 16-7**B**). In some, as in Turner's syndrome, short stature will become increasingly obvious in the postnatal period because the growth rate is slowed. In others, such as those with fetal malnutrition, the growth rate is rapid enough so that the child does not fall further behind the normal for his age. At puberty these children usually have a moderate delay in skeletal and sexual maturation, but eventually reach a height that is slightly below or within the lowest range of normal.

Newborns with thyroid deficiency are extremely difficult to recognize at birth. The baby's length and weight are usually slightly above average. Unexplained hyperbilirubinemia, an unusually large anterior fontanel or difficulty in maintaining a normal body temperature may suggest this diagnosis. If the infant has a goiter, further investigation of thyroid function is mandatory. During the first week of life, the newborn has mild physiological hyperthyroidism manifested by an elevated serum thyroxine, elevated T_3 resin uptake, and an increased radioactive iodine uptake. Measures of thyroid function made in early infancy should take this physiological phenomenon into account.

Growth Retardation in Infancy and Childhood

Most growth defects become apparent before the child is 10 years old; of these, endocrine defects form the smallest portion. As suggested previously, any condition that affects nutrition or normal cellular activity will inhibit growth.

Endocrine abnormalities, because their effects are continuous, slow growth in a way that can be demonstrated on the velocity chart or by showing on the growth grid that the child's growth pattern gradually falls toward or below the third percentile channel.

Most chronic diseases of childhood impair growth. In many of these, such as cyanotic congenital heart disease or cystic fibrosis, the underlying disease and mechanism of growth defect are readily apparent. In other disorders such as chronic renal disease, the underlying condition may not be so easy to detect. Therefore, children with a retarded growth rate should be carefully investigated for renal disease of various forms from chronic pyelonephritis to genetically determined renal tubular defects. Investigation of these patients involves repeated urinalyses (including pH and specific gravity), urine cultures, blood urea nitrogen, serum electrolytes, pH, and bicarbonate content. A urinary amino-acid chromatogram is occasionally helpful. Roentgenographic studies, including an intravenous pyelogram and voiding cystogram, are frequently indicated. Changes characteristic of renal osteodystrophy may be noted in roentgenograms of the knees and wrists.

Malabsorption may also be difficult to recognize in some patients. At the Hospital for Sick Children, Toronto, we have seen several children with growth failure who were considered to have an endocrine defect but who, on investigation, had celiac disease. These children usually have relatively low weights compared to their heights. The history may reveal that the stools have been bulky, pale, frothy, and foul, but the parents may not have noted any of these signs. The child usually has a prominent abdomen and a loss of subcutaneous fat, especially over the buttocks. This appearance contrasts with that in children with growth failure due to endocrine causes, who generally have normal or increased body fat. Routine hematological tests will usually show some degree of iron-deficiency anemia. Any of these leads would indicate a need for complete investigation for malabsorption.

Children who fail to thrive frequently have mental retardation, although the relationship between the physical and mental retardation may be obscure. Some of these patients have neurological defects, and in these, difficulty in feeding or recurrent infection may explain the growth deficiency. In some others, growth retardation seems to be of cerebral origin. By creating small hypothalamic lesions in experimental animals, Reichlin produced dwarfism. Stimulation of specific cerebral areas has been found to cause secretion of growth-hormone-releasing hormone (GHRH). A similar mechanism might operate in children with short stature and neurological disease. Growth-hormone secretion can be demonstrated in these children but the response to stimulatory tests may be incomplete, irregular, or inconsistent.

Several metabolic disorders that affect growth begin or become more apparent during infancy and childhood. In addition to the mucopolysaccharidoses, various forms of glycogen storage disease, some aminoacidopathies and many of the conditions discussed previously under growth failure in intrauterine life may present for the first time during infancy or even in later childhood. Screening tests for metabolic diseases include blood and urine amino-acid chromatograms, urine for reducing substances and mucopolysaccharides, serum calcium, phosphorus, alkaline phosphatase, pH, and total carbon-dioxide content. The blood-sugar response to glucagon or epinephrine should be determined in suspected glycogen-storage disease.

Some nonendocrine disorders such as malabsorption have secondary effects on hormonal function, but two conditions, malnutrition and emotional deprivation, have a major impact on the endocrine system.

Malnutrition

Malnutrition may take many forms. Specific deficiencies of minerals and vitamins may affect endocrine function—e.g., iodide lack leads to compensatory thyroid hyperplasia; vitamin D or calcium deficiency leads to secondary hyperparathyroidism.

In underdeveloped countries, growth failure is commonly seen in two types of malnutrition. Kwashiorkor is due to prolonged protein deficiency in the presence of a fairly adequate intake of total calories, largely in the form of carbohydrate. In addition to severe growth retardation, these children have depigmented skin and hair, edema, severe hypoalbuminemia, anemia, and hepatomegaly. In these individuals, fasting growth hormone serum levels are usually elevated and fall quickly after protein is added to the diet. In marasmus due to total caloric restriction, children have wasting of muscles and hypoalbuminemia. Fasting growth-hormone levels are usually elevated but not to the marked degree seen in kwashiorkor. Pimstone *et al.* have found an inverse relationship between serum albumin and growth hormone levels, but this relationship probably reflects the malnutrition rather than suggesting that hypoalbuminemia acts as a stimulus to growth hormone secretion.

In Canada, malnutrition due to caloric deprivation is uncommon; its presence usually suggests a secondary cause such as malabsorption or an-

Fig. 16-7. Russell-Silver syndrome.

A. Height of this 7½-year-old boy is 105 cm and weight 11.6 kg. The triangular facies is typical. After full gestation, his birth weight was 2.1 kg. He has asymmetry of face, trunk, and limbs.

B. Growth chart of female child with classic Russell-Silver syndrome. Note that the height curve (*heavy solid black line*) is well below the third percentile but runs parallel to it until the age of puberty. Although she is small, her growth is progressive; hence, she does not have an underlying endocrine abnormality.

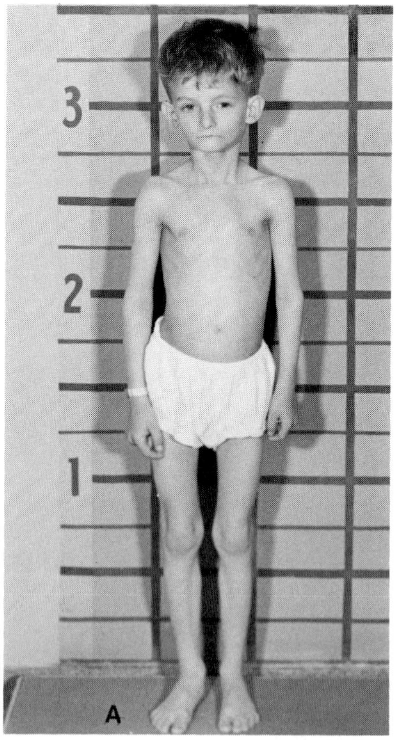

orexia nervosa. In such children, the serum growth-hormone level is usually normal or may be increased; an increase probably reflects action of growth hormone in conserving body protein and maintaining blood sugar during periods of starvation. In some of these conditions, the child may not show a normal rise in growth-hormone levels after stimulation by arginine or insulin-induced hypoglycemia.

Thyroid function studies in malnutrition have usually been within the normal range. Some series have shown minor variations in tests of thyroid function, but these differences are probably due to such factors as the iodide content of the diet or changes in thyroxine-binding proteins.

Emotional Deprivation (Psychosocial Deprivation)

In the past few years, we have become increasingly aware that decreased growth rate in a child may be due to disturbances in the child's home environment.[8] Children so affected are usually seen in the preschool period. In addition to growth retardation, they have an increased appetite, polydipsia, and a tendency to drink unusual fluids. In the hospital, they show personality disorders; they withdraw early from other people but gradually form "clinging relationships" to the attending staff.

Physically they have some characteristics of

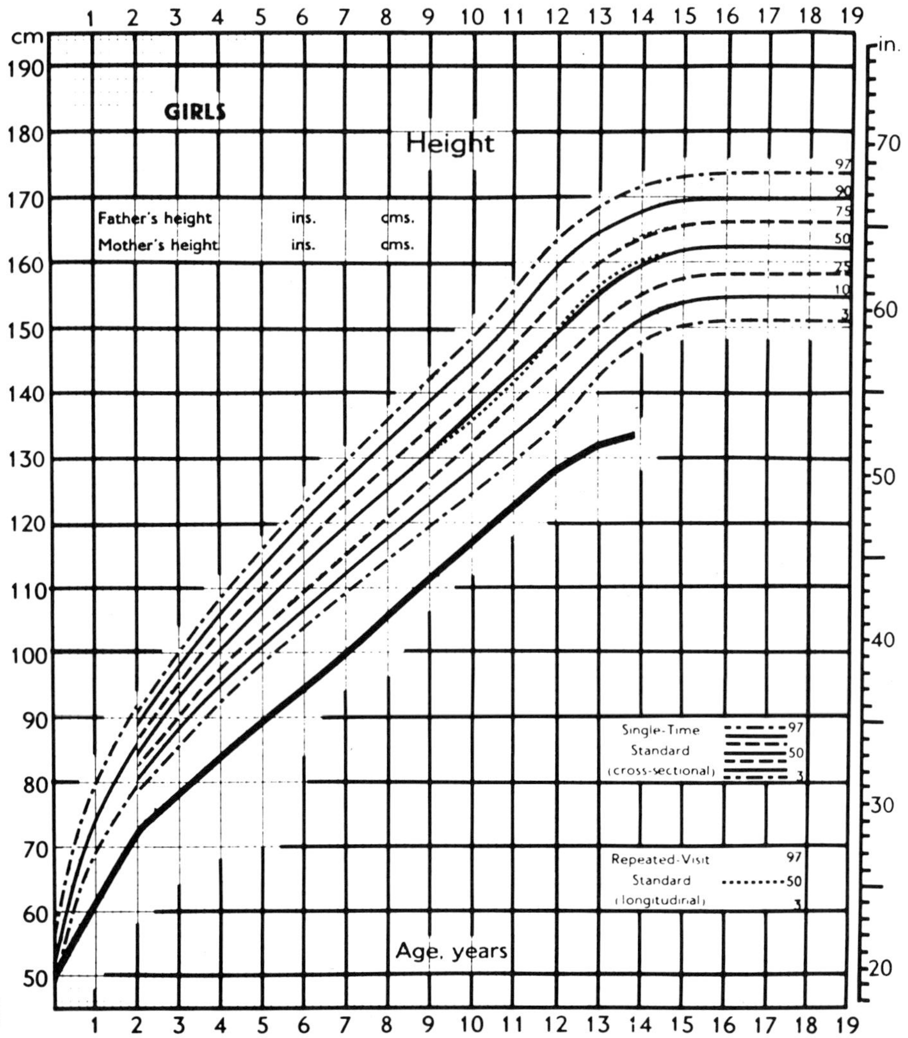

B

hypopituitarism and a similar delay in growth pattern. The abdomen, however, is often prominent, and body weight is decreased as much as, or more than, the height, a feature unusual in hypopituitarism (Fig. 16-8). On roentgenographic studies, they frequently show a decreased bone age but not to the same extent as children with congenital hypopituitarism or hypothyroidism.

Serum growth hormone levels may be decreased in emotional deprivation. Adrenocorticotropic function, measured by the Metopirone test, may be subnormal. The children may exhibit evidence of intestinal malabsorption and decreased urine-concentrating capacity, which is never as complete as in diabetes insipidus.

These children improve remarkably when placed in a new environment such as a hospital ward. Although most normal children do not gain readily when hospitalized, these children put on weight and often show a rapid improvement in personality and in physical health. With this clinical improvement, growth-hormone secretion returns quickly to normal although adrenocorticotropic function may not recover for several months. When a warm, meaningful social relationship is established, growth accelerates. When roentgenograms of the skull are taken after a few months, the sutures may be split as a result of increased growth of the brain. This finding should not be mistaken for increased intracranial pressure due to an expanding lesion.

Specific Endocrine Abnormalities

Hypothyroidism

Thyroid deficiency, beginning at birth, produces the clinical picture known as cretinism. The deficiency may be due to absence or incomplete development of the thyroid gland or to a defect in hormone production. Patients with defective production usually have a goiter because defective feedback to the pituitary results in increased TSH secretion, which causes the thyroid to hypertrophy. The enlargement, however, may not be recognized during infancy.

As noted previously, the baby with thyroid deficiency has a normal or slightly increased size at birth. Some have hyperbilirubinemia, which is due to slow development of the hepatic enzyme, bilirubin glucuronyl transferase, needed to convert lipid-soluble bilirubin (indirect-reacting) to the water-soluble glucuronide of bilirubin (direct-reacting). The associated jaundice usually clears after 4 or 5 weeks, but at this time other features of cretinism are usually apparent. In the hospital, the baby may have had difficulty in maintaining a normal temperature. During the first few weeks

Fig. 16-8. Emotional deprivation. A. This 3-year-old child's appearance is typical of emotional deprivation. The wasted limbs and distended abdomen provide a physique similar to that seen in celiac disease.

B. Growth chart of the child with deprivation syndrome. The height curve (*heavy solid black line*) shows that growth improved during periods of hospitalization but velocity slowed after she returned to the home environment.

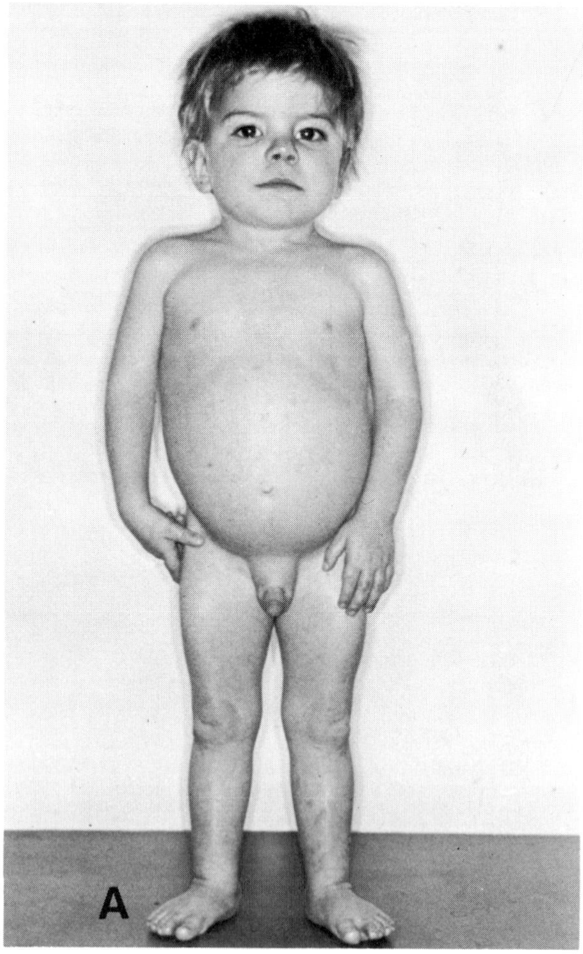

the mother will notice that the infant is sluggish or sleepy and difficult to feed. His appetite is decreased, and because of an enlarged tongue and thick pharyngeal tissues, he may have episodes of choking. His cry becomes hoarse, and his breathing may be noisy. The baby is usually constipated. In the untreated baby, a perceptive mother will notice delay in the baby's developmental milestones, such as sitting, walking, and talking. Dentition will also be delayed.

When the infant is examined at 4–5 weeks, the clinical features of cretinism are quite obvious: coarse facial features, puffiness of the eyelids, and an enlarged, protruding tongue (Fig. 16-9). A prominent unbilical hernia is usually present. Because of mild anemia and hypercarotenemia, the infant's complexion is sallow. The nasal bridge is poorly developed. The baby retains infantile body proportions and growth is markedly slowed. The skin is usually mottled and cold due to the poor peripheral circulation. Cardiac rate is slow and pulse pressure is low. Clinically, there is no cardiac enlargement; however, because a murmur may have been heard over the precordium, a mistaken diagnosis of congenital heart disease is occasionally made. The cry will be hoarse, and the infant frequently has some respiratory difficulty. The delay in skeletal maturation becomes more obvious with increasing age because the anterior fontanelles remain widely patent. The

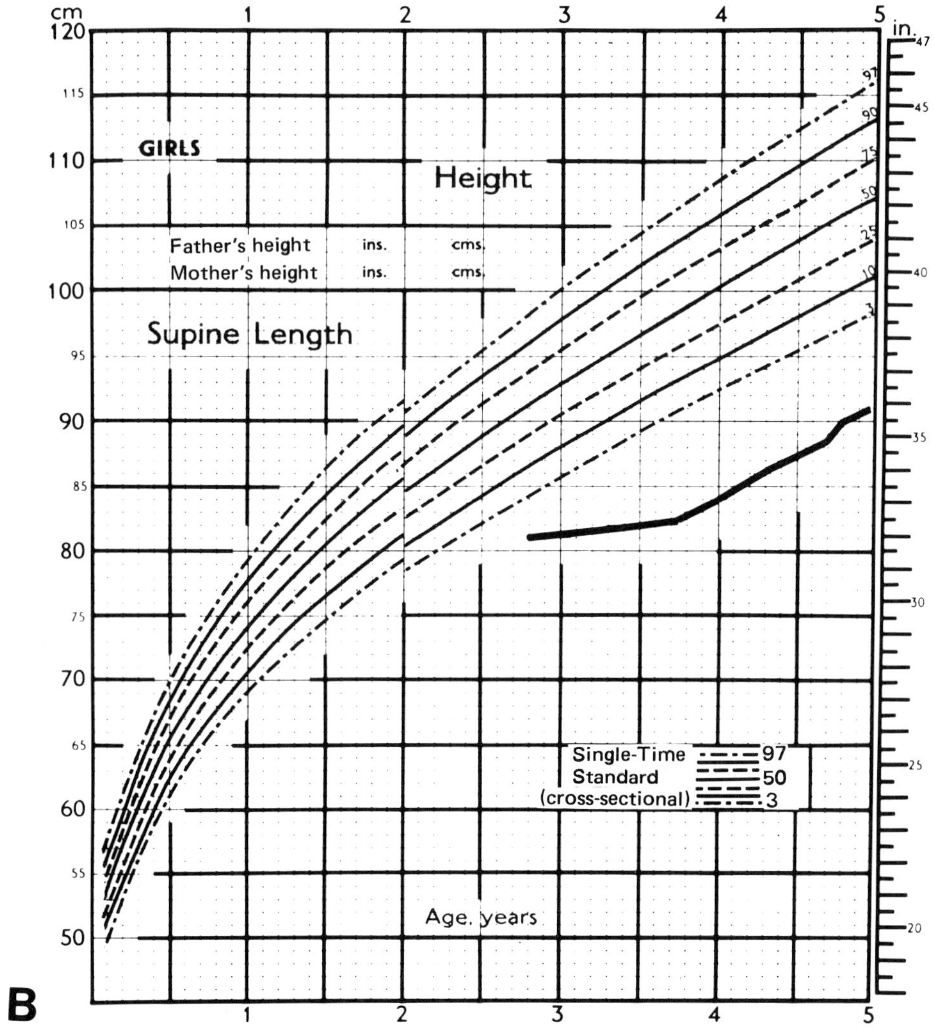

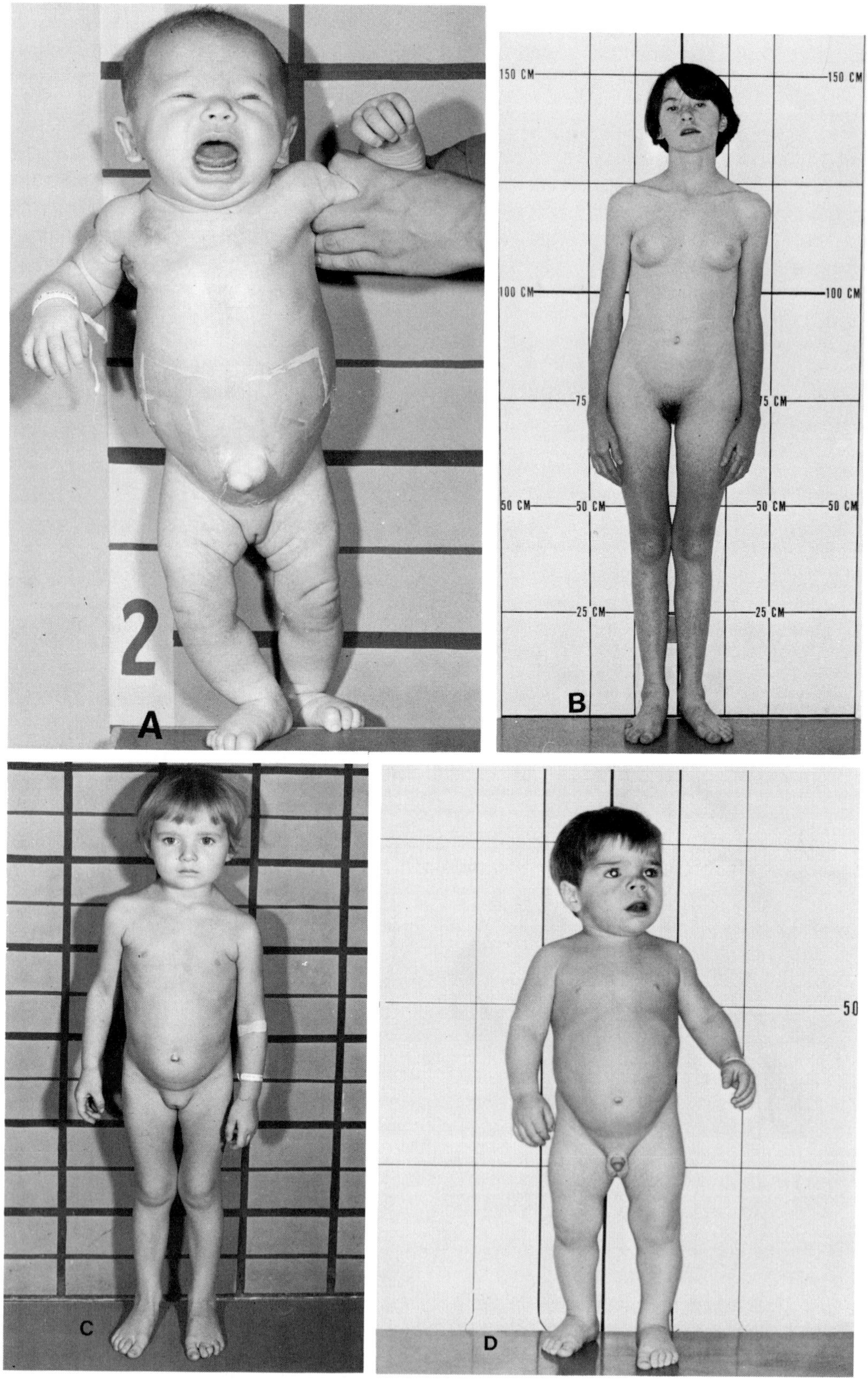

2
A
150 CM
150 CM
100 CM
100 CM
75
75 CM
50 CM
50 CM
50 CM
50 CM
25 CM
25 CM
B
C
50
D

reflexes may show a characteristic delay in the relaxation phase. Unless he is treated, the mental retardation demonstrated on developmental assessment will increase as the child grows older.

In partial hypothyroidism, the clinical features are less obvious and the defect is difficult to recognize (Fig. 16-9**C**). With increasing age, however, growth slows and the relatively slower limb growth results in infantile body proportions. Slow skeletal maturation is reflected in delayed closure of sutures and slow eruption of teeth. Constipation often continues as a prominent symptom, and the mother may complain that the child's skin is dry.

In partial congenital hypothyroidism, mental retardation may not be obvious. The child is often doing school work at, or above, average level when the condition is finally recongized. On formal testing of intelligence, however, the child's psychometric rating may be at the lower end of normal or even below. Such children unfortunately often fall behind in school after they have been made euthyroid.

In making the diagnosis of hypothyroidism during infancy and childhood, roentgenograms will demonstrate a delay in skeletal maturation that is often greater than that reflected in linear growth or weight. At the age of 6 months, the athyrotic cretin may have no epiphyseal centers at the knee; these should be present at birth. In some, the epiphyses that do appear are crenated or stippled; this radiographic finding, "epiphyseal dysgenesis," is more commonly noted in cretins with partial deficiency or in those who have been partially treated. In older children with mild degrees of hypothyroidism, the significant finding may be metaphyseal dysplasia associated with some delay of skeletal maturation. The metaphyseal area, which is thickened and more dense than usual, is slightly irregular.

The principal laboratory tests used to diagnose hypothyroidism have been outlined in Chapter 5, The Thyroid. In all cases of hypothyroidism, the serum thyroxine level will be low. In athyrotic cretinism, the levels are usually reported as less than 1 $\mu g/100$ ml. The serum T_3 resin uptake will also be low. Serum levels of protein bound iodine (PBI) and butanol-extractable iodine (BEI) will be low in these patients, but these tests are less specific than measurement of the serum thyroxine. Radioactive iodine uptakes are not done routinely in infants, but when done, are low. In partial thyroid agenesis, these tests will fall between the normal and athyrotic ranges.

In cretinism due to a metabolic defect of thyroid-hormone synthesis—goitrous cretinism (Fig. 16-9**D**), the serum thyroxine and T_3 resin uptake are low; in most types the radioactive iodine uptake will be normal or increased. The serum PBI may be normal or elevated, and the use of the PBI as a single screening test may lead to a misdiagnosis.

Growth Hormone Deficiency

Etiology. Growth-hormone (somatotropin) deficiency, a rare but important cause of short stature, may be genetic, either as a selective (isolated) deficiency or in association with a lack of other adenohypophyseal hormones. Both types of deficiency seem to be inherited as mendelian recessives. Congenital absence of the pituitary, which is rare, is usually associated with anencephaly. Two newborns encountered at the Hospi-

Fig. 16-9. Thyroid deficiency.

A. At 9 months of age this girl with athyrotic cretinism is only 53 cm (21 inches) long and weighs 6.1 kg (13.5 lb). Note disproportionately small lower limbs, umbilical hernia, and coarse facies.

B. This same child at 14 years. Her physique is within normal limits but her intellect reflects modest impairment.

C. This 4-year-old girl with partial hypothyroidism has short stature as the only obvious stigma of her deficiency. She was 89 cm (35 inches) tall and had relatively short lower limbs. Her only functioning thyroid tissue was at the base of the tongue (lingual thyroid). PBI was 2.4 $\mu g/100$ ml. Her skeletal maturation was retarded to two years.

D. A 3-year-old boy with cretinism due to a defect in thyroid-hormone synthesis. His height, 78 cm, is that of a normal 18-month-old child. The thyroid gland was not palpably enlarged, and diagnosis was delayed because serum PBI and BEI levels were normal.

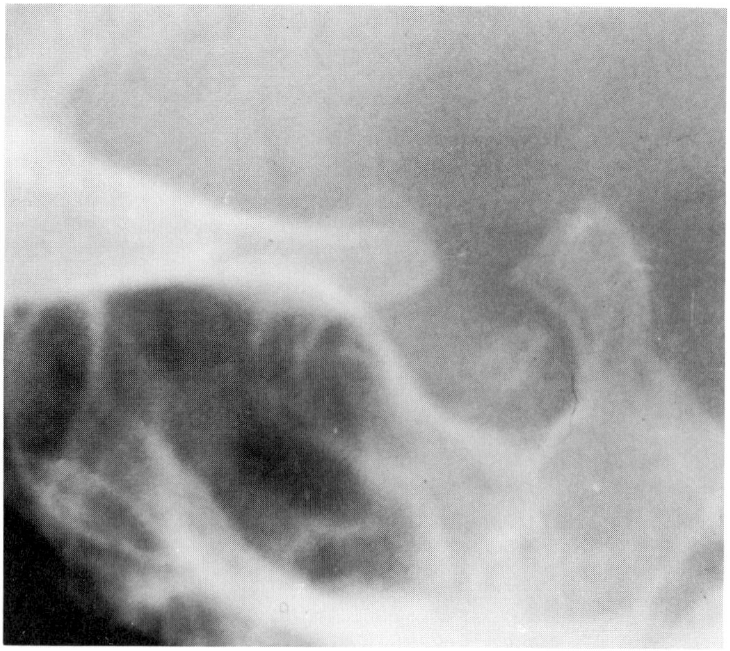

Fig. 16-10. Calcification in the pituitary fossa. This lesion, in a 15-year-old girl with adenohypophyseal deficiency, has remained unchanged since early childhood. The original lesion was presumed to be hemorrhagic infarction of the gland in the perinatal period.

tal for Sick Children had perinatal destruction of the hypophysis with hemorrhagic infarction of the pituitary; both of these infants died in shock. Another patient, who presented during childhood with pituitary insufficiency, had calcification in the pituitary fossa that had been unchanged over several years. This probably represented calcium deposition in an old area of hemorrhagic infarction (Fig. 16-10). The frequency with which children with idiopathic insufficiency are found to have been born by breech delivery suggests that perinatal pituitary damage may produce "idiopathic" hypopituitarism in later childhood.

Although craniopharyngioma is the most common cause of acquired hypopituitarism in childhood, occasionally other tumors in this area or histiocytosis may be responsible. Head injury, apart from that which occurs during delivery, is not a common cause. Congenital or acquired lesions of the hypothalamus may, by interfering with the production or release of growth hormone, produce secondary growth-hormone deficiency. The positive response to thyrotropin-releasing factor reported in a large percentage of children with "idiopathic" hypopituitary dwarfism indicates that hypothalamic deficiency rather than a primary pituitary disorder is the problem in these children.[2]

In "pseudo" growth-hormone deficiency, the hormone is secreted in normal or increased amounts but is not biologically effective (Fig. 16-11). This disorder takes at least two forms: In one, the child produces normal or increased amounts of growth hormone as measured by radioimmunoassay, but the material appears to be biologically inactive.* In the other, normal growth hormone is produced in normal amounts, but the end organ does not respond to it.[13]

Clinical Features. Except for growth failure, growth-hormone deficiency produces few signs or symptoms. The infant may have episodes of hypoglycemia, especially when he has multiple anterior-pituitary deficiencies.

The pattern of growth in anterior pituitary deficiency that begins at birth is illustrated in Figure 16-12**A**, the growth curve of a boy with multiple anterior pituitary deficiencies and that of his normal twin brother. Since these boys were identical twins, we postulate that, in one, the pituitary was damaged during a perinatal accident

* See Appendix: Addendum 1 to Chapter 16.

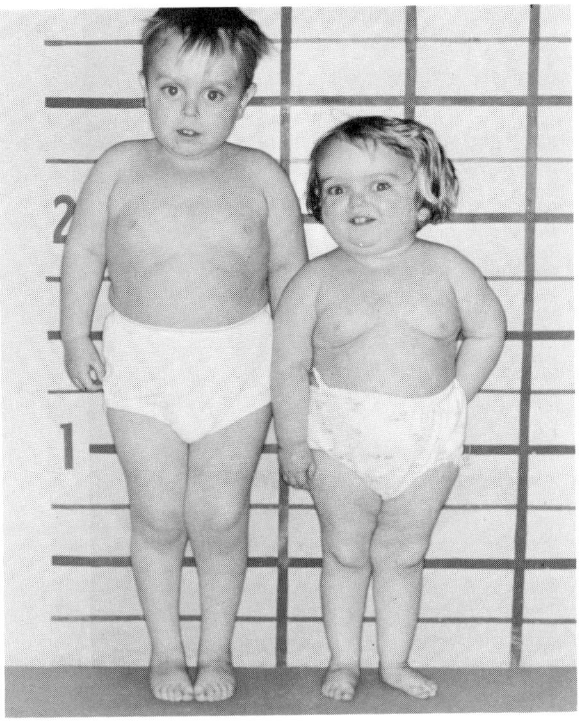

Fig. 16-11. "Pseudo" growth-hormone deficiency. Boy aged 6 with height of 79 cm and his sister aged 4 with height of 63 cm. Although these children show the features of growth-hormone deficiency, serum growth-hormone levels were high, as measured by radioimmunoassay.

although we cannot rule out a developmental defect. In children with such deficiency, growth decelerates after the first few months of life, but the child's short stature is often not recognized until near the end of the preschool period. Growth then continues at a slow pace and gradually falls off below the third percentile channel (Fig. 16-12**B**). If other anterior pituitary hormones are also deficient, the epiphyses will remain open and growth will continue until middle life. In isolated growth-hormone deficiency, however, the epiphyses fuse, and, after an initial slight growth spurt at the time of puberty (which is delayed), the individual remains very short. Because the child with hypopituitarism usually has a greater deficiency of height than weight, he has some degree of obesity. Muscular development, strength, and stamina are frequently slightly decreased.

In addition to recording the growth pattern, the physician must take a detailed history to assess possible etiological factors leading to hypopituitarism. The family history may suggest a genetic disorder. The history of a complicated delivery, such as a breech or twins, especially if associated with signs of neonatal brain damage—e.g., convulsions, spells of apnea, etc.—should be recorded in detail because this may point to perinatal pituitary damage. In later life, history of head injury or symptoms of a hypothalamic-pituitary tumor may provide significant clues. Symptoms of posterior-pituitary insufficiency suggest an acquired lesion in this area.

If the individual with pituitary deficiency has little or no thyrotropin and, hence, inadequate thyroid function, his physical appearance may be altered. Some patients have a sallow complexion and poor peripheral circulation—features that suggest hypothyroidism. Furthermore, these children are alert, and their facies suggest both immaturity and aging, a paradox that is peculiar to hypopituitarism.

Unless the child has suffered cerebral damage from hypoglycemia or from the lesion that produced the hypopituitarism, his intelligence is normal.

Laboratory Diagnosis. The diagnosis of growth-hormone deficiency is confirmed by the use of the radioimmunoassay for circulating growth hormone. Levels in affected patients will be nondetectable or very low and do not rise during any stimulatory test, such as insulin-induced hypoglycemia or arginine infusion.* Investigation should also be carried out to determine the adequacy of secretion of other anterior and posterior pituitary hormones. Thyroid deficiency, emotional deprivation, nutritional disturbances, and other generalized diseases should be treated before accepting low growth-hormone responses as evidence of permanent growth-hormone deficiency. In doubtful cases, the tests for growth-hormone secretion should be repeated after other associated conditions have been adequately treated for some months. The tests for pituitary function are outlined in an addendum to Chapter 4.

Insulin secretion after a glucose load or

* See Appendix: Addendum 2 to Chapter 16.

arginine infusion is decreased in hypopituitarism (see Fig. 5, Chap. 4 which shows the normal insulin and growth-hormone responses in a prolonged glucose tolerance test). The finding of low insulin levels during a glucose tolerance test or arginine infusion, therefore, supports the diagnosis of growth-hormone deficiency. This finding is especially helpful in diagnosing "pseudo" growth-hormone deficiency, in which the growth-hormone levels are normal or high while the insulin secretion is low. Contrariwise, the finding of normal or high levels of circulating insulin makes the diagnosis of growth-hormone deficiency unlikely and suggests that the physician should repeat earlier tests that showed an apparently inadequate growth-hormone response.

Roentgenographic Studies. In multiple adenohypophyseal deficiency, skeletal maturation is decreased to a degree more appropriate to the height age than the chronological age. The bones are slight and the skull is thin, unlike the bone structure seen in hypothyroidism, which usually produces a more marked retardation of skeletal maturation. In isolated growth-hormone deficiency, skeletal maturation shows less retardation,

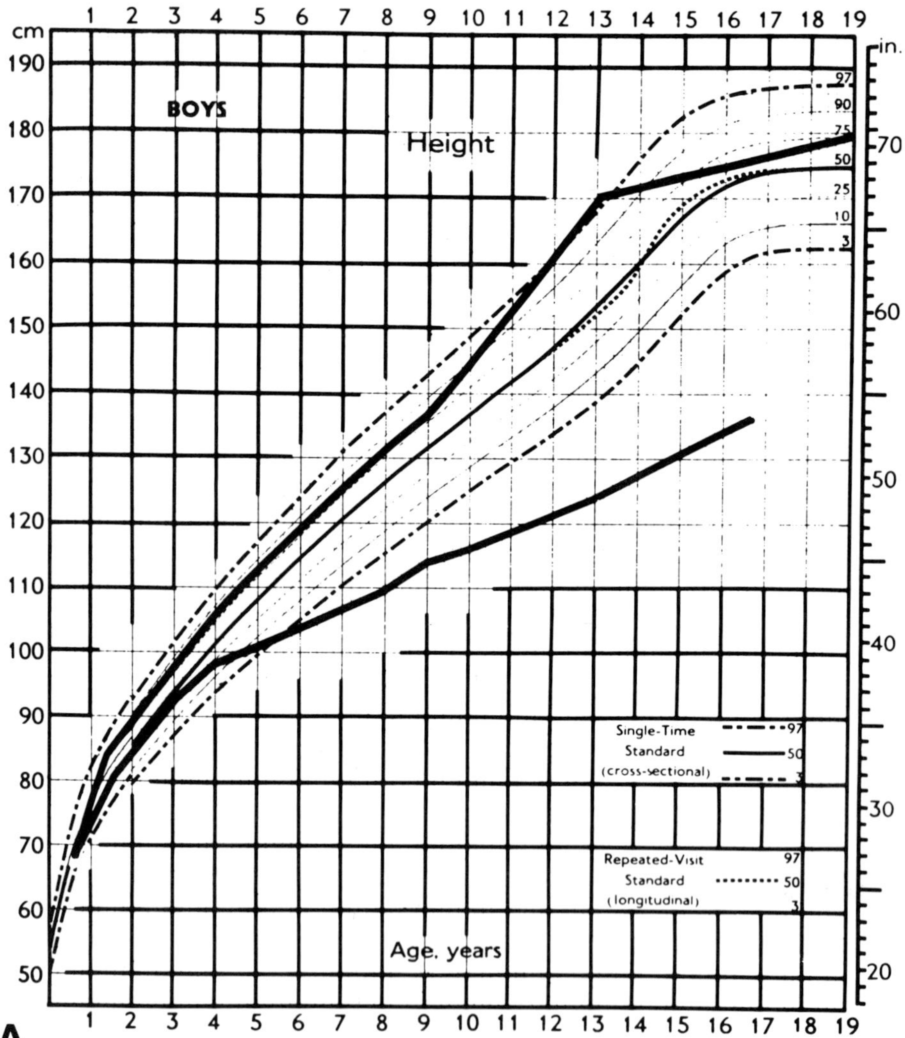

A

and the bone age is usually between the height age and the chronological age.

Adrenal Glucocorticoids and Growth

Cortisone or its analogues, administered for chronic diseases such as bronchial asthma, rheumatoid arthritis, or ulcerative colitis, commonly cause impaired growth in children. The impairment may be due in part to the underlying disease, but the glucocorticoids do markedly suppress growth. In these children, physical signs of glucocorticoid excess are usually evident, and, radiographically, they have delayed skeletal maturation and commonly osteoporosis.

Spontaneous Cushing's syndrome can produce the same type of growth failure. If a child develops truncal obesity and his growth rate slows, the physician should consider this diagnosis (Fig. 16-13). In this condition, however, the adrenal produces variable amounts of androgen; if the amounts are large enough, muscular wasting and growth failure may be less marked. These children will have pubic hair and other evidence of the androgen produced in the adrenal cortex. In

Fig. 16-12. Anterior pituitary deficiency and growth failure.

A. Growth chart of uniovulatory twins, one of whom was affected by adenohypophyseal deficiency, probably from perinatal infarction. For the first 18 months the growth of both twins was almost identical, and only late in the preschool period did the difference in height become noticeable.

B. The twins at 17 years of age. Note the immature appearance of the affected twin and the body proportions, which are in keeping with his "height-age"—approximately 9.5 years.

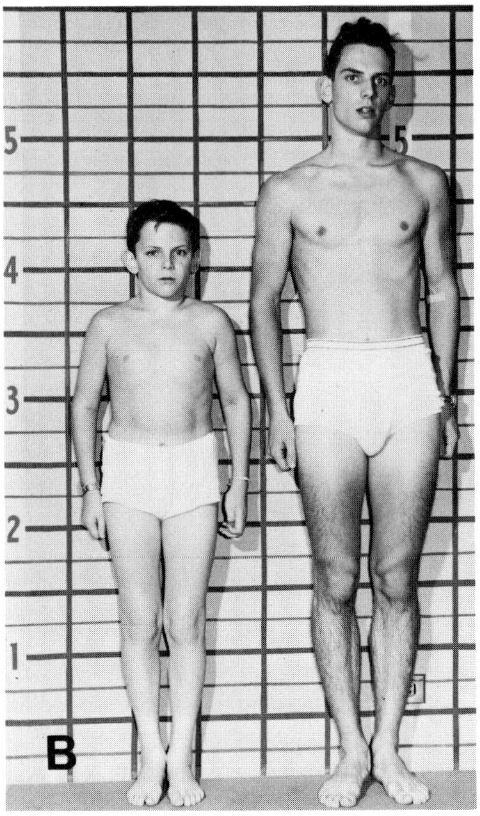

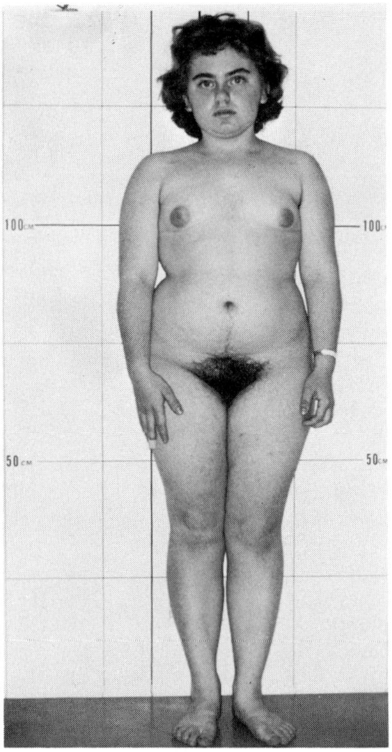

Fig. 16-13. Cushing's syndrome due to bilateral adrenal hyperplasia. The clinical picture in this 13-year-old girl—reduced growth rate, obesity, and signs of virilization—should suggest Cushing's syndrome. After treatment, "catch-up" growth occurs, but adult height is often less than would be expected from the patient's genetic background.

males, the testes remain small. Tests for Cushing's syndrome are outlined in Chapter 7.

Miscellaneous Conditions

In certain syndromes short stature is associated with endocrine abnormalities.

Turner's Syndrome. This chromosomal abnormality has been previously mentioned as a cause of intrauterine growth failure. The typical infant is easily recognized: a phenotypic female with neck webbing, a low hairline at the nape of the neck, low-set ears, arms with wide carrying angles, widespread nipples with a shield-like chest, and frequently short fourth metacarpals and scoliosis (Fig. 16-14**A**). A high arched palate and small chin produce a typical facial appearance. Coarctation of the aorta and renal abnormalities are common. Some have mild mental retardation, and specific perceptual handicaps may lead to learning difficulties and slow school progress. Roentgenograms of the skeleton often show osteoporosis with defects at the wrists and knees.

The diagnosis is supported by finding that sex-chromatin masses are absent on buccal smear and by dermatoglyphic studies that show an increased dermal ridge count. The diagnosis is confirmed by chromosomal analysis of cells cultured from blood or skin, which usually shows a 45,XO karyotype (Chapter 11).

Atypical cases are common. Apart from short stature, the other physical features may be absent in some instances and, rarely, sexual development may proceed normally. These persons usually have mosaicism of the karyotype. Others may have an isochromosome abnormality or other

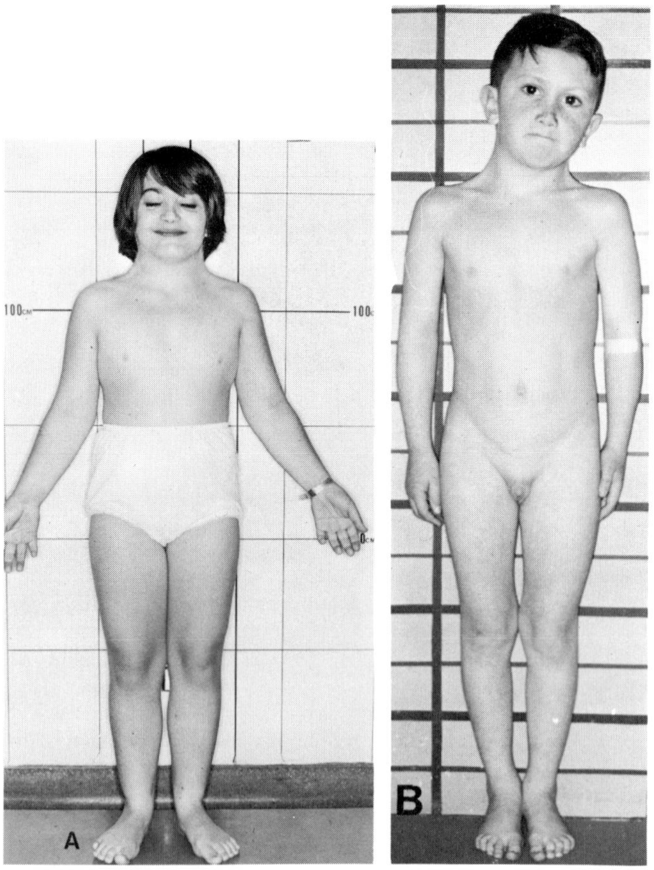

Fig. 16-14. Turner's syndrome.

A. This 15-year-old girl has the typical features of Turner's syndrome—webbing of the neck, short stature (126 cm), wide carrying angles, and widely-spaced, immature nipples. Her karyotype was 45,XO.

B. Turner's syndrome in a phenotypic male at age 9 years and 111 cm in height. His chromosome pattern was mosaic, with a mixture of cells showing a 45,XO and 46,XY karyotype. One testis was removed in infancy after strangulation. The left testis was undescended. Coarctation of the aorta was repaired in early infancy.

chromosome defect: There may be a total of 46 chromosomes in some cells, and the buccal smear may be misleading because some of the cells have sex-chromatin masses. In rare cases, a male phenotype can occur with XY,XO mosaicism but usually this karyotype is associated with a female habitus (Fig. 16-14**B**).

Noonan's Syndrome. Children with Noonan's syndrome,[6] like those with Turner's, have marked growth retardation and webbing of the neck (Fig. 16-15). They have normal chromosome karyotypes and differ, in several respects, from patients with Turner's. Males are frequently affected. Their eyes have an antimongoloid slant; they have moderate degrees of mental deficiency, and secondary sexual development is usually normal but delayed.

Pseudohypoparathyroidism. Children with pseudohypoparathyroidism have dwarfism, typical rounded facies, short metacarpals, and usually some degree of mental deficiency. Roentgenograms of the skull may show intracranial calcification. In pseudohypoparathyroidism, the serum calcium level is low and inorganic phosphate is elevated. In pseudopseudohypoparathyroidism, which is probably a variant of pseudohypoparathyroidism, serum calcium and phosphorus levels are normal. The physical characteristics of pseudohypoparathyroidism probably reflect an inherited syndrome rather than an endocrine disorder. This condition is described in more detail in Chapter 6.

Laurence-Moon-Biedl Syndrome. In addition to short stature, these children are obese and have polydactyly, retinitis pigmentosa, and mental retardation. They occasionally have diabetes insipidus and, as they grow older, may develop diabetes mellitus.

Prader-Willi Syndrome. In addition to their short stature, these children have muscular hypotonia, obesity, mental retardation, and a typical facies. Males have poorly developed genitalia and undescended testes. After 12 years of age, they frequently develop the adult type of diabetes mellitus.[3]

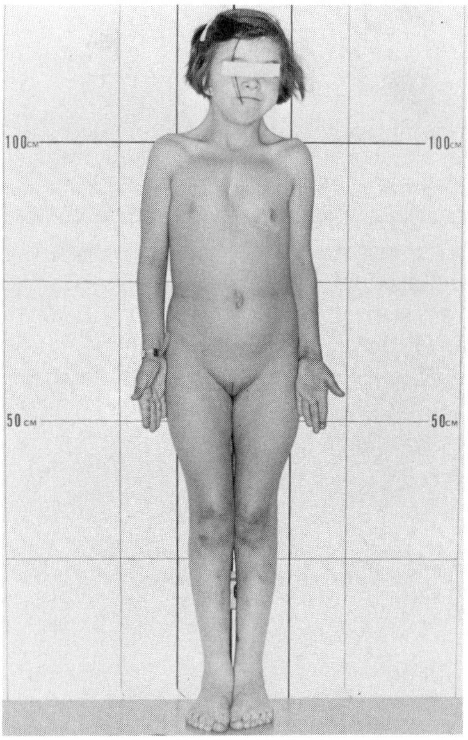

Fig. 16-15. Noonan's syndrome. In this 12½-year-old girl, short stature, webbed neck, and wide carrying angles give a superficial resemblance to Turner's syndrome. However, she has an antimongoloid slant to her eyes and pectus excavatum. She also had pulmonary atresia and a low dermal ridge count. Chromosome studies showed a normal female pattern (46,XX).

Growth Retardation in Adolescence

Most short individuals consult the doctor in their early or midteens. The causes of short stature in this period are numerous, but as in the younger child, endocrine abnormalities are relatively infrequent. The growth-retarding effects of the various nonendocrine causes, such as regional ileitis, renal disease, rheumatoid arthritis, or asthma, may only become apparent after 12 years of age. A few patients with mild bony dysplasias may also be seen for the first time at this age and, in them, radiographic studies will confirm the diagnosis. However, the most common causes of short stature in the teenager are: (1) delayed onset of puberty with its associated growth spurt; (2) familial constitutional short stature.

Delayed Adolescence

Sexual maturation and its associated growth spurt normally occurs later in boys than in girls. If puberty is delayed in a boy, the difference between his growth and that of his fellows rapidly becomes apparent and arouses his concern and that of his parents, particularly if he has always been a little shorter than his friends. Frequently, the father had a similar growth pattern. The endocrine function of such a child is usually normal, and his skeletal maturation, reflected in his bone age, is slightly less than normal.

The gonadotropic "triggering" of normal puberty may be delayed as a physiological variant, or rarely the gonadotropins may be permanently absent. These conditions must be distinguished, and in this, the physical examination helps. In delayed puberty, the testes and scrotum are usually normal structurally but are smaller than in the normal pubescent boy. When gonadotropins are permanently absent, the testes are often incompletely descended and may be smaller than those of an infant. The external genitalia are poorly developed even for the prepubertal male, and the patient develops a eunuchoid habitus. When gonadotropin is insufficient or absent, there is no pubertal growth spurt in the early teens but, because the epiphyses remain open and growth hormone and other factors continue to stimulate bone growth, the individual eventually becomes taller than average. In some cases, tests for growth-hormone secretion will be indicated to rule out a pituitary disorder causing a combined gonadotropin and growth hormone deficiency.

Genetic Short Stature

These young people come to the physician in their teens because they have become increasingly conscious of the social handicap imposed by short stature. In males the social norm requires an eventual height of at least 5 feet 6 inches (167 cm). If the boy is normal physically, the diagnosis of genetic short stature can usually be made from a careful family history. Skeletal maturation is usually normal unless the onset of puberty is also delayed. Those who have an equivocal family history and delayed puberty should have tests of growth-hormone secretion. Most teenagers with congenital growth-hormone deficiency have a distinctive growth pattern characterized by a gradual decline below the third percentile on the growth grid. This decline becomes more marked in the early teens because the expected adolescent growth spurt does not take place. Acquired growth-hormone deficiency, however, may be more difficult to distinguish from genetic short stature, and the physician, if he suspects a pituitary lesion, should investigate the patient's anterior pituitary function fully.

Endocrine Disorders

Thyroid Deficiency

In the adolescent, the most common cause of thyroid deficiency is chronic lymphocytic (Hashimoto's) thyroiditis. Rare causes are destruction of the gland from other types of inflammatory disease, and postirradiation or postthyroidectomy deficiency. Excess iodides and certain other drugs may cause a goiter and hypothyroidism. In constitutionally disposed individuals, deficient iodide intake may also induce goiter and, rarely, thyroid deficiency. Finally, cystinosis, a rare metabolic disease, may destroy the thyroid. In young people, mild congenital disorders of thyroid-hormone production may not become apparent until the usual age of puberty. These individuals usually have an associated goiter. In intrathyroid iodine metabolism, the site of the defect is often before "organification" and can be identified by the perchlorate flushing test.

In juvenile myxedema, the clinical findings depend on the duration and the degree of insufficiency. Commonly, the parents notice that the child has constipation, dryness of skin, and general lassitude. These children do not grow during the period of expected growth spurt and often gain weight despite their small appetites. They are short, often with a disproportionate shortness of limbs; they have sallow complexions, slight facial puffiness, dry skin and hair, slight obesity with supraclavicular fat pads, and delayed dentition (Fig. 16-16). A goiter may be present or not, depending on etiology. Sexual development is usually delayed but some females develop precociously with irregular episodes of vaginal bleed-

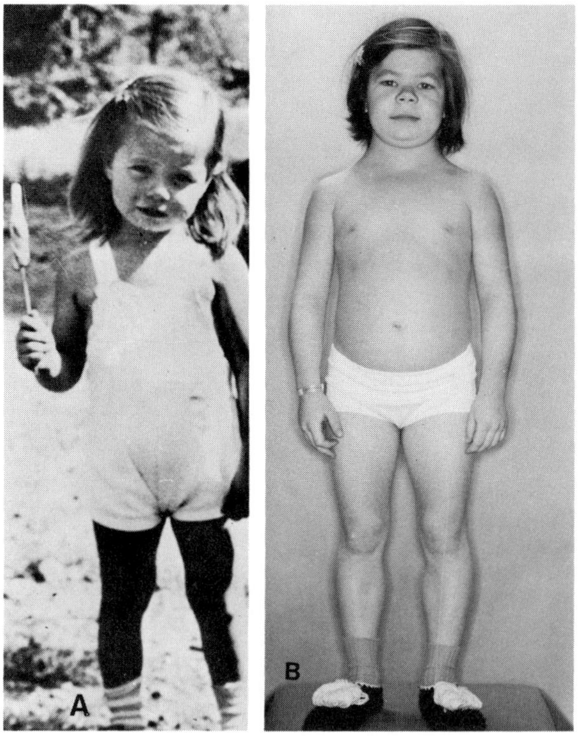

Fig. 16-16. Juvenile myxedema. A. At 2 years of age, this girl shows no signs of cretinism. Growth and physical appearance were normal up to 7 years of age. School progress was not affected by her hypothyroidism. **B.** The same girl at 13 years of age after she developed juvenile myxedema.

ing. This pseudopuberty associated with hypothyroidism has rarely been reported in males. The cause of the precocity is unknown but has been postulated as due to an overlap stimulation of pituitary gonadotropins along with the increased TSH production caused by primary hypothyroidism. Other theories include a possible loss of gonadotropin-inhibiting factor or a possible inefficiency of the hepatic enzymes that conjugate estrogens prior to excretion. In patients with chronic thyroiditis, thyroid antibodies will be elevated. Chapter 5 contains a more complete discussion of juvenile myxedema.

Growth Hormone Deficiency

If growth failure is due to growth-hormone deficiency and appears late in childhood, the child probably has an acquired lesion of the pituitary-hypothalamic region, usually a craniopharyngioma but, less commonly, other tumors, histocytosis, granulomatous lesions, inflammatory diseases, or trauma is the cause. Almost always in these individuals, an associated defect of gonadotropin secretion leads to cessation or delay in puberty. They also have a variable degree of thyrotropin and adrenocorticotropin insufficiency. The child with craniopharyngioma may also have posterior pituitary insufficiency.

To investigate these patients, the physician must carry out the radiographic and laboratory studies referred to earlier in this chapter.

Sexual Precocity

Children who have lesions of the hypothalamic-pituitary area, adrenal cortex, or gonads that produce sexual precocity have an early growth spurt, but their epiphyses close prematurely. By the expected age of puberty, they will be short

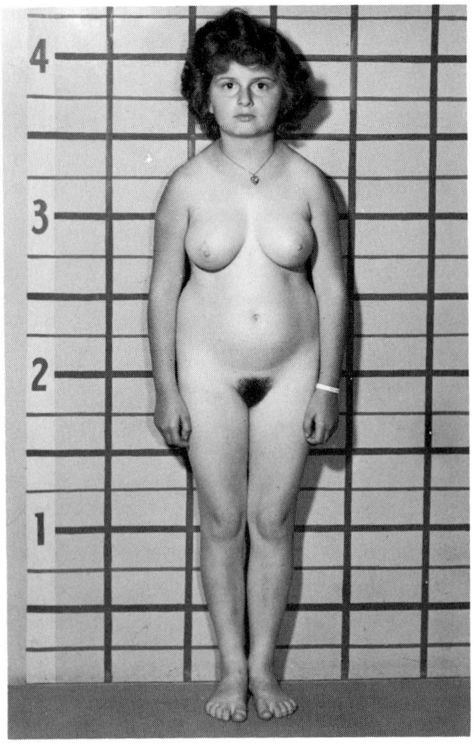

Fig. 16-17. Sexual precocity. A 9-year-old girl with sexual precocity due to hypothalamic tumor. Skeletal maturation was 13 years. This child had an adult height of 140 cm (55 inches) at 11 years.

and, because their epiphyses are fused, will have no further growth (Fig. 16-17).

Diabetes Mellitus

The short stature associated with an enlarged liver and delayed puberty (Mariac's syndrome) results from poor diabetic control. To ensure optimal growth and secondary sexual development, the diabetic child must be carefully managed throughout childhood and adolescence.

Other Lesions

Many of the endocrine and nonendocrine conditions that cause growth failure in infancy and childhood may also develop during adolescence. Such children must be carefully investigated to detect underlying systemic disease, especially that of the urinary tract. Dermatoglyphic studies and chromosome analyses are often useful, especially in the short female who has anomalies suggestive of Turner's syndrome. Spontaneous Cushing's syndrome, rare at any period in childhood, is more common in the adolescent.

Management of Patients with Short Stature

Specific therapy is available for only a small number of short patients. However, regardless of whether treatment is necessary or available, certain aspects of management are useful in all such children.

Therapy for Systemic or Generalized Nonendocrine Disease

The first principle in the management of children and adolescents with short stature is this: "Make an accurate diagnosis." If the child has a generalized systemic disease that can be treated, he will make a satisfactory growth response. In some cases the child may grow with increased velocity during a "catch-up" period and eventually achieve a normal stature—e.g., after a congenital heart defect is corrected or a recurrent urinary infection is successfully treated. In other situations, if the underlying disease cannot be completely cured, growth will be subnormal but improved—e.g., cystic fibrosis. However, in some conditions such as rheumatoid arthritis, treatment with corticosteroids may slow linear growth.

Nutritional Treatment

Regardless of the cause of growth failure, the patient's diet must be carefully assessed. He cannot grow unless he can tolerate and absorb adequate quantities of all required food. In nutritional deficiency, a full diet alone will produce rapid growth without other treatment. In such conditions as hypothyroidism or hypopituitarism, the child will not achieve his full growth response unless, in addition to replacement therapy, his intake of calories, protein, and other essential nutritional elements are increased.

Hormonal Therapy

The general rule is this: Correct the specific deficiencies with the specific hormones.

Hypothyroidism

Cretins should receive replacement doses of either l-thyroxine or desiccated thyroid. Treatment should be started promptly, given in adequate dosage, and continued without interruption.

In infants under 6 months of age, the initial dose of l-thyroxine 0.025 mg daily, is increased by 0.025 mg at 6 to 10-day intervals until the total daily dose reaches 0.075 mg. At 6 to 9 months, 0.1 mg is the usual daily dosage, and from 9 to 18 months, 0.15 mg. Increases are made over the next 3 or 4 years until the usual optimal dosage, between 0.25 and 0.3 mg daily, is reached. During adolescence a further increase may be required. The corresponding starting dose of desiccated thyroid is 15 mg daily with increases of 15 mg increments every 6 to 10 days until a dose of 45 mg is reached in young infants. At 6 to 9 months 60 mg is usually tolerated, and from 9 to 18 months, 90 mg. The usual daily dose after 18 months is gradually increased to 150–180 mg daily.

If the child is given too much thyroid hormone, he develops diarrhea, tachycardia, tremors, excess sweating, irritability, and wakefulness. If these symptoms appear, the dose should be reduced slightly.

We must emphasize that the optimal dosage for treatment is assessed on the basis of clinical response. The signs of hypothyroidism disappear, and after a "catch-up" growth spurt, the child subsequently reaches a normal growth rate. The growth chart and yearly radiographs for skeletal maturation provide useful guidelines to adequate treatment. Laboratory tests are less useful indexes. The child on adequate desiccated thyroid therapy will usually have a serum thyroxine level and PBI in the normal range (serum thyroxine of 4–11 μg/100 ml and PBI of 4–8 μg/100 ml). If l-thyroxine is used in treatment, these values will be slightly higher when the child is receiving optimal therapy.

The treated infant will increase his activity and will progress through the various maturational milestones that will bring his development closer to normal. The athyrotic cretin, however, may have a permanent intellectual deficit because he did not have enough thyroid in utero. This deficit will, of course, be accentuated if treatment is delayed, inadequate, or interrupted in early life. Treatment started late produces a good growth response (Fig. 16-18), but the child's intellectual ability does not improve significantly. In some instances, the older, severely retarded cretin may be easier to manage if the thyroid dosage is kept at a lower level.

The same principles apply in children with juvenile hypothyroidism or those in whom partial thyroid insufficiency has been diagnosed late in childhood (Fig. 16-19**A** & **B**). The initial daily dose of l-thyroxine could, in these children, be increased to 0.05 mg, or desiccated thyroid 30 mg. The dose of l-thyroxine is raised by increments of 0.05 mg (30 mg of desiccated thyroid) every 1-2 weeks until reaching the usual dose of 0.25–0.3 mg daily (150–180 mg of desiccated thyroid).

If on thyroid replacement the patient does not have an adequate increase in growth, the dosage and potency of the thyroid preparation should be checked. Finally, the child's hypothyroidism may be secondary, i.e., associated with anterior pituitary deficiency, in which case his growth will not respond to thyroid treatment alone.

Hypopituitarism

The child with hypopituitarism must receive all necessary hormones, that is, those from the adrenal and thyroid, growth hormone, and, ultimately, sex hormones. In the child with anterior-pituitary deficiency, the physician must ensure that his adrenal cortex is producing adequate amounts of corticoids. In this respect, it is sometimes difficult to decide whether he needs continual maintenance therapy with hydrocortisone or similar preparations. Infants and children who, while under observation, have had a hypoglycemic episode should be on a maintenance dose of hydrocortisone (or analogue). Since cortisone interferes with growth, the dose should be kept as low as possible, usually between 10 and 25 mg of corti-

A

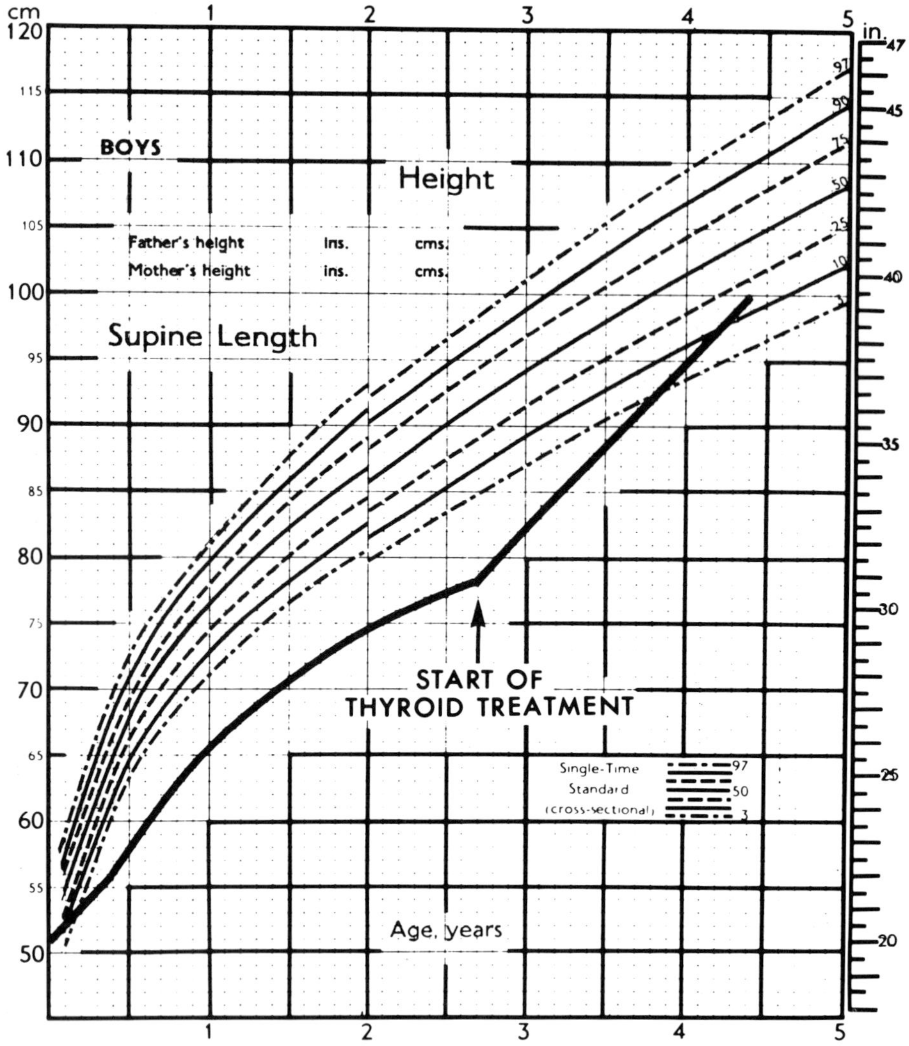

Fig. 16-18. Results of treatment for hypothyroidism. In the growth chart of the boy shown in Figure 16-9**D**, the *heavy solid line* depicts his rapid growth spurt after he started on thyroid replacement.

sone daily. However, whether the child is on maintenance therapy or not, he will not respond adequately to stress (operations, accidents, or serious illness) because he cannot produce additional adrenocorticotropic hormone. Therefore, when they come under severe stress, all patients with adrenocorticotropic insufficiency must receive intravenous hydrocortisone promptly; this is especially true if, because of associated illness, they cannot take cortisone by mouth. These patients should wear a bracelet or carry other identification that warns of this urgent need for steroids; this "built-in" alert system may prevent a tragedy.

Most children with anterior-pituitary deficiency require thyroid supplements but they usually require a lower dose of l-thyroxine or desiccated thyroid than those with primary hypothyroidism. Requirements will often increase during growth hormone treatment.

To achieve full growth, children with pituitary deficiency need human growth hormone. The dos-

Fig. 16-19A. A 16-year-old goitrous cretin. Skeletal maturation was 8 years. **Fig. 16-19B.** The same patient at age 17, 1 year after he started on thyroid replacement. The marked change in his physical appearance was associated with an increase of 8 cm in stature.

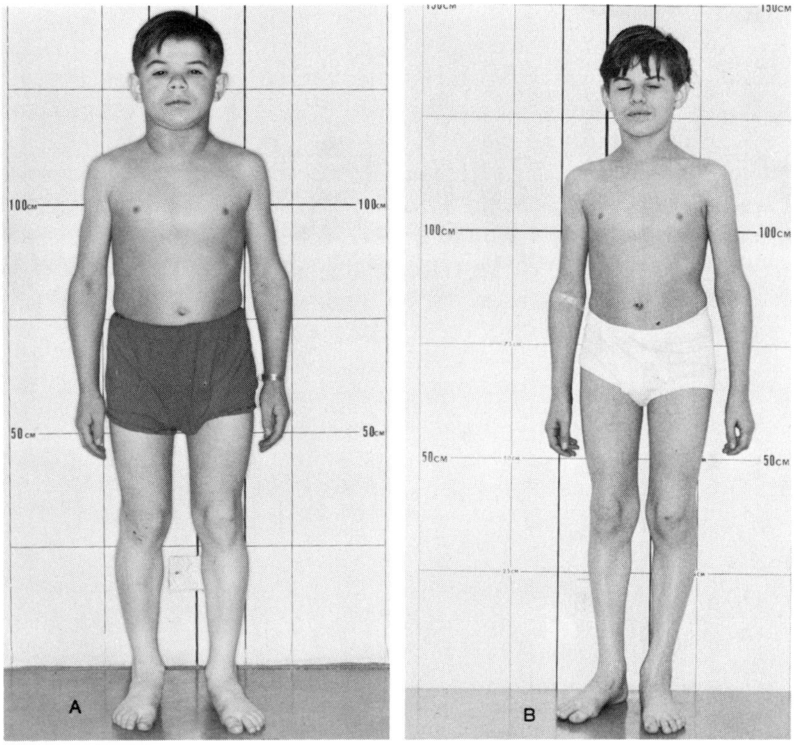

age, which is the same in isolated growth-hormone deficiency as it is when the anterior pituitary hormones are also lacking, is empirical: 2–5 units intramuscularly 3 times each week. Young children respond adequately on the lower dosage but older children or teenagers will need 5 units 3 times a week to achieve full growth. Growth is usually greatest during the first 6–12 months of treatment. Some children may not respond or may become resistant as a result of antibody production. After a waiting period, these patients may again respond to growth hormone treatment.

To achieve his full growth before his epiphyses fuse, the teenager with adenohypophyseal deficiency needs sex hormone replacement, but this should be postponed until he reaches the late teens. The physician should remember that the optimal growth spurt requires the synergistic effects of adequate thyroid, androgen, and growth hormone. Females usually need small doses of androgens along with the replacement of female sex hormones. The use of human gonadotropins to produce a more adequate sexual development is discussed in Chapter 10, The Ovary.

Diabetes insipidus is fairly common in patients with pituitary deficiency due to craniopharyngioma or other tumors, and vasopressin replacement is usually advisable. These patients often respond to chlorpropamide; however, this drug must be used with great caution because it produces hypoglycemia, and the long-term effects are unknown. Because he is deficient in adrenocorticotropic and growth hormones, the child with anterior pituitary deficiency can only respond in a limited way to hypoglycemia, and if his blood sugar is below the normal range, chlorpropamide should not be used.

Delayed Puberty

If the teenager with short stature and associated delayed sexual development has normal pituitary function, the physician need only reassure him. However, each patient's physical, sexual, and psychosocial development must be assessed carefully because, in some patients, the physician may provoke an emotional crisis by withholding treatment. In many, and especially in older teenage boys, pubertal development should be initiated with testosterone or human chorionic gonadotropin, a course which often seems to stimulate endogenous gonadotropin production and further maturity.

Before initiating such treatment, the patient should be carefully assessed in regard to physical, intellectual and emotional maturity. A radiograph of the wrists should be done to estimate skeletal maturation. In some cases, more complete investigation of pituitary function is indicated. With small, incompletely descended testes and no signs of secondary sexual development in a 14-year-old boy, the diagnosis of hypogonadotropic hypogonadism should be considered as a possible cause. Lack of sense of smell would suggest a diagnosis of Kallman's syndrome. Primary testicular defects may also present such a picture, but in this case the gonadotropins would be elevated.

If human chorionic gonadotropin (HCG) is used for treating delayed adolescence, the dose used is 2000 units intramuscularly three times a week for three months. The alternative approach is to give testosterone sublingually in a dose of 10 mg b.i.d. or t.i.d. (or I.M. long-acting testosterone in a dose of 200 mg every 2 weeks for a period of three months). Either hormone course may be repeated once, or occasionally twice, if progress remains at an unsatisfactory level. Failure of response, however, might indicate some abnormality which requires specialized investigation. In short, immature boys some clinicians prefer to use an androgenic anabolic agent such as fluoxymesterone in a dose of 5 mg b.i.d. for a similar three-month course.

Other Conditions

Children with sexual precocity require special consideration because their advanced physical and sexual development may have precipitated emotional and social problems. Because their skeletal maturation is also advanced, suppression of excess sex hormone production may prevent early epiphyseal fusion and eventual short stature. Congenital adrenal hyperplasia due to enzymatic blocks in hydrocortisone production can be suppressed by adrenocortical steroids. Children with isosexual true precocious puberty have been treated with such agents as medroxyprogesterone (Provera). This program, which involves intramuscular injections over a long period, has not produced a completely normal growth pattern.

The management of diabetes mellitus or insipidus, ovarian dysgenesis, and other endocrine disorders that may be associated with decreased growth, are discussed in the appropriate sections of this book.

Nonspecific Hormone Treatment

Several androgen derivatives have been used to treat children with short stature because their anabolic effects stimulate linear growth. However, the use of these agents is controversial. All have an androgenic effect and, hence, must be used with caution in young children, especially females. They have the same potential toxicity as oral testosterone—that is, they may produce cholestatic jaundice. The main objection to their use, however, is that these agents also increase the rate of skeletal maturation; thus these hormones may produce an immediate gain in stature at the expense of the child's eventual height.

At present, I believe that there are few indications for treatment with these androgen derivatives. The child with a chronic disease such as asthma or cystic fibrosis is a possible exception because he has grossly retarded skeletal maturation and poor muscular development. In this situation, the "anabolic agent" may improve the child's general health as well as stimulate his growth. Treatment should be given for a 3-month course and repeated if indicated by permanent small size and a delay of maturation.

Psychological Problems and Their Management

As noted previously, emotional deprivation can cause severe growth deficits. If the physician establishes with certainty that emotional deprivation is the principal cause of retarded growth, he must place the child in a new environment until his growth and emotional development catch up to the normal level. Some of these children have a growth-hormone or adrenocorticotropic deficit

condition is not recognized and treated in early infancy, the child's intelligence will be permanently impaired.

In many cases the child with short stature will be in good health; if so, it is usually better to reassess the child's progress 6 months later than begin an extensive and usually unproductive immediate investigation. During this period, the physician can measure the velocity of growth and, if it is decreased, he knows the child has a disorder that requires further study.

Children and adolescents with growth problems can be helped only if the physician makes an accurate diagnosis and carefully assesses the numerous endocrine and nonendocrine factors that are involved. In addition to specific hormone treatment, patients with endocrine disorders require adequate nutrition and a stable home environment. Many of these patients need psychological support, and in several types of growth problems, genetic counseling is most important.

References

1. Cheek, D. B. Cellular growth—hormones, nutrition and time: Borden award address, October 1967. *Pediatrics 41*:30–46, 1968.
2. Costom, B. H., Grumbach, M. M., and Kaplan, S. Effect of thyrotropin-releasing factor on serum thyroid-stimulating hormone: An approach to distinguishing hypothalamic from pituitary forms of idiopathic hypopituitary dwarfism. *J Clin Invest 50:* 2219–2225, 1971.
3. Dunn, H. G. The Prader-Labhart-Willi syndrome: Review of the literature and report of nine cases. *Acta Paediatr Scand* [*Suppl*] 186, 1968.
4. Greulich, W. W., and Pyle, S. I. *Radiographic Atlas of Skeletal Development of the Hand and Wrist,* 2d ed. Stanford, Stanford Univ. Press, 1959.
5. Laron, Z., Pertzelan, A., and Karp, M. Pituitary dwarfism with high serum levels of growth hormone. *Isr J Med Sci 4:*883–894, 1968.
6. Noonan, J. A. Hypertelorism with Turner phenotype: A new syndrome with associated congenital heart disease. *Am J Dis Child 116:*373, 1968.
7. Pimstone, B. L. Barbezat, G. Hansen, J. D. L., and Murray, P. Studies on growth hormone secretion in protein-calorie malnutrition. *Am J Clin Nutr 21:*482–487, 1968.
8. Powell, G. F., Brasel, J. A., and Blizzard, R. M. Emotional deprivation and growth retardation simulating idiopathic hypopituitarism. I. Clinical evaluation of syndrome. *N Engl J Med 276:*1271–1283, 1967.
9. Powell, G. F., Brasel, J. A., Raiti, S., and Blizzard, R. M. Emotional deprivation and growth retardation simulating idiopathic hypopituitarism. II. Endocrinologic evaluation of syndrome. *N Engl J Med 276:*1279–1283, 1967.
10. Prader, A. Testicular size: Assessment and clinical importance. *Triangle 7:*240–243, 1966.
11. Reichlin, S. Growth and the hypothalamus. *Endocrinology 67:*760–773, 1960.
12. Rimoin, D. L., Merimee, T. J., and McKusick, V. A. Growth hormone deficiency in man: An isolated recessively inherited defect. *Science 152:*1635–1637, 1966.
13. Rimoin, D. L., Merimee, T. J., Rabinowitz, D., McKusick, V. A., and Cavalli-Sforza, L. L. Growth hormone in African pygmies. *Lancet 2:*523–526, 1967.
14. Russell, A. A syndrome of "intra-uterine" dwarfism recognizable at birth with cranio-facial dysostosis, disproportionately short arms and other anomalies (5 examples). *Proc R Soc Med 47:*1040–1044, 1954.
15. Silver, H. K., Kiyasu, F., George, J., and Deamer, W. C. Syndrome of congenital hemihypertrophy, shortness of stature, and elevated urinary gonadotropins. *Pediatrics 12:*368–375, 1953.
16. Sotos, J. F., Dodge, P. R., Muirhead, D., Crawford, J. D., and Talbot, N. B. Cerebral gigantism in childhood. *N Engl J Med 271:*109–116, 1964.
17. Tanner, J. M. *Growth at Adolescence.* Oxford, Blackwell Sci., 1962.
18. Tanner, J. M., Whitehouse, R. H., and Takaishi, M. Standards from birth to maturity for height, weight, height velocity and weight velocity in British children, 1965. *Arch Dis Child 41:*454–471, 613–635, 1966.
19. Wettenhall, H. N. B., and Roche, A. F. Tall girls' assessment and management. *Aust Paediatr J 1:*210–216, 1966.
20. Winter, J. S. D., and Faiman, C. Pituitary-gonadal relations in male children and adolescents. *Pediatr Res 6:*126–135, 1972.

17

Hormones and Cancer

John D. Bailey

Although the connection between various malignancies and the endocrine system is complex, some aspects of this relationship have long been recognized. Early in the 19th century, it was observed that orchiectomy caused regression of the prostate and, on the basis of this observation, Huggins and his colleagues, in 1941, suggested this procedure might ameliorate advanced prostatic carcinoma. Castration was also recommended as a treatment for breast carcinoma late in the 19th century. This chapter presents a brief summary of present views of the relationships between hormones and cancer.

Some malignancies of the endocrine glands produce normal or abnormal amounts of their appropriate hormones, or in some instances, abnormal hormones. Sometimes the higher control of some endocrine malignancies may be maintained, but this control is usually partially lost or may be lost completely, giving rise to completely autonomous tumors. The therapy of certain malignancies in tissues normally susceptible to hormonal influences, such as the breast, uterus, or prostate gland, is based on this relationship. For example, withdrawing the normal hormone often brings improvement, as in castration for cancer of the prostate, whereas giving the opposite hormone may bring additional benefit, as in estrogen treatment for prostate cancer. Finally, an interesting group of nonendocrine tumors produce hormones which will be discussed in some detail below.

Hormone-Dependent Tumors

Although many endocrine tumors are autonomous, some malignant tumors of the endocrine glands remain partly dependent on higher stimulatory or inhibitory influences. This dependence may be temporary or may persist. Some ACTH-producing tumors of the adenohypophysis may be held in check (and thus remain occult) because the stimulated adrenal cortices produce excessive cortisol; this excess of circulating cortisol, by a feedback mechanism, inhibits the further growth of the ACTH-producing tumor. It is evident that the "set point" is too "high"—i.e., it takes a very large amount of cortisol to even partially inhibit the ACTH-producing tumor. Thus, when both adrenal glands are removed from a patient with this form of Cushing's syndrome, his only source of cortisol is his medication; the plasma cortisol is now not high enough to inhibit the growth of the ACTH-producing tumor. Consequently, the physiological circulating cortisol level in this situation cannot prevent the pituitary tumor from expanding further, and the ACTH and melanocyte-stimulating hormone (MSH) also increase. It is tempting to speculate that the original cause of the ACTH-secreting tumor might be an increase in corticotropin-releasing hormone (CRH) of the hypothalamus.

In certain susceptible animals, the experimental induction of long-standing hypothyroidism may lead to a TSH-secreting pituitary tumor, which initially depends on the level of thyroxine, subsequently becomes autonomous, and then may be transplanted even to a euthyroid animal. Only one (possible) pituitary TSH-secreting tumor has been reported in man, but this was not hormone-dependent.

Some thyroid carcinomas also retain a variable degree of dependence on TSH although this dependence may not persist indefinitely. Papillary and follicular thyroid carcinomas may thus be dependent—a state which has a definite therapeutic value; in such cases, the administration of thyroxine (which suppresses TSH) may at least partially retard the growth of the tumor.

Rarely, tumors of other endocrine glands may also be dependent although, of course, many endocrine malignancies are virtually autonomous. These tumors have been discussed individually in the appropriate chapters.

Malignancies in Tissues Susceptible to Hormonal Influence

Several tissues in which malignancies occur may be considered as end-organs for various hormones, most significantly the breast, uterus, and prostate; in such malignancies, the administration of hormones may have an adverse or a beneficial effect. It is now common knowledge that carcinoma of the breast may sometimes be aggravated by estrogen and sometimes retarded by androgen therapy. "Endocrine surgery"—i.e., oophorectomy, adrenalectomy, and/or hypophysectomy—is also used in the treatment of breast carcinoma and its metastases. In general, each of these procedures may retard the growth of metastases in cancer of the breast. The criteria for the selection of the patients who will benefit most from such procedures are less than perfect. Sometimes, however, some patients with metastatic carcinoma of the breast show striking improvement with regression of bony metastases after such procedures. However, this is always temporary, and endocrine surgery provides only palliation of metastatic carcinoma.

Carcinoma of the prostate is also influenced by the hormonal milieu. Androgens may aggravate carcinoma of the prostate, whereas orchidectomy and/or estrogen may bring remarkable and prolonged benefit.

Objective regression of metastatic carcinoma of the endometrium has been reported after progesterone therapy.

Since, in all of these examples, the growth of tumor tissue does not depend solely on hormonal influences, endocrine therapy is never wholly satisfactory, and sooner or later, the tumors escape completely.

Endocrine Tumors That Produce Hormones

Many (but not all) endocrine tumors are "active"—i.e., they produce hormones. Many such tumors produce either an excessive amount of a given hormone or group of hormones or at least a limited amount of hormone. Such diseases as acromegaly may be produced by adenomas or carcinomas of the pituitary gland, and several prolactin-secreting tumors of the pituitary have now been reported. ACTH-producing pituitary tumors can cause Cushing's syndrome. Thyroid cancer may produce either thyroxine or, in the case of medullary thyroid carcinoma, calcitonin. Parathyroid carcinomas generally produce parathyroid hormone, and choriocarcinomas produce chorionic gonadotropins and occasionally a TSH-like polypeptide. Tumors of the islet cells of the pancreas may produce excessive insulin or gastrin. Generally, only one cell type becomes malignant, and thus the tumor often produces only one hormone.

In short, tumors of each endocrine gland may produce excessive amounts of the appropriate hormone, limited amounts of hormone, or even none at all. They are independent and thus tend to produce excessive amounts of the hormone, or not enough—i.e., they often do not respond to normal physiological stimulation.

Often specific antineoplastic agents—e.g., dichlorodiphenyl-dichloroethane (o,p,DDD)—inhibit both the growth of adrenal cortical carcinoma and the production of adrenal cortical hormones. Methotrexate often inhibits the growth of choriocarcinomas, thereby reducing the production of chorionic gonadotropin. In other instances, specific drugs may inhibit the production of the specific hormone, yet not interfere with the growth of the tumor.

Nonendocrine Neoplasms Producing Hormones

In recent years, considerable attention has been given to a group of neoplasms producing humoral substances which resemble, or are indistinguishable from, hormones. These tumors may produce specific syndromes, and an increasing number of these syndromes are being described. These disorders are of immediate interest to the clinician because symptoms due to an excess of hormone should lead him to search for a malignant tumor.

The mechanisms of production of these syndromes have not been completely elucidated. Two major hypotheses have been advanced to explain these disorders.

Hypotheses Concerning Origin

Genetic Hypothesis

All cells of an organism presumably contain the same DNA information and are originally capable of synthesizing an unlimited number of proteins. With cellular differentiation, the function of a cell becomes restricted to the production of only a small number of proteins. Normally, repression of the regulator genes causes the structural gene to release messenger ribonucleic acids. During the period of neoplasia, derepression might occur, and the ability to synthesize a certain protein—e.g., a hormone—might be restored. If this were true, the hormone produced by the neoplasm should be similar to, or identical to, the natural hormones.

Aberrant Protein Synthesis

During neoplasia, the abnormal cells may contain new or altered DNA and would then synthesize one or more kinds of abnormal or "disfigured" proteins. Various other proteins having no apparent effect may be produced by such tumors. These neoplasms may then be recognized only by the anatomical disturbance created. From this hypothesis, we would expect that, in most instances, the hormones produced by the neoplasms would be different from the natural hormones.

Which Hypothesis?

It has not yet been demonstrated which hypothesis is correct. The evidence from patients with neoplasms causing hypoglycemia or hyperthyroidism supports the latter hypothesis, because the "hormone" in these cases differs immunologically (and presumably chemically) from the natural hormone. On the other hand, observations on neoplasms that cause hypercalcemia, Cushing's syndrome, and erythremia favor the first hypothesis, because in these the tumor product seems to be identical to the natural hormone.

Abnormalities Associated with Tumors Producing Inappropriate Hormones

The most important humoral syndromes associated with neoplasms are the following: hyperadrenocorticism, hypercalcemia, hypoglycemia, erythremia, hyperthyroidism, precocious puberty, inappropriate secretion of antidiuretic hormone, and atypical carcinoid syndrome.

Hyperadrenocorticism

By 1966, about 150 patients with Cushing's syndrome had been described who had neoplasms in nonendocrine tissues. Liddle *et al.* have now called this disorder the "ectopic ACTH syndrome." Eighty per cent of these neoplasms have been one of three cell types: bronchogenic carcinoma (small, or "oat cell"—undifferentiated), thymic carcinoma, and pancreatic carcinoma. In rare instances, other carcinomas have also produced Cushing's syndrome, including carcinoma of the ovary, prostate, thyroid, kidney, salivary glands, testes, breast, stomach, colon, and gallbladder.

Clinical Manifestations. Cushing's syndrome associated with nonendocrine neoplasia may develop coincidentally with the other clinical manifestations of the nonendocrine tumor. However, the hyperadrenocorticism may develop as early as 4 years before the neoplasm is recognized. In other cases, the neoplasm may have been diagnosed for some time before the Cushing's syndrome became evident. Curiously, although plasma ACTH levels are extremely high, the classic clinical symptoms of Cushing's syndrome may be absent, presumably because the disease has been of short duration; thirst, hypertension, and muscular weakness due to hypokalemic alkalosis are often the major manifestations. Liddle *et al.* reported that, of 36 patients with hyperadrenocorticism of all types, 19 had excessive amounts of *pituitary* ACTH, 8 had primary adrenocortical tumors, and 9 had the ectopic ACTH syndrome. Of these 9, only 2 had the classic appearance of Cushing's syndrome. Therefore, the physician should evaluate all cancer patients who have edema, hypokalemia, or abnormal glucose tolerance with this syndrome in mind. The diagnosis is often difficult. Of course, plasma cortisol and urinary cortisol metabolites are elevated. In Cushing's syndrome due to excess *pituitary* ACTH, urinary levels of 17-hydroxycorticoids range from slightly above to three times normal, whereas, in the ectopic ACTH syndrome, they are usually very greatly elevated. In Cushing's disease due to excessive *pituitary* ACTH, 17-ketosteroid excretion is sometimes normal; it is usually greatly elevated in the ectopic ACTH syndrome. In Cushing's syndrome of pituitary origin, large doses of dexamethasone will suppress ACTH and lower plasma and urinary 17-hydroxycorticoids, but in the ectopic ACTH syndrome they usually do not have this effect. Primary adrenocortical tumors are not suppressed by dexamethasone, but in these instances the plasma ACTH is low.

In the ectopic ACTH syndrome, the tumor elaborates a polypeptide that has ACTH activity. Liddle *et al.* have analyzed the tumor ACTH in great detail and found that, in its biological actions and chemical and immunological properties, this "hormone" did not differ significantly from pituitary ACTH. Thus, tumor ACTH seems virtually identical with pituitary ACTH. When the neoplasm is effectively treated, the Cushing's syndrome goes into remission. If the neoplasm cannot be treated, the Cushing's syndrome can be repressed by bilateral adrenalectomy.

Hypercalcemia

Hypercalcemia is found with a great variety of neoplasms, including carcinoma, sarcoma, and lymphomas. In most such cases, the hypercalcemia proves to be due to bony metastases, but in many carefully studied patients, the hypercalcemia developed in the absence of bony metastases.[9] Such patients characteristically have a high serum calcium and a low serum phosphorus and, in other studies of calcium and phosphorus metabolism, are indistinguishable from those with primary hyperparathyroidism. When the neoplasm is removed, the serum calcium returns to normal, demonstrating that the neoplasm has caused the hypercalcemia. In contrast, patients with widespread bony metastases and hypercalcemia usually have elevated serum phosphorus levels. Any patient with a neoplasm who complains of polyuria, anorexia, constipation, lethargy, or fatigue, or who is comatose should be regarded as having this syndrome until proved otherwise. Probably, serum calcium should be determined periodically in all patients with neoplasms.

In most patients who have cancer and hypercalcemia, the parathyroid glands (when they are examined) are normal, indicating that the patients did not have primary hyperparathyroidism and were not elaborating a substance which stimulated the parathyroid gland. Munson *et al.* have extracted from these tumors the substance which causes the hypercalcemia and believe it is identical to parathyroid hormone in its clinical, physical, and immunologic properties. Others, however, have found immunologic differences between the tumor product and true parathyroid hormones.

Treatment. In patients with such neoplasms, the hypercalcemia may often induce severe debility and even cause death. In some, the serum calcium levels can be reduced by increasing water and salt intake. Others may require sodium sulphate, phosphate, chelating agents, or even hemodialysis. Obviously, suppression or extirpation of the neoplasm will alleviate the hypercalcemia, and where possible, this is the treatment of choice.

Hypoglycemia

More than 100 patients have now been described who had hypoglycemia in association with a nonpancreatic tumor.[12] About two-thirds of these have mesenchymal tumors, particularly fibrosarcomas, most of which have been in the abdomen, often behind the peritoneum. Eighteen percent of these tumors have been within the thorax. All have been large, weighing from 800 to 10,000 gm. In addition to these mesenchymal tumors, a small number of hepatic carcinomas and adrenal carcinomas, and smaller numbers of miscellaneous tumors have been associated with hypoglycemia.

The mechanism by which the hypoglycemia is produced is unknown. However, the tumor probably produces an insulin-like substance that is immunologically distinct from true insulin.[11, 12] Some have suggested that the tumor absorbs large amounts of glucose, but most attempts have failed to demonstrate increased glucose absorption specific to the tumor. Excess insulin-like substance circulating without regard to physiological requirements produces prolonged fasting hypoglycemia; this, in turn, depresses the beta cells, often producing a diabetic glucose tolerance curve. The nature of the tumor product that causes the hypoglycemia is unknown; however, some evidence suggests that it may be related to the metabolic products of tryptophan.

Erythremia

Erythremia (erythrocytosis) associated with neoplasms has been described in about 200 patients. The tumors are generally renal carcinomas, but cerebellar hemangioblastomas, benign renal lesions such as adenomas or cysts, and a variety of other neoplasms may cause erythremia. Often, the neoplasms are occult, and a specific search must be made for these tumors. Whereas patients with polycythemia rubra vera usually have enlarged spleens, leukocytosis, and thrombocytosis, those with associated tumors do not. Polycythemia occurs in about 1.3–4.5% of patients with renal tumors, and in 9–20% of those with cerebellar hemangiomas.

This polycythemia appears to be a response to an "erythropoietin-like" material elaborated by the tumor. In over 60 patients, the polycythemia disappeared when the tumor was resected. Several workers have performed bioassays on tumor tissue or cyst fluid from patients with these disorders, and have found high levels of erythropoietin activity. This erythropoietin-like substance has many of the chemical properties of true erythropoietin. However, a small group of patients with hepatomas, urinary fibromas, and ovarian tumors have polycythemia but no demonstrable erythropoietin-like material.

Hyperthyroidism

Eighteen patients have now been described who had benign or malignant neoplasms containing trophoblastic cells and a peculiar form of hyperthyroidism[7, 10]; 17 were women who had choriocarcinomas or hydatidiform moles, and one was a man with a metastatic testicular teratocarcinoma.

In each of these patients, the urinary gonadotropin elaborated by the tumor was more than one million mouse units per 24 hours. Characteristically, these patients have few or no clinical symptoms and few physical findings attributable to hyperthyroidism; nevertheless, laboratory studies indicated marked abnormalities of thyroid function.

Elevated plasma TSH is found by bioassay but not on radioimmunoassay. Neither the tumor gonadotropin nor human chorionic gonadotropin had an intrinsic TSH-like activity. When the neoplasm was treated, the abnormalities of thyroid function disappeared.

The increased thyroid function associated with neoplasms which contain trophoblastic elements appears to be due to a TSH-like substance elaborated by the tumor. Although this material is extracted by the same techniques used to extract pituitary TSH and has similar biological activities, it appears to be different immunologically from both pituitary TSH and from chorionic gonadotropin. It is not an immunoglobulin and thus has no relationship to long-acting thyroid stimulator (LATS).

Water Retention (Inappropriate Secretion of Antidiuretic Hormone)

Inappropriate secretion of ADH may also be associated with a neoplasm; it is characterized by hyponatremia, a persistently hyperosmotic urine, and failure to conserve sodium.[1] This syndrome, which is identical to that caused by continuous administration of antidiuretic hormone, has been attributed to a vasopressin-like substance elaborated by certain neoplasms. The first such patients were described by Schwartz *et al.;* since then, over 25 have been reported.[1] The most common tumor causing this syndrome has been oat-cell bronchogenic carcinoma. On bioassay, extracts of oat-cell carcinomas and the urine of these patients contained large amounts of antidiuretic substance. While tumor extracts and vasopressin bear some chemical similarity, the material may not be identical to vasopressin.

Large amounts of 9-α-fluoro-hydrocortisone appear to alleviate the symptoms completely, but it is not clear how this occurs. The improvement might be due to a decrease in the elaboration of the antidiuretic substance, or to direct renal effects which compensate for the antidiuretic action. Such patients may also be treated by limiting their water intake, because, with water deprivation, vasopressin produces few symptoms.

Gonadotropin Formation

Precocious sexual development due to a gonadotropin-like material elaborated by hepatoblastomas constitutes a rare syndrome. All such patients have been boys ranging in age from 1 to 8 years. None of the neoplasms contained teratoid or trophoblastic elements that could have produced the gonadotropin.[3]

In the adult, benign and malignant placental tumors elaborate gonadotropin similar to that produced by the normal placenta. Hundreds of such patients have been reported. Teratomas of the ovary, testes, or pineal, which also elaborate gonadotropins, develop in adults and children. In three men with adrenocortical carcinoma, a woman with carcinoma of the breast, and another woman with malignant melanoma, the tumor elaborated a gonadotropin. A few patients with carcinoma of the lung have also elaborated large amounts of gonadotropin. At present, it is uncertain whether the material elaborated by these nontrophoblastic neoplasms is identical to chorionic gonadotropin or to one of the pituitary gonadotropins.

Atypical Carcinoid Syndrome

This term has been used to designate the syndrome associated with excessive production of serotonin, 5-hydroxytryptophan, and possibly histamine by a neoplasm *other* than a small intestinal carcinoid. The striking feature of this syndrome is an extraordinary, vivid, fiery, violet-red flush, often lasting several days. These attacks are accompanied by severe anxiety, disorientation, fever, nausea, and vomiting, wheezing, marked diaphoresis, and periorbital and facial edema.

About 25 patients have been described who had bronchial adenomas and the atypical carcinoid syndrome.[3,5] In other patients the syndrome was associated with a pancreatic duct-cell carcinoma, an islet-cell carcinoma (which also produced hypoglycemia), a bronchogenic oat-cell carcinoma, a gastric carcinoma, and a neuroblastoma.

In some of these patients, urinary histamine excretion is increased. In addition, the tryptophan metabolites excreted differ from those in the typical carcinoid syndrome. In the typical syndrome, 5-hydroxytryptamine (serotonin) is almost completely metabolized to 5-hydroxyindoleacetic acid (5-HIAA). In the atypical syndrome, 5-HIAA excretion is again increased, but the excretion of serotonin and 5-hydroxytryptophan is also elevated. Presumably, the tumor elaborates 5-hydroxytryptophan and metabolizes it to 5-HIAA and serotonin in other tissues. This alternate metabolic route may be important in treatment, because in a patient with *atypical* carcinoid syndrome, a decarboxylase inhibitor (α-methyl dopa) decreased the severity of symptoms by preventing metabolism of 5-hydroxytryptophan. However, this action would have no effect on the typical carcinoid syndrome. The vitamin B_6 antagonist, 4-deoxypyridoxine, has also been used to treat the atypical syndrome because the enzymatic decarboxylation of 5-hydroxytryptophan to 5-hydroxytryptamine requires pyriodoxol phosphate as cofactor.

Production of Two or More Humoral Factors by a Single Neoplasm

A number of tumors have been described that apparently produce more than one hormone[3]—e.g., a non-beta-cell carcinoma of the islet of Langerhans produced ACTH, MSH, and gastrin. A hepatoma caused hypercalcemia, erythremia, and hypoglycemia. Another hepatoma caused both hypoglycemia and polycythemia, and still another islet-cell tumor produced both hypoglycemia and carcinoid syndrome. Other examples of tumors producing more than one hormone have been described.

References

1. Lebacq, E., and Delaere, J. Origin of antidiuretic substances and explanation of hypernatriuresis in the Schwartz-Bartter syndrome. *Ann Endocrinol 26:* 375–382, 1965.
2. Liddle, G. W., Givens, J. R., Nicholson, W. C., and Island, D. P. The ectopic ACTH syndrome. *Cancer Res 25:*1057–1061, 1969.
3. Lipsett, M. B. Humoral syndromes associated with cancer. *Cancer Res 25:*1068–1073, 1965.
4. Lipsett, M. B., Odell, W. D., Rosenberg, L. E., and Waldmann, T. A. Humoral syndrome associated with non-endocrine tumors. *Ann Intern Med 61:* 733–756, 1964.
5. Melman, K. L., Sjoerdsma, A., and Mason, D. T. Distinctive clinical and therapeutic aspects of the syndrome associated with bronchial carcinoid tumors. *Am J Med 39:*568–581, 1965.
6. Munson, P. L., Tashjian, A. J., Jr., and Levine, L. Evidence for parathyroid hormone in non-parathyroid tumors associated with hypercalcemia. *Cancer Res 25:*1062–1067, 1965.
7. Odell, W. D., Hertz, R., Ross, G. T., Hammond, C. H., and Lipsett, M. B. Endocrine abnormalities associated with trophoblastic neoplasms. *Clin Obstet Gynecol 10:*290–302, 1967.
8. Schwartz, W. B., Bennett, W., Curelop, S., and Bartter, F. C. A syndrome of renal sodium loss and hyponatremia probably resulting from inappropriate secretion of antidiuretic hormone. *Am J Med 23:*529–542, 1957.
9. Sherwood, L. M., O'Riroden, J. L. H., Aurbach, G. D., and Potts, J. T. J. Production of parathyroid hormone by non-parathyroid tumors. *J Clin Endocrinol Metab 27:*140–146, 1967.
10. Steigbigel, N. H., Oppenheim, J. J., Fishman, L. M., and Carbone, P. P. Metastatic embryonal carcinoma of the testes associated with elevated plasma TSH-like activity and hyperthyroidism. *N Engl J Med 271:*345–349, 1964.
11. Unger, R. H. The riddle of tumor hypoglycemia. *Am J Med 40:*325–330, 1966.
12. Volpé, R., Evans, J., Clarke, D. W., Forbath, N., and Ehrlich, R. Evidence favoring the sarcomatous origin of an insulin-like substance in a case of fibrosarcoma with hypoglycemia. *Am J Med 38:*540–553, 1966.

Appendix

Addenda to Chapters 1, 2, 3, 4, 5, 10, 13, 16

Since the manuscript for this book was prepared, many significant changes have occurred in endocrinology. To update the text the following brief addenda describe the most important of these advances. Also included is information supplemental to the material in the text. These addenda are keyed into the text at the appropriate places by asterisked footnotes.

Addendum to Chapter 1

The target-cell enzyme, e.g., adipose-tissue lipase, is probably activated by cyclic AMP through the intervention of a cyclic AMP-dependent protein kinase. The two subunits of this kinase—the one regulatory and the other catalytic—are combined in the resting state. When the intracellular concentration of cyclic AMP increases, it interacts with the regulating subunit, altering its shape and liberating the catalytic subunit. Through a phosphorylation reaction, the free catalytic subunit, in the presence of ATP, converts the inactive enzyme to its active form. The sequence of membrane activation by hormone binding, which leads to an increased cellular cyclic AMP level and activation of a protein kinase, has been demonstrated for a number of hormonal reactions including glucagon-activated glycogenolysis, ACTH-stimulated steroidogenesis, and parathyroid-hormone-stimulated calcium transport in the renal tubule.

Prostaglandins are a group of ubiquitous membrane-associated lipids composed of 20 fatty acids containing a cyclopentane ring. Prostaglandins may increase cyclic AMP levels in many tissues, probably by modulation of adenyl-cyclase activity. The final effect of prostaglandins on hormone synthesis or hormone-mediated events may be either stimulation or inhibition, depending on the circumstances and the type of prostaglandin tested.

Addendum to Chapter 2

The two catecholamines, dopamine and norepinephrine, and the indoleamine, serotonin, appear to exert important influences on the secretion of hypothalamic releasing hormones. These neurotransmitters act in the "hypophysiotropic" area of the ventral hypothalamus to stimulate or inhibit the activity of the "transducer" neurons that manufacture the releasing hormones. Pharmacologic alteration of neurotransmitter function leads to changes in releasing-factor activity. The monoamine precursor, l-dopa, which, unlike the catecholamines, easily crosses the blood-brain barrier, has been used in the treatment of galactorrhea to stimulate the synthesis of dopamine and norepinephrine, which increase the release of prolactin inhibitory factor into the portal circulation.

References

1. Frohman, L. A. Clinical neuropharmacology of hypothalamic releasing factors. *N Engl J Med 286:*1391, 1972.
2. Weldon, V. V., Gupta, S. K., Haymond, M. W., Pagliara, A. S., Jacobs, L. S., and Daughaday, W. H. The use of L-dopa in the diagnoses of hyposomatotropism in children. *J Clin Endocrinol Metab 36:*42, 1973.

Addendum to Chapter 3

Diabetes Insipidus (DI) Diagnosis

The most useful test is complete water deprivation for 8 hours to induce hyperosmolality. In true DI, the serum osmolality will increase from 285 to more than 300 mOsm/kg of body weight. The urine osmolality will remain less than 400 mOsm/kg.

Procedure for 8-Hour Fluid Deprivation Test

This test is best carried out during the daytime from 8 A.M. to 4 P.M. using the following protocol:

7:00 A.M.	Light breakfast to include either one glass of juice (or milk) or one cup of tea (or coffee)
7:30 A.M.	Void urine: discard
8:00 A.M.	Weigh patient: record Urine sample (clearly labeled with time) for osmolality; 5 ml is required. Discard remainder of complete void. Serum sample—for osmolality (10 ml of clotted blood), clearly labeled with time Plasma electrolytes
10:00 A.M. Noon* 2:00 P.M. 4:00 P.M.	Weigh patient and obtain appropriate samples for serum and urine osmolalities and plasma electrolytes—all clearly labeled with time

* Lunch may consist of one or two sandwiches but no fluid.

Precautions

1. The test may have to be terminated prematurely in some patients with severe diabetes insipidus who develop intolerable thirst.

2. The test must be terminated if the patient has lost 5% of the initial body weight. Fluid depletion beyond this amount can lead to serious circulatory disturbances.

Determination of Vasopressin Responsiveness

In patients with true DI (established by their abnormal response to the 8-hour fluid deprivation) the following protocol may be used to distinguish nephrogenic from hypothalamic–pituitary DI. The fluid deprivation during the night can be used to confirm the previous daytime test.

At midnight	Discontinue food and fluid
7:00 A.M.	Void urine on arising: discard
7:30 A.M.	Light breakfast of 100 ml of orange juice and two slices of toast and jam
8:00 A.M.	Urine sample for osmolality (5 ml) Serum sample for osmolality (10 ml)
8:30 A.M.	Hydrate, using 20 ml of water per kg body weight, in three divided doses over 1 hr. Bladder should be emptied every ½ hour until 1 P.M. and urine volume recorded
10:00 A.M. 10:30 A.M. 11:00 A.M.	Urine and serum samples for osmolalities
11:00 A.M.	0.1 U of aqueous vasopressin is given I.V.
11:30 A.M. Noon 12:30 P.M. 1:00 P.M.	Urine and serum samples for osmolalities

Response to vasopressin occurs within the first hour, indicated by decreased urine flow and increased urine osmolality to above 400 mOsm/kg.

Table 3-A1. Preparations Used in Treatment of Diabetes Insipidus

Drug	*Duration of action (hr)*	*Supply*	*Approximate dose*
Pitressin (vasopressin) tannate in oil	36–48	1-cc vial (5 units)	1 cc IM 3 times a week
Hydrochlorothiazide (check for hypokalemia during treatment)	24	50 mg	50 mg each morning
Chlorpropamide (check for hypoglycemia during treatment)	12–24	100 mg 250 mg	125 to 500 mg daily in 1 or 2 doses

Addenda to Chapter 4

Addendum 1. Suggested Protocol for Investigation of Patients with Suspected Pituitary or Hypothalamic Dysfunction

Day 1

Complete blood count, urinalysis, ECG
Serum thyroxine, PBI
T_3 uptake
^{131}I capsule for 24-hour uptake
24-hour urine collection for gonadotropins

Day 2

Serum Ca, PO_4, alkaline phosphatase
Fasting blood sugar (FBS)
Electrolytes and BUN
Complete 24-hour ^{131}I uptake
24-hour urine collection for gonadotropins
EEG and echogram

Day 3

FBS, fasting serum, and urine osmolality
Plasma cortisol (8:00 A.M. and 12 midnight)
24-hour urine for 17-OHCS and 17-KS
Brain scan
X-rays—skull, chest
Tomographs of pituitary fossa

Day 4

24-hour urine for 17-OHCS and 17-KS
FBS
Electrolytes and BUN
Ophthalmology consultation (visual fields/acuity)
Start 200-gm CHO diet

Day 5

Metopirone, 750 mg q4h × 6 doses
24-hour urine for 17-OHCS and 17-KS
Record blood pressure q4h

Day 6

24-hour urine for 17-OHCS and 17-KS
Start TSH stimulation protocol if initial thyroid function tests are low
Record blood pressure q4h

Day 7

Oral glucose tolerance test (acromegaly)
(The patient should receive a diet containing not less than 200 gm of carbohydrate for at least 3 days before the test.)

Day 8

Arginine infusion test

L-Arginine Infusion

THEORY: Intravenous infusion of L-arginine, an essential amino acid, in normal subjects is followed by increased plasma levels of growth hormone (HGH) and immunoreactive insulin. In some normal men the above response may only be obtained if the individual is pre-treated with estrogens. In patients with acromegaly, the plasma HGH response to L-arginine infusion is variable; in some it may increase, in others it may fall transiently while in a third group there is no change. The test is most useful in identifying hypopituitarism and in the investigation of dwarfed patients with multiple hormone deficiencies or with isolated growth hormone deficiency. In these cases the low fasting (or absent) plasma levels of HGH fail to rise in response to L-arginine. The response may also be reduced in patients with simple obesity.

Procedure

1. The patient is fasted from 12 midnight. On the morning of the test the patient is allowed up to pass urine before commencing the procedure.
2. 30 minutes before the test starts an indwelling catheter is inserted into an antecubital vein, connected to a disposable 3-way stopcock, and a slow I.V. infusion of normal saline is used to keep the vein open.
3. All tubes for HGH samples are clearly labeled with time and placed on ice.
4. At zero time the following blood samples are withdrawn:
   5 ml heparinized (HGH and insulin)
   5 ml blood sugar
5. 30 G of L-arginine monohydrochloride (R-gene, R Cutter) dissolved in 600 ml distilled water is then infused over a 30 minute interval into the I.V. tubing already set up.
6. Blood samples are then withdrawn at the following times after starting the arginine infusion:
   5 ml heparinized for HGH — at 15, 30, 45, 60, 90 and 120 min
   5 ml blood glucose

Precautions

1. Owing to the simultaneous stimulation of insulin secretion by L-arginine a moderate degree of hypoglycemia may occur between 30 and 60 minutes after the start of the infusion. At this time the patient may complain of slight dizziness and/or sweating.

2. A syringe containing 20 ml 50% glucose should be ready and if the symptoms of hypoglycemia become more pronounced, the test is abandoned and the 50% glucose given I.V.

3. A doctor or nurse familiar with the test *MUST* be present throughout this procedure.

4. On completion of the test, the patient should be given a large CHO meal.

Day 9

Insulin stimulation test

Insulin Hypoglycemia

THEORY: The administration of insulin in doses sufficient to lower the blood glucose to one-half the initial fasting concentration is followed, in normal subjects, by a fivefold or greater increase in plasma HGH. The maximal increase occurs 15–30 minutes after the nadir in blood glucose concentration is reached and persists for one to two hours. The response of acromegalics to insulin-induced hypoglycemia is variable. Some patients show a small rise in HGH: some a fall: and others show no significant change. In patients with hypopituitarism, in spite of extreme sensitivity to insulin with more marked falls in blood sugar, there is little or no detectable HGH in the plasma before or during the insulin-induced hypoglycemia.

Procedure

1. The patient is fasted overnight from 12 midnight and is kept in bed on the morning of the test. Patient may get up to void and be weighed at 7.00 A.M.
2. Thirty minutes before starting the test an indwelling catheter is inserted into an antecubital vein, attached to a disposable 3-way stopcock, and kept open with a very slow saline infusion.
3. All tubes for HGH samples are clearly labeled with time and placed on ice.
4. After 30 minutes samples of blood are withdrawn as follows:
   5 ml heparinized (for HGH)
   5 ml into blood sugar tube.
5. Regular insulin is then injected I.V. into the opposite arm in the following dose:
   a) Acromegalic or diabetic patients—0.2–0.3 U/kg body weight
   b) Hypopituitary patients—0.05–0.10 U/kg body weight
   c) Other patients without evidence of gross pituitary disease, 0.15 U/kg body weight.
6. 5 ml heparinized blood samples and samples for blood sugar are taken then at the following times after insulin injections 15, 30, 45, 60, 90 and 120 minutes.

Precautions

1. A doctor or nurse familiar with the test MUST be present throughout the whole procedure.

2. A syringe containing 20 ml 50% glucose must be available.

3. Most patients experience slight sweating and/or dizziness at about 20–30 minutes after the insulin injection. Should these symptoms become more severe, the test is abandoned and the 50% glucose injected I.V. at once.

4. Follow the test with a large CHO meal.

The arginine and insulin stimulation tests are done somewhat differently in children. See Appendix to chapter on Hormones and Growth for details.

Day 10

Start cortisone replacement (if indicated)
Air encephalogram

Day 11

Finish

The following investigations will be necessary in certain patients:

Bone age (X-rays—wrists, elbows, knees)
IVP
Old tuberculin test (if sarcoid is suspected)
Serum proteins (if sarcoid is suspected)
Diabetes insipidus protocol (see Chapter 3, Addendum)

The following drugs may NOT be used, as they interfere with one or more of the tests:

All phenothiazines
Librium, Valium
Barbiturates
Chloral hydrate
Laxatives
Antibiotics
Salicylates (Darvon may be used as an analgesic)
Dilantin

A rapid one day outpatient investigation of pituitary insufficiency may soon be feasible using serial injections of insulin to induce hypoglycemia, TRH and LHRH. These substances stimulate the release of growth hormone and ACTH (insulin), prolactin and thyrotropin (TRH), FSH and LH (LHRH).

Addendum 2. Tests Used in Pituitary Insufficiency

Gonadotropic Hormones FSH and LH (ICSH)

The most useful test, bioassay for urinary gonadotropins, differentiates between primary and secondary gonadal failure. A 24-hour urine sample is dialyzed to remove toxic substances. Aliquots are injected into immature female mice, and the uterine weight is then determined. If the urine contains gonadotropins, the ovaries will be stimulated, and the uterus will grow as a result of the estrogen secreted by the ovaries. In the rat, increase in ovarian weight may also be used as a bioassay. Both these assays measure a combination of FSH and LH. The patient who has hypogonadism of pituitary origin has no gonadotropin in the urine. In primary gonadal failure, the patient may excrete more than 100 mouse units in 24 hours (normal range, 5–50 mouse units). Radioimmunoassay for HFSH and HLH is replacing the bioassay in many centers, particularly for the detection of low levels (see Table 3, Chapter 15).

Thyrotropin Deficiency

Diagnosis. Do baseline function studies (serum thyroxine, T_3-resin uptake, radioiodine thyroid uptake), then repeat after stimulating the gland for 3 days with thyroid stimulating hormone (TSH) 10 units intramuscularly daily. In pituitary hypothyroidism, TSH stimulation produces significant increase in values of thyroid radioiodine uptake, serum thyroxine, and T_3-resin uptake. Human (TSH) radioimmunoassay is not yet sensitive enough to detect this hormone in all normal adults, but appears to be very promising in the diagnosis of primary hypothyroidism; in these patients, TSH levels are usually elevated when the serum thyroxine is only slightly reduced. TRH will distinguish hypothalamic from hypopituitary hypopituitarism.

ACTH Deficiency

See appendix to Chapter 7 for ACTH stimulation test and Metopirone test. ACTH radioimmunoassay has been difficult and is still in the experimental stage.

Addendum 3. Drugs Used in Pituitary Insufficiency

Androgen Deficiency

Long-acting testosterone injections—e.g., testosterone cyclopentylpropionate 100 mg/cc, 4 cc intramuscularly once a month. Jaundice is not a complication of this treatment.

Linguets of methyl testosterone, 10 mg 3 times daily; these are held against the cheek or under the tongue until absorbed into the systemic circulation. In susceptible individuals, this route of administration may produce jaundice, probably because part of the dose is swallowed and absorbed into the portal circulation.

Defective Spermatogenesis

No satisfactory treatment.

Undescended Testes

Human chorionic gonadotropin (HCG) may be used in a dose of 1000 units 3 times a week for 6 weeks by intramuscular injection. Treatment is given before the age of 5, after mechanical obstruction to descent has been excluded. Operation should be scheduled for the end of this period if the testes have not fully descended into the scrotum. If the testes are not palpable, measurement of serum testosterone levels before and after this stimulation will distinguish anorchia or gonadal unresponsiveness from gonadotropin deficiency.

Estrogen and Progesterone Deficiency

This disorder may be corrected by one of the many sequential birth control agents now available. More physiologic replacement involves gradually increasing doses of an estrogen—e.g., mestranol for 21 days (from 10 to 50 μg daily)—plus a progestational agent for the third week—e.g., Provera, 10 mg daily. This program produces or restores secondary sexual characteristics and induces predictable withdrawal bleeding. (See also Addendum to Chapter 10.)

Stimulation of Ovulation

Clomiphene citrate, 50–150 mg daily for 5 days beginning on Day 5 of the cycle, will usually induce ovulation, about 5 days after stopping the clomiphene. This therapy sometimes precipitates multiple pregnancy or ovarian cyst formation.

Sequential human FSH and HCG administration should be reserved for special clinics. The FSH is extracted from menopausal urine or human pituitary glands obtained at necropsy (FSH from other species is not effective). HCG, which has an LH-like action, is used to stimulate ovulation after FSH has brought the graafian follicle(s) to the point of rupture.

Thyrotropin Deficiency

Treatment. L-thyroxine, 0.2–0.3 mg daily, depending on body weight. If the patient also has adrenal insufficiency, this should be corrected before thyroxine is given, otherwise the increase in metabolism may precipitate an adrenal crisis.

Corticotropin Deficiency

Prednisone, 2.5 mg to 5 mg at 8 A.M. and 2.5 mg at 4 P.M. replaces the glucocorticoid deficiency under normal circumstances. Dosages should be increased during stressful illnesses. The first symptom of adrenal insufficiency is usually nausea.

Addenda to Chapter 5

Addendum 1

Oppenheimer has indicated that more than 90% of circulating T_3 may derive from the peripheral deiodination of T_4, and has also suggested that T_3 may be overwhelmingly the active hormone.

Addendum 2

Even in the absence of TBG, T_3 is approximately three to five times more potent than T_4 when administered over long periods (in contrast to the acute effect of these agents).

Addendum 3. Major Tests of Thyroid Function

Basal Metabolic Rate (BMR)

This measure of the body's oxygen consumption under basal conditions was, until two decades ago, the most commonly used test of thyroid function. However, because it only correlates with the final assessment of thyroid activity in about 50% of cases, it is no longer widely used.

Protein-Bound Iodine (PBI)

This, the most commonly used test of thyroid function, has a normal range of 4–8 μg/100 ml. Because it measures the iodine bound to protein and in the normal state, almost all of this is thyroxine iodine, PBI is a good measure of the circulating thyroxine. PBI may be elevated as a result of iodine contamination. Furthermore, abnormal iodoproteins produced in certain thyroid diseases, although they are not metabolically active, are measured in the PBI. PBI is also altered by changes in thyroxine-binding proteins: A rise in thyroxine-binding globulin, as in estrogen therapy or pregnancy, produces a rise in the PBI, and a fall in this globulin will depress the serum PBI.

Serum Thyroxine (T_4)

Several techniques measure the total serum thyroxine but the most useful are those which involve progressive displacement of thyroxine from protein-binding sites. These techniques are not affected by iodine contamination, and do not measure iodoproteins. The normal range of serum thyroxine is 4–11 μg/100 ml. Serum thyroxine is now supplanting PBI as the most commonly used test of thyroid function.

Resin Uptake of ^{131}I-Triiodothyronine (T_3 Resin Uptake)

The T_3 resin uptake complements serum thyroxine because it is an indirect measure of the amount of *unsaturated* thyroxine-binding globulin. T_3 resin uptake (normal range, 25–35%) has supplanted the qualitatively similar erythrocyte uptake of ^{131}I-T_3 because it is technically easier to perform. When unsaturated thyroxine-binding sites are increased (as in myxedema, pregnancy, estrogen therapy), T_3 resin uptake falls *below* 25%. Most of the added triiodothyronine is then retained by the thyroxine-binding globulin, leaving much less to be picked up by the resin. Conversely, when unoccupied thyroxine-binding sites are decreased (e.g., hyperthyroidism, lack of TBG), the T_3 resin uptake is elevated about 35%. Because there is a considerable overlap between normal and abnormal values, this test should never be interpreted alone, but should be run conjointly with the serum thyroxines.

Radioactive Iodine Uptake

Radioactive iodine uptake by the thyroid gland, a useful and popular procedure, has many variations: the most common is the 24-hour uptake. The normal range varies from city to city, depending largely on the average dietary intake of iodine. In Southern Ontario, the 24-hour ^{131}I uptakes range normally between 10% and 35%.

Elevated uptakes may be found in conditions other than hyperthyroidism, such as iodine deficiency, the rebound phase after subacute thyroiditis, or after thyroid or antithyroid drug administration, or in certain enzymatic defects of the thyroid. Conversely, uptake may be suppressed in conditions other than hypothyroidism—e.g., after iodine contamination or the administration of antithyroid drugs.

Other Tests Employing ^{131}I

These tests measure secretion rate, or the incorporation of ^{131}I into the PBI (PB^{131}I) and suffer from many of the same drawbacks. Radioactive-iodine uptake (the Werner suppression test) may be used in addition to standard tests when a diagnosis of hyperthyroidism is in question. This test is based on the observation that, in normal persons or those with nontoxic goiters, triiodothyronine suppresses pituitary thyrotropin and thus suppresses thyroid function; this in turn suppresses radioactive iodine uptake. Thus, giving triiodothyronine, 75–100 μg daily for 10 days, to a person with nontoxic goiter will lower radioactive iodine uptake to less than 50% of its initial value within 10 days. In hyperthyroidism, however, thyroid function cannot be suppressed by triiodothyronine, and the uptake remains at its previous level.

Thyroid Scanning

Using thyroid scanning by rectilinear scanning devices or by gamma camera, the physician can determine the size and shape of the thyroid gland and can detect hyperfunctioning nodules or those with reduced function.

Thyroid Autoantibodies

Estimates of thyroid autoantibodies have limited value in the diagnosis of Hashimoto's thyroiditis (see text, Chapter 5).

Other Tests of Interest

Free thyroxine can be estimated, but is not yet a common diagnostic laboratory procedure. Estimation of *thyroxine-binding globulin capacity* and the capacity of the other binding proteins is generally reserved as a research procedure.

Kinemometry records the Achilles tendon reflex on electrocardiographic paper. The reflex is characteristically slowed in hypothyroidism, and more rapid in hyperthyroidism. This test is exceedingly simple, but there is considerable overlap between normals and those with either hyperthyroidism or hypothyroidism. Total *serum triiodothyronine* estimation may prove to be of considerable value because some patients with hyperthyroidism produce an excess of triiodothyronine without a proportionate increase in thyroxine. Conversely, some patients who are mildly hypothyroid have a very low serum thyroxine, whereas their serum total triiodothyronine remains within normal limits, or only slightly reduced.

Long-Acting Thyroid Stimulator (LATS)

This test, performed by mouse bioassay, is positive in most (but not all) patients with Graves' disease. This technique is not generally available in most hospital laboratories.

Plasma Thyrotropin Levels

Methods for determining these levels are now readily available and are most useful in distinguishing between primary and secondary hypothyroidism —i.e., high in primary hypothyroidism and low in secondary hypothyroidism.

TRH Stimulation Test

In patients with hypothyroidism associated with hypothalamic disease, the pituitary may still be able to respond to thyrotropin-releasing hormone (TRH) with increased output of TSH, measured by radioimmunoassay. To distinguish between "secondary" hypothyroidism due to pituitary disease and "hypothalamic" hypothyroidism (the "tertiary" form), give 200 μg of TRH intravenously and measure TSH levels at 20 and 60 minutes.

Addendum 4

With various new modifications, the normal range for the T_3 resin uptake will vary widely. It is perhaps preferable to express the results as a percentage of unity, i.e., the normal range will then be 0.8–1.2. When one multiplies this result by the serum thyroxine, the product will be "the effective T_4 (ET_4)." The ET_4 has the advantage that it is not subject to variations in TBG capacity and the ET_4 can be interpreted in much the same manner as a free T_4, itself a much more difficult procedure.

Addendum 5

In most sporadic goiters in adolescents and adults, no specific metabolic defect can be demonstrated, presumably because it is of minor degree.

Addendum 6

Refetoff and his colleagues have described a family whose members have a deficiency in the peripheral tissue utilization of thyroid hormones. This resulted in clinical signs of mild hypothyroidism, the presence of a goitre, high serum T_4 values, high ^{131}I thyroidal uptakes, and high serum TSH levels.

Addendum 7. Major Drugs in Thyroid Disease

Antithyroid Drugs

Drugs used for the treatment of hyperthyroidism fall into one of two major types: the thioureas and imidazoles. The most common thiourea, propylthiouracil, blocks the oxidation of iodide to iodine, and suppresses the coupling enzymes which produce thyroxine. Initial dosages of 600 mg/day in divided doses may be gradually reduced after the patient reaches a euthyroid state, and can be adjusted to maintain him there. Major side effects are rare; these include agranulocytosis (in about 0.7% of patients), dermatitis, and other less common toxic reactions.

The most common members of the imidazole group are carbimazole and methimazole. The initial daily dosages of these vary between 30 and 60 mg/day, with later maintenance dosages in the range of 5–20 mg/day.

Addendum 8

Possible mechanisms involved in the pathogenesis of Graves' disease have been summarized extensively in a recent publication (Volpé, R., Edmonds, M. W., Lamki, L., Clarke, P. V. and Row, V. V. The pathogenesis of Graves' disease—a disorder of delayed hypersensitivity? *Proc Mayo Clin,* November 1972).

Addendum 9

Vitiligo is also very common.

Addendum 10

Recently we have reported the presence of cell-mediated immunity in this disorder, using the migration inhibition factor test (Munro, R., Row, V. V., and Volpé, R. Cell-mediated immunity in the exophthalmos of Graves' disease as manifested by the migration inhibition factor test. *Proceedings of the 48th Meeting of the American Thyroid Association, Chicago, Illinois, September 20–23, 1972*).

Addendum 11

The recent demonstration that cell-mediated immunity is a factor in the pathogenesis of exophthalmos has led to a revival of orbital radiation as therapy, and considerable success has now been reported in active cases.

Addendum 12

It has now been established that cell-mediated immunity is a factor in Hashimoto's thyroiditis (Laryea, E., Row, V. V. and Volpé, R. The effect of blood leucocytes from patients with Hashimoto's disease on human thyroid cells in monolayer culture. *Clin Endocrinol,* January 1973).

Addendum 13. Thyroid Hormone Therapy

Thyroid hormone is used as replacement in primary or secondary hypothyroidism, and as a suppressant in all types of nontoxic goiter, and in some types of thyroiditis—particularly Hashimoto's thyroiditis. After surgical extirpation of most types of goiter (other than that causing hyperthyroidism), thyroid hormone should be used to prevent recurrent goiter. After the removal of primary thyroid carcinoma, thyroid hormone should be given in subtoxic doses, to suppress maximally the secretion of pituitary thyrotropin.

Thyroid hormone is available as desiccated thyroid, synthetic L-thyroxine (T_4), synthetic L-triiodothyronine (T_3), and a combination of synthetic T_4 and T_3 in a single preparation. Desiccated thyroid is cheap and generally acceptable to most patients. In severe disease or in elderly hypothyroid patients, the initial dosage should be in the order of 15–30 mg/day, and gradually increased, whenever possible, to a maintenance dosage of 120–180 mg/day. However, the reader should note that desiccated thyroid is assayed as organic iodine rather than as thyroxine; hence, it sometimes varies in potency, even to a profound degree.

Because of this variation, L-thyroxine is now used in its place and indeed is an effective agent—0.1 mg of T_4 corresponds to 60 mg of desiccated thyroid. T_4, because it is supplied in a relatively purified form, does not vary in potency. However, physiologic doses of T_4 tend to raise serum protein-bound iodine or serum thyroxine levels; hence one must learn to disregard these levels during thyroxine therapy.

Triiodothyronine, an equally effective agent, is much more potent—milligram for milligram, than is thyroxine. T_3 has a much more rapid, but much shorter action, than thyroxine. Accordingly, it should not be used for long-term replacement or suppressive therapy, but in those situations where a rapid effect is desirable. T_3 may also be useful when quick responses to changes in dose are important—e.g., in patients with angina, in whom it may be desirable to decrease the dosage suddenly. Twenty-five micrograms of T_3 are roughly equivalent to 0.1 mg of thyroxine. During T_3 therapy, the serum thyroxine on PBI remains low or falls.

Recently a new preparation has combined T_4 and T_3 in a 9:1 ratio. This agent, which seems to have no pharmacologic benefit over either drug given separately, has the doubtful advantage of maintaining serum PBI or serum T_4 in the normal range as physiologic replacement proceeds.

Addendum to Chapter 10

Prologue to Gynecological Therapy

It is impossible to provide the reader with a complete list of the agents presently available for the treatment of disturbances of the hypothalamic–pituitary–ovarian axis, because these preparations are continually undergoing modification in composition, dosage, and combinations. Basically, they are divided into drugs used *topically,* such as vaginal creams or suppositories, or administered *orally*.

The six basic areas of application are: (1) inhibition of ovulation; (2) stimulation of ovulation; (3) substitution of ovarian sex hormones; (4) inhibition of lactation; (5) relief of menopausal symptoms; and (6) control of disturbed menstrual patterns. These agents are described in the following paragraph, or are listed in the accompanying tables.

Estrogens. Three main types of estrogens are available commercially: the natural conjugated, the synthetic "pure" estrogen, and synthetic compounds with estrogenic activity. When the physician uses the agents in the second group, the "pure" estrogens, he knows precisely what he is administering.

Estrogenic compounds are available both orally and in the form of topical vaginal cream or suppository. The dosage in the oral preparation varies in accordance with the indication (i.e., for oral contraceptive purposes versus relief of menopausal symptoms).

The oral administration of an estrogenic compound is customarily combined with a progestin, either with the two compounds in each tablet or in sequential form wherein estrogen is given alone for 14 days, then combined with some form of progestin (see Tables 10-A3a and 10-A4a.). Oral estrogen preparations have also been used in combination with testosterone as intramuscular and oral preparations, in some instances for the relief of menopausal symptoms. Although popular with some physicians, there are many who would concur that testosterone given to the female of any age is not physiological.

Progestogens. Progestins are chemical agents that, when administered, produce secretory changes in the endometrium of the experimental animal. Two basic types exist: the progesterone-like chemicals which contain 21-carbon atoms like progesterone itself; secondly, the testosterone derivatives which contain 19- or 18-carbon atoms (19-nor agents).

The testosterone derivatives of the 19- or 18-carbon atom group are most useful and most used as part of the oral contraceptive "package" (see Table 10-A3a). In the human, these agents produce endometrical atrophy and therefore should not be used to develop the uterus and endometrium. These agents are also valuable in the treatment of menopausal symptoms, when estrogens are contraindicated. However, before stimulating ovulation with the agents described in Table 10-A5a (Ovulatory Agents), the endometrium should be prepared through the sequential administration of increasing doses of a "pure" (synthetic) estrogen, followed by a combination of estrogen and a 21-carbon progestational agent. The C-21 carbon progestational preparations have an anabolic rather than a catabolic effect on the endometrium—unlike the 19- or 18-carbon atom testosterone-like derivatives. Such a regimen creates a more receptive intauterine environment, favoring implantation in the event of success with stimulation of ovulation and fertilization.

Some of the indications for the use of estrogen therapy, with the accompanying side effects and

Table 10-A1. Estrogen Therapy: Indications, Side Effects, and Contraindications

Indications
- Substitution therapy to induce growth and development of hypoplastic genitalia and secondary sex characteristics
- Functional uterine bleeding for initial hemostasis and replacement when hypoestrogenism is cause
- Peri- and postmenopausal replacement
- Diseases of vulva and vagina due to estrogen deficiency (e.g., senile vaginitis and vulvovaginitis of infancy)
- Suppression of lactation and relief of breast engorgement
- Advanced breast carcinoma in postmenopausal women

Side effects
- Gastrointestinal disturbances
- Leukorrhea and predisposition to Trichomonas vaginitis
- Metabolic:
  - Plasma proteins:
    - Increase in thyroid-binding globulin
    - Increase in cortisol-binding globulin (transcortin)
    - Increase in transferrin
  - Carbohydrate metabolism:
    - Increase in glucose intolerance caused by peripheral resistance to insulin
  - Liver: cholestasis
  - Plasma lipids: increase in plasma triglycerides
  - Water and electrolytes: increase in salt and water retention
  - Calcium: stabilization of bone mass
- Thromboembolism:*
  - Vasculitis
  - Increase in platelet adhesiveness
  - Increase in hematocrit
  - Increase in clotting factors
- Neoplasia:
  - Increase in fibroid growth
  - Aggravation of existing cancer target organs

Contraindications
- Existing malignancy, especially in target organ
- Endometriosis
- Severe hepatic disease
- History of thromboembolism in past
- Serious cardiovascular disease

Indications for therapy with estrogens and androgens
- Severe menopausal symptoms not controlled with estrogen alone
- Osteoporosis; delayed union of fractures in elderly
- Postpartum breast engorgement and suppression of lactation

Side effects of estrogens and androgens
- All estrogenic side effects, plus:
- Virilization and hirsutism
- Edema

Contraindications to therapy with estrogens and androgens
- Malignancy of breast or genital tract
- Cardiac or renal disease because of increased salt and water retention
- Preexisting signs and symptoms of virilization, hirsutism, or androgenicity

* These effects may explain deep vein thrombosis; pulmonary embolus; myocardial infarction; cerebrovascular accidents and transient ischemic attacks; vascular headaches (? migraine); ophthalmological problems.

contraindications, are outlined in Table 10-A1 and those for progestin therapy, with indications, side effects, and contraindications, in Table 10-A2. The indications, side effects, and contraindications of the use of combined therapy (i.e., estrogen plus a progestin) are listed in Table 10-A3a and those associated with the use of sequential therapy in Table 10-A3b.

The currently used ovulatory agents and their indications, side effects, and contraindications are listed in Tables 10-A4a and 10-A4b.

Table 10-A2. Progestogen (Progestin) Therapy: Indications, Side Effects and Contraindications

Indications

- Amenorrhea: estrogen essential in primary amenorrhea and may be necessary in secondary amenorrhea
- Functional uterine bleeding, especially in juvenile anovulatory hemorrhage
- Contraception: oral products combined with estrogen; parenteral products used alone for long-term contraceptive effect
- Progesterone withdrawal test: a clinical test for early pregnancy. Only 17-acetoxy and retroprogesterone should be used, to avoid virilization of fetus by testosterone derivative
- Threatened and recurrent abortions: to help maintain a pregnancy, especially when there is evidence of progesterone deficiency
- Endometrium: progesterone may be combined with estrogen and given continuously for 6–12 months to induce a pseudopregnancy
- Primary dysmenorrhea

Side effects

- Pure progestional agents:
  - Premenstrual molimina: lethargy, tiredness, malaise, depression, excitability, irritability; pelvic congestion, constipation, acne, dilation and aching of varicose veins
  - Liver: may be cholestatic, like estrogen
  - Thromboembolism: increased blood stasis, secondary smooth muscle dilation, especially in varicose veins
  - "Atypical" cervical hyperplasia—benign condition presenting as cervical polyp, erosion, hyperplasia
  - Libido generally decreased
  - Salt and water metabolism: salt dissipation; aldosterone antagonist, therefore increased Na excretion; protein catabolist, therefore increased potassium excretion
- Testosterone derivatives:
  - All above except decrease in libido and effects on salt and water metabolism
  - Weight gain: water retention and appetite stimulation
  - Amenorrhea after completion of therapy (hypothalamic hypersuppression)
  - Hirsutism and acne
  - Libido generally increased
  - Depression, irritability, and emotional response
  - Fetal masculinization
  - Increase in serum lipids and lipoproteins

Contraindications

- Liver disease or dysfunction
- Testosterone derivatives must *not* be used in:
  - Cases of known or suspected pregnancy
  - Hirsutism or virilization
  - Oligomenorrhea due to hypothalamic–pituitary dysfunction
- Advantages of therapy must be carefully weighed against risks involved in:
  - Diabetes mellitus
  - Cardiovascular and thromboembolic disorders and hypertension
  - Psychotic disorders, especially depressions
  - Epilepsy
  - Asthma
  - Migraine
- Malignancy of genital tract and other target organs

Table 10-A3a. Combination Products Available

Name and manufacturer*	Dose (mg)	Estrogen Type	Estrogen Dose (mg)	Progestin Type	Progestin Dose (mg)
Ortho-Novum	1/50	Mestranol	0.05	Norethindrone	1.0
(Ortho)	1/80		0.08		1.0
	2		0.10		2.0
	5		0.075		5.0
	10		0.6		10.0
Norinyl†	1	Mestranol	0.05	Norethindrone	1.0
(Syntex)	1+80		0.08		1.0
			0.10		2.0
Lyndiol-22‡ (Organon)		Mestranol	0.075	Lynestrenol	2.5
Enovid	5	Mestranol	0.075	Norethynodrel	5.0
(Searle)	10		0.15		9.85
Enovid-E (Searle)	2.5	Mestranol	0.10	Norethynodrel	2.5
Ovulen	0.5	Mestranol	0.10	Ethynodiol diacetate	0.5
(Searle)	1.0		0.10		1.0
Norlestrin§	1.0	Ethinyl estradiol	0.05	Norethindrone acetate	1.0
(Parke-Davis)	2.5		0.05		2.5
Ovral (Wyeth)		Ethinyl estradiol	0.05	Norgestrel	0.25
Novinol (Desbergers)		Mestranol	0.10	Norethynodrel	2.5
Demulen (Searle)		Ethinyl estradiol	0.05	Ethynodiol diacetate	1.0

* Regimen for all products listed is 21 days, beginning on Day 5 of cycle, except as noted.
† Also supplied as 28-day packet with 7 days of placebo. Note: This product is off the Canadian market.
‡ A 22-day packet.
§ Available in 20- or 21-day regimens, also as a 28-day packet with 7 days of placebo.

Table 10-A3b. Combination Therapy: Indications, Side Effects, and Contraindications

Indications
- Contraception
- Amenorrhea of 3 months' minimum duration
- Dysmenorrhea of 3 months' minimum duration
- Functional uterine bleeding of 3 months' minimum duration
- Endometriosis for 9 months continuous
- Lactation suppression post partum (high dose for 5 days)
- Menopausal syndrome

Side effects
- Gastrointestinal upset: nausea, vomiting, abdominal bloating
- Breakthrough bleeding, spotting
- Decreased menstrual flow; amenorrhea
- Edema
- Chloasma, melasma
- Breast changes: tenderness, enlargement, secretion
- Weight change: increase or decrease
- Cervical erosion, hyperplasia, polypoid lesions
- Decreased lactation
- Cholestatic jaundice
- Migraine headaches: may worsen or improve
- Hypertension
- Depression, irritability
- Thromboembolic episodes
- Metabolic effects:
  - Plasma globulins:
    - Increased thyroid-binding globulin (hence increased PBI)
    - Decreased T_3 uptake
    - Increased total T_4
    - Increased transcortin (hence, increased total plasma cortisol and decreased 17-KS and 17-OHCS in urine)
    - Increased transferrin (hence, increased serum Fe and total iron-binding capacity)
  - Carbohydrate metabolism: diabetogenic
  - Plasma lipids: increased plasma triglycerides
- Hypothalamic–pituitary hypersuppression—i.e., pro-

Table 10-A3b (Continued)

longed amenorrhea and anovulation after cessation of therapy	Undiagnosed vaginal bleeding
Contraindications	Breast feeding (possible transmission of agent to child)
History of thrombophlebitis, pulmonary embolism, cerebrovascular accident, exophthalmos, migraine	Incomplete epiphyseal closure when further growth is desired
Liver dysfunction or disease	Ocular lesions associated with vascular disease
Known or suspected malignancy of breast or genital tract	Suspected or confirmed pregnancy
	Fibroids (estrogen component causes rapid enlargement)

Table 10-A4a. Sequential Products Available

	Estrogen		*Progestin*		
Name & manufacturer	*Type*	*Dose (mg)*	*Type*	*Dose (mg)*	*Regimen*
Ortho-Novum S.Q. (Ortho)	Mestranol	0.08	Norethindrone	2	Estrogen × 14 days, then both × 7 days
Norquen (Syntex)	Mestranol	0.08	Norethindrone	2	Estrogen × 14 days, then both × 7 days
Oracon (Mead Johnson)	Ethinyl estradiol	0.10	Dimethisterone	25	Estrogen × 16 days, then both × 5 days
Secrovin (B.D.H.)	Ethinyl estradiol	0.10	Dimethisterone	25	Estrogen × 16 days, then both × 5 days
Miniquen (Searle)	Mestranol	0.10	Ethynodiol diacetate	0.5	Estrogen × 11 days, then both × 10 days

Table 10-A4b. Sequential Therapy: Indications, Side Effects, and Contraindications

Indications
- Contraception
- Dysfunctional uterine bleeding
- Dysmenorrhea
- Menopausal syndrome

Side effects
- Same as for combined preparations, with the following important differences:
  - Progestational side effects are minimized
  - Estrogenic side effects are maximized
  - Hypersuppression syndrome occurs less frequently
  - Breakthrough bleeding more common
  - Higher failure rate as a contraceptive

Contraindications
- Same as for combined products

Table 10-A5a. Ovulatory Agents

Preparation	*Content*	*Dose*	*Route*	*Mode of action*	*Regimen*
Clomid (Merrell)	Clomiphene citrate	50 or 100 mg	Oral	Antiestrogenic—a competitive inhibitor Acts on an intact hypothalamic-pituitary-ovarian axis, which is potentially functional to increased LH release and synthesis, plus a transient increased FSH release May stimulate steroidogenic systems of ovary	50–100 mg daily for 5 days from Day 5 to Day 9 if patient has menstrual or withdrawal bleeding Effectiveness may be increased by: (1) endometrial priming in estrogen-deficient patients, with incremental sequential preparation for a few cycles before clomiphene; (2) simultaneous use of low-dose estrogen (e.g., 10–20 μg ethinyl estradiol Days 1–22; (3) HCG in a single dose between Days 12 and 15 or a series of doses given every 2 days between Days 11 and 16
A.P.L. (Ayerst)	Human chorionic gonadotropin	1,000 I.U./ml (10-cc vials)	I.M.	A source of LH activity	May be given (1) with clomiphene, as noted above; (2) together with HPG, as noted below; (3) following a course of HPG
Pregnyl (Organon)	Human chorionic gonadotropin	10,000 I.U. & 10 ml. diluent	I.M.		
Pergonal (Cutter)	Postmenopausal gonadotropin from urine	75 I.U. FSH activity per vial	I.M.	Potentially functional ovaries and uterus required Action is that of FSH	75–100 I.U. (2 vials) daily for 8–10 days; 24 hr after last dose, give 5,000 I.U. HCG
Human pituitary gonadotropin*	HPG extracted from human pituitaries	5–10 mg (approx. 100 I.U. FSH activity)		Same as for Pergonal	Pergonal and HCG may be given together for 7–8 days

* Not yet available in Canada, even for investigation.

Table 10-A5b. Ovulatory Agents: Indications, Side Effects, and Contraindications

Indications for use of clomiphene citrate
- Induction of ovulation in:
  - Primary infertility due to ovulatory dysfunction
  - Primary or secondary amenorrhea
  - Lactation-amenorrhea syndrome
  - Dysfunctional uterine bleeding and a desire for pregnancy
  - Endometrial hyperplasia and carcinoma in situ of endometrium
  - Gynecomastia

Side effects of clomiphene citrate
- Vasomotor instability (especially hot flushes)
- Midcycle abdominal pain (mittelschmerz or ovarian cyst)
- Ovarian hyperstimulation leading to ovarian cysts with or without ascites, etc.
- *Rarely:*
  - Skin rash
  - Galactorrhea
  - Depression
  - Thinning of hair
  - Visual spots and intensification and prolongation of after-images
  - Multiple pregnancy

Contraindications to use of clomiphene citrate
- Pregnancy
- Liver disease or dysfunction
- Presence of large ovarian cysts (Stein-Leventhal ovaries); start with a very low dose—e.g., 25 mg
- Abnormal bleeding not yet diagnosed

Indications for use of HCG (A.P.L. or Pregnyl)
- Infertility
- Amenorrhea
- Chronic cystic mastitis
- Numerous uses also in males

Indications for use of PMG (Pergonal) or HPG
- Primary infertility in the following cases:
  - Endogenous gonadotropins low or absent
  - As secondary therapy in patients who have failed to conceive with several trials of clomiphene citrate

Side effects with use of PMG or HPG
- All due to overstimulation of the ovaries, as manifested by:
  - Superovulation and multiple pregnancy
  - Hyperstimulation syndrome
  - Thromboembolic phenomena

Addendum to Chapter 13

The presence of circulating antibodies to insulin is helpful in detecting persons who are taking insulin surreptitiously.

Addenda to Chapter 16

Addendum 1

The lack of growth hormone response in Laron-type dwarfism has been shown to be associated with an absence of somatomedin. Somatomedin (sulfation factor) is a polypeptide produced in the liver and possibly the kidneys. This substance acts as a mediator of the growth promoting effect of growth hormone on cartilage.

References

1. Daughaday, W. H. *Am J Med 50*:277–280, 1971.
2. Daughaday, W. H., Hall, K., Raben, M. S., Salmon, W. D., Den Brande, J. L. and Van Wyk, J. J. *Nature 235*: 170, 1972.

Addendum 2. Tests Used for Growth Hormone Secretion

Arginine Stimulation Test

Intravenous arginine in a dose of 0.5 mg/kg/body weight (maximum 30 gm) will stimulate growth hormone secretion in most normal children. Since there are few side effects, it is a useful screening test for suspected growth hormone deficiency.

Procedure

1. Fast the patient from 2400 hours (midnight). Water may be given before the test begins.
2. 0.800 (8 A.M.). Start intravenous normal saline and maintain intravenous rate at a level just sufficient to keep the needle open.
3. Take baseline fasting blood samples for growth hormone, insulin, and glucose determinations at 15 and 30 minutes after the intravenous is started.
4. The arginine infusion should be supervised by a doctor. Because the arginine solution is slightly acidic, it must be buffered before administration. Twelve ml of sodium bicarbonate solution containing approximately 10.5 mEq of soda bicarbonate should be added to a 50 ml bottle of 25% l-arginine monochloride. Thirty-eight ml of normal saline is added to the 62 ml of combined solution to bring a total volume of 100 ml. The concentration of arginine used is 12.5%. The arginine is infused intravenously at a dose of 0.5 gm of arginine/kg/body weight given over a 30-minute period. Zero time is taken at the moment that the arginine infusion begins.
5. Collect blood samples for growth hormone, insulin, and glucose determinations at 30 minutes, 60 minutes and 90 minutes after the arginine infusion begins. A nurse should be in attendance with the patient throughout the test.
6. Some patients develop vomiting and headache during, and for a short period following, the infusion. This may be accompanied by mild hypoglycemia. If significant symptoms occur, the test should be discontinued and glucose added to the intravenous.
7. It is important to label all samples carefully and to remove the serum promptly to be frozen for the hormone determinations.

Insulin Tolerance Test

Insulin-induced hypoglycemia stimulates growth hormone secretion. The test has been standardized by widespread use, and lack of response to this test provides strong confirmatory evidence of growth hormone deficiency. Because of possible severe hypoglycemic reactions, the test should be limited to testing patients who are suspected of growth hormone deficiency and do not respond to other stimulatory tests such as the arginine infusion.

In children who are suspected to have growth hormone deficiency, the dose of regular (Toronto) insulin should be 0.05 unit/kg given intravenously. If the child has a previous history of spontaneous hypoglycemia or documented blood sugars in the hypoglycemic range, a smaller dose (0.025 unit/kg) should be used. If the dose does not produce satisfactory hypoglycemia (blood sugar fall of greater than 50% or to below 40 mg %), the test should be repeated using 0.1 unit/kg.

Procedure

1. Fast the patient from 2400 hours (midnight). Water may be given until the test begins.
2. 0.800 hours (8 A.M.). Start intravenous normal saline and maintain intravenous rate at a level just sufficient to keep the needle open.
3. Take fasting baseline blood samples for growth hormone and glucose determinations at 15 minutes and 30 minutes after the intravenous is started.
4. The doctor should carefully measure the dose of regular (Toronto) insulin on the basis of 0.05 unit/kg/body weight, and this is given intravenously. Record zero time at injection. The patient must be carefully monitored by the doctor for the next 60 minutes. A nurse should also be in attendance throughout the entire test.
5. Hypoglycemia usually occurs with mild symptoms of hunger, weakness, sweating or mild headache at 20 to 40 minutes after the insulin injection. These symptoms are usually transient, but in some patients, and especially those with hypopituitarism, there is a more severe hypoglycemia. With any disturbance of the sensorium, the test should be terminated immediately with administration of intravenous 50% glucose. The syringe loaded with

50% glucose should be available throughout the test.

6. Collect blood samples for growth hormone and glucose determination at 10, 20, 30, 60, 90, and 120 minutes after the insulin injection has been given.
7. The blood samples should be sent to the laboratory immediately for blood sugar determinations and removal of serum to freeze for the growth hormone assays. Adrenocorticotropic response to insulin-induced hypoglycemia can be tested by serum cortisol-determination done on blood samples taken at 0 and 60 minutes.

Addendum 3

Diethylstilbestrol, 3 to 5 mg, is given until the epiphyses fuse, which may take 6 months to 2 years. On the first 4 days of every month, a progestational agent, e.g., norethindrone (Norlutin) 5 mg, is also given to build up a secretory endometrium, and thus allow for periodic progesterone withdrawal bleeding.

Addendum 4

Recently several workers have reported that diethylstibestrol may induce carcinogenesis when given in large doses over several years. Furthermore, female children of mothers given this hormone have developed cancer of vagina in their teens. These findings provide a further contraindication to hormonal treatment of excessive height.

Index

Page numbers set in *italics* indicate illustrations. Page numbers followed by the letter "t" indicate tabular material.

73–74–75–76–77–78—10–9–8–7–6–5–4–3–2–1